Bibliometric Studies and Worldwide Research Trends on Global Health

Bibliometric Studies and Worldwide Research Trends on Global Health

Editors

Francisco Manzano Agugliaro
Esther Salmerón-Manzano

MDPI • Basel • Beijing • Wuhan • Barcelona • Belgrade • Manchester • Tokyo • Cluj • Tianjin

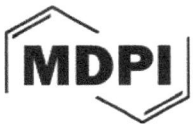

Editors
Francisco Manzano Agugliaro
University of Almeria
Spain

Esther Salmerón-Manzano
Universidad Internacional de La Rioja (UNIR)
Spain

Editorial Office
MDPI
St. Alban-Anlage 66
4052 Basel, Switzerland

This is a reprint of articles from the Special Issue published online in the open access journal *International Journal of Environmental Research and Public Health* (ISSN 1660-4601) (available at: http://www.mdpi.com).

For citation purposes, cite each article independently as indicated on the article page online and as indicated below:

LastName, A.A.; LastName, B.B.; LastName, C.C. Article Title. *Journal Name* **Year**, *Article Number*, Page Range.

ISBN 978-3-03943-094-9 (Hbk)
ISBN 978-3-03943-095-6 (PDF)

© 2020 by the authors. Articles in this book are Open Access and distributed under the Creative Commons Attribution (CC BY) license, which allows users to download, copy and build upon published articles, as long as the author and publisher are properly credited, which ensures maximum dissemination and a wider impact of our publications.

The book as a whole is distributed by MDPI under the terms and conditions of the Creative Commons license CC BY-NC-ND.

Contents

About the Editors vii

Esther Salmerón-Manzano and Francisco Manzano-Agugliaro
Bibliometric Studies and Worldwide Research Trends on Global Health
Reprinted from: *Int. J. Environ. Res. Public Health* **2020**, *17*, 5748, doi:10.3390/ijerph17165743 . . . 1

Fan Li, Hao Zhou, De-Sheng Huang and Peng Guan
Global Research Output and Theme Trends on Climate Change and Infectious Diseases: A Restrospective Bibliometric and Co-Word Biclustering Investigation of Papers Indexed in PubMed (1999–2018)
Reprinted from: *Int. J. Environ. Res. Public Health* **2020**, *17*, 5228, doi:10.3390/ijerph17145223 . . . 7

José Antonio Garrido-Cardenas, Belén Esteban-García, Ana Agüera, José Antonio Sánchez-Pérez and Francisco Manzano-Agugliaro
Wastewater Treatment by Advanced Oxidation Process and Their Worldwide Research Trends
Reprinted from: *Int. J. Environ. Res. Public Health* **2020**, *17*, 170, doi:10.3390/ijerph17010170 . . . 21

Fen Qin, Jing Du, Jian Gao, Guiying Liu, Yonggang Song, Aifu Yang, Hong Wang, Yuan Ding and Qian Wang
Bibliometric Profile of Global Microplastics Research from 2004 to 2019
Reprinted from: *Int. J. Environ. Res. Public Health* **2020**, *17*, 5639, doi:10.3390/ijerph17165639 . . . 41

Bach Xuan Tran, Giang Hai Ha, Long Hoang Nguyen, Giang Thu Vu, Men Thi Hoang, Huong Thi Le, Carl A. Latkin, Cyrus S.H. Ho and Roger C.M. Ho
Studies of Novel Coronavirus Disease 19 (COVID-19) Pandemic: A Global Analysis of Literature
Reprinted from: *Int. J. Environ. Res. Public Health* **2020**, *17*, 4095, doi:10.3390/ijerph17114095 . . . 57

Hai Thanh Phan, Giap Van Vu, Giang Thu Vu, Giang Hai Ha, Hai Quang Pham, Carl A. Latkin, Bach Xuan Tran, Cyrus S.H. Ho and Roger C.M. Ho
Global Mapping of Research Trends on Interventions to Improve Health-Related Quality of Life in Asthma Patients
Reprinted from: *Int. J. Environ. Res. Public Health* **2020**, *17*, 3540, doi:10.3390/ijerph17103540 . . . 73

Giap Van Vu, Giang Hai Ha, Cuong Tat Nguyen, Giang Thu Vu, Hai Quang Pham, Carl A. Latkin, Bach Xuan Tran, Roger C. M. Ho and Cyrus S. H. Ho
Interventions to Improve the Quality of Life of Patients with Chronic Obstructive Pulmonary Disease: A Global Mapping during 1990–2018
Reprinted from: *Int. J. Environ. Res. Public Health* **2020**, *17*, 3089, doi:10.3390/ijerph17093089 . . . 87

Giang Thu Vu, Bach Xuan Tran, Chi Linh Hoang, Brian J. Hall, Hai Thanh Phan, Giang Hai Ha, Carl A. Latkin, Cyrus S.H. Ho and Roger C.M. Ho
Global Research on Quality of Life of Patients with HIV/AIDS: Is It Socio-Culturally Addressed? (GAP$_{RESEARCH}$)
Reprinted from: *Int. J. Environ. Res. Public Health* **2020**, *17*, 2127, doi:10.3390/ijerph17062127 . . . 101

Giang Thu Vu, Bach Xuan Tran, Roger S. McIntyre, Hai Quang Pham, Hai Thanh Phan, Giang Hai Ha, Kenneth K. Gwee, Carl A. Latkin, Roger C.M. Ho and Cyrus S.H. Ho
Modeling the Research Landscapes of Artificial Intelligence Applications in Diabetes (GAP$_{RESEARCH}$)
Reprinted from: *Int. J. Environ. Res. Public Health* **2020**, *17*, 1982, doi:10.3390/ijerph17061982 . . . 115

Bach Xuan Tran, Long Hoang Nguyen, Ngoc Minh Pham, Huyen Thanh Thi Vu, Hung Trong Nguyen, Duong Huong Phan, Giang Hai Ha, Hai Quang Pham, Thao Phuong Nguyen, Carl A. Latkin, Cyrus S.H. Ho and Roger C.M. Ho
Global Mapping of Interventions to Improve Quality of Life of People with Diabetes in 1990–2018
Reprinted from: *Int. J. Environ. Res. Public Health* **2020**, *17*, 1597, doi:10.3390/ijerph17051597 . . . **129**

Esther Salmerón-Manzano, Jose Antonio Garrido-Cardenas and
Francisco Manzano-Agugliaro
Worldwide Research Trends on Medicinal Plants
Reprinted from: *Int. J. Environ. Res. Public Health* **2020**, *17*, 3376, doi:10.3390/ijerph17103376 . . . **143**

Bach Xuan Tran, Son Nghiem, Clifford Afoakwah, Carl A. Latkin, Giang Hai Ha, Thao Phuong Nguyen, Linh Phuong Doan, Hai Quang Pham, Cyrus S.H. Ho and
Roger C.M. Ho
Characterizing Obesity Interventions and Treatment for Children and Youths during 1991–2018
Reprinted from: *Int. J. Environ. Res. Public Health* **2019**, *16*, 4227, doi:10.3390/ijerph16214227 . . . **163**

Marta Gómez-Galán, Ángel-Jesús Callejón-Ferre, José Pérez-Alonso, Manuel Díaz-Pérez and Jesús-Antonio Carrillo-Castrillo
Musculoskeletal Risks: RULA Bibliometric Review
Reprinted from: *Int. J. Environ. Res. Public Health* **2020**, *17*, 4354, doi:10.3390/ijerph17124354 . . . **175**

Clara Martinez-Perez, Cristina Alvarez-Peregrina, Cesar Villa-Collar and
Miguel Ángel Sánchez-Tena
Current State and Future Trends: A Citation Network Analysis of the Academic Performance Field
Reprinted from: *Int. J. Environ. Res. Public Health* **2020**, *17*, 5352, doi:10.3390/ijerph17155352 . . . **223**

Mila Cascajares, Alfredo Alcayde, José Antonio Garrido-Cardenas and
Francisco Manzano-Agugliaro
The Contribution of Spanish Science to Patents: Medicine as Case of Study
Reprinted from: *Int. J. Environ. Res. Public Health* **2020**, *17*, 3638, doi:10.3390/ijerph17103638 . . . **247**

Minxi Wang, Ping Liu, Rui Zhang, Zhi Li and Xin Li
A Scientometric Analysis of Global Health Research
Reprinted from: *Int. J. Environ. Res. Public Health* **2020**, *17*, 2963, doi:10.3390/ijerph17082963 . . . **271**

Pilar Aparicio-Martinez, Alberto-Jesus Perea-Moreno, María Pilar Martinez-Jimenez, María Dolores Redel-Macías, Manuel Vaquero-Abellan and Claudia Pagliari
A Bibliometric Analysis of the Health Field Regarding Social Networks and Young People
Reprinted from: *Int. J. Environ. Res. Public Health* **2019**, *16*, 4024, doi:10.3390/ijerph16204024 . . . **291**

About the Editors

Francisco Manzano-Agugliaro, full professor at the Engineering Department in the University of Almeria (Spain), received his MS in Agricultural Engineering and completed his PhD in Geomatics at the University of Cordoba (Spain). He has published over 160 papers in JCR journals (https://orcid.org/0000-0002-0085-030X), H-index 26. His main interests are energy, sustainability, scientometrics, water, and engineering. He has been the supervisor of 27 PhD theses. He has also been the Vice Dean of the Engineering Faculty (2001–2004); the Director of Central Research Services (2016–2019); PhD Program Coordinator for Environmental Engineering (2000 to 2012), Greenhouse Technology, Industrial and Environmental Engineering (from 2010); and General Manager of Infrastructures (from 2019) at University of Almeria. He has won the following awards: Top Reviewer in Cross-Field—September 2019 (Web of Science), 2019 Outstanding Reviewer Award (*Energies*), 2019 Winner of *Sustainability* Best Paper Awards.

Esther Salmerón-Manzano is a lecturer at the Faculty of Law in the Universidad Internacional de la Rioja (Spain) and Lecturer at Law Department of University of Almeria (Spain). She received her MS degree in Law and completed her PhD in Law at the University of Almeria (Spain). She has published over 16 papers in JCR journals (https://orcid.org/0000-0003-3019-3539), H-index 5. Her main interests are laws and emerging technologies, and contract law. She has been the supervisor of 25 bachelor's and master's Final Reports. She is Academic Director of the master's degree in legal consultancy for companies and the master's degree in family law at Universidad Internacional de la Rioja (Spain).

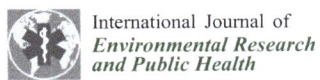 International Journal of
*Environmental Research
and Public Health*

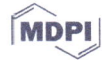

Editorial

Bibliometric Studies and Worldwide Research Trends on Global Health

Esther Salmerón-Manzano [1] and Francisco Manzano-Agugliaro [2,*]

[1] Faculty of Law, Universidad Internacional de La Rioja (UNIR), Av. de la Paz, 137, 26006 Logroño, Spain; esther.salmeron@unir.net
[2] Department of Engineering, University of Almeria, ceiA3, 04120 Almeria, Spain
* Correspondence: fmanzano@ual.es; Tel.: +34-950-015346; Fax: +34-950-015491

Received: 6 August 2020; Accepted: 7 August 2020; Published: 9 August 2020

Abstract: Global health, conceived as a discipline, aims to train, research and respond to problems of a transboundary nature in order to improve health and health equity at the global level. The current worldwide situation is ruled by globalization, and therefore the concept of global health involves not only health-related issues but also those related to the environment and climate change. Therefore, in this Special Issue, the problems related to global health have been addressed from a bibliometric approach in four main areas: environmental issues, diseases, health, education and society.

Keywords: COVID-19; asthma; pulmonary disease; HIV/AIDS; diabetes; medicinal plants; musculoskeletal risks; obesity; microplastics; climate change; wastewater treatment; patents; social networks

1. Introduction

Science aims to answer questions, and from a pragmatic approach, science can be understood as a resolution of problems in our society. Science cannot be considered an independent activity, and therefore, it must be remembered that prior studies have been carried out in any given scientific field. Combining scientific aspects with documental aspects gives rise to a certain type of scientific work: scientometric, bibliometric, and informetric studies. These take different titles according to the final approach of the work, such as the following: examining the scholarly literature, evolution, and new trends; worldwide research trends; mapping of the knowledge base; visualizing the knowledge structure; analysis of global research; publication trends; knowledge domain visualization. Scientific literature is losing its relevance more and more quickly, but the aging of literature is not uniform for all scientific subjects. This means that being up to date in a scientific field requires bibliometric studies through which new trends are revealed when undertaking scientific studies of interest to the community. Two topics of special interest to society today are environmental research and public health, and within these larger topics are sub-topics related to global health. Global health, in a broad context, refers to improving health worldwide, reducing disparities, and protecting against global threats that do not consider national borders. This Special Issue aims to provide a global view of all of these global health issues, and through bibliometric studies, we believe that this objective can be achieved. Therefore, articles reviewing the state of the art in any of these fields, bibliometric or scientometric studies, and research articles dealing with a global perspective are welcome.

2. Publications Statistics

The summary of the call for papers for this Special Issue on the 28 manuscripts submitted: rejected (12; 43%) and published (16; 67%).

The submitted manuscripts come from many countries and are summarized in Table 1. For this statistic only the first affiliation of the authors has been considered, in which it gives the opportunity to observe 66 authors from nine countries. Note that it is common for a manuscript to be signed by more than one author and for authors to belong to different affiliations. The average number of authors per published manuscript in this Special Issue was seven authors.

Table 1. Statistics of authors by country.

Country	Authors
Spain	20
China	18
Vietnam	6
USA	2
Singapore	2
Canada	1
Sweden	1
Australia	2
UK	1
Total	53

3. Authors' Affiliations

There are 23 different affiliations of the authors. Note that only the first affiliation per author has been considered. Table 2 summarizes the authors and their first affiliations.

Table 2. Authors and affiliations.

Author	First Affiliation	References
Martinez-Perez, C.	Universidad Europea de Madrid	[1]
Alvarez-Peregrina, C.	Universidad Europea de Madrid	[1]
Villa-Collar, C.	Universidad Europea de Madrid	[1]
Sánchez-Tena, M. Á.	Universidad Europea de Madrid	[1]
Li, F.	China Medical University	[2]
Zhou, H.	China Medical University	[2]
Huang, D. S.	China Medical University	[2]
Guan, P.	China Medical University	[2]
Hoang, M. T.	Duy Tan University	[3]
Le, H. T.	Hanoi Medical University	[3]
Cascajares, M.	University of Almería	[4]
Alcayde, A.	University of Almería	[4]
Pham, H. Q.	Duy Tan University	[5]
Salmerón-Manzano, E.	University of Almería	[6]
Vu, G. V.	Hanoi Medical University	[7]
Nguyen, C. T.	Duy Tan University	[7]
Wang, M.	Chengdu University of Technology	[8]
Liu, P.	Chengdu University of Technology	[8]
Zhang, R.	Chengdu University of Technology	[8]
Li, Z.	Chengdu University of Technology	[8]
Li, X.	Chengdu University of Technology	[8]
Hall, B. J.	Johns Hopkins University	[9]
Hoang, C. L.	Nguyen Tat Thanh University	[9]
McIntyre, R. S.	University of Toronto	[10]
Pham, N. M.	Curtin University	[11]
Vu, H. T. T.	Hanoi Medical University	[11]

Table 2. Cont.

Author	First Affiliation	References
Nguyen, H. T.	National Institute of Nutrition	[11]
Esteban-García, B.	University of Almería	[12]
Agüera, A.	University of Almería	[12]
Sánchez-Pérez, J. A.	University of Almería	[12]
Nghiem, S.	Griffith University	[13]
Afoakwah, C.	Griffith University	[13]
Doan, L.P.	Nguyen Tat Thanh University	[13]
Aparicio-Martinez, P.	University of Cordoba	[14]
Perea-Moreno, A. J.	University of Cordoba	[14]
Martinez-Jimenez, M. P.	University of Cordoba	[14]
Redel-Macías, M. D.	University of Cordoba	[14]
Vaquero-Abellan, M.	University of Cordoba	[14]
Pagliari, C.	University of Edinburgh	[14]
Gómez-Galán, M.	University of Almería	[15]
Callejón-Ferre, Á. J.	University of Almería	[15]
Pérez-Alonso, J.	University of Almería	[15]
Díaz-Pérez, M.	University of Almería	[15]
Carrillo-Castrillo, J. A.	University of Seville	[15]
Qin F.	Dalian University of Technology Library	[15]
Du J.	Liaoning Ocean and Fisheries Science Research Institute	[15]
Gao J.	Dalian University of Technology Library	[15]
Liu G.	Liaoning Ocean and Fisheries Science Research Institute	[15]
Song Y.	Liaoning Ocean and Fisheries Science Research Institute	[15]
Yang, A.	Technology Center of Dalian Customs District	[16]
Wang H.	Ocean University of China	[16]
Ding, Y.	Dalian University of Technology Library	[16]
Wang Q.	Ocean University of China	[16]
Tran, B. X.	Hanoi Medical University	[3,5,7,9–11,13]
Ha, G. H.	Duy Tan University	[3,5,7,9–11,13]
Nguyen, L. H.	Vietnam National University	[3,11]
Vu, G. T.	Nguyen Tat Thanh University	[3,5,7]
Latkin C. A.	Johns Hopkins University	[3,5,7,9–11,13]
Ho, C.S.H.	National University Hospital	[3,5,7,9–11,13]
Ho, R.	National University of Singapore	[3,5,7,9–11,13]
Phan, H. T.	Hanoi Medical University	[5,9,10]
Vu, G. T.	Nguyen Tat Thanh University	[5,9,10]
Pham, H. Q.	Duy Tan University	[7,10,11,13]
Nguyen, T.P.	Nguyen Tat Thanh University	[11,13]
Garrido-Cardenas, J. A.	University of Almería	[4,6,12]
Manzano-Agugliaro, F.	University of Almería	[4,6,12]

4. Topics

Table 3 summarizes the research conducted by the authors in this Special Issue, by identifying the areas to which they report. It was noted that they have been grouped into four main lines of research: environmental issues, diseases, health and society. They have mainly explored the issue of disease research, these have been: COVID-19, asthma, pulmonary disease, HIV/AIDS, and diabetes. Related to health, they were: medicinal plants, musculoskeletal risks, and obesity. The environmental issues were related to: microplastics, climate change, and wastewater treatment. Finally, research related to education and society: academic performance, patents, bibliometric analysis, and social networks and young people.

Table 3. Topics for worldwide research trends on global health.

Bibliometric Studies	Number of Manuscripts	References
Environmental issues	3	[2,12,16]
Diseases	6	[3,5,7,9–11]
Health	3	[6,13,15]
Education and society	4	[1,4,8,14]

Author Contributions: The authors all made equal contributions to this article. All authors have read and agreed to the published version of the manuscript.

Funding: This research received no external funding.

Conflicts of Interest: The authors state that there are no conflict of interest.

References

1. Martinez-Perez, C.; Alvarez-Peregrina, C.; Villa-Collar, C.; Sánchez-Tena, M.Á. Current State and Future Trends: A Citation Network Analysis of the Academic Performance Field. *Int. J. Environ. Res. Public Health* **2020**, *17*, 5352. [CrossRef] [PubMed]
2. Li, F.; Zhou, H.; Huang, D.S.; Guan, P. Global Research Output and Theme Trends on Climate Change and Infectious Diseases: A Restrospective Bibliometric and Co-Word Biclustering Investigation of Papers Indexed in PubMed (1999–2018). *Int. J. Environ. Res. Public Health* **2020**, *17*, 5228. [CrossRef] [PubMed]
3. Tran, B.X.; Ha, G.H.; Nguyen, L.H.; Vu, G.T.; Hoang, M.T.; Le, H.T.; Latkin, C.A.; Ho, C.S.H.; Ho, R. Studies of Novel Coronavirus Disease 19 (COVID-19) Pandemic: A Global Analysis of Literature. *Int. J. Environ. Res. Public Health* **2020**, *17*, 4095. [CrossRef] [PubMed]
4. Cascajares, M.; Alcayde, A.; Garrido-Cardenas, J.A.; Manzano-Agugliaro, F. The Contribution of Spanish Science to Patents: Medicine as Case of Study. *Int. J. Environ. Res. Public Health* **2020**, *17*, 3638. [CrossRef] [PubMed]
5. Phan, H.T.; Vu, G.V.; Vu, G.T.; Ha, G.H.; Pham, H.Q.; Latkin, C.A.; Tran, B.X.; Ho, C.S.H.; Ho, R. Global Mapping of Research Trends on Interventions to Improve Health-Related Quality of Life in Asthma Patients. *Int. J. Environ. Res. Public Health* **2020**, *17*, 3540. [CrossRef] [PubMed]
6. Salmerón-Manzano, E.; Garrido-Cardenas, J.A.; Manzano-Agugliaro, F. Worldwide Research Trends on Medicinal Plants. *Int. J. Environ. Res. Public Health* **2020**, *17*, 3376. [CrossRef] [PubMed]
7. Vu, G.V.; Ha, G.H.; Nguyen, C.T.; Vu, G.T.; Pham, H.Q.; Latkin, C.A.; Tran, B.; Ho, R.; Ho, C.S. Interventions to Improve the Quality of Life of Patients with Chronic Obstructive Pulmonary Disease: A Global Mapping During 1990–2018. *Int. J. Environ. Res. Public Health* **2020**, *17*, 3089. [CrossRef] [PubMed]
8. Wang, M.; Liu, P.; Zhang, R.; Li, Z.; Li, X. A Scientometric Analysis of Global Health Research. *Int. J. Environ. Res. Public Health* **2020**, *17*, 2963. [CrossRef] [PubMed]
9. Vu, G.T.; Tran, B.X.; Hoang, C.L.; Hall, B.J.; Phan, H.T.; Ha, G.H.; Latkin, C.A.; Ho, C.S.; Ho, R. Global research on quality of life of patients with HIV/AIDS: Is it socio-culturally addressed? (GAPRESEARCH). *Int. J. Environ. Res. Public Health* **2020**, *17*, 2127. [CrossRef] [PubMed]
10. Vu, G.T.; Tran, B.X.; McIntyre, R.S.; Pham, H.Q.; Phan, H.T.; Ha, G.H.; Latkin, C.A.; Ho, R.; Ho, C.S. Modeling the Research Landscapes of Artificial Intelligence Applications in Diabetes (GAPRESEARCH). *Int. J. Environ. Res. Public Health* **2020**, *17*, 1982. [CrossRef] [PubMed]
11. Tran, B.X.; Nguyen, L.H.; Pham, N.M.; Vu, H.T.T.; Nguyen, H.T.; Phan, D.H.; Ha, G.H.; Phan, H.Q.; Nguyen, T.P.; Latkin, C.A.; et al. Global Mapping of Interventions to Improve Quality of Life of People with Diabetes in 1990–2018. *Int. J. Environ. Res. Public Health* **2020**, *17*, 1597. [CrossRef] [PubMed]
12. Garrido-Cardenas, J.A.; Esteban-García, B.; Agüera, A.; Sánchez-Pérez, J.A.; Manzano-Agugliaro, F. Wastewater treatment by advanced oxidation process and their worldwide research trends. *Int. J. Environ. Res. Public Health* **2020**, *17*, 170. [CrossRef] [PubMed]
13. Tran, B.X.; Nghiem, S.; Afoakwah, C.; Latkin, C.A.; Ha, G.H.; Nguyen, T.P.; Doan, L.P.; Pham, H.Q.; Ho, C.S.; Ho, R. Characterizing Obesity Interventions and Treatment for Children and Youths During 1991–2018. *Int. J. Environ. Res. Public Health* **2019**, *16*, 4227. [CrossRef] [PubMed]

14. Aparicio-Martinez, P.; Perea-Moreno, A.J.; Martinez-Jimenez, M.P.; Redel-Macías, M.D.; Vaquero-Abellan, M.; Pagliari, C. A bibliometric analysis of the health field regarding social networks and young people. *Int. J. Environ. Res. Public Health* **2019**, *16*, 4024. [CrossRef] [PubMed]
15. Gómez-Galán, M.; Callejón-Ferre, Á.J.; Pérez-Alonso, J.; Díaz-Pérez, M.; Carrillo-Castrillo, J.A. Musculoskeletal Risks: RULA Bibliometric Review. *Int. J. Environ. Res. Public Health* **2020**, *17*, 4354. [CrossRef] [PubMed]
16. Qin, F.; Du, J.; Gao, J.; Liu, G.; Song, Y.; Yang, A.; Wang, H.; Ding, Y.; Wang, Q. Bibliometric Profile of Global Microplastics Research from 2004 to 2019. *Int. J. Environ. Res. Public Health* **2020**, *17*, 5639. [CrossRef]

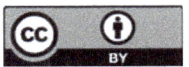

© 2020 by the authors. Licensee MDPI, Basel, Switzerland. This article is an open access article distributed under the terms and conditions of the Creative Commons Attribution (CC BY) license (http://creativecommons.org/licenses/by/4.0/).

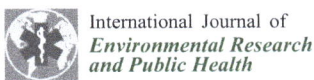 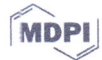

Article

Global Research Output and Theme Trends on Climate Change and Infectious Diseases: A Restrospective Bibliometric and Co-Word Biclustering Investigation of Papers Indexed in PubMed (1999–2018)

Fan Li [1], Hao Zhou [2,3], De-Sheng Huang [2,4] and Peng Guan [2,*]

1. School of Medical Informatics, China Medical University, Shenyang 110122, China; fanli@cmu.edu.cn
2. Department of Epidemiology, School of Public Health, China Medical University, Shenyang 110122, China; zhouhao@cipuc.edu.cn (H.Z.); dshuang@cmu.edu.cn (D.-S.H.)
3. Department of Impression Evidence Examination Technology, Criminal Investigation Police University of China, Shenyang 110854, China
4. Department of Mathematics, School of Fundamental Sciences, China Medical University, Shenyang 110122, China
* Correspondence: pguan@cmu.edu.cn

Received: 26 June 2020; Accepted: 14 July 2020; Published: 20 July 2020

Abstract: Climate change is a challenge for the sustainable development of an international economy and society. The impact of climate change on infectious diseases has been regarded as one of the most urgent research topics. In this paper, an analysis of the bibliometrics, co-word biclustering, and strategic diagram was performed to evaluate global scientific production, hotspots, and developing trends regarding climate change and infectious diseases, based on the data of two decades (1999–2008 and 2009–2018) from PubMed. According to the search strategy and inclusion criteria, a total of 1443 publications were found on the topic of climate change and infectious diseases. There has been increasing research productivity in this field, which has been supported by a wide range of subject categories. The top highly-frequent major MeSH (medical subject headings)/subheading combination terms could be divided into four clusters for the first decade and five for the second decade using a biclustering analysis. At present, some significant public health challenges (global health, and travel and tropical climate, etc.) are at the center of the whole target research network. In the last ten years, "Statistical model", "Diarrhea", "Dengue", "Ecosystem and biodiversity", and "Zoonoses" have been considered as emerging hotspots, but they still need more attention for further development.

Keywords: climate change; infectious diseases; bibliometric analysis; co-word analysis; biclustering; strategic diagram

1. Introduction

It has been firmly established that the Earth is warming, which is shown by the increase in the average ocean temperature and air temperature, and in the melting of snow and ice. Global climate change is one of the most widely discussed topics, not only in the field of climate science or policy making, but also in a range of health researches [1,2]. It can affect human health via different pathways of complexity, directness, and scale [3–5]. A better understanding of the human health dimensions of climate change is necessary for protecting people from climate-sensitive hazards and the development of a sustainable coping strategy [6–9]. In particular, the direct and indirect impact of climate change on infectious diseases has been regarded as one of most urgent research topics [10–12].

It has been well accepted by the academic community that climate change could not only affect the pathogens' ecology and the transmission dynamics of infectious diseases, but also the development of health promotion-related policy and the implementation process of the Sustainable Development Goals [13–15].

In the above-mentioned background, over the past several decades, there has been a large increase in scientific investigations about climate change and infectious diseases [14–16]. For example, the effect of global warming on vector-borne diseases, especially malaria, has been actively investigated [17–22]. The temperature can directly affect the biology of vectors and parasites, and increased precipitation may lead to an increase in the number and quality of breeding sites, and affect the availability of resting sites [23–26]. The temporal and spatial changes in climatic variables might affect the vectors, intermediate hosts, and, consequently, the risk of disease transmission [27,28]. Evidence has also indicated the impact of inter-annual and inter-decadal climate change on vector-borne diseases, which should be explored not only in a continental basis, but also in regional and local basis [29,30].

Bibliometrics is a kind of research method that analyzes bibliographic information using quantitative indicators, and has been widely employed for the statistical analysis of the bibliographic materials in a particular field [31,32]. In view of the impressive progress on climate change and infectious diseases, the quantitative and qualitative assessment of the scientific output will help to know the history, publication trends, research interest, and maturity degree of this field. Thus, the primary aim of the present work was to map the research output and theme trends in climate change and infectious diseases in the last 20 years (from 1999 to 2018), using the bibliometric indicators of production, word co-occurrence biclustering analysis, and strategic diagram. It is anticipated that this kind of reference can help the researchers in this field to prevent repeated work, avoid wasting resources, and know the research trends in the future. For the sake of shorthand, in the following section "this field" refers to "the field related to climate change and infectious diseases".

2. Materials and Methods

2.1. Data Collection

The data from 1999 until 2018 were retrieved from PubMed of the National Library of Medicine on the web (http://www.ncbi.nlm.nih.gov/pubmed), with the medical subject headings (MeSH) terms "Climate Change", "Climate", "Meteorological Concepts", "Weather", and "Communicable Diseases"; the key words "Meteorological" and "Infectious diseases" in the title and abstract fields; and the Boolean combinations of these words as the retrieval strategy (for details of the retrieval strategy, see Table S1 in Supplementary Materials). The literature type was limited to journal articles. All publications were saved as two files, in the format of XML and MEDLINE, separately. Two independent researchers filtered the downloaded records manually according to the inclusion and exclusion criteria, after reviewing the titles and abstracts, and even, in some cases, the full text of the records. If they disagreed, the third person would judge whether a record was relevant. The included records were journal articles concerning both climate change and infectious diseases. The exclusion criteria were the following: (1) books, retracted publications, and bibliographies; (2) records of which the topic was related to political climate, social climate, economic climate, financial climate, organizational climate, etc.; and (3) repeated records.

Aiming to map the knowledge structure and theme trends of climate change and infectious diseases in the last 20 years, two periods of 10 years each were established, namely: 1 January 1999–31 December 2008, and 1 January 2009–31 December 2018. Furthermore, the comparative analysis for articles published in the two periods was conducted from the perspectives of bibliometric indicators and topics.

2.2. Data Analysis

Bibliographic Items Co-occurrence Matrix Builder (BICOMB), provided by Professor Cui from China Medical University [33], and Microsoft Excel were employed to determine the annual number of publications, most active journals, distribution of journals' publication places, and the frequency of major MeSH/subheading combination terms. In the following section, "major MeSH/Subheading combination term" is referred to as "term" for short. The publication time of an article in this study was the final publication time, which meant that the information about the volume, pages, or serial article number had been released.

A research hotspot refers to a focus of research where researchers have conducted a lot of studies and published many related papers. By obtaining the frequencies and relationship of the words reflecting the content of the articles in a field, the hotspots of the field can usually be identified [34]. In this study, based on the principle for the g-index of the word frequency, a proper threshold (g) was set for the number of terms in order to generate a list of highly-frequent terms and a term-article matrix [35]. Egghe put forward a g-index used to reflect the contribution value of high-quality papers (i.e., highly cited papers) to a scientist. Similarly, a co-word analysis is used to select highly-frequent words to reflect the hotspots of a certain research field, so the g-index can also reflect the contribution value of highly-frequent words to all of the words in a given field [36]. Zhang et al. and Yang et al. have proved the simplicity and effectiveness of the g-index in selecting highly-frequent words in their empirical studies [35,37]. The method for the determination of the number, g, is as follows: firstly, all major MeSH/subheading combination terms were sorted in descending order of frequency; i was the sequence number of each term; when i was equal to g, the cumulative frequency of the first g terms was not less than g^2, while that of the first $(g + 1)$ terms was less than $(g + 1)^2$. Then, the first g terms were considered as high-frequency terms [37]. If there were multiple terms with the frequency equal to that of the gth term, these terms were also identified as the highly-frequent terms. Next, a binary matrix with highly-frequent term-source article was created from BICOMB. By using the software "gCLUTO" (Graphical Clustering Toolkit, developed by Rasmussen et al. from University of Minnesota)) version 1.0 (University of Minnesota, Minneapolis, MN, USA), the matrix was imported for further biclustering [38]. The parameters in gCLUTO—repeated bisection for the clustering method, cosine for similarity function, and I^2 for criterion function of clustering—were set based on those appropriate for the biclustering analysis of the literature. In order to gain the optimal number of clusters, the procedure for biclustering was repeated with different numbers of clusters. The biclustering result of the term-article matrix was presented through the visualization format of a mountain and matrix. With the aid of semantic relationships between the MeSH/subheading combination terms, and the content of the representative articles in each cluster, the basic framework of research hotspots on climate change-related infectious diseases was drawn and analyzed.

Moving forward, every hot research topic was put into the strategic diagram to show the relational patterns inside each cluster and among all of the clusters, so that the current status and evolutionary trends of this field could be revealed. In 1988, Law et al. proposed a strategic diagram to describe the internal linkages in the research domains and inter-domain interactions [39]. The strategic diagram is manifested as a two-dimensional chart, with the horizontal axis representing the centrality (the average value of external links, and external links refer to the sum of times that every term in a given cluster and every term in other clusters co-occur in the same article) and the vertical axis standing for the density (the average value of internal links, and internal links are the sum of times that every pair of terms in a given cluster co-occur in the same article) [40]. The centrality is used to judge the degree to which each term is connected with the terms in the other clusters, which can indicate the degree that one theme affects the others. The greater the number and intensity of links between a subject domain and other subject domains, the more central the subject domain becomes in the whole research work. The density is used to measure the closeness degree of the internal terms inside the same cluster, indicating the strength of relations that make terms into a cluster, i.e., the ability of one theme to maintain and develop itself [41]. Based on the results of the co-word clustering analysis and co-occurrence matrix of the highly-frequent terms, the density and the centrality were calculated for each cluster. The origin of coordinate is the average value of all centralities and that of all densities. With the help of the content, as well as the centrality and density of each cluster, the development status of the hot research topics in the two decades was presented by strategic diagrams, from which the evolutionary trend of the global research on climate change and infectious diseases was analyzed and discussed.

3. Results

3.1. Growth and Journals of the Relevant Publications

Based on our search strategy and on the inclusion and exclusion criteria, 1443 journal articles were retrieved in PubMed on the topic of climate change and infectious diseases from 1999 to 2018. The annual number of related articles grew exponentially from only 18 in 1999, to the maximum, 147 in 2017, as shown in Figure 1, where an exponential trend line could be added (the degree of fitting, R^2, is 0.83). For the two periods, 1999–2008 and 2009–2018, there were 368 and 1075 journal articles involved, respectively, which were then subjected to a comparative analysis.

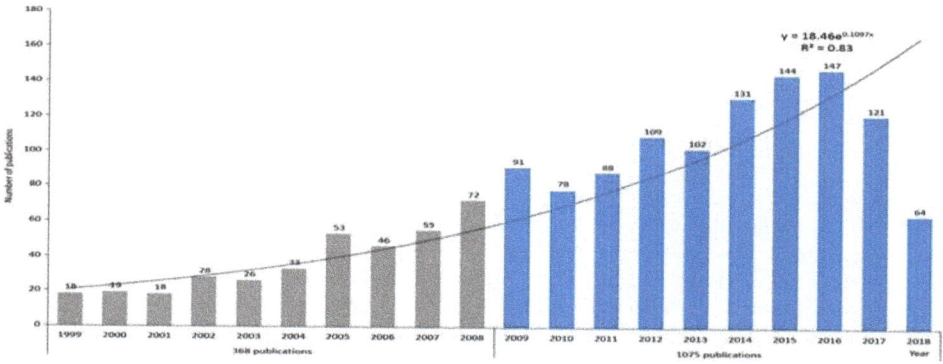

Figure 1. Temporal distribution of research output about climate change and infectious diseases (PubMed sourced).

Altogether, 521 journals were involved in the field (1999–2008: 226 journals; 2009–2018: 407 journals). The United States and England were always two major publication places of journals publishing relevant articles in the two decades, as illustrated in Figure 2. The third publication places were France in the first decade and the Netherlands in the second decade. Table 1 displays the top ten productive journals for each period, as well as their languages, publication places, and number of publications. In 1999–2008, the top three most active journals were *Emerging Infectious Diseases*, *Journal of Travel Medicine*, and *Annals of the New York Academy of Science*, whereas in the latter ten years, *PLoS One*, *International Journal of Environmental Research and Public Health*, and *Epidemiology and Infection* were the most popular.

Table 1. Most active journals of publications on climate change and infectious diseases in PubMed (1999–2008 and 2009–2018).

Period	Rank	Most Active Journals	Languages	Publication Places	Number of Publications	Percentage (%)
1999–2008	1	Emerging Infectious Diseases	English	United States	11	2.99
	2	Journal of Travel Medicine	English	England	9	2.45
	3	Annals of the New York Academy of Sciences	English	United States	6	1.63
	4	International Journal of Health Geographics	English	England	6	1.63
	5	Medecine Tropicale: Revue du Corps de Sante Colonial	French	France	6	1.63
	6	Proceedings of the National Academy of Sciences of the United States of America	English	United States	5	1.36
	7	Epidemiology and Infection	English	England	5	1.36
	8	Revue Scientifique et Technique (International Office of Epizootics)	English, French, Spanish	France	5	1.36
	9	Nature	English	England	5	1.36
	10	New South Wales Public Health Bulletin	English	Australia	5	1.36
	Total				63	17.12
2009–2018	1	PLoS One	English	United States	64	5.93
	2	International Journal of Environmental Research and Public Health	English	Switzerland	31	2.87
	3	Epidemiology and Infection	English	England	25	2.32
	4	BMC Infectious Diseases	English	England	23	2.13
	5	PLoS Neglected Tropical Diseases	English	United States	23	2.13
	6	Przeglad Epidemiologiczny	English, Polish	Poland	18	1.67
	7	Proceedings of the National Academy of Sciences of the United States of America	English	United States	18	1.67
	8	Communicable Diseases Intelligence Quarterly Report	English	United States	17	1.58
	9	Emerging Infectious Diseases	English	United States	17	1.58
	10	Global Health Action	English	United States	16	1.48
	Total				252	23.35

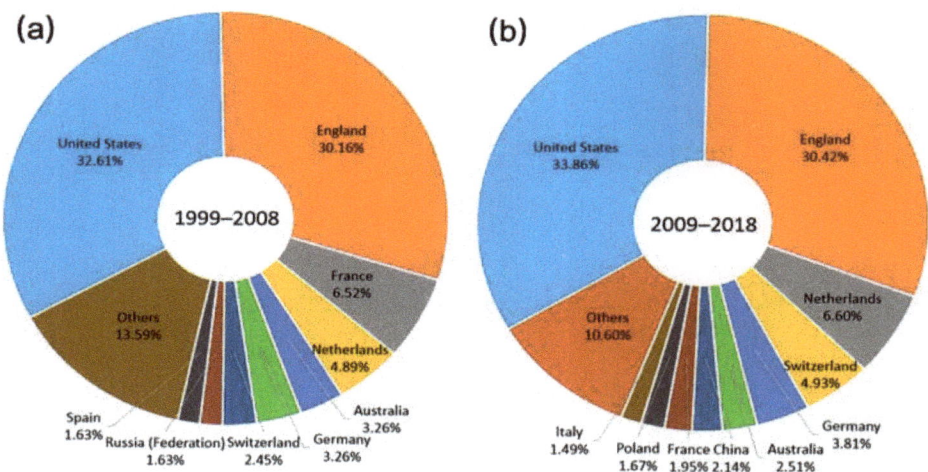

Figure 2. Publication places of journals publishing articles on climate change and infectious diseases. (**a**) Publication places of journals publishing relevant articles from 1999 to 2008; (**b**) publication places of journals publishing relevant articles from 2009 to 2018.

3.2. Highly-Frequent MeSH/Subheading Combination Terms and Their Cluster Pattern

From the articles included, 26 and 39 high-frequency major MeSH/subheadings combination terms were extracted for the first and second decade, respectively, based on the method for the g-index of the word frequency mentioned above, with a cumulative frequency percentage of 32.95% and 37.39%, respectively (Tables S2 and S3 in Supplementary Materials). Furthermore, these terms were subject to a co-word biclustering analysis to reveal the research hotspots for climate change and infectious diseases in the past two decades.

The high-frequency terms were classified into four clusters for the first decade and five for the second decade using the biclustering analysis, as presented in Figures 3 and 4. These two figures also show the mountain and matrix visualization of these terms. In the mountain visualization, each 3D peak labeled by the cluster number contains a cluster of terms, of which the location on the plane, volume, height, and color are used to portray information about a cluster. The distance between two peaks on the plane reflects the relative similarity of two clusters. There is positive correlation between the peak's height and the cluster's internal similarity. The volume of a peak is positively correlated with the number of terms classified into a cluster. In addition, the peak's color represents the internal standard deviation of a cluster's terms. Blue represents a high internal standard deviation of the objects inside, whereas red represents a low internal standard deviation. In the matrix visualization, the high-frequency terms are listed on the right side. The number before each term represents its serial number (See Tables S2 and S3). The top and left hierarchical trees display the relationships among the included articles and those among the high-frequency terms, by which the themes of all of the clusters have been able to identify and summarize, and insights into the representative articles of each cluster could be attained as well. The hotspots of climate change and infectious diseases revealed by the cluster analysis of high-frequency terms during the two periods are presented in Table 2.

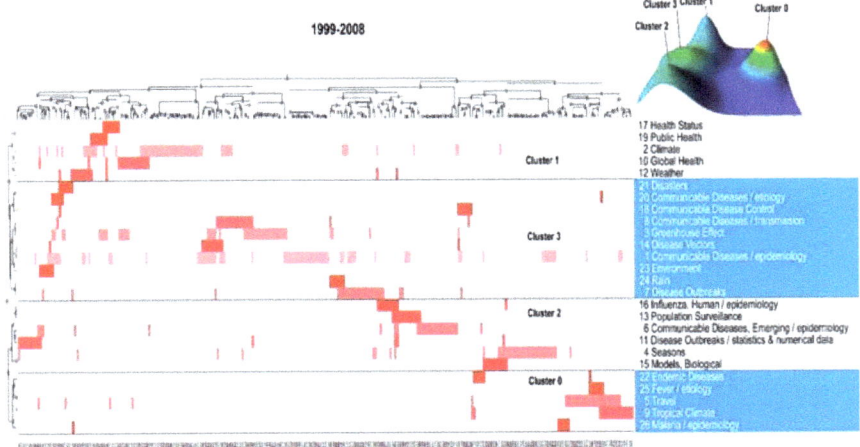

Figure 3. Mountain and matrix visualization of biclustering of highly-frequent major medical subject headings (MeSH)/subheading combination terms and articles on climate change and infectious diseases from 1999 to 2008.

Table 2. Hotspots of climate change and infectious diseases explored by biclustering analysis of high-frequency major MeSH/subheading combination terms in 1999–2008 and 2009–2018.

Period	Cluster	Term * No.	Cluster Analysis
1999–2008	0	22, 25, 5, 9, 26	1. Fever, malaria, and endemic diseases; 2. Travel and tropical climate
	1	17, 19, 2, 10, 12	1. Global health 2. Public health
	2	16, 13, 6, 11, 4, 15	1. Human influenza and emerging communicable diseases 2. Season 3. Biological models
	3	21, 20, 18, 8, 3, 14, 1, 23, 24, 7	1. Etiology, transmission, and control of communicable diseases 2. Greenhouse effect, disasters, environment, and rain
2009–2018	0	36, 4, 10, 15, 19, 35	1. Gastroenteritis and hand, foot, and mouth disease 2. Disease outbreaks 3. Environment
	1	18, 32, 39, 30, 22, 7, 11	1. Temperature and rain 2. Diarrhea, malaria, and dengue
	2	24, 12, 21, 31, 20, 5, 2, 1, 28	1. Travel and tropical climate 2. Epidemiology, transmission, and methods, organization, and administration of communicable diseases 3. Global health
	3	34, 23, 17, 8, 3, 9, 27, 29	1. Human influenza and epidemics 2. Statistical and biological model 3. Season
	4	26, 25, 13, 37, 38, 6, 16, 14, 33	1. Greenhouse effect 2. Ecosystem and biodiversity 3. Public health 4. Emerging communicable diseases and zoonoses

* Term refers to the high-frequency major MeSH/subheading combination term.

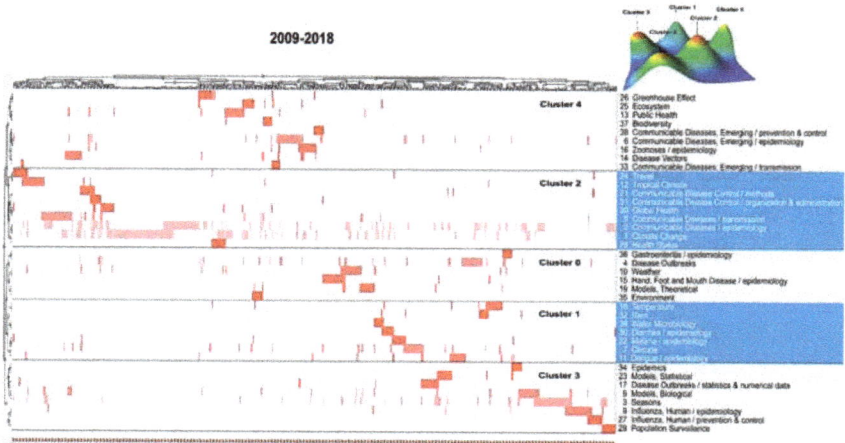

Figure 4. Mountain and matrix visualization of biclustering of highly-frequent major MeSH/subheading combination terms and articles on climate change and infectious diseases from 2009 to 2018.

3.3. Trends of Research Themes

A strategic diagram can generally represent the structure of a research field, in which all of the research hotspots are placed in the four quadrants of the coordinate graph, based on the values of the centrality and density, thus describing the research status and trend of each hotspot. The density is used to determine the closeness of the terms within each cluster of hotspots. It represents the self-sustainability of each cluster of hotspot, i.e., stability [41]. The centrality spot measure the closeness between the terms of each cluster and those in the other cluster, indicating the degree of mutual influence of one cluster of a hotspot and the other clusters. The greater the centrality of one cluster of hotspot, the more central it tends to be in the entire research field [42]. Therefore, the clusters in Quadrant 1 are the relative core and stable themes (strongly connected with other clusters and having intense internal relationships). The clusters located within Quadrant 2 represent peripheral but already well-developed themes. The clusters in Quadrant 3 are both peripheral and unstable. The clusters in Quadrant 4 are central but not stable, yet they are becoming mature or are vanishing to some extent [39]. Typically, analyses are the most interested in the new and exciting topics in Quadrant 4.

Based on the results of the co-word biclustering analysis and the co-occurrence matrix of high-frequency terms, we calculated the centrality and density of each cluster and drew two strategic diagrams on research hotspots for the two decades. Then, we analyzed the basic framework, alteration, and trend of research hotspots on climate change and infectious diseases in the world (Figure 5).

Four clusters from 1999 to 2008 are scattered in the four quadrants, i.e., Cluster 1 in Quadrant 1, Cluster 2 in Quadrant 2, Cluster 0 in Quadrant 3, and Cluster 3 in Quadrant 4. Cluster 1, global and public health, is considered as the motor theme (of which centrality and density are both high). In the decade from 2009 to 2018, Cluster 2 lies in Quadrant 1, Cluster 0 in Quadrant 2, and the rest of three clusters (Clusters 1, 3, and 4) lie in Quadrant 3, while no cluster is in Quadrant 4. The contrast of the clusters and their positions in the strategic diagrams between the two 10-year periods can also be visualized in Figure 5, showing the trend and alteration of the hot research themes.

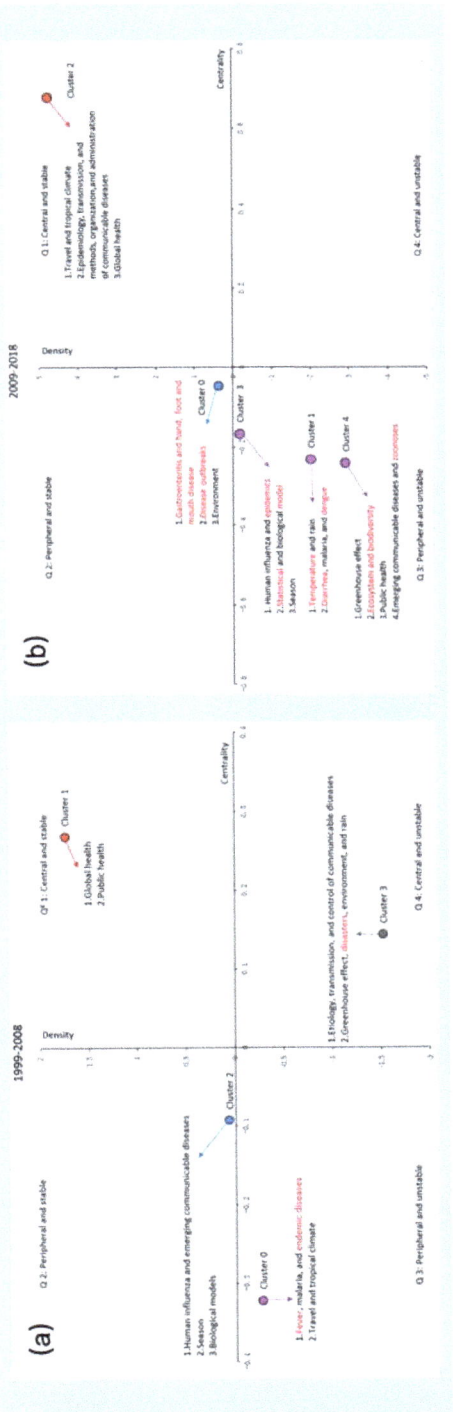

Figure 5. Strategic diagrams of hotspots in research output on climate change and infectious diseases from 1999 to 2008 and from 2009 to 2018. (**a**) Strategic diagrams of hotspot from 1999 to 2008; (**b**) strategic diagrams of hotspots from 2009 to 2018. $^\text{€}$ Q stands for quadrant. Clusters inside each strategic diagram refer to the clustering results shown in Table 2. The descriptions indicated by arrows are the hotspots of each cluster. The words in the red font represent the exclusive hotspot research topics in the first decade or the second decade.

4. Discussion

In the context of global warming, academic communities have paid increasing attention to the direct and indirect effects of climate change on the appearance and spread of infectious diseases. The relationship between climate change and infectious diseases has become an important research field, which requires the systematic analysis of the knowledge structure and theme trends. In this study, the bibliometric analysis, co-word biclustering analysis, and strategic diagram on the scientific productions from the quantitative and content's points of view were integrated to investigate the knowledge structure and evolution of this field in the past 20 years.

4.1. Principal Findings

To the authors' knowledge, for the first time, an evaluation is reported on the research status and trend of climate change and infectious diseases around the world in the last two decades. The quantitative study clearly shows the exponentially rapid growth of the relevant publications, focusing on the topic of climate change and infectious diseases from 1999 to 2018. The articles published in the last decade (2009–2018) are nearly threefold of those in the previous decade (1999–2008).

According to the summarized distribution data of journals, the number of journals is almost twice as much in the last decade as in the previous decade, demonstrating that more and more journals began to publish articles regarding climate change and infectious diseases. It is also notable that comprehensive journals, for example, *Nature* and *PLoS One*, have shown interest in collecting papers in this field, confirming that the research on climate change-related infectious diseases had been supported by a wide range of subject categories. In the last two decades, however, the publication places of relevant journals were mainly developed countries or regions, such as The United States, England, Switzerland, and France.

As expected, this study provided some hints of the recent research hotspots in the field of climate change and infectious diseases. A co-word biclustering analysis was performed to reveal the research hotspots in the field, where there were four big clusters (nine subclass topics) and five big clusters (15) found in 1999 to 2008 and 2009 to 2018, respectively. Some topics, such as travel and tropic climate, global health, public health, environment, rain, biological model, and the greenhouse effect, have always been interesting for researchers. Human influenza, malaria, and emerging communicable diseases are the consistently concerned infectious diseases. From 1999 to 2008, hotspots like disasters, fever, and endemic diseases were not the same hotspots from 2009 to 2018. In the last ten years, researchers have begun to pay attention to some new hotspots, e.g., statistical model, diseases outbreaks, ecosystem, and biodiversity (Table 2 and Figure 5). Specifically, research on statistical models have become a hotspot, probably due to the development of data science, as well as new statistical methodology, such as deep learning, and their recent application in medicine [43]. Meanwhile, gastroenteritis; hand, foot, and mouth disease; diarrhea; dengue; and zoonoses are new foci among the research field of climate-sensitive communicable diseases. Hand, foot, and mouth disease, in particular, is a type of communicable disease emerging in recent decades. Although occurring much later in some countries like China, where it was originally seen in 1981, this disease is very prevalent, and often leads to outbreaks among children [44,45]. Therefore, researchers have begun to carry out related studies from multiple perspectives. In the aspect of its correlation with climate, a considerable amount of journal articles (32 articles) have been published within the last decade, according to the analysis of this study.

In parallel, the strategic diagram was employed to interpret the trends in themes during the two periods. Global health locates in Quadrant 1 all the time, indicating it is mature, but is indeed the eternal core theme of the whole body of literature. The topic on malaria is always in Quadrant 3, demonstrating that it is neither mature nor a core topic in the whole related field, and thus needs further investigation.

During the second decade (2009–2018), "Travel and tropical climate" within Quadrant 1, previously considered as the undeveloped and peripheral theme, progressed well and become the core of the relevant field. New hotspots of "gastroenteritis and hand, foot, and mouth disease" and "disease outbreaks" have become mature in the last ten years, although they are still on the edge of the whole field. Other new hotspots, like "Statistical model", "Diarrhea", "Dengue", "Ecosystem and biodiversity", and "Zoonoses", are far from the research core, and do not connect closely with other subfield studies within the overall research network, and thus are neither mature nor the central topics in this field. They need more attention from researchers. However, research on some meteorological factors, such as "Greenhouse effect" and "Rain", remain unstable or undeveloped, and have shifted from the central to the edge of the whole research field.

4.2. Limitations and Future Work

This present study has several potential limitations, which might encourage further research efforts. These include the research output of the target field being only represented by the publications in a single database. Bias could arise in terms of an underestimation or unbalanced estimation of each subfield. However, PubMed, as used in this study, is a world-renowned authoritative bibliographic database for biomedicine, from which the relevant literature could represent the research status on climate-related infectious diseases well, to certain degree. The second potential limitation is that as climate change and infectious diseases are closely related to national security and defense, due to their direct or indirect military applications, it is possible that part of the publications were not open to the public research community, thus they could not be included in the present bibliometric study for analysis. However, based on the open publications, the tendency and hotspots in the field can still be drawn. We plan to utilize diverse databases for further analyses in future studies.

5. Conclusions

While there is rising global attention to climate change, there is also increased research productivity in the field of climate change-related infectious diseases, which has been supported by a wide range of subject categories. At present, some significant public health challenges (global health, travel and tropical climate, etc.) are at the center of the whole target research network. "Statistical model", "Diarrhea", "Dengue", "Ecosystem and biodiversity", and "Zoonoses" were considered as emerging hotspots during the last ten years, but they still need more attention for further development. The present study provides the academic community and policymakers with baseline information in this field. Additionally, it provides a framework of the bibliometric analysis, co-word biclustering analysis, and strategic diagram on the scientific productions from a quantitative and contents points of view. The framework can assist the researchers to clarify the history, development, and trend in themes in the target field.

Supplementary Materials: The following are available online at http://www.mdpi.com/1660-4601/17/14/5228/s1: Table S1: Search strategy for retrieval of literature on climate change and infectious diseases from PubMed; Table S2: High-frequency major MeSH/Subheading combination terms from the included articles on climate and infectious diseases in 1999–2008; Table S3: High-frequency major MeSH/Subheading combination terms from the included articles on climate and infectious diseases in 2009–2018.

Author Contributions: Conceptualization, F.L. and P.G.; methodology, F.L. and P.G.; software, F.L.; validation, H.Z., D.-S.H. and P.G.; formal analysis, F.L. and H.Z.; investigation, F.L. and H.Z.; resources, F.L., D.-S.H. and P.G.; data curation, F.L.; writing (original draft preparation), P.G.; writing (review and editing), F.L., H.Z. and D.-S.H.; visualization, F.L.; supervision, P.G.; project administration, P.G.; funding acquisition, F.L., D.-S.H. and P.G. All of the authors have read and agreed to the published version of the manuscript. All authors have read and agreed to the published version of the manuscript.

Funding: This research was funded by the National Natural Science Foundation of China, grant numbers 71974199 and 71573275; the Science Foundation of Liaoning Provincial Department of Education of China, grant number JCRW2020006; and the Liaoning Natural Science Foundation of China, grant number 2020-MS-159.

Conflicts of Interest: The authors declare no conflict of interest.

References

1. McMichael, C. Human mobility, climate change, and health: Unpacking the connections. *Lancet Planet Health* **2020**, *4*, e217–e218. [CrossRef]
2. Gartin, M.; Larson, K.L.; Brewis, A.; Stotts, R.; Wutich, A.; White, D.; du Bray, M. Climate change as an involuntary exposure: A comparative risk perception study from six countries across the global development gradient. *Int. J. Environ. Res. Public Health* **2020**, *17*, 1894. [CrossRef]
3. Wu, X.; Lu, Y.; Zhou, S.; Chen, L.; Xu, B. Impact of climate change on human infectious diseases: Empirical evidence and human adaptation. *Environ. Int.* **2016**, *86*, 14–23. [CrossRef]
4. Filho, W.L.; Scheday, S.; Boenecke, J.; Gogoi, A.; Maharaj, A.; Korovou, S. Climate change, health and mosquito-borne diseases:Trends and implications to the pacific region. *Int. J. Environ. Res. Public Health* **2019**, *16*, 5114. [CrossRef] [PubMed]
5. Liu, J.; Wu, X.; Li, C.; Xu, B.; Hu, L.; Chen, J.; Dai, S. Identification of weather variables sensitive to dysentery in disease-affected county of China. *Sci. Total Environ.* **2017**, *575*, 956–962. [CrossRef]
6. Smith, J.; Taylor, E.M. What is next for NTDs in the era of the sustainable development goals? *PLoS Negl. Trop. Dis.* **2016**, *10*, e0004719. [CrossRef] [PubMed]
7. Helm, D. Climate policy: The Kyoto approach has failed. *Nature* **2012**, *491*, 663–665. [CrossRef] [PubMed]
8. Rogelj, J.; McCollum, D.L.; Reisinger, A.; Meinshausen, M.; Riahi, K. Probabilistic cost estimates for climate change mitigation. *Nature* **2013**, *493*, 79–83. [CrossRef]
9. Altizer, S.; Ostfeld, R.S.; Johnson, P.T.; Kutz, S.; Harvell, C.D. Climate change and infectious diseases: From evidence to a predictive framework. *Science* **2013**, *341*, 514–519. [CrossRef]
10. McMichael, A.J.; Woodruff, R.E.; Hales, S. Climate change and human health: Present and future risks. *Lancet* **2006**, *367*, 859–869. [CrossRef]
11. Dora, C.; Haines, A.; Balbus, J.; Fletcher, E.; Adair-Rohani, H.; Alabaster, G.; Hossain, R.; de Onis, M.; Branca, F.; Neira, M. Indicators linking health and sustainability in the post-2015 development agenda. *Lancet* **2015**, *385*, 380–391. [CrossRef]
12. Kilpatrick, A.M.; Randolph, S.E. Drivers, dynamics, and control of emerging vector-borne zoonotic diseases. *Lancet* **2012**, *380*, 1946–1955. [CrossRef]
13. Axelsen, J.B.; Yaari, R.; Grenfell, B.T.; Stone, L. Multiannual forecasting of seasonal influenza dynamics reveals climatic and evolutionary drivers. *Proc. Natl. Acad. Sci. USA.* **2014**, *111*, 9538–9542. [CrossRef]
14. Patz, J.A.; Frumkin, H.; Holloway, T.; Vimont, D.J.; Haines, A. Climate change: Challenges and opportunities for global health. *J. Am. Med. Assoc.* **2014**, *312*, 1565–1580. [CrossRef] [PubMed]
15. Shuman, E.K. Global climate change and infectious diseases. *N. Engl. J. Med.* **2010**, *362*, 1061–1063. [CrossRef] [PubMed]
16. Konrad, S.K.; Miller, S.N. A temperature-limited assessment of the risk of Rift Valley fever transmission and establishment in the continental United States of America. *Geosp. Health* **2012**, *6*, 161–170. [CrossRef] [PubMed]
17. Massad, E.; Coutinho, F.A.; Lopez, L.F.; Da, S.D. Modeling the impact of global warming on vector-borne infections. *Phys. Life Rev.* **2011**, *8*, 169–199. [CrossRef]
18. Ramasamy, R.; Surendran, S.N. Possible impact of rising sea levels on vector-borne infectious diseases. *BMC Infect Dis.* **2011**, *11*, 18. [CrossRef]
19. Hertig, E. Distribution of Anopheles vectors and potential malaria transmission stability in Europe and the Mediterranean area under future climate change. *Parasites Vectors* **2019**, *12*, 18. [CrossRef]
20. Xiang, J.; Hansen, A.; Liu, Q.; Tong, M.X.; Liu, X.; Sun, Y.; Cameron, S.; Hanson-Easey, S.; Han, G.S.; Williams, C.; et al. Association between malaria incidence and meteorological factors: A multi-location study in China, 2005–2012. *Epidemiol. Infect* **2018**, *146*, 89–99. [CrossRef]
21. Hongoh, V.; Gosselin, P.; Michel, P.; Ravel, A.; Waaub, J.P.; Campagna, C.; Samoura, K. Criteria for the prioritization of public health interventions for climate-sensitive vector-borne diseases in Quebec. *PLoS ONE* **2017**, *12*, e0190049. [CrossRef] [PubMed]
22. Tong, M.X.; Hansen, A.; Hanson-Easey, S.; Cameron, S.; Xiang, J.; Liu, Q.; Liu, X.; Sun, Y.; Weinstein, P.; Han, G.S.; et al. Perceptions of malaria control and prevention in an era of climate change: A cross-sectional survey among CDC staff in China. *Malar J.* **2017**, *16*, 136. [CrossRef] [PubMed]

23. Moore, S.; Shrestha, S.; Tomlinson, K.W.; Vuong, H. Predicting the effect of climate change on African trypanosomiasis: Integrating epidemiology with parasite and vector biology. *J. R. Soc. Interface* **2012**, *9*, 817–830. [CrossRef]
24. Thai, K.T.; Anders, K.L. The role of climate variability and change in the transmission dynamics and geographic distribution of dengue. *Exp. Biol. Med. (Maywood)* **2011**, *236*, 944–954. [CrossRef] [PubMed]
25. Bai, Y.L.; Huang, D.S.; Liu, J.; Li, D.Q.; Guan, P. Effect of meteorological factors on influenza-like illness from 2012 to 2015 in Huludao, a northeastern city in China. *PeerJ* **2019**, *7*, e6919. [CrossRef]
26. Bai, X.H.; Peng, C.; Jiang, T.; Hu, Z.M.; Huang, D.S.; Guan, P. Distribution of geographical scale, data aggregation unit and period in the correlation analysis between temperature and incidence of HFRS in mainland China: A systematic review of 27 ecological studies. *PLoS Negl. Trop. Dis.* **2019**, *13*, e0007688. [CrossRef]
27. Cheng, Q.; Jing, Q.; Spear, R.C.; Marshall, J.M.; Yang, Z.; Gong, P. Climate and the timing of imported cases as determinants of the dengue outbreak in Guangzhou, 2014: Evidence from a mathematical model. *PLoS Negl. Trop. Dis.* **2016**, *10*, e0004417. [CrossRef]
28. Dicko, A.H.; Percoma, L.; Sow, A.; Adam, Y.; Mahama, C.; Sidibe, I.; Dayo, G.K.; Thevenon, S.; Fonta, W.; Sanfo, S.; et al. A spatio-temporal model of African animal trypanosomosis risk. *PLoS Negl. Trop. Dis.* **2015**, *9*, e0003921. [CrossRef] [PubMed]
29. Githeko, A.K.; Lindsay, S.W.; Confalonieri, U.E.; Patz, J.A. Climate change and vector-borne diseases: A regional analysis. *Bull. WHO* **2000**, *78*, 1136–1147.
30. Randolph, S.E. Tick-borne encephalitis virus, ticks and humans: Short-term and long-term dynamics. *Curr. Opin. Infect Dis.* **2008**, *21*, 462–467. [CrossRef]
31. Mas-Tur, A.; Guijarro, M.; Carrilero, A. The influence of the circular economy: Exploring the knowledge base. *Sustainability* **2019**, *11*, 4367. [CrossRef]
32. Chantre-Astaiza, A.; Fuentes-Moraleda, L.; Muñoz-Mazón, A.; Ramirez-Gonzalez, G. Science mapping of tourist mobility 1980–2019. technological advancements in the collection of the data for tourist traceability. *Sustainability* **2019**, *11*, 4738. [CrossRef]
33. Cui, L.; Liu, W.; Yan, L.; Zhang, H.; Hou, Y.; Huang, Y.; Zhang, H. Development of a text mining system based on the co-occurrence of bibliographic items in literature databases. *New Technol. Libr. Inf. Serv.* **2008**, *4*, 70–75.
34. Li, F.; Li, M.; Guan, P.; Ma, S.; Cui, L. Mapping publication trends and identifying hot spots of research on Internet health information seeking behavior: A quantitative and co-word biclustering analysis. *J. Med. Internet Res.* **2015**, *17*, e81. [CrossRef]
35. Zhang, S.; Liu, C.; Chang, Y. Selection research of keywords in co-word clustered based on the g-index of word frequency—Taking educational technology master thesis as an example. *Mod. Educ. Technol.* **2013**, *23*, 53–57.
36. Egghe, L. Theory and practise of the g-Index. *Scientometrics* **2006**, *69*, 131–152. [CrossRef]
37. Yang, A.; Ma, X.; Zhang, F.; Xue, W. Application research of g-index in the topic words of co-word analysis. *J. Intell.* **2012**, *74*, 52–55.
38. Rasmussen, M.; Karypis, G. gCLUTO: An Interactive Clustering, Visualization, and Analysis System. CSE/UMN Technical Report: TR# 04–021. 2004. Available online: http://glaros.dtc.umn.edu/gkhome/node/174 (accessed on 25 May 2004).
39. Law, J.; Bauin, S.; Courtial, J.P.; Whittaker, J. Policy and the mapping of scientific change: A co-word analysis of research into environmental acidification. *Scientometrics* **1988**, *14*, 251–264. [CrossRef]
40. Guo, D.; Chen, H.; Long, R.; Lu, H.; Long, Q. A co-word analysis of organizational constraints for maintaining sustainability. *Sustainability* **2017**, *9*, 1928. [CrossRef]
41. Callon, M.; Courtial, J.P.; Laville, F. Co-word analysis as a tool for describing the network of interactions between basic and technological research: The case of polymer chemsitry. *Scientometrics* **1991**, *22*, 155–205. [CrossRef]
42. Bauin, S.; Michelet, B.; Schweighoffer, M.G.; Vermeulin, P. Using bibliometrics in strategic analysis: "understanding chemical reactions" at the CNRS. *Scientometrics* **1991**, *22*, 113–137. [CrossRef]
43. Xu, Q.; Gel, Y.R.; Ramirez, R.L.; Nezafati, K.; Zhang, Q.; Tsui, K.L. Forecasting influenza in Hong Kong with Google search queries and statistical model fusion. *PLoS ONE* **2017**, *12*, e0176690. [CrossRef] [PubMed]

44. Zhao, D.; Wang, L.; Cheng, J.; Xu, J.; Xu, Z.; Xie, M.; Yang, H.; Li, K.; Wen, L.; Wang, X.; et al. Impact of weather factors on hand, foot and mouth disease, and its role in short-term incidence trend forecast in Huainan City, Anhui Province. *Int. J. Biometeorol.* **2017**, *61*, 453–461. [CrossRef] [PubMed]
45. Wu, X.; Hu, S.; Kwaku, A.B.; Li, Q.; Luo, K.; Zhou, Y.; Tan, H. Spatio-temporal clustering analysis and its determinants of hand, foot and mouth disease in Hunan, China, 2009–2015. *BMC Infect Dis.* **2017**, *17*, 645. [CrossRef] [PubMed]

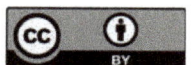

© 2020 by the authors. Licensee MDPI, Basel, Switzerland. This article is an open access article distributed under the terms and conditions of the Creative Commons Attribution (CC BY) license (http://creativecommons.org/licenses/by/4.0/).

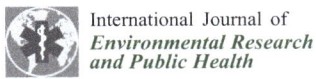

Article

Wastewater Treatment by Advanced Oxidation Process and Their Worldwide Research Trends

José Antonio Garrido-Cardenas [1,*], Belén Esteban-García [2,3], Ana Agüera [2], José Antonio Sánchez-Pérez [2,3] and Francisco Manzano-Agugliaro [4]

1. Department of Biology and Geology, University of Almeria, 04120 Almeria, Spain
2. Solar Energy Research Centre (CIESOL), Joint Centre University of Almería-CIEMAT, 04120 Almería, Spain; abgarcia@ual.es (B.E.-G.); aaguera@ual.es (A.A.); jsanchez@ual.es (J.A.S.-P.)
3. Department of Chemical Engineering, University of Almería, 04120 Almeria, Spain
4. Department of Engineering, ceiA3, University of Almeria, 04120 Almeria, Spain; fmanzano@ual.es
* Correspondence: jcardena@ual.es

Received: 26 November 2019; Accepted: 23 December 2019; Published: 25 December 2019

Abstract: *Background*: Water is a scarce resource and is considered a fundamental pillar of sustainable development. The modern development of society requires more and more drinking water. For this cleaner wastewater, treatments are key factors. Among those that exist, advanced oxidation processes are being researched as one of the sustainable solutions. The main objective of this manuscript is to show the scientific advances in this field. *Methods*: In this paper, a systematic analysis of all the existing scientific works was carried out to verify the evolution of this line of research. *Results*: It was observed that the three main countries researching this field are China, Spain, and the USA. Regarding the scientific collaboration between countries, three clusters were detected—one of Spain, one of China and the USA, and one of Italy and France. The publications are grouped around three types of water: industrial, urban, and drinking. Regarding the research, 15 clusters identified from the keywords analyzed the advanced oxidation process (alone or combined with biological oxidation) with the type of wastewater and the target pollutant, removal of which is intended. Finally, the most important scientific communities or clusters detected in terms of the number of published articles were those related to the elimination of pollutants of biological origin, such as bacteria, and of industrial nature, such as pesticides or pharmaceutical products.

Keywords: reclaimed water; advanced oxidation process; microorganisms; concern emergent contaminant; worldwide

1. Introduction

Water is the core of sustainable development, but it is a limited resource. The world population growth and climate change have given rise to an alarming decline of freshwater resources and their availability, thus posing a major challenge worldwide. In the last 35 years, the frequency and the intensity of droughts have drastically increased due to the effect of global warming. The number of people and areas affected by water scarcity increased almost 20% in summer of 2017 in Europe [1]. This trend is expected to continue, causing concern across the European Union (EU) and neighboring countries and giving place to important environmental and economic consequences.

Excessive water extraction for agricultural irrigation and for industrial applications [2] is one of the chief menaces to the aquatic ecosystems in the EU, while provision of healthy water is a critical condition for development of economic sectors that depend on water. In response to this problem, hydric resources should be managed more efficiently. A feasible alternative is to apply environmentally sustainable treatments to wastewater to recover them for future purposes. Water reuse is a process with few adverse environmental impacts when compared with desalination or water transfers and offers economic and social benefits. Nowadays, even though water reuse could never solve by itself water scarcity issues, it can help to improve the quality and quantity of the planet's water supplies.

Although usefulness of treated water is a recognized practice in some EU countries with hydric stress (Greece, Malta, Italy, Cyprus, Portugal, and Spain), only a small fraction of this recycled effluent is reused in them. Additionally, the lack of harmonization regarding permit uses, monitored parameters, and limiting values increases environmental and health risks, which are the main obstacles in carrying out these practices. This non-agreement has caused each member state (MS) to adopt its own guidelines for different water reuse purposes [3].

The World Health Organization (WHO) and the Directive 2015/1787 that amends Directive 98/83/EC on the quality of water intended for human consumption recommend a risk management framework with the aim of developing an approach with minimum quality requirements not only for aquifer recharge and agricultural irrigation but also for drinking, recreational, and recycled water [4]. Countries such as Australia developed their own guidelines for water recycling (NHMRC-NRMMC, 2006). The "Australian Guidelines for Water Recycling" provide a common framework for management of reclaimed water quality and uses, including aquifer recharge and agricultural irrigation. In 2012, the United States Environmental Protection Agency (USEPA) included a wide range of reuse applications [5] and improved these roles. Three years later, in 2015, the International Organization for Standardization (ISO) issued the "Guidelines for treated wastewater use for irrigation projects" [6], including agricultural uses [7]. These roles incorporate limit values of parameters that ensure environmental and health safety of water reuse in irrigation. Spain also has its own regulation. The Royal Decree 1620/2007, established by the Spanish government (National Water Council, Spain's communities, and local authorities) on 7 December 2007, manages the reuse of reclaimed water in this country. This Royal Decree overturns all other regulations included in articles 272 and 273 of Public Water Resources Domain Regulations. This decree establishes that the water analyses must be carried out in laboratories, which have a quality control system in accordance with general requirements for the competence of testing and calibration laboratories (UNE- ISO/IEC 17025). The microorganisms monitored are intestinal nematodes, *Escherichia coli*, and *Legionella spp*. The main physical-chemical characteristics controlled are turbidity, suspended solids, nitrates, phosphorus, nitrogen, and dangerous substances such as heavy metals.

However, the situation has changed since 12 February 2019 with a European Parliament legislative resolution of the European Parliament and of the Council regarding the proposal for a regulation on minimum requirements for treated water reuse. This regulation sets EU-wide standards that reclaimed water would need to meet in order to be used for agricultural irrigation. In this report are national regulations on water reuse already published by some EU countries as well as a risk analysis carried out by MS for guaranteeing safe use of the treated water. In order to reuse reclaimed water in crop irrigation, different physical-chemical and microbiological steps have been proposed depending on type of crops. Requirements differ according to four water quality classes defined based on the type of crop and irrigation practice and include microbiological parameters (presence of pathogen organisms: *Escherichia coli*, *Legionella spp*., and intestinal nematodes) and physico-chemical variables [turbidity, biochemical oxygen demand (BOD5), and total suspended solids (TSS)]. In addition, member states should implement programs to monitor environmental matrices in order to establish the impact of reclaimed water on ecosystems, soils, and crops and to assess health risks. For agricultural irrigation, the monitoring programs of the environmental matrices are described in the ISO guidelines (ISO 16075, 2015). These samplings should be carried out taking into account the minimum requirements concerning the frequency of testing in order to establish a risk management plan. In this way, the potential additional hazards may be addressed.

The choice of the best treatment for reclaiming wastewater with the aforementioned requirements depends on its later purpose. Consideration should be given to adding the chemical procedures applied and the residual products resulting from the treatment. This prevents contamination and salting problems from affecting freshwater sources. Therefore, lower cost, robust, and more effective processes to decontaminate and disinfect wastewater are required without endangering human health or stressing the environment by the treatment itself, mainly in sub-developed countries. In this context, advanced oxidation processes (AOPs) are considered a highly competitive technology regarding water treatments for the removal of organic pollutants classified as bio-recalcitrant and for the inactivation of pathogen microorganisms not treatable by conventional techniques. AOPs were first suggested for drinking water treatments in 1980 (NHMRC-NRMMC, 2011). In later years, they were widely studied as oxidizing treatments applied to different wastewaters. AOPs are defined as the oxidation processes related to the generation of reactive oxygen species (ROS) such as hydroxyl radicals (HO) in enough quantity to produce reclaimed effluents. HO· radicals have high redox potential (2.8 eV) and are non-selective [8]. They are capable of attacking organic compounds through four pathways: hydrogen abstraction, combination or addition of radicals, and electron transfer [9]. Their reaction with organic contaminants generates carbon radicals (R· or R·−HO), which may be transformed to organic peroxyl radicals (ROO) with O_2. All the radicals further react accompanied by the formation of other reactive species such as super oxide ($O_2·−$) and hydrogen peroxide, leading to chemical destruction and, in certain cases, the mineralization of water target pollutants. When an AOP is applied as a tertiary treatment, HO· radicals are generated in situ due to their short lifetime by different procedures, including a mixture of oxidizing agents (ozone and hydrogen peroxide), ultrasound (US) or irradiation (UV), and catalysts [10]. The most frequent catalyst is titanium dioxide (TiO_2). When the TiO_2 particles are illuminated by UV light, they are excited and generate valence band holes where HO· are produced in contact with water [11]. However, the recycling and the recovery of these suspended TiO_2 particles become cumbersome and expensive, making the use of suspended systems not viable. As an alternative, new systems have been developed using this immobilized catalyst [12,13]. However, the combination of hydrogen peroxide with Ultraviolet-C light (UVC) radiation results in a most effective procedure for yielding HO· [14]. On the other hand, the use of iron species as free catalysts for producing HO in Fenton processes has widely been studied, but its application on wastewater such as tertiary treatments in real conditions is restricted since the optimal pH is 2.8. For this reason, studies have proposed three modified Fenton process: heterogeneous Fenton, photo-Fenton, and electro-Fenton [15]. In order to carry out the photo-Fenton reaction, the traditional Fenton system is exposed to the UV light with the aim of improving the photo-reduction of dissolved ferric iron (Fe^{3+}) to ferrous iron species (Fe^{2+}). In the electro-Fenton reaction, the two Fenton reagents can be produced with electrochemical procedures [16]. Another HO· and hydrogen peroxide generation system is the water sonolysis [17]. This treatment is less studied in wastewater because the initial operational costs are very high, and the treated volumes are very small in comparison with other methods. Not only are HO· oxidant agents, but they are also sulphate radicals. These species are highly reactive, and they have a short life cycle. Therefore, the HO can be generated from them at alkaline conditions.

As has been described previously, HO· radicals, generated during the application of AOPs on secondary effluents are able to remove wastewater toxic products and transform them to non-dangerous pollutants, providing a solution for wastewater treatment [10,18]. Besides oxidation by HO, other simultaneous reactions can take place during the treatments with AOP, giving rise to destruction of target compounds in wastewater. The function of these non-radical oxidative mechanisms in the pollutant removal may be insignificant or dominant depending on the reaction conditions and the applied AOP type.

In recent years, small concentrations of inorganic, organic, and mineral compounds in the aquatic environment have increased noticeably, mainly by human activities such as excessive and rapid industrialization, urban encroachment, and improved agricultural operations. One feasible option for eliminating organic pollutants from wastewater is the application of AOPs or their combinations with other treatments. These methods have been commonly recognized as being highly capable for removing recalcitrant contaminants or being used as pretreatment to transform contaminants into shorter-chain compounds that can be treated after by traditional biological processes. One AOP or a combination must be appropriately selected for remediation of a specific industrial or urban wastewater, considering factors such as wastewater characteristics, technical applicability, regulatory requirements, economical aspects, and long-term environmental impacts.

AOPs such as photocatalysis and photo-Fenton have been proposed as tertiary treatments for urban effluents due to their ability to detoxify wastewater streams containing persistent contaminants. The treatment of industrial wastewater (IWW) effluents is a very complex challenge due to the broad array of substances and high concentrations that it can contain. Treatment by activated sludge is more efficient and less expensive for removing high concentrations of organic compounds. However, there are some circumstances where AOPs may offer some advantages. AOPs typically have a small footprint and can be easily integrated with other treatment processes. They could be used to remove non-biodegradable substances that persist after biological treatment. In fact, some IWWs are toxic or bio-recalcitrant to activated sludge treatment due to the high dissolved organic carbon (DOC) concentration. It was proven that AOPs can be used to partially degrade toxic compounds for obtaining effluents with more biodegradables prior to the biological process [19]. In this way, studies about combined AOPs and biological technologies for treating some complex IWWs have greatly increased in recent years [18,20,21]. For that, the reuse of IWW as a harmless hydric resource under adequate sanitary conditions is a real possibility. According to this, novel treatments based on AOPs and their combination with conventional treatments are being evaluated, covering an extensive range of IWWs generated from different processing industries. Olive oil production is one of the major agronomic activities in the Mediterranean region [22]. However, the high phenolic toxicity of resulting effluents generated serious environmental issues in these places, making it necessary to find a suitable treatment in order to diminish the environmental impact of their discharge. A possible solution is to apply a treatment with active sludge as pre-treatment to enhance the biodegradability of IWW [23], since processes such as electrochemical oxidation [24], Fenton oxidation [25,26], and ozonation [27,28] can only reach partial decontamination even after extended times. Another industry that obtains large amounts of IWW is the winery industry, as Europe is the main producer of this drink. In scientific literature, some studies demonstrated high efficiency on organic matter removal by ozone [24,25] or photo-Fenton processes [29,30], pointing out the process combination to improve traditional techniques. If attention is paid to textile industries, they generate a negative environmental impact due to discharge of dyes and chemicals in stream water. In recent years, research has reported that these industrial wastewaters must be treated in the first place by applying a biological system and after with AOP oxidation to complete the treatment of textile IWWs. AOPs such as ozone, UV/H_2O_2, TiO_2-assisted photocatlysis ozonation, or Fenton, photo-Fenton, hydrogen peroxide, and electro-oxidation processes have been evaluated to treat these types of IWW with promising results [18].

In addition to industrial effluents, it is also recognized that municipal wastewater treatment plants (MWWTPs) represent a relevant reserve of environmental water contamination. The total charge of organic pollutants discharged by MWWTPs depends on the number of residents and the pollution received from local industries connected to the urban sanitary system. A wide variety of toxic residues (chemicals or biological products) are generated daily by different sectors, which can be classified as hazardous or toxic due to the possible adverse effects that can generate (neurotoxicity, endocrine disruption, cancer) [31]. Among the contaminants present in WWTP effluents are personal care products, pharmaceuticals, pesticides, gasoline additives, flame retardants, drugs, plasticizers, and a long list of chemicals commonly identified as "contaminants of emerging concern (CECs)" [32,33]. These compounds are found at ng/L–μg/L concentrations in MWWTP effluents, but they are not regulated. WWTPs are considered as the main pathway of entry of CECs to the environment. During the water treatment processes, or once in the natural environment, these compounds can also be transformed by a variety of chemical, photochemical, or biological processes that lead to the formation of transformation products (TPs), which can eventually be more persistent or dangerous than the original compounds [34,35]. The inefficient removal of CECs by MWWTPs is a serious limitation for water reuse in regard to the safety/sustainability of reuse practices such as irrigation in agriculture or gardens and golf courses [36]. Therefore, the regulations do not permit that the biologically treated wastewater can be directly reused because of its content of health hazard micropollutant. These dangerous products can be accumulated in vegetables and soils with great impact on drinking water resources and food security [37]. This situation requires the development of alternative remediation technologies to limit the discharge of these compounds in the environment. Numerous scientific studies were recently reported proving the effective removal of micropollutants contained in actual urban wastewater [38,39]. Membrane bioreactors technology (MBR) combining conventional activated sludge (CAS) treatment with a membrane filtration system was reported as an alternative to increase the effluent quality decreasing the membrane cost [40,41]. On the contrary, MBR is not available operational technology for eliminating micropollutants due to membrane-fouling control. In this way, membrane aeration, permeability loss, and membrane replacements are factors with high operation costs [42]. In this sense (and to replace MBR technology), some authors have proposed the use of solar AOPs as tertiary treatments for CECs removal due to the use of solar energy diminish investments costs [43], resulting in WW treatments that are simple, robust, and inexpensive. Among the AOPs, the more studied is the heterogeneous photocatalysis using TiO_2 as a catalyst. However, it was demonstrated that it is not effective because long treatment times are necessary for total elimination of microcontaminants [10]. Another AOP that produced low microcontaminant degradation is the solar photo-Fenton working at neutral pH [44]. In order to avoid the iron precipitation in neutral pH conditions, chelating agents are needed for keeping the catalyst in solution. Commonly, the complexing agents exist in the WW but are removed during secondary biological treatment or drinking water treatment phases. In nature, there is a wide range of agents that can be very useful for keeping the dissolved iron in the course of the solar photo-Fenton process and to stabilize the free radical production [45–47].

Wastewater effluents contain not only harmful inorganic and organic compounds but also pathogen microorganisms. Chlorination, UV-C radiation, and ozone are treatments traditionally used for microorganisms' inactivation in WWTPs. WW disinfection mainly focuses on specific groups of bacteria included in the water reuse regulations for different uses, which include total and fecal coliforms, *Crystosporidium* sp., or *Legionella* sp. The addition of chlorine substances (chlorine gas, sodium hypochlorite, or calcium hypochlorite) is the most cost-effective treatment and has proven to be lethal against a wide range of wastewater pathogens microorganisms. Microorganisms' inactivation is reached by different cellular oxidation mechanisms and inhibition of enzymatic activity together with the damage of the cell membrane [48]. In relation to the WW disinfection under UV-C radiation, it was demonstrated that the photons were absorbed by the microorganisms' genetic material (DNA), thus avoiding the cellular replication. In addition, the accumulated UV-A energy per unit of treated water volume dose (QUV), in terms of kJ/L, is a key parameter to monitor the microorganism inactivation under UV radiation in the function of treatment time when the system is photo-limited [49]. Nonetheless, the interest in ozone treatments is increasing since this chemical has the power to inactivate microbial cells and to decrease the load of organic chemicals [46,50].

Currently, AOPs are shown as alternative technologies due to their ability to destroy a broad variety of contaminants and to kill microorganisms from WW. However, these treatments are being investigated in order to diminish associated operational costs and ensure the feasibility. The main AOPs studied for water purification are TiO_2, photocatalysis, UV/O_3, UV/H_2O_2, Fenton, and photo-Fenton [51]. In order to evaluate their feasibility, model microorganisms of fecal contamination are selected due to their great immunity to most water disinfection methods conventionally applied. Among them, the most common are *Escherichia coli* (*E. coli*), *Cryptosporidium* sp., or *Bacillus* sp. These microorganisms are extremely dangerous to human health. *E. coli* can hydrolyze conjugated estrogens by sulfatase and glucuronidase enzyme. Regarding protozoan microorganisms, *Cryptosporidium* is known for its resistance to chlorination processes, causing intestinal infections in the human population [10]. On the other hand, *Bacillus* sp. is a facultative anaerobic bacteria that can live with a low amount of dissolved oxygen. There are many *Bacillus* species existing in nature—some of them have a high wastewater purification ability to decompose highly concentrated organic matter in a short time, and they secrete a large quantity of enzymes that can decompose excess sludge. However, other species are toxic if they appear in the treated water after secondary treatments, and tertiary processes such as chlorination are not capable of inactivating them [52].

The use of UV radiation combined with H_2O_2 or TiO_2 increases the efficiency of the inactivation process. The action mechanism of microorganism inactivation by UV differs from the pathogen inactivation by UV/H_2O_2. When both WW disinfection techniques are compared, the treatment times are shorter when the combined process is applied [53]. Another type of UV radiation is UV-C, which has been demonstrated to be more effective than UVA/TiO_2 or UV/sono-chemical treatments since it has a great disinfectant power, obtaining an inactivation reduction of 6-log in 10 min of treatment time. However, the photo-reactivation of bacteria occurred at 72 h after the end of the applied process [54]. Another effective, solar driven AOP is the photo-Fenton process. When the pH values are increased, the ferrous iron solubility decreases, leading to its precipitation as Fe^{3+} hydroxides. This fact can be an issue when the photo-Fenton process is selected for disinfecting wastewater, thus the survival of the majority of the monitored pathogens decreases or even dies at acidic pH (pH < 3). In order to deal with this blockage and evaluate the inactivation of pathogen organisms by the photo-Fenton process, several studies were performed at pH over 4, where microbes are able to survive [49,55,56]. In order to inactivate microbial cells for photocatalysis by TiO_2, a critical fact is the internal cellular damage produced by acts of reactive oxygen species (ROS), such as HO·, just as for photocatalysis by TiO_2. This effect on vital compounds of the cell begins with the photon absorbance through the plasmatic membrane of microorganisms causing lethal physical damage followed by an oxidative attack by hydroxyl radicals on the cellular walls, generating oxidative stress and pores and causing loss of their permeability [55]. This circumstance is dependent on the amount of HO· and the availability of iron along the photocatalytic treatment.

Nonetheless, current microbial pathogen identification methods in WW have reported the presence of a widespread range of other microbes. These organisms are considered "emerging pathogens" with an inherent alarm to the population due to their appearance in reclaimed waters and discharged waters to the environment. An example of emerging pathogens is the antibiotic-resistant bacteria (ARB). The presence of antibiotics in effluents has increased in the past year. In particular, urban [56] and hospital wastewaters [57] are among common ARB spread and anthropogenic sources into the aquatic world. Finding an effective and advanced technology to remove antibiotic compounds from treated water has been a major study focus for many years. Mechanical procedures such as nanofiltration and ultrafiltration after a traditional activated sludge have demonstrated that the removal of antibiotics increased by up to 30% [58], but these techniques do not remove microcontaminants; they only transfer them from one point to another. For this reason, the AOPs can be applied to clean the effluent containing pharmaceutical products as an environmentally friendly process by using reusable catalysts and solar light. TiO_2 photocatalysis, Fenton, and photo-Fenton processes have emerged as promising wastewater treatment technologies.

Presence of ARBs in the WWTP effluents discharged into aqueous ecosystems or reused for irrigation in agriculture indicates that disinfection routine practices do not successfully control the spread of these pathogen organisms into the environment. ARBs are frequently found in WW effluents from hospitals, MWWTPs, and wastewater from cattle (known as "grey waters"). Currently, the main conventional disinfection methods are chlorination, application of ozone, and UV-C. Regarding chlorine compounds, it is reported in bibliography that ARB inactivation rates are not lower than those of total heterotrophic microorganisms, and even the proportion of numerous ARBs can be raised after adding chlorine compounds [59].

Accordingly, the external and the internal mechanisms of how the chlorination process affords to increase the concentrations of ARB and antibiotic resistant gene (ARG) in WW remains uncertain, hence more studies in this field are mandatory. Concerning UV-C radiation effects, the available information indicates that this treatment is not effective in the death of ARB and the removal of ARG under UV-doses around 30 mJ/cm^2, which are commonly used. When mJ/cm^2 is increased, the microorganism inactivation rate is increased too, thus achieving the total log reduction. According to the studies found in literature, inactivation of 4–5 log of cell ARB requires low UV-doses from 10–20 mJ/cm^2 in comparison with those required for eliminating ARG (UV-doses from 200 to 400 mJ/cm^2). This indicates that chlorination and UV treatments may not produce an important impact over concentrations of ARB and ARG in WW, although the ways of elimination of these biological products are not clear. On the other hand, the effect of ozonation on ARB has been evaluated in few investigations. They reported that this method is not feasible for killing ARB or eliminating ARG. Nevertheless, other treatments are being considered in order to improve the efficacy of wastewater disinfection and to overcome numerous drawbacks of the aforementioned conventional technologies, decreasing the associated operational expenditures as well. AOPs driven under solar light such as Fenton and photo-Fenton processes have been evaluated on WW for inactivating ARB and ARG. The results extracted from these studies confirmed its lethal power on natural ARB from MWWTPs secondary effluents. Conversely, and depending on the type of resistant gene, its efficacy is lower when the ARG concentrations are analyzed, obtaining total damage in some monitored AG [60–62]. The presence and the spread of resistant microorganisms in the effluents from MWWTPs disposed into reused effluents are some of the biggest threats to humanity associated with the domestic use of wastewater. These facts reveal the inefficacy of traditional wastewater treatments and disinfection processes for controlling the spread of pathogenic microorganisms and microbial resistance into the aquatic environments. Nowadays, although some research is being carried out to control the spread of ARB and ARG in aquatic environments, the biological procedures to effectively deactivate these microorganisms remain unclear. These studies pave the way to addressing this challenge.

The objective of this work was to review the state of the art of scientific publications on wastewater and advanced oxidation. In this way, it is possible to establish the true state of research in this topic, defining trends and tracing possible lines of work for the development of future research. To this end, an extensive bibliometric analysis was carried out, and scientific communities were established based on the keywords defined in each article.

2. Materials and Methods

Web of Science (WoS) and Scopus are the most important databases of scientific literature. However, there are works comparing them and concluding that using Scopus, the largest database of peer-reviewed scientific articles in the world, is the best option [63]. Studies determine that, while 54% of Scopus titles are indexed in WoS [64], 84% of WoS titles are also indexed in Scopus. Thus, comparative studies conclude that it is much more effective to use Scopus than WoS in bibliometric analysis. Therefore, in bibliography, a large number of bibliometric works using this database can be found [64,65]. Scopus contains almost 40,000 titles belonging to more than 10,000 publishers, and the analysis of these allow the scientific community to identify where, who, when, and how research is taking place in a given scientific area. Therefore, Scopus was the database chosen by us to carry out this analysis.

In the present analysis, a full search of the Elsevier Scopus database was conducted using [TITLE-ABS-KEY (Wastewater and "advanced oxidation")] as the search query. This resulted in 3208 documents obtained between 1990, the year of first publication, and 2018, the last full year from Scopus database. If the search criteria are modified, the results obtained can be significantly different Similarly, continuous updates or modifications of the database may also result in certain differences in the result obtained. On the other hand, it must also be taken into account that some of the elements analyzed are the keywords entered by the author or the editor, and these do not always fit the subject matter of the articles. These small anomalies do not invalidate the methodology, and Scopus is considered the best option in bibliometric analysis.

In analyzing the keywords, it was considered that there are terms mentioning the same concept. For example, ozonation and ozonization. Therefore, these keywords were considered as one. On the other hand, keywords that do not contribute to the analysis, such as "article", were discarded The items analyzed were: evolution of scientific output, publication distribution by countries and institutions, and keywords. The software tool VOSviewer (http://www.vosviewer.com/) was used in the detection of scientific communities. These scientific communities are represented in graphs, and they are studied as nodes that establish connections between them giving rise to complex networks that determine the relationships within the whole.

3. Results and Discussion

3.1. Progression of Scientific Output

The search returned 3208 documents. More than 90% of these documents are written in English, but there are also articles written in other languages, such as Spanish, French, Russian, or Chinese. No document from Scopus was excluded. Figure 1 shows the evolution of the number of documents on wastewater and advanced oxidation since 1990. As can be seen, the topic is of recent interest, because only in the last 30 years has the advanced oxidation in wastewater treatment been used.

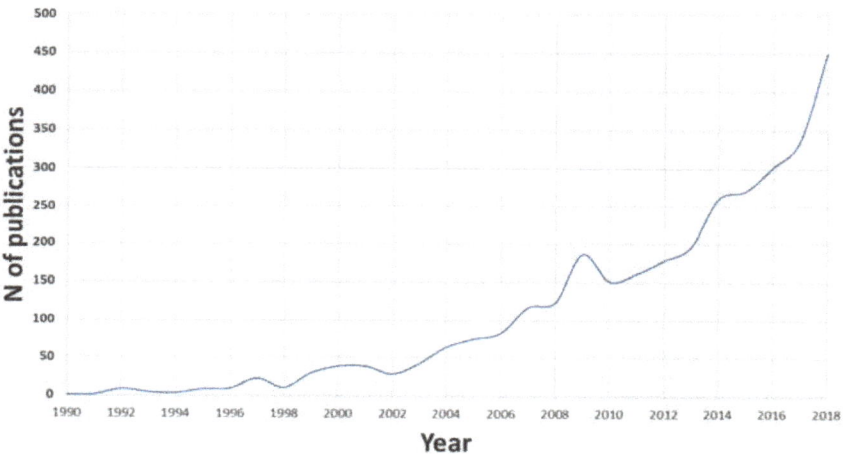

Figure 1. Trend of the number of publications per year in wastewater and advanced oxidation from the years 1990–2018.

There has been continuous growth since the first year analyzed, but this occurs at two speeds. In the period 1990–2002, there is a slow growth in the number of annual publications, while in the period 2002–2018, the growth is much greater with a publication intensity greater than 25 articles per year, reaching the absolute maximum in the year 2018 with 450 articles published.

3.2. Publication Distribution by Countries and Institutions

Figure 2 shows, in a funnel chart, the distribution by country of the scientific production on wastewater and advanced oxidation. Thirteen countries have published at least 100 articles on this subject in the period under review. Of these, China stands out with 508 articles. It is followed, in this order, by Spain, the USA, and India, with 200–400 publications. The rest of the countries have published between 100 and 200 documents. China's water pollution has increased in the last 40 years due to population and industrialization growth. Compared with the European Union and the United States standards, China's wastewater discharge standards still have shortcomings, and there exist many challenges in this field. For this reason, the Chinese government is putting more effort into exploring new wastewater treatments [66]. In the United States, the potential use of municipal reclaimed water in the power sector has led to an increase in the number of publications about wastewater reclamation treatments. The implementation of technologies capable of supplying reclaimed water for electric power plants is a major challenge for this developed country [67]. As it is presented in Figure 2, Spain holds second place in the ranking with 371 publications related to the studies about advanced oxidation treatments applied to wastewater. In recent years, the changes of legislation at the European level have been a point of departure for increasing the investigation in this area, especially in countries with a huge water scarcity, such as Spain.

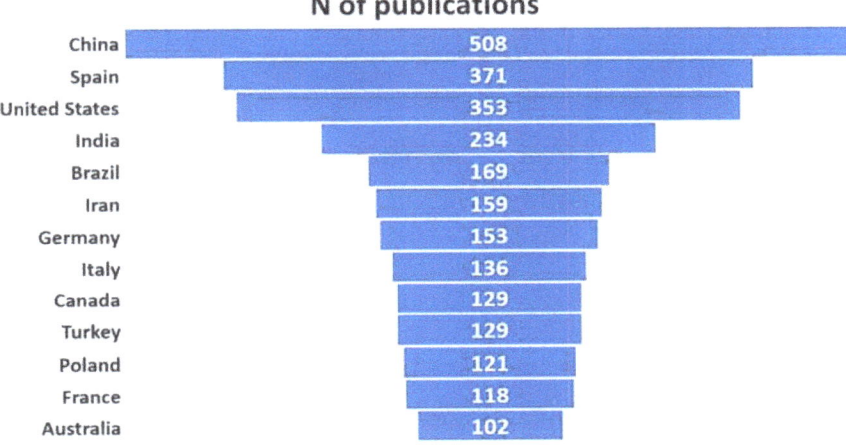

Figure 2. Representation of the countries with the highest number of publications on wastewater and advanced oxidation.

A total of 87 countries have published at least one article in this scientific field. However, the 13 most important countries account for almost 85% of all publications. In Figure 3, the countries with at least one publication are represented in a color-coded world map.

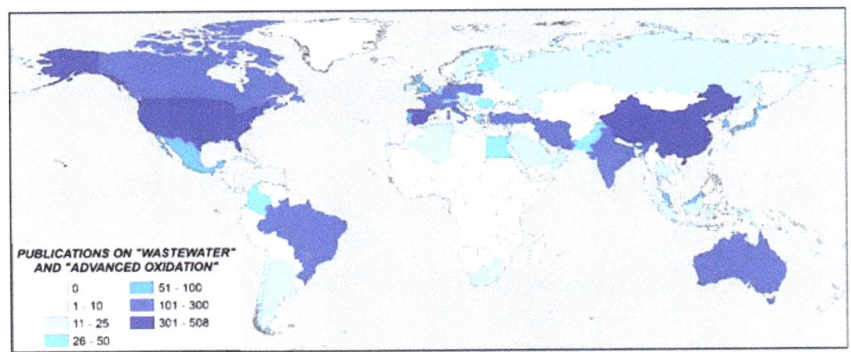

Figure 3. World map representing the scientific production by countries.

Figure 4 shows an analysis of the relations established between the different countries based on articles published by several countries. In the analysis of communities, each node represents a country, and from this, there are as many lines of union as there are relations at the level of publications with other countries. The size of each node refers to the number of publications carried out in that country, and the thickness of each union line refers to the number of collaborations carried out with another country. It can be observed that, in the analysis, there are three clusters, each identified with a color. The largest cluster is represented in red and is dominated by China. The USA also plays a very important role in this cluster. The rest of the countries belonging to the cluster are Australia, Canada, India, South Korea, Taiwan, Malaysia, and Iran. The second cluster, represented in green, is formed by European and Latin American countries. The central role is occupied by Spain, and the rest of the countries are the United Kingdom, Switzerland, Poland, Germany, Portugal, Brazil, and Mexico. The third cluster is made up of France, Italy, Turkey, and Japan and is represented in blue.

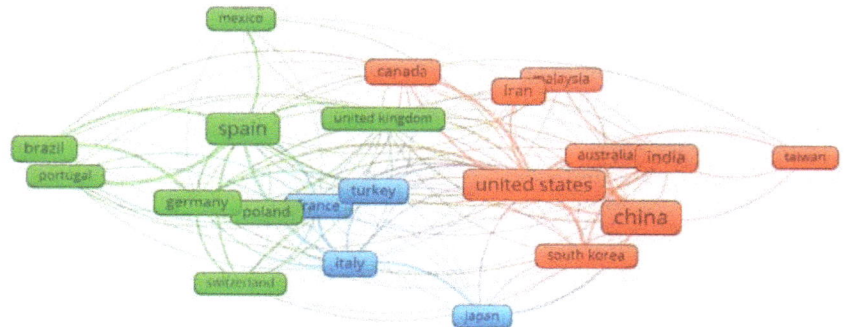

Figure 4. Graph of the analysis of communities by country representing the relations established with other countries.

Figure 5 shows the institutions with more than 25 publications on wastewater and advanced oxidation. Of these, five are Spanish (CIEMAT-Plataforma Solar de Almería, Universitat de Barcelona, Universidad de Almeria, Universidad de Extremadura, and Universidad de Granada), four are Chinese (Ministry of Education China, Tsinghua University, Chinese Academy of Sciences, and Harbin Institute of Technology), three are Turkish (Istanbul Teknik Üniversitesi, Middle East Technical University METU, and Boğaziçi Üniversitesi), and there is an institution of Brazil (Universidade de Sao Paulo), Italy (Università di Salerno), Portugal (Universidade do Porto), Switzerland (Swiss Federal Institute of Technology EPFL), India (Institute of Chemical Technology), France (CNRS Centre National de la Recherche Scientifique), and Poland (Lodz University of Technology). It is striking that, of the 20 institutions with the highest number of publications, none are American, despite the fact that the USA is the third country, after China and Spain, with the highest number of publications in wastewater and advanced oxidation. This is because, while in other countries such as Switzerland, the majority of research in this field is carried out in a single institution, in the USA, the research is not led by a single center. There are many institutions spread all over the country that publish in this scientific field without highlighting, as far as the number of publications is concerned, any of them.

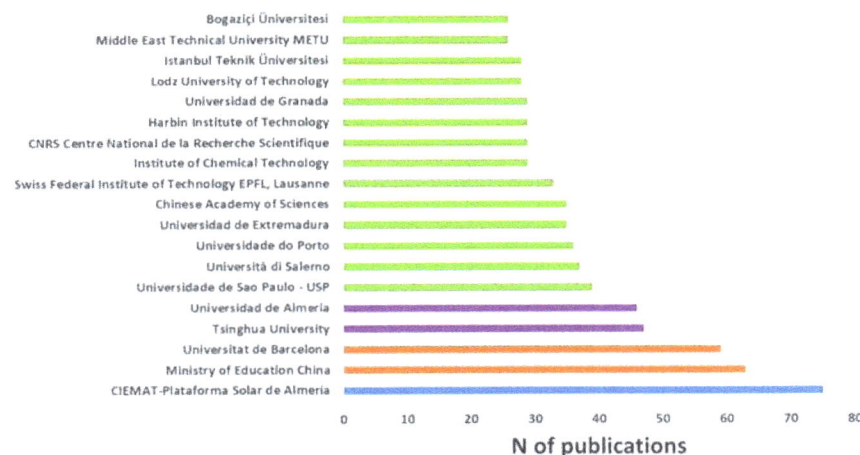

Figure 5. Main institutions related to scientific production in wastewater and advanced oxidation.

3.3. Keyword Analysis

In order to carry out the analysis of the keywords, the data were previously cured, eliminating irrelevant terms and unifying terms that allude to the same concept. This analysis allowed us to establish the true state of research in a topic, defining trends and tracing possible lines of work for the development of future research. Figure 6 is a cloud-word showing the 32 keywords that appear in more than 300 publications in this area. The size of each keyword represents the relative proportion of each term to the total number of words.

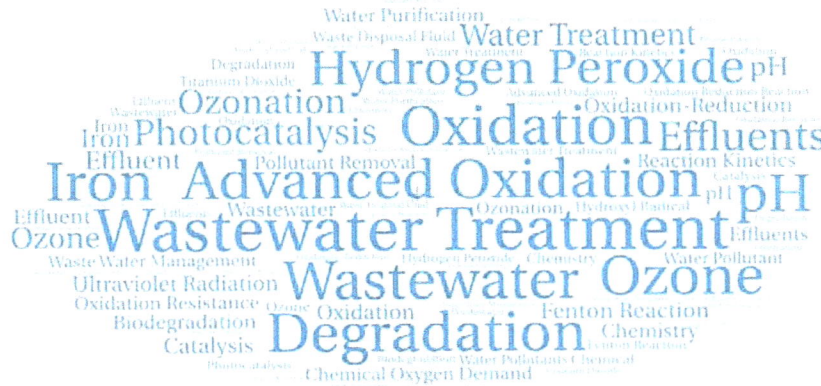

Figure 6. Cloud-word with the more representative keywords.

Among the 160 keywords that appear in more than 80 publications, many of them allude to water-related parameters such as pH, temperature, total organic carbon, or organic matter, and many others refer to water pollutant compounds such as phenols, sulfur compounds, aromatic compounds, or antibiotics.

On the other hand, a large number of articles appear around keywords related to three water types—industrial, urban, and drinking water—with 1357, 786, and 468 articles, respectively. Figure 7 shows the relative importance that each of the 20 most important countries, in terms of the number of publications, attaches to each of these types of water.

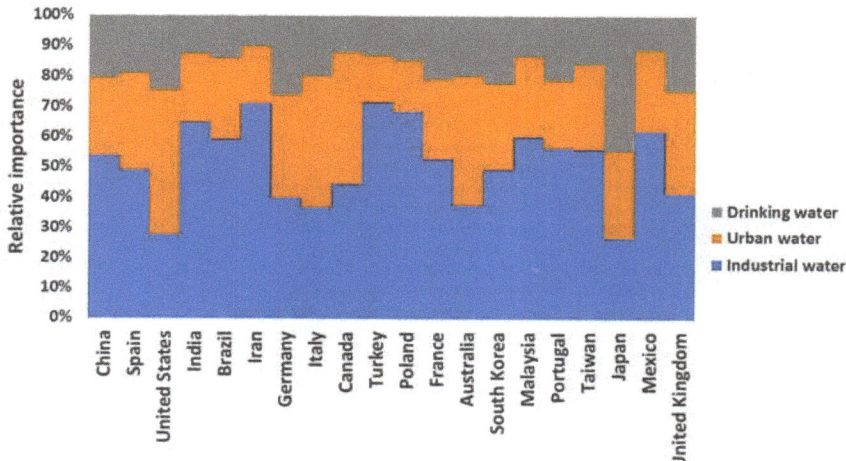

Figure 7. Relative importance given by each country to each type of water.

It can be observed that, on average, the greatest importance is given to industrial water with 50%, then urban water with 30%, and finally drinking water with approximately 20%. However, if we look in detail at the data for each country, there are countries such as the United States in which the main concern is focused on urban water. Research in Australia also places the greatest importance on urban water. In contrast, urban water has very little relative importance in the research of countries such as Poland, whose research focuses on the study of industrial water. Finally, special consideration should be given to the data obtained in Japan, where almost half of the articles focus on drinking water. This fact is especially important when looking at the year 2011, when the Great East Japan Earthquake occurred, leading to the Japanese Prime Minister declaring the state of nuclear emergency. From that moment on, the Ministry of Health, Labour and Welfare, Japan (MHLW) showed its great concern for the healthiness of tap water and defined a series of indications [68].

The analysis of the keywords by means of the detection of scientific communities allowed us to group the publications in clusters of functions of the keywords used. Figure 8 shows the 15 communities that appeared in the analysis carried out, identifying each cluster with a color. The size of each cluster refers to the importance of the keywords around which the cluster is built, and the thickness of the lines of union between two clusters refers to the number of interactions established between two different communities. In each cluster, there is a variable number of keywords, but it was detected that, in all cases, there are always keywords referring to three aspects related to the analysis we carried out: AOP treatment, wastewater, and targets. Thus, in Table 1, each cluster is identified with the color with which it appears in Figure 8 and with the set of keywords that appear grouped around the three aspects mentioned above.

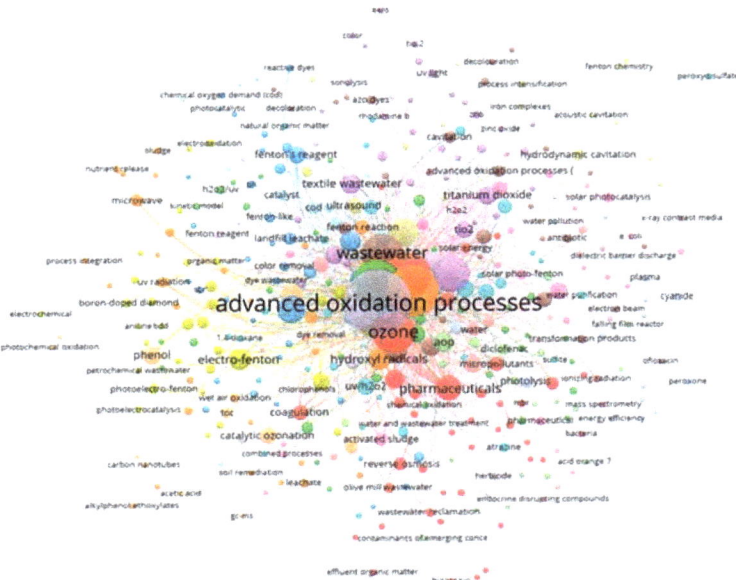

Figure 8. Scientific communities grouped in clusters based on the analysis of keywords in publications on wastewater and advanced oxidation.

Table 1. Summary of different advanced oxidation processes (AOPs) associated with target wastewater and compounds.

Cluster	Color	AOP Treatments	Wastewater	Targets
1	Red	Ozone, ozone/UV, TiO$_2$,	Hospital, olive mill, petroleum refinery	Pharmaceuticals, bacteria
2	Dark Green	Electrochemical, H$_2$O$_2$/UV, heterogeneous photocatalysis, TiO$_2$	Textile industrial, paper industrial	Bisphenol a, formaldehydo, lignin, pharmaceuticals, pesticides, antibiotic resistant bacteria, endocrine disruptors
3	Dark Blue	Fenton	Coking, textile, paper industrial, oil refinery, winery	Endocrine disruptors, acetaminophen, colors, COD
4	Dark Yellow	Electro-Fenton, anodic oxidation, sonoelectrochemistry	Industrial textile, petrochemical	Organic pollutants, organic matter, dyes
5	Dark Purple	TiO$_2$, Fenton, photo-Fenton, UV	Livestock, winery, textile	Persistent organic pollutants
6	Cyan	Electrolysis, Fenton, ozone, peroxy- and peroxymonodisulfate, UV/persulfate, UV/H$_2$O$_2$, UV/TiO$_2$, zero-valent ion	Saline	COD, 1,4-dioxane, atrazine, dyes
7	Dark Orange	Electro-Fenton, Fenton, microwave, ozonization, UV radiation, wet air oxidation	Dyeing	Phenols, heavy metals
8	Brown	Cavitation, ionizing radiation	Oily	Emerging contaminants, azo dyes
9	Pink	H$_2$O$_2$, photo-Fenton, UV,	Slaughterhouse, urban	*E. coli*, pharmaceuticals, COD
11	Green	Ozonation, UV/Fenton	Municipal	Pharmaceuticals
12	Blue	H$_2$O$_2$, UV, UV/H$_2$O$_2$	Textile	Pesticides, nitrate, nitrite, dyes
13	Yellow	Ultrasound, hydrodynamic cavitation, Fenton, photo-Fenton, TiO$_2$	Pharmaceutical	Paracetamol, phenol,
14	Purple	Fenton, sonolysis, ultrasonic radiation	Papermaking	Herbicides, organic pollutant, COD
15	Light Blue	Solar irradiation	Drinking, tannery	COD, dyes
16	Orange	Ozonation	Drinking, tannery	Phenol, COD

Table 1 presents 15 clusters identified from the keywords analyzed relating the AOP treatments (alone or combined with biological oxidation) with the type of wastewater and the target pollutant of which removal is intended. From this, several conclusions can be drawn. On the one hand, ozone-based treatments are mainly used for pharmaceutical removal in a wide range of water matrices, from drinking water (cluster 16) to hospital or olive mill wastewater (cluster 1) [69]. Fenton and assisted Fenton processes find application in complex media such as industrial wastewater from different industrial sectors to remove dyes (cluster 4 and cluster 7), COD, and several persistent organic pollutants (cluster 9 and 14). Among the radiation based AOPs, heterogeneous photocatalysis (TiO$_2$) has been widely studied for industrial wastewater treatment (cluster 13), although hydrogen peroxide-based treatments such as photo-Fenton and H$_2$O$_2$/UVC gained attention for municipal wastewater to remove micropollutants (mainly pharmaceuticals) as well as water and wastewater disinfection (cluster 9 and 12).

Finally, if an analysis is carried out on the importance of keywords in time, two periods can be identified. The first period extends from 2005 to 2008 (Figure 9), while the second period extends from 2010 to 2016 (Figure 10).

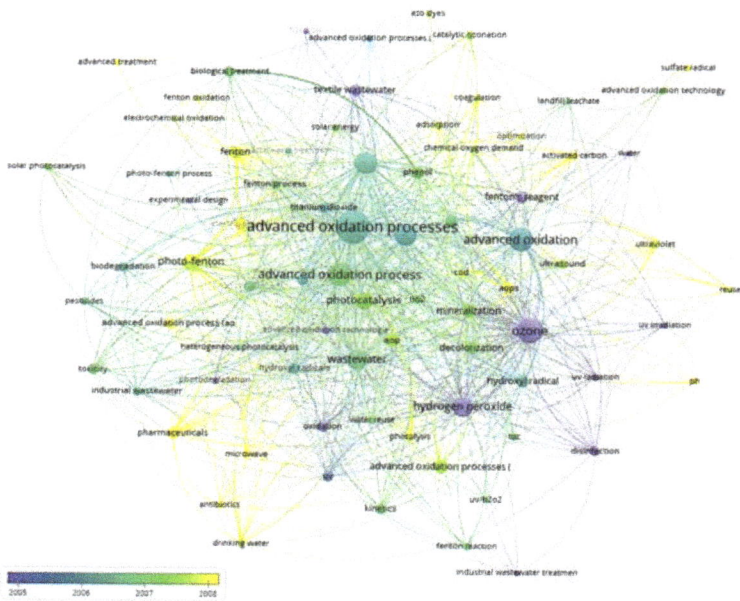

Figure 9. First period of evolution in advanced oxidation for wastewater treatment (2005–2008).

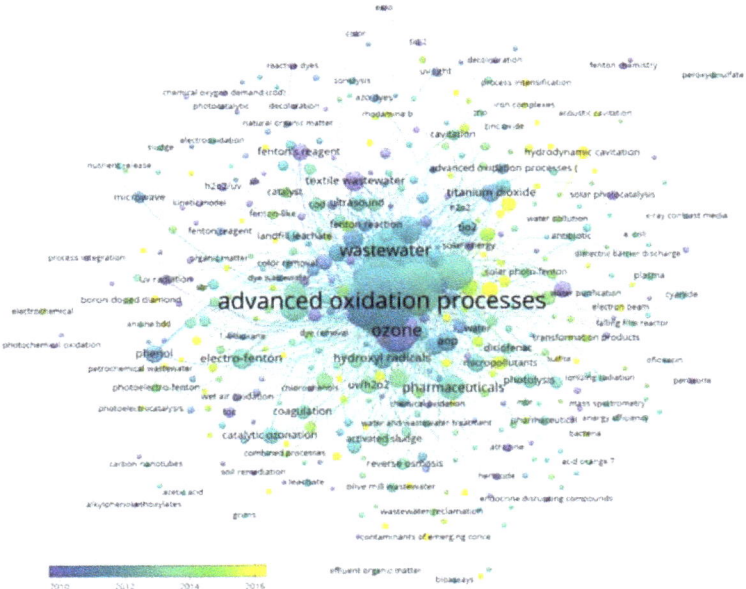

Figure 10. Second period of evolution in advanced oxidation for wastewater treatment (2010–2016).

In the first period, in its beginning toward the year 2005, there were numerous articles that presented keywords such as ozone, hydrogen peroxide, or UV irradiation. Then, mid-term was when advanced oxidation processes, solar energy, or biodegradation stood out. Finally, these lost their leading role to keywords related to the processes of Fenton and microwave, photo-Fenton, drinking water, or pharmaceuticals. This trend was confirmed in the second period, with the Fenton gaining prominence as it progressed at the end of this period, highlighting, above all, solar photo-Fenton.

4. Conclusions

Analyzing the number of publications on wastewater and advanced oxidation from 1990 to 2018, a great increase in the evolution is shown, demonstrating the growing scientific interest in this research area. The evolution in the number of publications is especially outstanding from the year 2002 onwards. This growing interest is likely due to the growing need to solve the problem of water purification in all points of the planet. However, the trend regarding the number of publications was not the only item studied. Other variables also received our attention. Thus, it was shown how China and Spain are the countries that publish the largest number of scientific publications in this area, and how five of their institutions (two Chinese and three Spanish) lead the scientific production on wastewater and advanced oxidation, with the CIEMAT-Solar Platform of Almeria leading the ranking. The analysis of the keywords allowed us to establish different scientific communities, focusing each of them on different AOP treatments, type of wastewater, and the target pollutant to remove. The most important scientific communities in terms of the number of published articles are those related to the elimination of pollutants of biological origin, such as bacteria, and of industrial nature, such as pesticides or pharmaceutical products. The treatments mostly present in these articles are those related to ozone/UV, heterogeneous photocatalysis, and H_2O_2/UV. The following points are worthy of special attention for future research in the advanced oxidation field:

(1) The current research in wastewater treatments with AOPs is mainly focused at a pilot scale in batch mode. The evaluation in real conditions in continuous flow mode is mandatory for large-scale implementation.

(2) Strengthening the investigation on the removal of contaminants of emergent concern and bacterial inactivation for wastewater reuse using different AOPs.
(3) Contamination caused by antibiotics and ARBs/ARGs should be highlighted as a worldwide health and environmental concern. In-depth research about removal mechanisms of antibiotics and ARBs/ARGs using AOPs is required.

Author Contributions: Conceptualization, J.A.G.-C. and F.M.-A.; methodology, J.A.G.-C., J.A.S.-P., A.A. and B.E-G.; formal analysis, J.A.G.-C. and F.M.-A.; investigation, J.A.G.-C., and B.E.-G.; writing—original draft preparation, J.A.G.-C. and B.E.-G.; writing—review and editing, F.M.-A., J.A.S.-P. and A.A. All authors have read and agreed to the published version of the manuscript.

Funding: This research received no external funding.

Conflicts of Interest: The authors declare no conflict of interest.

References

1. European Commission (EC). Water Scarcity & Droughts. 2018. Available online: https://ec.europa.eu/environment/water/quantity/about.htm (accessed on 8 June 2019).
2. Fernández-García, A.; Rojas, E.; Pérez, M.; Silva, R.; Hernández-Escobedo, Q.; Manzano-Agugliaro, F. A parabolic-trough collector for cleaner industrial process heat. *J. Clean. Prod.* **2015**, *89*. [CrossRef]
3. Paranychianakis, N.V.; Salgot, M.; Snyder, S.A.; Angelakis, A.N. Water reuse in EU states: Necessity for uniform criteria to mitigate human and environmental risks. *Crit. Rev. Environ. Sci. Technol* **2015**, *45*. [CrossRef]
4. WHO. *Guidelines for Drinking-Water Quality*; World Health Organization: Geneva, Switzerland, 2011; Available online: https://apps.who.int/iris/bitstream/handle/10665/44584/9789241548151_eng.pdf;jsessionid=AEEB237C93D4E479E95B9FF65B88AA8F?sequence=1 (accessed on 6 June 2019).
5. USEPA. *Guidelines for Water Reuse*; Office of Wastewater Management, Office of Water: Washington, DC, USA, 2012. Available online: https://www.epa.gov/sites/production/files/2019-08/documents/2012-guidelines-water-reuse.pdf (accessed on 6 June 2019).
6. ISO 16075. Guidelines for Treated Wastewater Use for Irrigation Projects—Part 1: The Basis of a Reuse Project for Irrigation. 2015. Available online: http://https://www.iso.org/standard/62756.html (accessed on 7 June 2019).
7. Bartzas, G.; Tinivella, F.; Medini, L.; Zaharaki, D.; Komnitsas, K. Assessment of groundwater contamination risk in an agricultural area in north Italy. *Inf. Process. Agric.* **2015**, *2*. [CrossRef]
8. Pignatello, J.J.; Oliveros, E.; MacKay, A. Advanced oxidation processes for organic contaminant destruction based on the fenton reaction and related chemistry. *Crit. Rev. Environ. Sci. Technol.* **2006**, *36*. [CrossRef]
9. Deng, Y.; Zhao, R. Advanced Oxidation Processes (AOPs) in Wastewater Treatment. *Curr. Pollut. Rep.* **2015**, *1*. [CrossRef]
10. Malato, S.; Fernández-Ibáñez, P.; Maldonado, M.I.; Blanco, J.; Gernjak, W. Decontamination and disinfection of water by solar photocatalysis: Recent overview and trends. *Catal. Today* **2009**, *147*. [CrossRef]
11. Choi, H.; Antoniou, M.G.; de la Cruz, A.A.; Stathatos, E.; Dionysiou, D.D. Photocatalytic TiO_2 films and membranes for the development of efficient wastewater treatment and reuse systems. *Desalination*. *Desalination* **2007**, *202*. [CrossRef]
12. Al-Dawery, S.K. Photo-catalyst degradation of tartrazine compound in wastewater using TiO_2 and UV light. *J. Eng. Sci. Technol.* **2013**, *8*, 683–691.
13. Da Silva, S.W.; Klauck, C.R.; Siqueira, M.A.; Bernardes, A.M. Degradation of the commercial surfactant nonylphenol ethoxylate by advanced oxidation processes. *J. Hazard. Mater.* **2015**, *282*. [CrossRef]
14. Mierzwa, J.C.; Rodrigues, R.; Teixeira, A.C.S.C. UV-Hydrogen Peroxide Processes, in: Advanced Oxidation Processes for Wastewater Treatment: Emerging Green Chemical Technology. *Sciencedirect* **2018**. [CrossRef]
15. Gernjak, W.; Krutzler, T.; Glaser, A.; Malato, S.; Caceres, J.; Bauer, R.; Fernández-Alba, A.R. Photo-fenton treatment of water containing natural phenolic pollutants. *Chemosphere* **2003**. [CrossRef]
16. Moreira, F.C.; Boaventura, R.A.R.; Brillas, E.; Vilar, V.J.P. Electrochemical advanced oxidation processes: A review on their application to synthetic and real wastewaters. *Appl. Catal. B Environ.* **2017**. [CrossRef]

17. Villeneuve, L.; Alberti, L.; Steghens, J.P.; Lancelin, J.M.; Mestas, J.L. Assay of hydroxyl radicals generated by focused ultrasound. *Ultrason. Sonochem.* **2009**. [CrossRef]
18. Oller, I.; Malato, S.; Sánchez-Pérez, J.A. Combination of Advanced Oxidation Processes and biological treatments for wastewater decontamination—A review. *Sci. Total Environ.* **2011**. [CrossRef] [PubMed]
19. Amor, C.; Marchão, L.; Lucas, M.S.; Peres, J.A. Application of advanced oxidation processes for the treatment of recalcitrant agro-industrial wastewater: A review. *Water* **2019**, *11*, 205. [CrossRef]
20. Ballesteros Martín, M.M.; Sánchez Pérez, J.A.; García Sánchez, J.L.; Casas López, J.L.; Malato Rodríguez, S. Effect of pesticide concentration on the degradation process by combined solar photo-Fenton and biological treatment. *Water Res.* **2009**. [CrossRef]
21. Zapata, A.; Malato, S.; Sánchez-Pérez, J.A.; Oller, I.; Maldonado, M.I. Scale-up strategy for a combined solar photo-Fenton/biological system for remediation of pesticide-contaminated water. *Catal. Today* **2010**. [CrossRef]
22. Rahmanian, N.; Jafari, S.M.; Galanakis, C.M. Recovery and removal of phenolic compounds from olive mill wastewater. *J. Am. Oil Chem. Soc.* **2014**. [CrossRef]
23. Kallel, M.; Belaid, C.; Mechichi, T.; Ksibi, M.; Elleuch, B. Removal of organic load and phenolic compounds from olive mill wastewater by Fenton oxidation with zero-valent iron. *Chem. Eng. J.* **2009**. [CrossRef]
24. Cañizares, P.; Lobato, J.; Paz, R.; Rodrigo, M.A.; Sáez, C. Advanced oxidation processes for the treatment of olive-oil mills wastewater. *Chemosphere* **2007**. [CrossRef]
25. Lucas, M.S.; Peres, J.A.; Li Puma, G. Treatment of winery wastewater by ozone-based advanced oxidation processes (O_3, O_3/UV and O_3/UV/H_2O_2) in a pilot-scale bubble column reactor and process economics. *Sep. Purif. Technol.* **2010**. [CrossRef]
26. García, C.A.; Hodaifa, G. Real olive oil mill wastewater treatment by photo-Fenton system using artificial ultraviolet light lamps. *J. Clean. Prod.* **2017**. [CrossRef]
27. Benitez, F.J.; Real, F.J.; Acero, J.L.; Garcia, J.; Sanchez, M. Kinetics of the ozonation and aerobic biodegradation of wine vinasses in discontinuous and continuous processes. *J. Hazard. Mater.* **2003**. [CrossRef]
28. Andreozzi, R.; Longo, G.; Majone, M.; Modesti, G. Integrated treatment of olive oil mill effluents (OME): Study of ozonation coupled with anaerobic digestion. *Water Res.* **1998**. [CrossRef]
29. Velegraki, T.; Mantzavinos, D. Solar photo-Fenton treatment of winery effluents in a pilot photocatalytic reactor. *Catal. Today* **2015**. [CrossRef]
30. Ioannou, L.A.; Fatta-Kassinos, D. Solar photo-Fenton oxidation against the bioresistant fractions of winery wastewater. *J. Environ. Chem. Eng.* **2013**. [CrossRef]
31. Genthe, B.; Le Roux, W.J.; Schachtschneider, K.; Oberholster, P.J.; Aneck-Hahn, N.H.; Chamier, J. Health risk implications from simultaneous exposure to multiple environmental contaminants. *Ecotoxicol. Environ. Saf.* **2013**. [CrossRef]
32. Rivera-Utrilla, J.; Sánchez-Polo, M.; Ferro-García, M.Á.; Prados-Joya, G.; Ocampo-Pérez, R. Pharmaceuticals as emerging contaminants and their removal from water. A review. *Chemosphere* **2013**. [CrossRef]
33. Bueno, M.J.M.; Gomez, M.J.; Herrera, S.; Hernando, M.D.; Agüera, A.; Fernández-Alba, A.R. Occurrence and persistence of organic emerging contaminants and priority pollutants in five sewage treatment plants of Spain: Two years pilot survey monitoring. *Environ. Pollut.* **2012**. [CrossRef]
34. Petrovic, M.; Eljarrat, E.; Lopez De Alda, M.J.; Barceló, D. Endocrine disrupting compounds and other emerging contaminants in the environment: A survey on new monitoring strategies and occurrence data. *Anal. Bioanal. Chem.* **2004**. [CrossRef]
35. Pérez-Estrada, L.A.; Malato, S.; Agüera, A.; Fernández-Alba, A.R. Degradation of dipyrone and its main intermediates by solar AOPs. *Catal. Today* **2007**. [CrossRef]
36. Christou, A.; Agüera, A.; Bayona, J.M.; Cytryn, E.; Fotopoulos, V.; Lambropoulou, D.; Manaia, C.M.; Michael, C.; Revitt, M.; Schröder, P.; et al. The potential implications of reclaimed wastewater reuse for irrigation on the agricultural environment: The knowns and unknowns of the fate of antibiotics and antibiotic resistant bacteria and resistance genes—A review. *Water Res.* **2017**. [CrossRef] [PubMed]
37. Martínez-Piernas, A.B.; Plaza-Bolaños, P.; García-Gómez, E.; Fernández-Ibáñez, P.; Agüera, A. Determination of organic microcontaminants in agricultural soils irrigated with reclaimed wastewater: Target and suspect approaches. *Anal. Chim. Acta* **2018**. [CrossRef] [PubMed]

38. Soriano-Molina, P.; Plaza-Bolaños, P.; Lorenzo, A.; Agüera, A.; García Sánchez, J.L.; Malato, S.; Sánchez Pérez, J.A. Assessment of solar raceway pond reactors for removal of contaminants of emerging concern by photo-Fenton at circumneutral pH from very different municipal wastewater effluents. *Chem. Eng. J.* **2019**. [CrossRef]
39. Rivas Ibáñez, G.; Casas López, J.L.; Esteban García, B.; Sánchez Pérez, J.A. Controlling pH in biological depuration of industrial wastewater to enable micropollutant removal using a further advanced oxidation process. *J. Chem. Technol. Biotechnol.* **2014**. [CrossRef]
40. Wijekoon, K.C.; Hai, F.I.; Kang, J.; Price, W.E.; Guo, W.; Ngo, H.H.; Nghiem, L.D. The fate of pharmaceuticals, steroid hormones, phytoestrogens, UV-filters and pesticides during MBR treatment. *Bioresour. Technol.* **2013**. [CrossRef]
41. Sánchez Peréz, J.A.; Carra, I.; Sirtori, C.; Agüera, A.; Esteban, B. Fate of thiabendazole through the treatment of a simulated agro-food industrial effluent by combined MBR/Fenton processes at µg/L scale. *Water Res.* **2014**. [CrossRef]
42. Gabarrón, S.; Ferrero, G.; Dalmau, M.; Comas, J.; Rodriguez-Roda, I. Assessment of energy-saving strategies and operational costs in full-scale membrane bioreactors. *J. Environ. Manag.* **2014**. [CrossRef]
43. Prieto-Rodríguez, L.; Oller, I.; Klamerth, N.; Agüera, A.; Rodríguez, E.M.; Malato, S. Application of solar AOPs and ozonation for elimination of micropollutants in municipal wastewater treatment plant effluents. *Water Res.* **2013**. [CrossRef]
44. Klamerth, N.; Malato, S.; Agüera, A.; Fernández-Alba, A. Photo-Fenton and modified photo-Fenton at neutral pH for the treatment of emerging contaminants in wastewater treatment plant effluents: A comparison. *Water Res.* **2013**. [CrossRef]
45. Lipczynska-Kochany, E.; Kochany, J. Effect of humic substances on the Fenton treatment of wastewater at acidic and neutral pH. *Chemosphere* **2008**. [CrossRef] [PubMed]
46. Zhang, L.; Zhu, Z.; Zhang, R.; Zheng, C.; Zhang, H.; Qiu, Y.; Zhao, J. Extraction of copper from sewage sludge using biodegradable chelant EDDS. *J. Environ. Sci.* **2008**. [CrossRef]
47. Yuan, Z.; VanBriesen, J.M. The Formation of Intermediates in EDTA and NTA Biodegradation. *Environ. Eng. Sci.* **2006**. [CrossRef]
48. Nybo, T.; Dieterich, S.; Gamon, L.F.; Chuang, C.Y.; Hammer, A.; Hoefler, G.; Malle, E.; Rogowska-Wrzesinska, A.; Davies, M.J. Chlorination and oxidation of the extracellular matrix protein laminin and basement membrane extracts by hypochlorous acid and myeloperoxidase. *Redox Biol.* **2019**. [CrossRef] [PubMed]
49. Ortega-Gómez, E.; Esteban García, B.; Ballesteros Martín, M.M.; Fernández Ibáñez, P.; Sánchez Pérez, J.A. Inactivation of natural enteric bacteria in real municipal wastewater by solar photo-Fenton at neutral pH. *Water Res.* **2014**. [CrossRef] [PubMed]
50. Rizzo, L.; Malato, S.; Antakyali, D.; Beretsou, V.G.; Đolić, M.B.; Gernjak, W.; Heath, E.; Ivancev-Tumbas, I.; Karaolia, P.; Lado Ribeiro, A.R.; et al. Consolidated vs new advanced treatment methods for the removal of contaminants of emerging concern from urban wastewater. *Sci. Total Environ.* **2019**. [CrossRef]
51. Giannakis, S.; Polo López, M.I.; Spuhler, D.; Sánchez Pérez, J.A.; Fernández Ibáñez, P.; Pulgarin, C. Solar disinfection is an augmentable, in situ-generated photo-Fenton reaction—Part 1: A review of the mechanisms and the fundamental aspects of the process. *Appl. Catal. B Environ.* **2016**. [CrossRef]
52. Lapara, T.M.; Alleman, J.E. Thermophilic aerobic biological wastewater treatment. *Water Res.* **1999**. [CrossRef]
53. Ndounla, J.; Pulgarin, C. Solar light (hv) and H2O2/hv photo-disinfection of natural alkaline water (pH 8.6) in a compound parabolic collector at different day periods in Sahelian region. *Environ. Sci. Pollut. Res.* **2015**. [CrossRef]
54. Nyangaresi, P.O.; Qin, Y.; Chen, G.; Zhang, B.; Lu, Y.; Shen, L. Effects of single and combined UV-LEDs on inactivation and subsequent reactivation of E. coli in water disinfection. *Water Res.* **2018**. [CrossRef]
55. Spuhler, D.; Andrés Rengifo-Herrera, J.; Pulgarin, C. The effect of Fe2+, Fe3+, H2O2 and the photo-Fenton reagent at near neutral pH on the solar disinfection (SODIS) at low temperatures of water containing Escherichia coli K12. *Appl. Catal. B Environ.* **2010**. [CrossRef]
56. Esteban García, B.; Rivas, G.; Arzate, S.; Sánchez Pérez, J.A. Wild bacteria inactivation in WWTP secondary effluents by solar photo-fenton at neutral pH in raceway pond reactors. *Catal. Today* **2018**. [CrossRef]

57. Rizzo, L.; Manaia, C.; Merlin, C.; Schwartz, T.; Dagot, C.; Ploy, M.C.; Michael, I.; Fatta-Kassinos, D. Urban wastewater treatment plants as hotspots for antibiotic resistant bacteria and genes spread into the environment: A review. *Sci. Total Environ.* **2013**. [CrossRef] [PubMed]
58. Sahar, E.; David, I.; Gelman, Y.; Chikurel, H.; Aharoni, A.; Messalem, R.; Brenner, A. The use of RO to remove emerging micropollutants following CAS/UF or MBR treatment of municipal wastewater. *Desalination* **2011**. [CrossRef]
59. Huang, J.J.; Hu, H.Y.; Wu, Y.H.; Wei, B.; Lu, Y. Effect of chlorination and ultraviolet disinfection on tetA-mediated tetracycline resistance of *Escherichia coli*. *Chemosphere* **2013**. [CrossRef]
60. Ferro, G.; Fiorentino, A.; Alferez, M.C.; Polo-López, M.I.; Rizzo, L.; Fernández-Ibáñez, P. Urban wastewater disinfection for agricultural reuse: Effect of solar driven AOPs in the inactivation of a multidrug resistant E. coli strain. *Appl. Catal. B Environ.* **2015**. [CrossRef]
61. Giannakis, S.; Le, T.T.M.; Entenza, J.M.; Pulgarin, C. Solar photo-Fenton disinfection of 11 antibiotic-resistant bacteria (ARB) and elimination of representative AR genes. Evidence that antibiotic resistance does not imply resistance to oxidative treatment. *Water Res.* **2018**. [CrossRef]
62. Giannakis, S.; Watts, S.; Rtimi, S.; Pulgarin, C. Solar light and the photo-Fenton process against antibiotic resistant bacteria in wastewater: A kinetic study with a Streptomycin-resistant strain. *Catal. Today* **2018**. [CrossRef]
63. Mongeon, P.; Paul-Hus, A. The journal coverage of Web of Science and Scopus: A comparative analysis. *Scientometrics* **2016**, *106*, 213–228. [CrossRef]
64. Gavel, Y.; Iselid, L. Web of Science and Scopus: A journal title overlap study. *Online Inf. Rev.* **2008**, *32*, 8–21. [CrossRef]
65. Garrido-Cardenas, J.A.; Mesa-Valle, C.; Manzano-Agugliaro, F. Human parasitology worldwide research. *Parasitology* **2018**, *145*, 699–712. [CrossRef] [PubMed]
66. Qu, J.; Wang, H.; Wang, K.; Yu, G.; Ke, B.; Yu, H.Q.; Ren, H.; Zheng, X.; Li, J.; Li, W.W.; et al. Municipal wastewater treatment in China: Development history and future perspectives. *Front. Environ. Sci. Eng.* **2019**. [CrossRef]
67. Cherchi, C.; Kessano, M.; Badruzzaman, M.; Schewab, K.; Jacangelo., J.G. Municipal reclaimed water for multi-purpose applications in the power sector. A review. *J. Environ. Manag.* **2019**. [CrossRef] [PubMed]
68. Ikemoto, T.; Magara, Y. Measures against impacts of nuclear disaster on drinking water supply systems in Japan. *Water Pract. Technol.* **2011**. [CrossRef]
69. Ochando-Pulido, J.M.; Victor-Ortega, M.D.; Hodaifa, G.; Martinez-Ferez, A. Physicochemical analysis and adequation of olive oil mill wastewater after advanced oxidation process for reclamation by pressure-driven membrane technology. *Sci. Total Environ.* **2015**. [CrossRef]

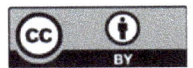

© 2019 by the authors. Licensee MDPI, Basel, Switzerland. This article is an open access article distributed under the terms and conditions of the Creative Commons Attribution (CC BY) license (http://creativecommons.org/licenses/by/4.0/).

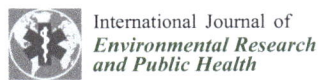 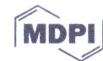

Article

Bibliometric Profile of Global Microplastics Research from 2004 to 2019

Fen Qin [1], Jing Du [2,*], Jian Gao [1], Guiying Liu [2], Yonggang Song [2], Aifu Yang [3], Hong Wang [1], Yuan Ding [1] and Qian Wang [4]

1. Dalian University of Technology Library, 2# Linggong Road, Ganjingzi District, Dalian 116024, China; qinfen@dlut.edu.cn (F.Q.); gaojian@dlut.edu.cn (J.G.); wanghong@dlut.edu.cn (H.W.); dingyuan@dlut.edu.cn (Y.D.)
2. Liaoning Ocean and Fisheries Science Research Institute, 50# Heishijiao Road, Shahekou District, Dalian 116023, China; liuguiying2006@126.com (G.L.); hyzjs_lnshky@163.com (Y.S.)
3. Technology Center of Dalian Customs District, 60# Changjiang East Road, Zhongshan District, Dalian 116001, China; yaf_dlhg@hotmail.com
4. Ocean University of China, 238# Songling Road, Laoshan District, Qiangdao 266100, China; wq13864223681@163.com
* Correspondence: marine_ln@sina.com; Tel.: +86-411-84691603

Received: 30 June 2020; Accepted: 29 July 2020; Published: 5 August 2020

Abstract: Microplastics (MPs) have generated worldwide attention due to their global distribution in the environment, and their potential harmful effects on human and animal health. To analyze MPs-related scientific publications from a global point of view, we created a bibliometric profile, by searching the Web of Science Core Collection database for the topic "microplastic* or (micro near/1 plastic*)", in publications dated from 2004 to 2019. The results revealed an increasing trend in publication output, and identified contributions of different countries and their collaborations, as well as influential authors and productive journals in the field of MPs research. Using co-citation network analysis in VOSviewer, we mined cited references for knowledge bases about analytical methods, potential sources and spatial distributions of MPs, the impacts of MPs on organisms, and the interaction of MPs with contaminants, as well as microorganisms. We also identified four global hotspots for MPs related research, using author keywords co-occurrence network analysis of all extracted publications, as well as Essential Science Indicators highly cited papers from Clarivate Analytics. Results of this study provide a valuable reference for ongoing MPs-related research, which may be of intrigue and awesome noteworthiness for relevant researchers.

Keywords: microplastics; bibliometric; network analysis; VOSviewer software; research hotspots

---

1. Introduction

Plastics used in our daily life and in a wide range of manufacturing processes provide numerous societal benefits, due to their lightweight, durable, and economic nature [1]. However, plastics are resistant to aging, and their refractory degradation makes plastic waste a serious environmental issue [2–4]. Microplastics (MPs), which are smaller items of plastic litter, are of increasing concern due to their ubiquitous global distribution in aquatic environments [5–7], and their close interactions with biota [8]. Although no universal definition of MP size exists, a diameter smaller than 5 mm is commonly accepted [9]. Examples of MPs include resin pellets, microbeads used for cosmetics or associated with industrial spillages (primary source) [10–12], or pieces broken off of larger plastic litter by ultraviolet radiation, oxidation, or mechanical abrasion (secondary source) [13]. Release of synthetic fibers by textile washing is another potential source of MPs [14].

As there has been increasing concern about MPs research, scholars have reviewed literatures in this domain covering different aspects. Initially, reviews of MPs research focused mainly on the marine environment. For example, Cole et al. discussed the sources and transfer of MPs into the marine environment, and assessed the spatial and temporal distribution of MPs in the worldwide marine environment [3], and they concluded that the fate of these MPs was still elusive. Wright et al. investigated the impacts of MPs on marine invertebrates [8]. Later, Horton et al. critically reviewed the presence, behavior, and fate of MPs in terrestrial environments, by evaluating studies of the extent of MPs pollution in freshwater, treated water sources, and even agriculture soil [15]. Recently, the biological effects of MPs have emerged as areas of interest. Researchers have summarized the potential health effects of MPs present in the food chain [16], and emphasized the interaction between MPs and microorganisms [17]. The authors of these reviews amassed, summarized, and extended the MPs-related research based on their long-term research experiences. To date, studies of the evolution of MPs-related scientific research from a global point of view over time were still insufficient. Bibliometric analysis, which takes advantage of bibliometric theory using mathematical and statistical approaches, is a method that can be used to address this knowledge gap. It has been applied to analyze pertinent literatures in various research fields [18–20], including environment-related fields [21]. With regard to MPs research, Ivar do Sul et al. summarized the common denominator between MPs and microbiology, using the bibliometric approach [22], and Barboza et al. evaluated research trends and future perspectives on MPs in the marine environment for the period 2004–2014, using the cross-disciplinary quantitative analysis method [23]. As MPs research has increased substantially since 2011, Zhang et al. conducted an in-depth statistical analysis of global MPs research, using the number of publications as a primary metric for productivity of countries, institution, authors and journals [24]. An up-to-date comprehensive review of the scientific literature, which interprets the influence and importance of different countries, authors and journals, as well as co-occurrence keywords analysis initiated in both extracted literatures from the database and Essential Science Indicators (ESI) highly cited papers from Clarivate Analytics; this is still needed to trace global research hotspots in MPs research.

In this study, we conducted an integrated bibliometric analysis of the literatures on MPs research published from 2004 to 2019. The initial time was set as 2004, because that year, Thompson et al. [25] coined the term "microplastics (MPs)" to define the smaller plastic litter. We used the analysis to identify influential countries, international collaborations, contributing authors, preferred journals, a knowledge base of MPs studies, and research hotspots. The results of our analysis provide a valuable picture of the status of current global MP research, and help illuminate the next steps for future studies.

2. Materials and Methods

2.1. Data Sources

The Web of Science Core Collection (WoSCC), which generates standardized and high-quality academic publication information, is used extensively for the bibliometric examination of the evolution of scientific issues [18,26,27]. On March 12, 2020, all original data were extracted from the online version of the WoSCC database (indexes: Science Citation Index-Expanded and Conference Proceeding Citation Index), using the TOPIC "microplastic* or (micro near/1 plastic*)" for the years 2004 to 2019. ESI highly cited individuals along with the number of their MPs-related publications and ESI highly cited papers were collected by the same TOPIC from Clarivate Analytics on the same day.

2.2. Data Screening

Initially, 3246 publications (after removal of duplications) were extracted using our data searching strategy, including some articles related to material science studies. The latter publications could not be removed simply by excluding some keywords in the data search (e.g., by using "not 'micro-plastic deformation behavior'" or "not 'micro-plasticity'"), because some studies of biodegradable polymers relate to both material science (composites modification) and our study objective (safe for environment), such as [28]. Thus, we conducted content analyses of titles and abstracts of all 3246 publications, and sometimes the full manuscripts were evaluated to exclude irrelevant publications. Ultimately, 2637 publications written in English or with an English abstract remained after the manual screening of four types of documents (articles, reviews, proceeding papers and book chapters). Because these types of documents contained novel concepts, none of them were excluded from our analysis, thus, these 2637 publications were all included in the bibliometric analysis. Moreover, a total of 395 ESI highly cited MPs-related papers were extracted from Clarivate Analytics.

2.3. Analytical Methods

2.3.1. Basic Bibliometric Analysis Method

The basic bibliometric analysis method used a range of indicators to identify distributed characteristics and structural patterns of the general bibliographic data for MPs ongoing work. For example, the year-wise distribution of research output demonstrated the developing trend of increasing work in the MPs discipline. The contribution of an individual country/academic researcher in the MPs scientific research field was ranked by how many times their publication was cited by others (non-self-citation, NSC), and other data recorded included their total number of publications (TNP), sum of times cited (STC), non-self-citation ratio (NSCR), number of publications cited by more than 100 and 50 times, and number of ESI highly cited publications. Preferred journals were identified as those that delivered academic articles and contributed to the development of the research field [29]. Both the journal impact factor (IF) and quartiles in relevant categories were derived from Journal Citation Report (JCR) 2018, and used to explore the publishing journal's influence in the MPs field and their interdisciplinary research areas. All bibliographic data were analyzed using Microsoft Excel 2016, and figures were created using GraphPad Prism (version 7.04, GraphPad Software Inc., San Diego, CA, USA) and VOSviewer software (version 1.6.9, Centre for Science and Technology Studies, Leiden University, Leiden, The Netherlands). We used the results of quantitative analysis of the evolution of literature, as well as the bibliometric indicators, to present a general informative overview of MPs research during the study time period.

2.3.2. Network Analysis Methods

VOSviewer is a free software tool based on the Java environment, that is suitable for constructing complex networks using large-scale data. Therefore, we used VOSviewer software (version 1.6.9) to conduct an in-depth network analysis to visualize the connections between various MFs-related items, and to explain their network structure.

Countries co-authorship network: We conducted the co-authorship analysis to identify collaboration networks among different countries in the MPs research field. The nodes represented countries contributing to MPs research, and the links between items implied cooperative relationships. The size of the node increased as the number of articles published by an individual country increased. The value of the links indicated the number of times a given country shared co-authorship with others. The strength of the link increased as the number of co-authorships increased.

Cited reference co-citation network: Analyzing a knowledge base in a certain research field can be conducted by co-citation network analysis for the cited references [18]. In our co-citation analysis, the nodes represented scientific references. The node size represented the number of times a reference was cited. The distance between two references indicated the correlation of the articles according to co-citation links, based on the assumption that more frequently co-cited references exhibited greater co-citation strength.

Author keywords co-occurrence network: The keywords that authors provided for their articles about MPs research represented their academic viewpoints. Thus, our author keywords co-occurrence analysis identified important terms in the MPs academic, as well as the research hotspots in the MPs discipline. The nodes represented high-frequency author keywords, and the size of an individual node represented how many times that keyword occurred. The link strength between two nodes indicated the number of articles in which two keywords occurred together.

3. Results and Discussion

3.1. Basic Bibliometric Analysis

3.1.1. Characteristics of Publication Output

The year-wise distribution of publication output revealed the progress of MPs research over time (Figure 1a). The number of publications related to MPs fluctuated slightly from 2004 to 2008, and the annual publications were all less than 100 until 2014. Obvious growth of MPs research began in 2014, when the first United Nations Environment Assembly of the United Nations Environment Programme (UNEP) issued the resolution UNEP/EA.1/L.8, which emphasized critical activities to address marine plastic debris and MPs challenges. Governments worldwide began a shared commitment to addressing MPs problems and to conducting the systematic research of many aspects of MPs [30–33]. The cumulative number of annual publications since 2004 follows an exponential model (Figure 1b), and the simulation results suggest that publications about MPs issues might increase to 1703 in 2020. On May 8, 2020, we collected data using the same TOPIC from the WoSCC database, for the time period spanning January 1, 2020 to April 30, 2020, and identified 442 relevant publications. This value was less than the expected value for one-third of the year 2020 (567), which may be a result of the significant disruption that is being caused by the COVID-19 pandemic.

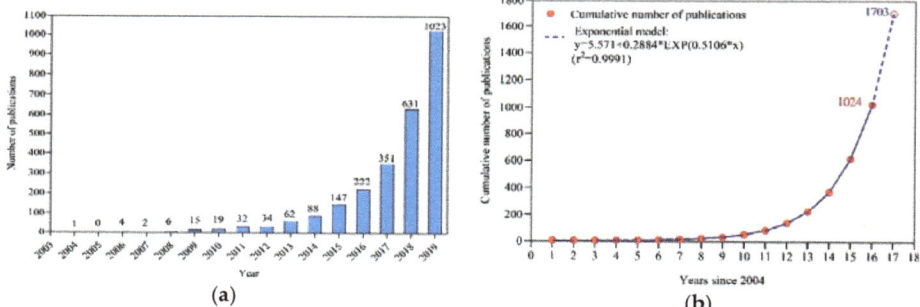

Figure 1. (a) Annual number of publications on microplastics (MPs) research from 2004 to 2019, retrieved from WOSCC; (b) The cumulative annual number of publications since 2004 follows an exponential model.

3.1.2. National Contribution Analysis

According to the author address information in the 2637 publications, 104 countries made contributions to MPs research during the study time period. Table 1 lists the top 10 countries by their NSC times of publications in MPs research field, as well as TNP (with ranking), STC (with ranking), NSCR, and the number of publications cited more than 100 and 50 times. Developed countries, including six European countries, two North American countries, and one Oceania country, along with a developing country (China) occupied leading positions in MPs research. England led the NSC index and was second for STC, which indicated that it produced high quality MPs research. The USA also performed well in the areas of research depth and influence, as it ranked first for STC and had 62 publications that were cited more than 100 times, and 107 publications that were cited more than 50 times. China had the most publications (459), but ranked seventh for NSC. Canada, the other five Europe countries, and Australia also performed well. The 10 countries listed in Table 1 contributed 92.8% of all publications, and the high NSCR values (89.38% on average) indicated that these countries had great external influence not only in numbers of studies but also in the quality of MPs-related publications.

Table 1. The top 10 countries for MPs research ranked by NSC; values for other criteria are given as well.

Rank	Country	NSC [1]	TNP (R) [2]	STC (R) [3]	NSCR [4]	≥100 [5]	≥50 [6]
1	England	23,182	282 (4)	25,376 (2)	91.3%	60	101
2	USA	23,166	381 (2)	25,472 (1)	90.9%	62	107
3	Germany	11,187	317 (3)	127,28 (3)	87.9%	37	76
4	France	10,015	179 (6)	107,83 (4)	92.9%	29	51
5	Netherlands	8369	157 (8)	9096 (6)	92.0%	30	52
6	Australia	8001	155 (9)	8496 (7)	94.2%	21	36
7	China	7491	459 (1)	10,315 (5)	72.6%	19	54
8	Canada	6050	129 (10)	6393 (8)	94.6%	17	28
9	Spain	5084	159 (7)	5504 (9)	92.4%	13	27
10	Italy	4703	230 (5)	5530 (10)	85.0%	15	28

[1] NSC: Non-self-citation; [2] TNP (R): Total number of publications (ranking); [3] STC(R): Sum of times cited (ranking).[4] NSCR: Non-self-citation ratio; [5] ≥100: the number of publications cited more than 100 times; [6] ≥50: the number of publications cited more than 50 times.

3.1.3. Author Contribution Analysis

According to the statistics, 8191 authors (without debugging repetitions of authors' names) have contributed to the increasing scientific knowledge about MPs. Table 2 lists the top 10 influential authors, ranked by the criteria of NSC on MPs issues, as well as their institution (the latest one), country, TNP, STC, and the number of ESI highly cited papers (NEHC). These data were manually debugged to improve the quality of analysis, as a single author may have different forms of abbreviations but with separately counted articles. Half of these influential authors are from European countries, which is in agreement with the known active participation of European countries in MPs-related research. Thompson, R.C. from England was the most productive and influential author, as his 48 publications were cited 11,617 times, and half of his publications were listed as ESI highly cited papers. Galloway, T.S. and Cole, M., from the University of Exeter, England, ranked second and fourth, respectively, with the ratio NEHC/TNP > 55%. Shi, H.H., who ranked ninth, was the most active MPs researcher in China, and 50% of his publications were included as ESI highly cited papers. Galgani, F.; Koelmans, A.A.; Thiel, M.; Rochman, C.M.; Shim, W.J. and Costa, M.F. also performed well with their MPs-related research, and contributed information about the MPs distribution in their regional marine environments, MPs analytical methods, hazardous chemical sorption of MPs, and release of MPs. These scholars were all listed as ESI highly cited researchers in the Ecology/Environment field, which indicated that their articles had significant influence on subsequent research.

Table 2. The top 10 authors for MPs research ranked by NSC; values for other criteria are given as well.

Rank	Author	Organization	Country	NSC	TNP	STC	NEHC [1]
1	Thompson, R.C.	University of Plymouth	England	11,371	48	11,617	24
2	Galloway, T.S.	University of Exeter	England	6616	31	6739	18
3	Galgani, F.	Ifremer [2]	France	4038	28	4110	10
4	Cole, M.	University of Exeter	England	3100	20	3178	11
5	Koelmans, A.A.	Wageningen University	Netherlands	2988	39	3173	12
6	Thiel, M.	Universidad Catolica del Norte	Chile	2570	18	2612	5
7	Rochman, C.M.	University of Toronto	Canada	1654	24	1696	5
8	Shim, W.J.	KIOST [3]	SouthKorea	1629	33	1767	5
9	Shi, H.H.	East China Normal University	China	1615	36	1761	18
10	Costa, M.F.	Federal University of Pernambuco	Brazil	1277	20	1347	1

[1] NEHC: Number of ESI highly cited papers; [2] Ifremer: Institut Français de Recherche pour l'Exploitation de la Mer; [3] KIOST: Korea Institute of Ocean Science Technology.

3.1.4. Journal Analysis

The 2637 publications were retrieved from 399 journals. Among them, most journals (384, 96.2%) published fewer than 20 articles about MPs. Table 3 shows the top 15 most productive journals in which more than 65% of publications related to MPs were published during the period 2004-2019. These journals were classified in six categories, and all placed in higher quartiles in category (Q1/Q2) according to the 2018 JCR report. Ten of the journals were grouped in the *Environmental Sciences* category and three were grouped in the *Marine and Freshwater Biology* category, which indicated that MPs in the aquatic environment was the research hotspot. *Mar Pollut Bull* published the most articles (536) and had the highest STC and NSC, but its NSCR was lower than that of the other 14 journals. *Environ Pollut*, with 327 articles, ranked second. *Water Res* ranked eighth for TNP, but had the highest IF (7.913) among the ten *Environmental Sciences* journals. *Sci Rep-UK* and *Plos One*, were grouped in the *Multidisciplinary Sciences* category, and *Trac-Trend Anal Chem* and *Analmethods-UK* were grouped in the *Chemistry, Analytical* category. Articles in *Environ Toxicol Chem* and *Ecotox Environ Safe*, which were classified in the *Toxicology* category, focused on the ecotoxicological effects of MPs.

Table 3. The top 15 productive journals that published articles about the MPs issue.

Rank	Journal	TNP	STC(R)	NSC(R)	NSCR	IF	Categories (Quartile)
1	Mar Pollut Bull	536	22,572(1)	18,544(1)	82.2%	3.782	Environmental Sciences (Q2); Marine and Freshwater Biology (Q1)
2	Environ Pollut	327	14,456(3)	12,711(3)	87.9%	5.714	Environmental Sciences (Q1)
3	Sci Total Environ	206	6082(4)	5534(4)	91.0%	5.589	Environmental Sciences (Q1)
4	Environ Sci Technol	172	14,466(2)	13,580(2)	93.9%	7.149	Environmental Sciences (Q1)
5	Chemosphere	90	2139(9)	2036(9)	95.2%	5.108	Environmental Sciences (Q1)
6	Environ Sci Pollut R	63	867(11)	835(11)	96.3%	2.914	Environmental Sciences (Q2)
7	Sci Rep-UK	63	3134(5)	3071(5)	98.0%	4.011	Multidisciplinary Sciences (Q1)
8	Water Res	49	2583(6)	2424(7)	93.8%	7.913	Environmental Sciences (Q1); Water resources (Q1)
9	Front Mar Sci	31	435(14)	425(14)	97.7%	3.086	Marine and Freshwater Biology (Q1)
10	Mar Environ Res	29	2467(7)	2431(6)	98.5%	3.445	Environmental Sciences (Q2); Marine and Freshwater Biology (Q1)
11	Trac-Trend Anal Chem	29	563(13)	551(13)	97.9%	8.428	Chemistry, Analytical (Q1)
12	Analmethods-UK	28	749(12)	739(12)	98.7%	2.378	Chemistry, Analytical (Q2)
13	Environ Toxicol Chem	28	1127(10)	1094(10)	97.0%	3.421	Environmental Sciences (Q2); Toxicology(Q2)
14	PlosOne	25	2430(8)	2399(8)	98.7%	2.776	Multidisciplinary Science(Q2)
15	Ecotox Environ Safe	21	304(15)	298(15)	98.0%	4.527	Environmental Sciences (Q1); Toxicology(Q1)

3.2. Network Analysis

3.2.1. Co-Authorship Network Analysis of Countries

Figure 2 illustrates the collaboration network of countries conducting MPs research from 2004–2019. The number of publications threshold was set at 30, and of the 104 countries considered, 29 met this threshold. The whole network consisted of 29 nodes (referred to as countries) and 306 links (total link strength = 1815). England and the USA were the most affiliated countries; their close international cooperation was indicated by 28 links and a total link strength of 353 and 369, respectively. They were followed by Germany (links = 27, total link strength = 274), France (links = 26, total link strength = 218), and the Netherlands (links = 25, total link strength = 239). Academic collaboration between China and the USA was far more frequent than that of any other two countries (link strength = 52), which may be attributed to the high number of Chinese postgraduates/visiting scholars studying or working on MPs research in the USA. Other countries had fewer academic exchanges, such as Turkey (links = 9, total link strength = 12), possibly due to the consequence of language and finance barriers.

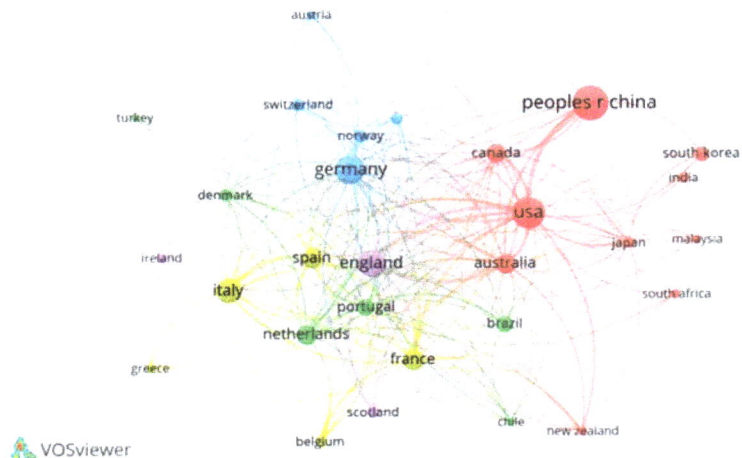

Figure 2. Co-authorship network diagram showing cooperation between countries (with a threshold of 30).

3.2.2. Co-CitationNetwork Analysis of Cited References

Of the 57,834 cited references from MPs articles published between 2004 and 2019, 713 references that were cited at least 30 times were used to create the co-citation network diagram (five clusters with different colors, Figure 3). Each cluster contained some core literatures with high citation rates and academic relationships, which revealed a knowledge base in the MPs research field.

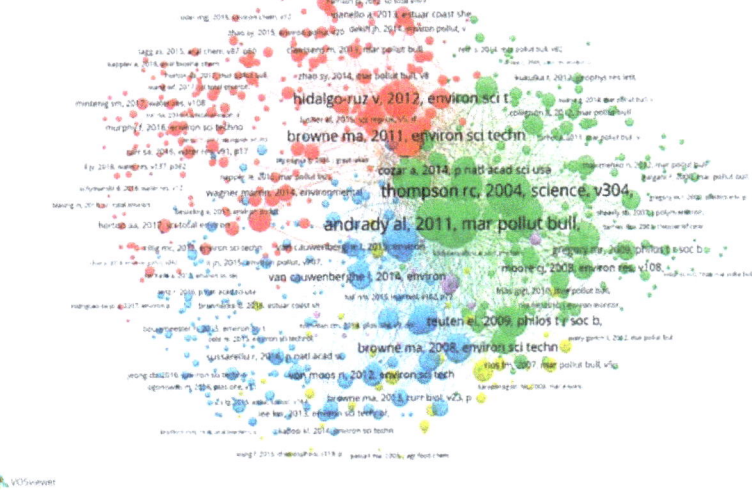

Figure 3. Co-citation network diagram of cited references from MPs articles cited a minimum of 30 times.

In cluster red, the references with the largest nodes were the articles by Browne et al. [34] and Hidalgo-Ruz et al. [35], published in *Environ Sci Technol*, both with 712 co-citations and total link strengths of 25,800 and 24,418, respectively. Browne et al. [34] was the first study to explore the global distribution of MPs, which formed the knowledge base for MPs spatial distribution research. Hidalgo-Ruz et al. [35] reviewed 68 studies, to compare the methodologies used for MPs identification and quantification from seawater and sediment samples, and they called for standardized sampling programs to develop a more comprehensive understanding of MPs distribution. This study undoubtedly formed the knowledge base for MPs analytical methods. In cluster green, the documents with the largest nodes were authored by Andray [36] (published in *Mar. Pollut. Bull.*) and Thompson et al. [25] (published in *Science*). These articles were co-cited 712 times and had total link strengths of 29,817 and 26,743, respectively, indicating that they played a crucial role in the MPs co-citation network structure. Thompson et al. [25] clearly defined the term "MPs" and initiated global research on them. Andray [36] discussed the mechanism by which MPs are derived from marine debris, forming the knowledge base for MPs sources. In cluster blue, the document with the largest node (712 co-citations, 23,574 total link strength) was the article authored by Wright et al. [8] and published in *Environ Pollut*. Additionally, the laboratory experiments conducted by Setälä et al. [37] and Mattsson et al. [38] confirmed that MPs could transfer through food chains, and that lower trophic organisms could be the vector. In cluster yellow, the document with the largest node was written by Teuten et al. [39], who examined the uptake and subsequent release of hydrophobic organic contaminants present on plastic debris. This study formed a knowledge base about the interaction of MPs with contaminants. In cluster purple, Zettler et al. [40] first described a microbial community as a "plasticphere", and called for research on the interaction between MPs and microorganisms.

3.2.3. Co-Occurrence Network Analysis of Author Keywords

(1) In Publications Extracted from WoSCC

There were 4957 unique author keywords recorded in extracted publications from WoSCC. Among them, 3785 words (76.4%) were only used once, 566 (11.4%) were used twice, and 178 (3.6%) were used three times. These author keywords emphasized the breadth of MPs-related research, but also indicated a lack of continuity in research focuses. Some author keywords had different forms, but the same meaning (e.g., "FT-IR Spectroscopy" and "FT-IR" manually standardized as "FT-IR"), so we manually standardized 299 author keywords (with a minimum of 5 occurrences) to 230 keywords, and used them for co-occurrence network analysis (Figure 4). "Microplastic" (the biggest dot, Occurrence = 1146) was the most frequently used author keyword (and was used as our search term). The keywords "marine environment pollution" (occurrence = 366), "marine debris" (occurrence = 296), "ingestion" (occurrence = 105), "nanoplastic" (occurrence = 89), "sediments" (occurrence = 88), "polystyrene" (occurrence = 69), "FT-IR" (occurrence = 66), "freshwater" (occurrence = 60), and "polyethylene" (occurrence = 57) ranked second to tenth in the author keywords analysis, during the period from 2004 to 2019. These keywords were used in a large number of articles dealing with the distribution of MPs in different environments (e.g., marine environment, sediments, and freshwater), the ingestion of MPs by organisms, analytical techniques and quantification of these particles, and the biological effects of exposure to polystyrene or polyethylene nanoplastic. Figure 4 shows that the author keywords provided for MPs articles formed different clusters (by color), which represented global hotspots in MPs-related field (see Section 3.3).

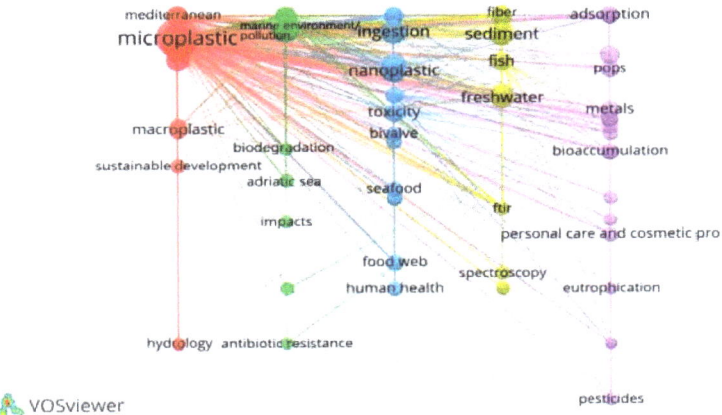

Figure 4. Co-occurrence network diagram of author keywords, appearing in a minimum of five publications between 2004 and 2019.

(2) In ESI highly Cited Papers

There were 859 unique author keywords recorded in 395 ESI highly cited papers of MPs research, among which a total of 26 author keywords (manually standardized) appeared at least five times. The co-occurrence network analysis of these 26 author keywords were shown in Figure 5. "Microplastic" (the biggest dot, Occurrence = 198) was undoubtedly the most frequently used author keyword in ESI highly cited papers of MPs research, followed by "marine environment pollution" (occurrence = 72), "marine debris" (occurrence = 59), "sediments" (occurrence = 40), "ingestion" (occurrence = 28), "freshwater" (occurrence = 24), "nanoplastic" (occurrence = 23), "fish" (occurrence = 21), "accumulation" (occurrence = 13), "mussels" (occurrence = 12), ranked second to tenth. Most of these keywords were the same as those in publications extracted from WoSCC, and they also contributed to exploring the global hotspots of MPs-related research in the next section.

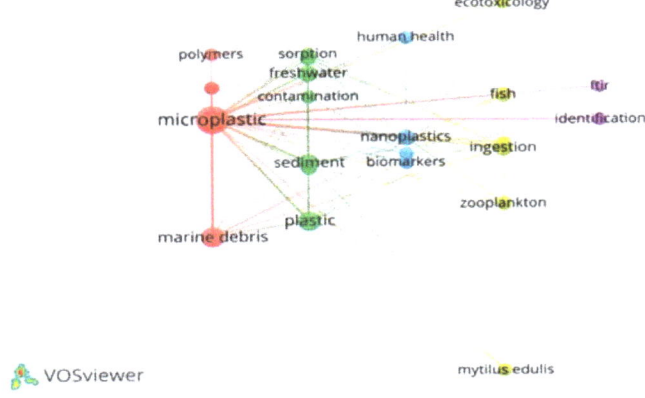

Figure 5. Co-occurrence network diagram of author keywords appearing in a minimum of five ESI highly cited papers, between 2010 and 2019.

3.3. Hotspots of MPs Research

3.3.1. MPs Sources and Spatial Distribution

Contributed keywords can be found in cluster red and green in Figures 4 and 5, including marine plastic pollution, marine debris, beach, surface water, Mediterranean, accumulation, etc.

To address the key MPs problems, the international community has already developed policy responses, such as the European Marine Strategy Framework Directive, which is an ambitious program aimed at preventing MPs pollution. The scientific literature related to sources, pathways, and distribution of MPs is already substantial and constantly growing. MPs have been observed in almost every habitat of the aquatic environment, including ocean surface water [41], the water column [42], beaches [43], subtidal and deep-sea sediments [44,45], and freshwater lakes [46]. However, how to integrate MPs monitoring into existing environmental monitoring programs with reliable quantification routines requires further work.

3.3.2. MPs Analytical Methods

Contributed keywords can be found in cluster yellow in Figure 4 and cluster purple in Figure 5, including identification, density separation, elutriation, sediment, spectroscopy, FT-IR, Raman, etc.

MPs analytical methods were developed to meet different purposes in MPs surveys, and can be divided into three steps: (1) sampling; (2) pretreatment for MPs extraction; and (3) qualitative and quantitative analysis. For sediment samples, high density solutions were commonly used to extract MPs, based on density separation [47]. In addition, elutriation columns proved to be useful tools with high extraction efficiency [48]. For seawater or water samples, selective sampling [49,50] and bulk sampling [51] methods were used in different studies, as were different pretreatment methods, such as enzyme digestion with subsequent filtration [49], and the sieve method [50]. For biota samples, the sampling methods always depended on the organisms being studied. For example, plankton trawls and nets were used to study the accumulation of MPs in plankton [52], whereas the dissection of different organs [53] was used for other target species. Digestion pretreatment methods for MPs extraction from biota samples have received a lot of attention, and many studies compared different digestion pretreatment methods, in pursuit of higher extraction efficiency [54]. For qualitative and quantitative analysis, MPs were usually measured and classified by shape, size, color, and chemical components. Most commonly, the extracted MPs were visually sorted under a microscope, and in some cases, the chemical components of MPs were determined by Raman spectroscopy [49], FT-IR micro-spectroscopy [51], and FT-IR [53]. It is notable that MPs analytical methods are now still debatable and have yet to be standardized.

3.3.3. The Interaction of MPs with Contaminants

Contributed keywords can be found in cluster purple in Figure 4 and cluster green in Figure 5, including sorption, heavy metals, polychlorinated biphenyls (PCBs), polycyclic aromatic hydrocarbons (PAHs), phthalates, persistent organic pollutants (POPs), etc.

Partitioning of contaminations to MPs has also been well documented. It has been evidenced that POPs [55], such as PCBs and PAHs, as well as heavy metals, can be adsorbed onto the surface of MP particles [56], and the sorption capacity is not only influenced by external factors, such as salinity, environment temperature, and weathering, but also by polymer type [57]. Additionally, contaminants adsorbed to MPs as well as MPs additives (e.g., phthalates, alkylphenols) can be desorbed from the surface of MPs during their transit through the digestive tract in organisms [58], which may have negative impacts on them [59]. The challenges of understanding MPs sorption/desorption behavior in different environments and their combined toxic effects on organisms require further research.

3.3.4. MPs Accumulation in Organisms and Their Potential Impact

Contributed keywords can be found in cluster blue in Figure 4 and cluster blue and yellow in Figure 5, including ingestion, biomarkers, mussel, fish, seafood, trophic transfer, food web, toxicity, human health, etc.

MPs have been detected in many wild aquatic organisms, such as beaked whale [53], lobster [60], crab [61], fish [62,63], bivalves [64–66], and zooplankton [52,67,68]. Laboratory experiments have shown that MPs can cause some physical harm to a diverse array of organisms upon ingestion [8]. Additional threats of MPs are their capacity to leach toxic additives such as monomers and plasticizers, and to be potential vectors for hydrophobic POPs, which may cause further health problems, such as endocrine disruption and even carcinogenesis to organisms upon ingestion [69]. To quantify the exposure risk from ingested MPs and to evaluate their potential eco-toxicological risk, scientists have studied the survival rate [70,71], growth [72], reproductive status [73,74] and gene expression [75] of target species. As biomarkers are useful indicators of exposure, they should be used to identify ecologically significant effects of MPs on sentinel species.

In recent years, the global presence of MPs and nanoplastics in foodstuff, drinking water, and air samples has been well documented. Consequently, human exposure to MPs via ingestion and inhalation is inevitable. Initial concern about human exposure to MPs focused on ingestion of MPs contaminated aquatic organisms. Evidence has shown that the consumption of entirely consumed organisms such as oysters and mussels may pose a higher risk of MPs exposure than consumption of eviscerated ones [76]. Other sources of human exposure to MPs include commercial salt and bottled drinks, as well as airborne MPs that can be inhaled [77]. Although MPs have been detected in human stool samples [78], nanoplastics reportedly might decrease the viability of human Caco-2 cells [79], and they can induce pro-inflammatory responses [80]—adverse effects of MPs on human health have not been reported to date. Thus, studies of the effects of MPs on human health are still urgently needed.

4. Conclusions

MPs, as an environmental pollutant, have become a global problem and they may pose a risk to human health. To summarize research progress and identify future research topics based on current hotspots, we conducted a bibliometric profile of MPs relevant research, using data from the WoSCC database for the period 2004–2019. We found that the scientific output of MPs-related research experienced rapid growth during the past 16 years, and that this booming research area has expanded into many related fields. Developed countries were important contributors to MPs research, as England, the USA, and Germany occupied the top three positions, based on the criterion of NSC. China was the only developing country in the top 10 national contributors. These influential countries foster close academic collaborations, as shown by the co-authorship network analysis of countries. However, more exchanges and cooperation between these countries and others are needed. We also found that Thompson RC, who defined the term "MPs", was the most productive author, as well as the most influential one. All of the top 10 authors identified based on the criterion of NSC were ESI highly cited researchers in the *Ecology/Environment* field, which highlights their significant influence on MPs-related research. Our results show that the issue of MPs is a multidisciplinary research field, because journals classified in six different categories contained MPs-related articles. The results of co-citation network analysis of cited references indicated that in-depth research laid a solid foundation for the MPs scientific field. The internal composition relationships of MPs studies were visualized by co-occurrence networks of author keywords, both in extracted publications and ESI highly cited papers, which identified the following research hotspots: potential sources and spatial distributions of MPs, analytical methods, the interaction of MPs with contaminants, and the impacts of MPs on organisms as well as human beings. Future MPs studies should focus on the following five aspects: (1) integration of MPs monitoring into existing environmental monitoring programs; (2) unified technical standards and reliable quantification routines; (3) sorption/desorption behavior of contaminants on MPs in different environments; (4) biological effects on sentinel species and molecular toxicology mechanisms; and (5) the effects of MPs exposure on human health.

Author Contributions: Conceptualization, F.Q., J.D. and H.W.; methodology and software, F.Q., J.G. and G.L.; formal analysis, J.D., J.G., G.L. and Y.S.; investigation, A.Y., Y.D. and Q.W.; resources, J.G., G.L. and H.W.; writing—original draft preparation, review and editing, F.Q., J.D. and H.W.; visualization, F.Q., Y.S. and A.Y.; funding acquisition, J.D. and H.W. All authors have read and agreed to the published version of the manuscript.

Funding: This research was funded by The Science and Technology Innovation Fund of Dalian, P.R. China, grant number 2019J13SN119; Key Laboratory of Huanghuai Water Environment and Pollution Control, Ministry of Education, P.R. China, grant number KFJJ-2017-11; Department of Ocean and Fishery of Liaoning Province, P.R. China, grant number 201808.

Acknowledgments: We would like to thank XianWen Wang of Dalian University of Technology for his technical support on VOSviewer software.

Conflicts of Interest: The authors declare no conflict of interest.

References

1. Phuong, N.N.; Zalouk-Vergnoux, A.; Poirier, L.; Kamari, A.; Châtel, A.; Mouneyrac, C.; Lagarde, F. Is there any consistency between the microplastics found in the field and those used in laboratory experiments? *Environ. Pollut.* **2016**, *211*, 111–123. [CrossRef] [PubMed]
2. Barnes, D.K.; Galgani, F.; Thompson, R.C.; Barlaz, M. Accumulation and fragmentation of plastic debris in global environments. *Philos. Trans. R. Soc. Lond. B Biol. Sci.* **2009**, *364*, 1985–1998. [CrossRef] [PubMed]
3. Cole, M.; Lindeque, P.; Halsband, C.; Galloway, T.S. Microplastics as contaminants inthe marine environment: A review. *Mar. Pollut. Bull.* **2011**, *62*, 2588–2597. [CrossRef] [PubMed]
4. Eerkes-Medrano, D.; Thompson, R.C.; Aldridge, D.C. Microplastics in freshwater systems: A review of the emerging threats, identification of knowledge gaps and prioritisation of research needs. *Water Res.* **2015**, *75*, 63–82. [CrossRef]
5. Derraik, J.G. The pollution of the marine environment by plastic debris: A review. *Mar. Pollut. Bull.* **2002**, *44*, 842–852. [CrossRef]
6. Ivar do Sul, J.A.; Costa, M.F. The present and future of microplastic pollution in the marine environment. *Environ. Pollut.* **2014**, *185*, 352–364. [CrossRef]
7. Wang, J.; Tan, Z.; Peng, J.; Qiu, Q.; Li, M. The behaviors of microplastics in the marine environment. *Mar. Environ. Res.* **2016**, *113*, 7–17. [CrossRef]
8. Wright, S.L.; Thompson, R.C.; Galloway, T.S. The physical impacts of microplastics on marine organisms: A review. *Environ. Pollut.* **2013**, *178*, 483–492. [CrossRef]
9. Arthur, C.; Baker, J.; Bamford, H. NOAA Technical Memorandum NOS-OR&R30. In Proceedings of the International Research Workshop On The Occurrence, Effects And Fate Of Microplastic Marine Debris, Tacoma, WA, USA, 9–11 September 2008; pp. 9–11.
10. Fendall, L.S.; Sewell, M.A. Contributing to marine pollution by washing your face: Microplastics in facial cleansers. *Mar. Pollut. Bull.* **2009**, *58*, 1225–1228. [CrossRef]
11. Napper, I.E.; Bakir, A.; Rowland, S.J.; Thompson, R.C. Characterisation, quantity and sorptive properties of microplastics extracted from cosmetics. *Mar. Pollut. Bull.* **2015**, *99*, 178–185. [CrossRef]
12. Eriksen, M.; Mason, S.; Wilson, S.; Box, C.; Zellers, A.; Edwards, W.; Farley, H.; Amato, S. Microplastic pollution in the surface waters of the Laurentian Great Lakes. *Mar. Pollut. Bull.* **2013**, *77*, 177–182. [CrossRef] [PubMed]
13. Browne, M.A.; Galloway, T.; Thompson, R. Microplastic-an emerging contaminant of potential concern? *Integr. Environ. Assess. Manag.* **2007**, *3*, 559–561. [CrossRef] [PubMed]
14. Cesa, F.S.; Turra, A.; Baruque-Ramos, J. Synthetic fibers as microplastics in the marine environment: A review from textile perspective with a focus on domestic washings. *Sci. Total Environ.* **2017**, *598*, 1116–1129. [CrossRef] [PubMed]
15. Horton, A.A.; Walton, A.; Spurgeon, D.J.; Lahive, E.; Svendsen, C. Microplastics in freshwater and terrestrial environments: Evaluating the current understanding to identify the knowledge gaps and future research priorities. *Sci. Total Environ.* **2017**, *586*, 127–141. [CrossRef] [PubMed]

16. van Raamsdonk, L.W.D.; van der Zande, M.; Koelmans, A.A.; Hoogenboom, R.L.A.P.; Peters, R.J.B.; Groot, M.J.; Peijnenburg, A.A.C.M.; Weesepoel, Y.J.A. Current insights into monitoring, bioaccumulation, and potential health effects of microplastics present in the food chain. *Foods* **2020**, *9*, 72. [CrossRef]
17. Lu, L.; Luo, T.; Zhao, Y.; Cai, C.H.; Fu, Z.W.; Jin, Y.X. Interaction between microplastics and microorganisms as well as gut microbiota: A consideration on environmental animal and human health. *Sci. Total Environ.* **2019**, *667*, 94–100. [CrossRef] [PubMed]
18. Zou, X.; Yue, W.L.; Vu, H.L. Visualization and analysis of mapping knowledge domain of road safety studies. *Accid. Analy. Prev.* **2018**, *118*, 131–145. [CrossRef]
19. Zhang, M.; Gao, M.; Yue, S.Y.; Zheng, T.L.; Gao, Z.; Ma, X.Y.; Wang, Q.H. Global trends and future prospects of food waste research: A bibliometric analysis. *Environ. Sci. Pollut. R.* **2018**, *25*, 24600–24610. [CrossRef]
20. Wang, L.; Zhao, L.; Mao, G.; Zuo, J.; Du, H. Way to accomplish low carbon development transformation: A bibliometric analysis during 1995–2014. *Renew. Sust. Energ. Rev.* **2017**, *68*, 57–69. [CrossRef]
21. Ruiz-Real, J.L.; Uribe-Toril, J.; Valenciano, J.D.P.; Gazqiez-Abad, J.C. Worldwide research on circular economy and environment: A bibliometric analysis. *Int. J. Environ. Res. Pub. Heath* **2018**, *15*, 2699. [CrossRef]
22. Ivar do sul, J.A.; Tagg, A.S.; Labrenz, M. Exploring the common denominator between microplastics and microbiology: A scientometric approach. *Scientometrics* **2018**, *117*, 2145–2157. [CrossRef]
23. Barboza, L.G.A.; Gimenez, B.C.G. Microplastics in the marine environment: Current trends and future perspectives. *Mar. Pollut. Bull.* **2015**, *97*, 5–12. [CrossRef]
24. Zhang, Y.; Pu, S.Y.; Lv, X.; Gao, Y.; Ge, L. Global trends and prospects in microplastics research: A bibliometric analysis. *J. Hazard. Mater.* **2020**, *400*, 123110. [CrossRef] [PubMed]
25. Thompson, R.C.; Olsen, Y.; Mitchell, R.P.; Davis, A.; Rowland, S.J.; John, A.W.G.; Mcgonigle, D.; Russell, A.E. Lost at sea: Where is all the plastic? *Science* **2004**, *304*, 838. [CrossRef] [PubMed]
26. Ji, L.; Liu, C.W.; Huang, L.C.; Huang, G.H. The evolution of resources conservation and recycling over the past 30 years: A biboliometric overview. *Resour. Conserv. Recy.* **2018**, *134*, 34–43. [CrossRef]
27. Mao, G.Z.; Huang, N.; Chen, L.; Wang, H.M. Research on biomass energy and environment from the past to the future: A bibliometric analysis. *Sci. Total Environ.* **2018**, *635*, 1081–1090. [CrossRef]
28. Su, B.B.; Hyeong, C.N.; Won, H.P. Electrospraying of environmentally sustainable alginate microbeads for cosmetic additives. *Int. J. Biol. Macromol.* **2019**, *133*, 278–283. [CrossRef]
29. Khudzari, J.M.; Kurian, J.; Tartakovsky, B.; Raghavan, G.S.V. Biboliometric analysis of global research trends on microbial fuel cells using Scopus database. *Biochem. Eng. J.* **2018**, *136*, 51–60. [CrossRef]
30. Avio, C.G.; Gorbi, S.; Regoli, F. Experimental development of a new protocol for extraction and characterization of microplastics in fish tissues: First observations in commercial species from Adriatic Sea. *Mar. Pollut. Bull.* **2015**, *111*, 18–26. [CrossRef]
31. Stolte, A.; Forster, S.; Gerdts, G.; Schubert, H. Microplastic concentrations in beach sediments along the German Baltic coast. *Mar. Pollut. Bull.* **2015**, *99*, 216–229. [CrossRef]
32. Avio, C.G.; Gorbi, S.; Milan, M.; Benedetti, M.; Fattorini, D.; d'Errico, G.; Pauletto, M.; Bargelloni, L.; Ragoli, F. Pollutants bioavailability and toxicological risk from microplastics to marine mussels. *Environ. Pollut.* **2015**, *198*, 211–222. [CrossRef] [PubMed]
33. Ma, Y.N.; Huang, A.; Cao, S.Q.; Sun, F.F.; Wang, L.H.; Guo, H.Y.; Ji, R. Effects of nanoplastics and microplastics on toxicity, bioaccumulation, and environmental fate of phenanthrene in fresh water. *Environ. Pollut.* **2016**, *219*, 166–173. [CrossRef] [PubMed]
34. Browne, M.A.; Crump, P.; Niven, S.J.; Teuten, E.; Tonkin, A.; Galloway, T.; Thompson, R. Accumulation of Microplastic on Shorelines Worldwide: Sources and Sinks. *Environ. Sci. Technol.* **2011**, *45*, 9175–9179. [CrossRef] [PubMed]
35. Hidalgo-Ruz, V.; Gutow, L.; Thompson, R.C.; Thiel, M. Microplastics in the marine environment: A review of the methods used for identification and quantification. *Environ. Sci. Technol.* **2012**, *46*, 3060–3075. [CrossRef]
36. Andrady, A.L. Microplastics in the marine environment. *Mar. Pollut. Bull.* **2011**, *62*, 1596–1605. [CrossRef]
37. Setälä, O.; Fleming-Lehtinen, V.; Lehtiniemi, M. Ingestion and transfer of microplastics in the planktonic food web. *Environ. Pollut.* **2014**, *185*, 77–83. [CrossRef]
38. Mattsson, K.; Ekvall, M.T.; Hansson, L.A.; Linse, S.; Malmendal, A.; Cedervall, T. Altered behavior, physiology, and metabolism in fish exposed to polystyrene nanoparticles. *Environ. Sci. Technol.* **2015**, *49*, 553–561. [CrossRef]

39. Teuten, E.L.; Rowland, S.J.; Galloway, T.S.; Thompson, R.C. Potential for plastics to transport hydrophobic contaminants. *Environ. Sci. Technol.* **2007**, *41*, 7759–7764. [CrossRef]
40. Zettler, E.R.; Mincer, T.J.; Amaral-Zettler, L.A. Life in the "Plastisphere": Microbial communities on plastic marine debris. *Environ. Sci. Technol.* **2013**, *47*, 7137–7146. [CrossRef]
41. Chae, D.H.; Kim, I.S.; Kim, S.K.; Song, Y.K.; Shim, W.J. Abundance and distribution characteristics of microplastics in surface seawaters of the Incheon/Kyeonggi coastal region. *Arch. Environ. Contam. Toxicol.* **2015**, *69*, 269–278. [CrossRef]
42. Cózar, A.; Echevarría, F.; González-Gordillo, J.I.; Irigoien, X.; Úbeda, B.; Hernández-León, S.; Palma, A.T.; Navarro, S.; García-de-Lomas, J.; Ruiz, A.; et al. Plastic debris in the open ocean. *Proc. Natl. Acad. Sci. USA* **2014**, *118*, 10239–10244. [CrossRef]
43. Turra, A.; Manzano, A.B.; Dias, R.J.S.; Mahiques, M.M.; Barbosa, L.; Balthazar-Silva, D.; Moreira, F.T. Three-dimensional distribution of plastic pellets in sandybeaches: Shifting paradigms. *Sci. Rep.* **2014**, *4*, 1–7. [CrossRef]
44. Vianello, A.; Boldrin, A.; Guerriero, P.; Moschino, V.; Rella, R.; Sturaro, A.; Da Ros, L. Microplastic particles in sediments of lagoon of Venice, Italy: First observations on occurrence, spatial patterns and identification. *Estuar. Coast. Shelf Sci.* **2013**, *130*, 54–61. [CrossRef]
45. Van Cauwenberghe, L.; Vanreusel, A.; Mees, J.; Janssen, C.R. Microplastic pollution indeep-sea sediments. *Environ. Pollut.* **2013**, *182*, 495–499. [CrossRef] [PubMed]
46. Wang, W.F.; Ndungu, A.W.; Li, Z.; Wang, J. Microplastics pollution in inland freshwaters of China: A case study inurban surface waters of Wuhan, China. *Sci. Total Environ.* **2017**, *575*, 1369–1374. [CrossRef]
47. Quinn, B.; Murphy, F.; Ewins, C. Validation of density separation for the rapid recovery of microplastics from sediment. *Anal. Methods-UK* **2016**. [CrossRef]
48. Kedzierski, M.; Tilly, V.L.; Bourseau, P.; Bellegou, H.; César, G.; Sire, O.; Bruzaud, S. Microplastics elutriation from sandy sediments: A granulometric approach. *Mar. Pollut. Bull.* **2016**, *107*, 315–323. [CrossRef]
49. Zhao, S.; Zhu, L.; Li, D. Microplastic in three urban estuaries, China. *Environ. Pollut.* **2015**, *206*, 597–604. [CrossRef]
50. Florian, F.; Camille, S.; Gael, P.; François, G.; Luiz, A.; Pascal, H. An evaluation of surface micro and meso plastic pollution in pelagic ecosystems of western Mediterranean Sea. *Environ. Sci. Pollut. R.* **2015**, *22*, 12190–12197. [CrossRef]
51. Song, Y.K.; Hong, S.H.; Jiang, M.; Han, G.M.; Shim, W.J. Occurrence and distribution of microplastics in the sea surface microlayer in Jinhae bay, South Korea. *Arch. Environ. Contam. Toxicol.* **2015**, *69*, 279–287. [CrossRef]
52. Desforges, J.P.W.; Galbraith, M.; Ross, P.S. Ingestion of microplastics by zooplankton in the Northeast Pacific Ocean. *Arch. Environ. Contam. Toxicol.* **2015**, *69*, 320–330. [CrossRef]
53. Lusher, A.L.; Hernandez-Millian, G.; O'Brien, J.; Berrow, S.; O'Connor, I.; Officer, R. Microplastic and macroplastic ingestion by a deep diving, oceanic cetacean: The True's beaked whale *Mesoplodon mirus*. *Environ. Pollut.* **2015**, *199*, 185–191. [CrossRef] [PubMed]
54. Dehaut, A.; Cassone, A.L.; Frère, L.; Hermabessiere, L.; Himber, C.; Rinnert, E.; Rivière, G.; Lambert, C.; Soudant, P.; Huvet, A.; et al. Microplastics in seafood: Benchmark protocol for their extraction and characterization. *Environ. Pollut.* **2016**, *215*, 223–233. [CrossRef] [PubMed]
55. Rios, L.M.; Moore, C.; Jones, P.R. Persistent organic pollutants carried by synthetic polymers in the ocean environment. *Mar. Pollut. Bull.* **2007**, *54*, 1230–1237. [CrossRef] [PubMed]
56. Holmes, L.A.; Turner, A.; Thompson, R.C. Adsorption of trace metals to plastic resin pellets in the marine environment. *Environ. Pollut.* **2012**, *160*, 42–48. [CrossRef] [PubMed]
57. Bakir, A.; Rowland, S.J.; Thompson, R.C. Competitive sorption of persistent organic pollutants onto microplastics in the marine environment. *Mar. Pollut. Bull.* **2012**, *64*, 2782–2789. [CrossRef]
58. Rochman, C.M.; Hoh, E.; Kurobe, T.; Teh, S.J. Ingested plastic transfers hazardous chemicals to fish and induces hepatic stress. *Sci. Rep.* **2013**, *3*, 3263. [CrossRef]
59. Rochman, C.M.; Kurobe, T.; Flores, I.; Teh, S.J. Early warning signs of endocrine disruption in adult fish from the ingestion of polyethylene with and without sorbed chemical pollutants from the marine environment. *Sci. Total Environ.* **2014**, *493*, 656–661. [CrossRef]
60. Murray, F.; Cowie, P.R. Plastic contamination in the decapod crustacean *Nephrops norvegicus* (Linnaeus, 1758). *Mar. Pollut. Bull.* **2011**, *62*, 1207–1217. [CrossRef]

61. Wójcik-Fudalewska, D.; Normant-Saremba, M.; Anastácio, P. Occurrence of plasticdebris in the stomach of the invasive crab *Eriocheir sinensis*. *Mar. Pollut. Bull.* **2016**, *113*, 306–311. [CrossRef]
62. Lusher, A.L.; McHugh, M.; Thompson, R.C. Occurrence of microplastics in the gastrointestinal tract of pelagic and demersal fish from the English Channel. *Mar. Pollut. Bull.* **2013**, *67*, 94–99. [CrossRef] [PubMed]
63. Jabeen, K.; Su, L.; Li, J.N.; Yang, D.Q.; Tong, C.F.; Mu, J.L.; Shi, H.H. Microplastics and mesoplastics in fish from coastal and fresh waters of China. *Environ. Pollut.* **2017**, *221*, 141–149. [CrossRef] [PubMed]
64. Mathalon, A.; Hill, P. Microplastic fibers in the intertidal ecosystem surrounding Halifax Harbor, Nova Scotia. *Mar. Pollut. Bull.* **2014**, *81*, 69–79. [CrossRef] [PubMed]
65. Van Cauwenberghe, L.; Janssen, C.R. Microplastics in bivalves cultured for human consumption. *Environ. Pollut.* **2014**, *193*, 65–70. [CrossRef]
66. Li, J.N.; Yang, D.Q.; Li, L.; Jabeen, K.; Shi, H.H. Microplastics in commercial bivalves from China. *Environ. Pollut.* **2015**, *207*, 190–195. [CrossRef] [PubMed]
67. Steer, M.; Cole, M.; Thompson, R.C.; Lindeque, P.K. Microplastic ingestion in fish larvae in the western English Channel. *Environ. Pollut.* **2017**, *226*, 250–259. [CrossRef]
68. Sun, X.X.; Li, Q.J.; Zhu, M.L.; Liang, J.H.; Zheng, S.; Zhao, Y.F. Ingestion of microplastics by natural zooplankton groups in the northern South China Sea. *Mar. Pollut. Bull.* **2017**, *115*, 217–224 [CrossRef]
69. Teuten, E.L.; Saquing, J.M.; Knappe, D.R.U.; Barlaz, M.; Jonsson, S.; Björn, A.; Rowland, S.J.; Thompson, R.C.; Galloway, T.S.; Yamashita, R.; et al. Transport and release of chemicals from plastics to the environment and to wildlife. *Philos. Trans. R. Soc. Lond. B Biol. Sci.* **2009**, *364*, 2027–2045. [CrossRef]
70. Au, S.Y.; Bruce, T.F.; Bridges, W.C.; Klaine, S.J. Responses of *Hyalella azteca* to acute and chronic microplastic exposures. *Environ. Toxicol. Chem.* **2015**, *34*, 2564–2572. [CrossRef]
71. Mazurais, D.; Ernande, B.; Quazuguel, P.; Severe, A.; Huelvan, C.; Madec, L.; Mouchel. O.; Soudant, P.; Robbens, J.; Huvet, A.; et al. Evaluation of the impact of polyethylene microbeads ingestion in European sea bass (*Dicentrarchus labrax*) larvae. *Mar. Environ. Res.* **2015**, *112*, 78–85. [CrossRef]
72. Besseling, E.; Wegner, A.; Foekema, E.M.; van Den, H.M.J.; Koelmans, A.A. Effects of microplastic on fitness and PCB bioaccumulation by the lugworm *Arenicola marina* (L.). *Environ. Sci. Technol.* **2013**, *47*, 593–600. [CrossRef] [PubMed]
73. Lee, K.W.; Shim, W.J.; Kwon, O.Y.; Kang, J.H. Size-dependent effects of micro polystyrene particles in the marine copepod *Tigriopus japonicas*. *Environ. Sci. Technol.* **2013**, *47*, 11278–11283. [CrossRef] [PubMed]
74. Cole, M.; Lindeque, P.; Fileman, E.; Halsband, C.; Galloway, T.S. The impact of polystyrene microplastics on feeding, function and fecundity in the marine copepod *Calanus helgolandicus*. *Environ. Sci. Technol.* **2015**, *49*, 1130–1137. [CrossRef] [PubMed]
75. Sussarellu, R.; Suquet, M.; Thomas, Y.; Lambert, C.; Fabioux, C.; Pernet, M.E.; Le, G.N.; Quillien, V.; Mingant, C.; Epelboin, Y.; et al. Oyster reproduction is affected by exposure to polystyrene microplastics. *Proc. Natl. Acad. Sci. USA* **2016**, *113*, 2430–2435. [CrossRef]
76. Carbery, M.; O'Connor, W.; Palanisami, T. Trophic transfer of microplastics and mixed contaminants in the marine food web and implications for human health. *Environ. Int.* **2018**, *115*, 400–409. [CrossRef]
77. Liu, C.; Zhang, Y.; Wang, L.; Deng, J.; Gao, Y.; Sun, H. Widespread distribution of PET and PC microplastics in dust in urban China and their estimated human exposure. *Environ. Int.* **2019**, *128*, 116–124. [CrossRef]
78. Schwabl, P.; Köppel, S.; Königshofer, P.; Bucsics, T.; Michael, T.; Reiberger, T.; Liebmann, B. Detection of various microplastics in human stool. *Ann. Intern. Med.* **2019**, *171*, 453–457. [CrossRef]
79. Wu, S.J.; Wu, M.; Tian, D.C.; Qiu, L.Q.; Li, T.T. Effects of polystyrene microbeads on cytotoxicity and transcriptomic profiles in human Caco-2 cells. *Environ. Toxicol.* **2020**, *35*, 495–506. [CrossRef]
80. Forte, M.; Iachetta, G.; Tussellino, M.; Carotenuto, R.; Prisco, M.; De falco, M.; Laforgia, V.; Valiente, S. Polystyrene nanoparticles internalization in human gastric adenocarcinoma cells. *Toxicol. Vitr.* **2016**, *31*, 126–136. [CrossRef]

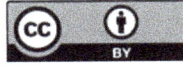

© 2020 by the authors. Licensee MDPI, Basel, Switzerland. This article is an open access article distributed under the terms and conditions of the Creative Commons Attribution (CC BY) license (http://creativecommons.org/licenses/by/4.0/).

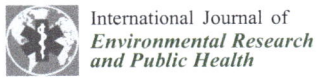 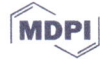

Article

Studies of Novel Coronavirus Disease 19 (COVID-19) Pandemic: A Global Analysis of Literature

Bach Xuan Tran [1,2,*], Giang Hai Ha [3,4], Long Hoang Nguyen [5], Giang Thu Vu [6], Men Thi Hoang [3,4], Huong Thi Le [1], Carl A. Latkin [2], Cyrus S.H. Ho [7] and Roger C.M. Ho [8,9]

1. Institute for Preventive Medicine and Public Health, Hanoi Medical University, Hanoi 100000, Vietnam; lethihuong@hmu.edu.vn
2. Bloomberg School of Public Health, Johns Hopkins University, Baltimore, MD 21205, USA; carl.latkin@jhu.edu
3. Institute for Global Health Innovations, Duy Tan University, Da Nang 550000, Vietnam; hahaigiang@duytan.edu.vn (G.H.H.); hoangthimen@duytan.edu.vn (M.T.H.)
4. Faculty of Pharmacy, Duy Tan University, Da Nang 550000, Vietnam
5. VNU School of Medicine and Pharmacy, Vietnam National University, Hanoi 100000, Vietnam; nhlong.smp@vnu.edu.vn
6. Center of Excellence in Evidence-based Medicine, Nguyen Tat Thanh University, Ho Chi Minh City 700000, Vietnam; giang.coentt@gmail.com
7. Department of Psychological Medicine, National University Hospital, Singapore 119074, Singapore; cyrushosh@gmail.com
8. Department of Psychological Medicine, Yong Loo Lin School of Medicine, National University of Singapore, Singapore 119228, Singapore; pcmrhcm@nus.edu.sg
9. Institute for Health Innovation and Technology (iHealthtech), National University of Singapore, Singapore 117599, Singapore
* Correspondence: bach.ipmph2@gmail.com; Tel.: +84-888288399

Received: 7 May 2020; Accepted: 3 June 2020; Published: 8 June 2020

Abstract: Novel coronavirus disease 19 (COVID-19) is a global threat to millions of lives. Enormous efforts in knowledge production have been made in the last few months, requiring a comprehensive analysis to examine the research gaps and to help guide an agenda for further studies. This study aims to explore the current research foci and their country variations regarding levels of income and COVID-19 transmission features. This textual analysis of 5780 publications extracted from the Web of Science, Medline, and Scopus databases was performed to explore the current research foci and propose further research agenda. The Latent Dirichlet allocation was used for topic modeling. Regression analysis was conducted to examine country variations in the research foci. Results indicate that publications are mainly contributed by the United States, China, and European countries. Guidelines for emergency care and surgical, viral pathogenesis, and global responses in the COVID-19 pandemic are the most common topics. There is variation in the research approaches to mitigate COVID-19 problems in countries with different income and transmission levels. Findings highlighted the need for global research collaborations among high- and low/middle-income countries in the different stages of pandemic prevention and control.

Keywords: scientometrics; content analysis; text mining; COVID-19

1. Introduction

Novel coronavirus disease 19 (COVID-19), caused by severe acute respiratory syndrome coronavirus 2 (SARS-CoV-2), is currently threatening millions of lives in the world. Since the first introduction at the end of 2019, this disease was officially declared as a global pandemic by the World Health Organization (WHO) on March 11, 2020 [1]. Until April 30, 2020, 185 countries/territories reported 3.2 million confirmed cases with 227,847 total deaths [2], and the highest-burden has been placed in European and American countries [1]. Serious health, social, and economic consequences of COVID-19 have been well-recognized [3–7], especially among the elderly with comorbidities, homeless individuals, and also residents who face financial, mental, and physical hardships due to social distancing policies [8].

Given that COVID-19 is a new threat without any antiviral therapies or vaccines, current measures to mitigate this crisis depend heavily on the national and regional preparedness and responses [9]. However, optimal strategies to cope with the complexity of this pandemic demand substantial scientific evidence. Recently, the WHO has issued technical guidance for countries/regions and research institutions, as well as having worked closely with global researchers to update the empirical evidence [10,11]. Efforts have been made around the globe to enhance the understanding of the COVID-19's dynamic transmission, develop effective vaccines and treatment regimes, as well as evaluating impacts of current responses on different populations' health and well-being [12]. As a result, in the last four months, the number of COVID-19-related publications has increased dramatically in various forms including articles, reviews, letters to editors, or preprint documents [13]. These contributions have proven the importance of scientific research in pandemic preparedness and helped governments to respond rapidly and effectively to the crisis [14].

The current growth body of literature has rapidly shaped our knowledge about COVID-19, but it also raises the need to identify the remaining research questions that should be prioritized [15]. However, there has been a lack of studies attempting to identify the country and regional variations in COVID-19-related research foci. Several systematic reviews have been conducted to examine the clinical characteristics of COVID-19 [16,17], or the effectiveness of specific COVID-19 treatment and policies [18–20]. However, these studies only focused on a specific aspect of COVID-19, as well as only reviewing a small volume of articles, which are unable to capture a comprehensive picture of global COVID-19 research. One potential solution to address these limitations is bibliometric analysis. By using systematically quantitative analyses for a vast amount of publications, this method is widely used to quantify the growth of research productivity, the most prolific countries and institutions, and the development of research contents [21–23]. In this paper, we used the bibliometric analysis with aims to explore the current research foci and their country variations regarding levels of income and COVID-19 transmission features. Findings of this study would potentially inform current knowledge gaps about COVID-19, as well as propose future research directions.

2. Materials and Methods

2.1. Searching Strategy and Study Selection

Information on COVID-19 and SARS-CoV-2-related documents published until 23 April 2020 were extracted from the Medline, Scopus, and Web of Science (WoS) databases. These databases allowed us to retrieve essential information for bibliometric analysis including title/abstract, keywords, number of citations, and authors' affiliations, which might not be available in other databases (such as Embase or Science Direct). We did not use preprint databases (e.g., bioRxiv, arXiv, or medRxiv) for searching process since publications in these databases have not undergone the peer-reviewed process, which might hinder their quality. The search terms and search queries for each online database were developed according to the WHO naming process for the virus and the disease it causes [24], and are presented in Tables A1–A3. Any English-language publications containing COVID-19 disease or SARS-CoV-2 virus published from December 2019 to 23 April 2020 were included. Document types such as corrections, data papers, reprints, or conference papers were excluded because they might be duplicated in peer-reviewed papers. Datasets of three databases were merged, and duplications were screened independently and removed by two researchers. A final dataset of 5780 papers was used for further analysis. The searching process was presented in Figure 1.

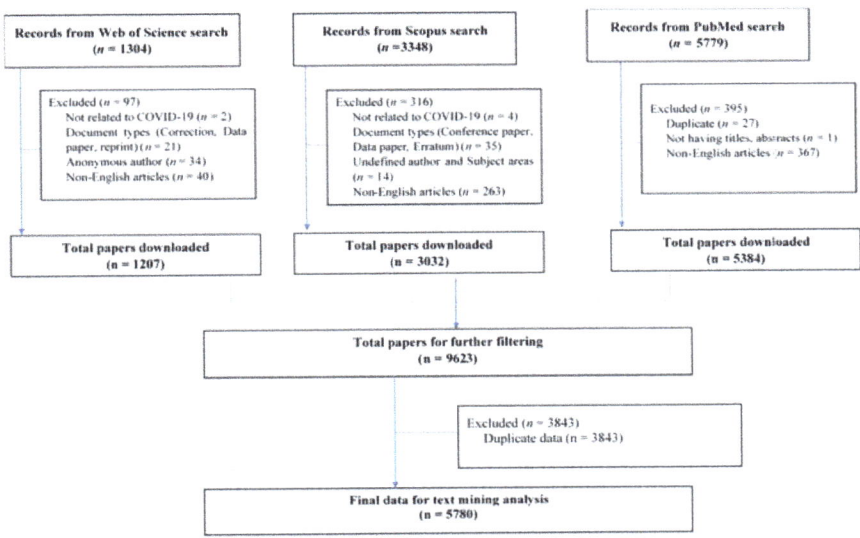

Figure 1. Selection process.

2.2. Data Analysis

In this paper, we extracted data on documents' title, abstract, keywords, citation, and authors' affiliation for analysis. As a document could be authored by scholars from different countries, we considered that all these countries contributed to the document preparation. Moreover, we decided to include both documents with, and without, abstracts for text analysis since the title of the document could partly reflect the document's topic. We first descriptively analyzed the number of publications in each country and presented these data by using Microsoft Excel's Map function. Then, we exported the top ten most cited publications for a detailed analysis of these papers' content.

We used the VOSviewer software (version 1.6.15, Centre for Science and Technology Studies, Leiden University, the Netherlands) to illustrate the networks of the co-occurrence of keywords and most frequent terms in title/abstract [25,26]. Then, we employed Latent Dirichlet allocation (LDA) to discover fifteen latent topics from the titles and abstracts of documents. This Bayesian model treats each document as a set of topics, and topics are probability distributed over a set of words and their co-occurrence [27]. Thus, the LDA technique can produce two outputs: (1) probability distributions of different topics per document (to acknowledge how many topics are created based on the given publications), and (2) probability distributions of unique words per topic (to define the topic) [27]. Because each title/abstract may contain a mixture of topics, the LDA outputs may not reflect a specific research field or discipline. However, experiences from previous work suggested that documents focusing on a particular theme would be more likely to be categorized in the same group. To assure the robustness in labeling each topic, we checked at least ten documents per topic to ensure that the theme's name could generally fit the content of documents.

Multivariable linear regression models were performed to examine the research foci of countries with different income classifications (low, low-middle, high-middle, and high income—according to the World Bank classifications) [28], and different COVID-19 transmission classifications (Pending, Sporadic case, Clusters of cases, Community transmission—according to the WHO classifications) [29]. The dependent variable was the share of publications in specific topic out of total publications in each country (%), while the main independent variables were income classifications and transmission classifications. The models were adjusted to the natural logarithm of gross domestic product (GDP) per capita, the number of COVID-19 cases, and the number of COVID-19 deaths per country. The latest data on GDP per capita and income classifications were collected from the World Bank database, while data on COVID-19 cases and deaths were extracted from WHO reports on 24 April 2020. A p-value of less than 0.05 was used to detect statistical significance.

3. Results

Figure 2 shows the research productivity of each country. A total of 115 countries produced 5780 publications in the searching period. It appears that scientific publications were mainly driven by the research hubs such as China, the United States, Canada, France, Italy, the United Kingdom, and India, which were also heavily hit by the COVID-19. In contrast, the majority of African countries had no more than 10 publications about COVID-19.

The list of ten most cited publications about SARS-CoV-2 and COVID-19 and their main findings are presented in Table 1. Reports on the clinical and laboratory characteristics of the confirmed cases are of the most interest, with six out of ten papers in the list. The most cited paper was a descriptive study about epidemiological and clinical features of 99 cases from Wuhan, China, which was believed to be the genesis of SARS-CoV-2.

Figure 3 presents the network of 200 keywords with a co-occurrence of at least 20 times. The keywords were assigned to three major clusters. Cluster 1 (blue) reveals some basic imaging techniques for the diagnosis of lung function impairments (tomography and thorax radiograph) in children, adolescents, and adults. Cluster 2 (red) refers to the major concerns of the world regarding COVID-19, such as prevention, medicine, and public health response. Cluster 3 (green) focuses on the biology of SARS-CoV-2, including the origin, the phylogenetic network, and the genomic, proteomic, and metabolomic characteristics of the virus.

Thematic analysis of 250 most frequent terms is presented in Figure 4. Major themes of current research on COVID-19 are (1) promising therapies for COVID-19 prevention and treatment, and their mechanisms (blue); (2) hot spots of the pandemic and governments' responses (red); and (3) clinical patterns and complications of COVID-19 (green).

Figure 5 shows the dendrogram analysis which indicates clustering of research areas in the WOS database. The research landscapes were the combination of several research areas. The first cluster was Infectious diseases and Pharmacology. This cluster has a close connection with Surgery and Gastroenterology (second cluster). The third cluster relates to treatment and diagnosis (such as Radiology, Hematology, Virology, Psychiatry, Gerontology, or Metabolism). The other clusters in COVID-19 research areas include (1) Critical care and Respiratory System (the fourth cluster), (2) Health care service and Health policy (the fifth cluster), (3) Microbiology and Immunology (the sixth cluster), (4) Oncology and Experimental Research (the seven cluster), and (5) Biology (the eight cluster).

The LDA results are presented in Table 2. Overall, researchers have devoted special attention to the biology of SARS-CoV-2 (Topics 3 and 4) and made an enormous effort on various aspects of clinical investigations, such as diagnostic tests for virus detection, clinical examination, and treatment for hospitalized patients (Topic 5, 7, 8, 9, 10, 11, and 15). Meanwhile, research on global and national responses to COVID-19 accounts for nearly a quarter of available publications (Topic 2, 12, and 13). Epidemiological characteristics of COVID-19 and psychological disorders during the epidemic are also of great interest (Topic 1, 6, and 14).

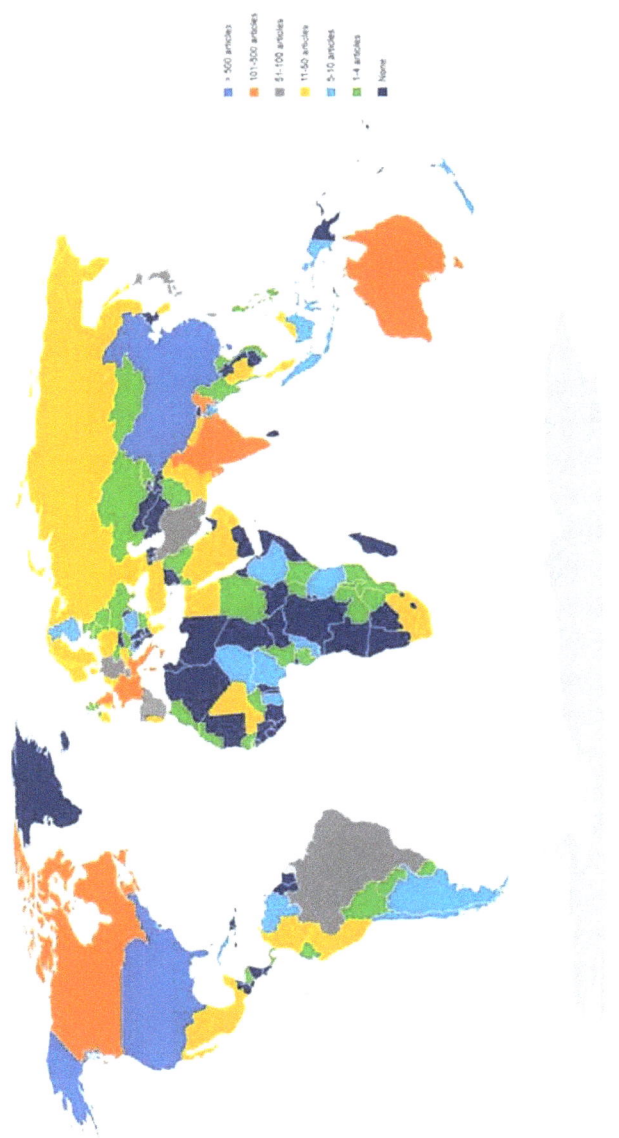

Figure 2. Number of publications per country

Table 1. Top ten most cited papers.

No.	Title	Journal (IF)	Number of Citations	Main Findings
01	Epidemiological and clinical characteristics of 99 cases of 2019 novel coronavirus pneumonia in Wuhan, China: a descriptive study	The Lancet (IF = 59.1)	319	• SARS-CoV-2 infection was of clustering onset, and more likely to affect older males with comorbidities. • Patients had clinical manifestations of fever, cough, shortness of breath, muscle ache, confusion, headache, sore throat, rhinorrhea, chest pain, diarrhea, and nausea and vomiting. • Imaging examination revealed bilateral pneumonia, multiple mottling, and ground-glass opacity. • Results confirmed that SARS-CoV-2 was transmitted through person-to-person contact.
02	A familial cluster of pneumonia associated with the 2019 novel coronavirus indicating person-to-person transmission: a study of a family cluster	The Lancet (IF = 59.1)	245	• Older patients (aged >60 years) had more systemic symptoms, extensive radiological ground-glass lung changes, lymphopenia, thrombocytopenia, and increased C-reactive protein and lactate dehydrogenase levels. • Phylogenetic analysis of showed that this is a novel coronavirus, which is closest to the bat severe acute respiratory syndrome (SARS)-related coronaviruses found in Chinese horseshoe bats.
03	Clinical characteristics and intrauterine vertical transmission potential of COVID-19 infection in nine pregnant women: a retrospective review of medical records	The Lancet (IF = 59.1)	75	• Clinical characteristics of COVID-19 pneumonia in pregnant women were similar to those reported for non-pregnant adult patients. • Fevers, cough, myalgia, sore throat, and malaise were also observed. • No neonatal asphyxia was observed in newborn babies.
04	Detection of 2019 novel coronavirus (2019-nCoV) by real-time RT-PCR	Eurosurveillance (IF = 7.4)	74	• The laboratory diagnostic workflow for detection of SARS-CoV-2 was described and validated.
05	Emerging coronaviruses: Genome structure, replication, and pathogenesis	Journal of Medical Virology (IF = 2.0)	51	• Available understanding on genome structure and replication, and functions proteins in coronaviral replication of coronaviruses (CoVs) were reviewed. • SARS-CoV-2 has a typical genome structure of CoV and belongs to the cluster of betacoronaviruses, including Bat-SARS-like (SL)-ZC45, Bat-SL ZXC21, SARS-CoV, and MERS-CoV.
06	CT imaging features of 2019 novel coronavirus (2019-NCoV)	Radiology (IF = 7.6)	51	• Typical CT findings included bilateral pulmonary parenchymal ground-glass and consolidative pulmonary opacities, sometimes with a rounded morphology and a peripheral lung distribution. • Lung cavitation, discrete pulmonary nodules, pleural effusions, and lymphadenopathy were absent. • All symptomatic patients had multifocal ground-glass opacities on chest CT, and 1 also had subsegmental areas of consolidation and fibrosis.
07	Presumed Asymptomatic Carrier Transmission of COVID-19	JAMA - Journal of the American Medical Association (IF = 51.3)	49	• All the symptomatic patients had increased C-reactive protein levels and reduced lymphocyte counts. • The coronavirus may have been transmitted by the asymptomatic carrier.
08	Breakthrough: Chloroquine phosphate has shown apparent efficacy in treatment of COVID-19 associated pneumonia in clinical studies	BioScience Trends (IF = 1.7)	48	• Chloroquine phosphate is superior to the control treatment in inhibiting the exacerbation of pneumonia, improving lung imaging findings, promoting a virus-negative conversion, and shortening the disease course according to the news briefing. • Severe adverse reactions to chloroquine phosphate were not noted in the patients in trial.
09	Genomic characterization of the 2019 novel human-pathogenic coronavirus isolated from a patient with atypical pneumonia after visiting Wuhan	Emerging Microbes and Infections (IF = 6.2)	46	• Genome of SARS-CoV-2 has 89% nucleotide identity with bat SARS-like-CoVZXC21 and 82% with that of human SARS-CoV. • Phylogenetic trees of their orf1a/b, Spike, Envelope, Membrane and Nucleoprotein clustered closely with those of the bat, civet, and human SARS coronaviruses.
10	Incubation period of 2019 novel coronavirus (2019-nCoV) infections among travellers from Wuhan, China, 20–28 January 2020	Eurosurveillance (IF = 7.4)	30	• The mean incubation period was estimated to be 6.4 days (95% credible interval: 5.6–7.7), ranging from 2.1 to 11.1 days (2.5th to 97.5th percentile).

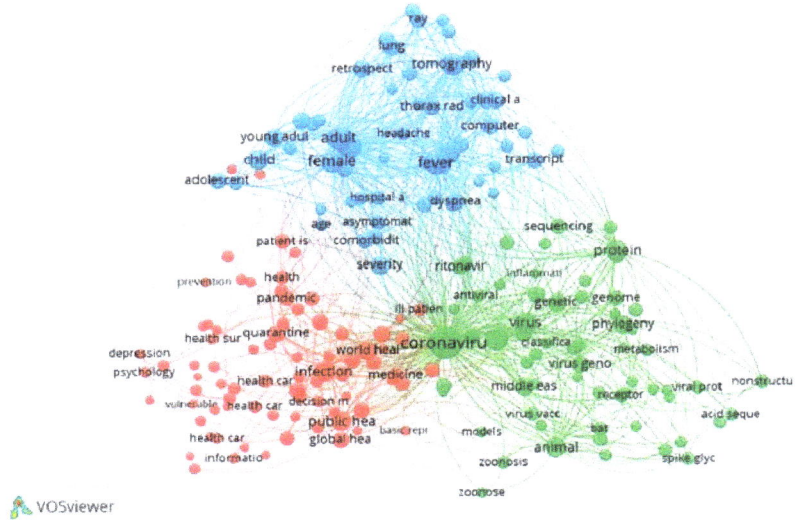

Figure 3. Co-occurrence analysis of keywords.

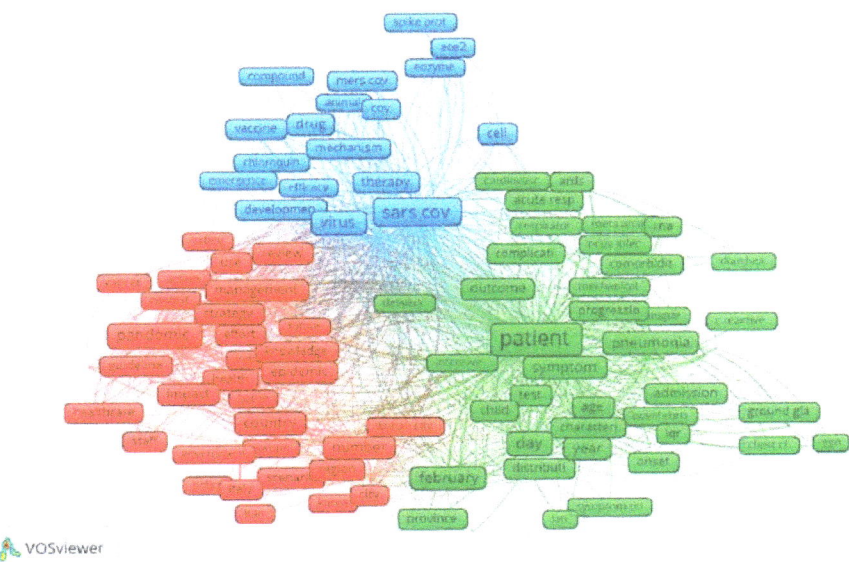

Figure 4. Co-occurrence analysis of the most frequent terms.

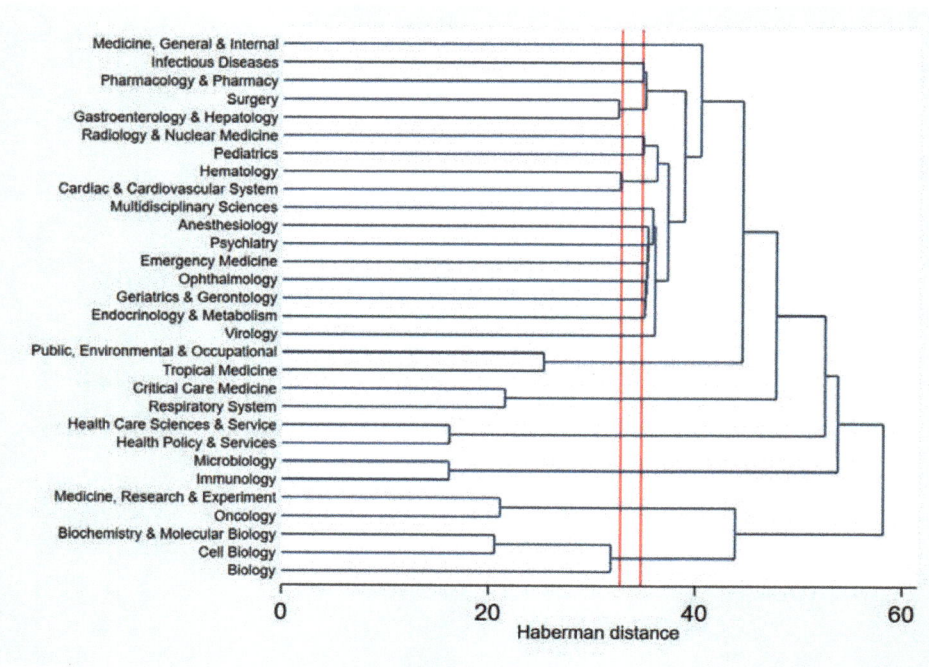

Figure 5. Dendrogram of research areas in WOS database.

Table 2. Fifteen topics about COVID-19 according to topic modeling.

Topic	Content	Top Ten Most Frequent Terms	n	%
Topic 1	Epidemiological reports on COVID-19 outbreaks in different countries.	Covid-19; cases; transmission; first; disease; coronavirus; march; countries; confirmed; and health.	295	5.1
Topic 2	Global and international health security and responses in COVID-19 pandemic crisis.	Health; covid-19; pandemic; public; global; response; community; world; emergency; and outbreak.	571	9.9
Topic 3	SARS-CoV-2 virus structure and molecular analysis.	Sars-cov-2; 2019-ncov; human; coronavirus; sars-cov; protein; virus; viral; spike; and receptor.	231	4.0
Topic 4	Distinguishes between old and novel coronavirus: origin, pathology, and pathogenesis.	Coronavirus; respiratory; novel; china; disease; sars-cov-2; severe; syndrome; acute; and outbreak.	611	10.6
Topic 5	Radiographic detection of COVID-19.	Covid-19; patients; symptoms; pneumonia; chest; clinical; disease; children; findings; and imaging.	310	5.4
Topic 6	Psychological disorders in COVID-19 epidemic: epidemiological characteristics and interventions.	Covid-19; health; mental; during; outbreak; study; social; psychological; anxiety; and media.	256	4.4
Topic 7	Clinical and laboratory examinations in hospitalized patients with COVID-19.	Patients; covid-19; clinical; severe; study; group; cases; disease; results; Wuhan	232	4.0
Topic 8	Comorbidities in patients with COVID-19.	covid-19; patients; disease; respiratory; severe; acute; infection; syndrome; article; and coronavirus.	474	8.2
Topic 9	Impacts of COVID-19 on pregnancy outcomes.	Covid-19; review; studies; evidence; women; pregnant; clinical; research; literature; and results.	156	2.7
Topic 10	Diagnostic values of SARS-CoV-2 tests and improvement strategies.	Sars-cov-2; positive; covid-19; viral; testing; detection; rt-pcr; samples; results; and negative.	234	4.1
Topic 11	Guidelines for emergency care and surgical management during COVID-19 pandemic.	Covid-19; pandemic; patients; during; management; cancer; hospital; recommendations; clinical; and surgery.	669	11.6
Topic 12	Global logistics concerns in COVID-19 prevention, treatment and care.	Covid-19; protective; transmission; healthcare; workers; equipment; personal; during; infection; and staff.	242	4.2
Topic 13	Medical education in COVID-19 pandemic.	Covid-19; pandemic; medical; education; medicine; during; response; lessons; students; and nursing.	561	9.7
Topic 14	COVID-19 epidemiological modelling and forecasting.	Covid-19; cases; china; epidemic; number; outbreak; model; Wuhan; measures; and confirmed.	292	5.1
Topic 15	Treatment interventions against COVID-19.	Covid-19; treatment; drugs; clinical; therapeutic; against; antiviral; sars-cov-2; therapy; and effective.	311	5.4

The country variations in research foci are shown in Table 3. High-income countries (HICs) showed less attention on research in epidemiological characteristics and interventions of psychological disorders in the COVID-19 pandemic (Topic 6) compared with countries with other income levels. Meanwhile, low-middle income countries were found to have a less interest in diagnostic values of SARS-CoV-2 tests and improvement strategies (Topic 10) compared to low-income countries. Treatment interventions for COVID-19 (Topic 15) attracted the interest of scientists among countries at all income levels, especially in HICs.

Table 3. Regression models to identify the research trend among countries with different income level and epidemic characteristics.

	World Bank Income Classification [1]			WHO COVID-19 Transmission Classification [2]		
Topic	Low-Middle Income Countries	High-Middle Income Countries	High Income Countries	Sporadic Cases	Clusters of Cases	Community Transmission
	Coef. (95%CI)	Coef. (95%CI)	Coef. (95%CI)	Coef. (95%CI)	Coef. (95%CI)	Coef. (95%CI)
Topic 1	4.7 (−4.7; 14.0)	6.8 (−6.9; 20.4)	14 (−6.4; 34.5)	−1.1 (−9.1; 6.9)	3 (−3.8; 9.7)	6.7 (−0.7; 14.1)
Topic 2	3.4 (−12.2; 18.9)	−7.1 (−29.8; 15.5)	−10.4 (−44.4; 23.6)	−5.3 (−18.6; 7.9)	−3 (−14.2; 8.3)	2.2 (−10.1; 14.4)
Topic 3	1 (−2.7; 4.7)	1.9 (−3.5; 7.3)	1.3 (−6.8; 9.4)	−0.9 (−4.1; 2.2)	1 (−1.7; 3.6)	0.2 (−2.7; 3.2)
Topic 4	2 (−9.0; 13.0)	3 (−13.1; 19.0)	8.2 (−15.8; 32.3)	1.2 (−8.2; 10.5)	6 (−2.0; 14.0)	5.2 (−3.4; 13.9)
Topic 5	−1 (−2.7; 0.8)	−0.8 (−3.4; 1.7)	−2.6 (−6.4; 1.2)	−1.5 (−2.9; 0.0)	−1 (−2.3; 0.3)	−1.4 (−2.8; 0.0)
Topic 6	−6.4 (−12.4; −0.4) *	−16.9 (−25.6; −8.1) *	−23.5 (−36.6; −10.4) *	4.6 (−0.5; 9.7)	1.3 (−3.0; 5.7)	2 (−2.7; 6.7)
Topic 7	−0.1 (−1.6; 1.3)	0.3 (−2.5; 3.8)	0.7 (−2.5; 3.8)	0 (−1.2; 1.2)	0.4 (−0.7; 1.4)	0.7 (−0.4; 1.9)
Topic 8	2.8 (−3.4; 9.1)	−0.2 (−9.3; 8.9)	3.4 (−10.3; 17.1)	−5.8 (−11.2; −0.5) *	−4.1 (−8.7; 0.4)	1.7 (−3.3; 6.6)
Topic 9	2.2 (−2.9; 7.2)	0.9 (−6.5; 8.3)	0.9 (−10.1; 12.0)	−0.3 (−4.6; 4.0)	2.1 (−1.6; 5.8)	2.5 (−1.5; 6.4)
Topic 10	−1.5 (−2.9; −0.1) *	−1.9 (−3.9; 0.1)	−2.7 (−5.6; 0.3)	−0.3 (−1.5; 0.8)	0.4 (−0.6; 1.4)	0 (−1.1; 1.0)
Topic 11	−10.2 (−20.9; 0.5)	−13.7 (−29.3; 1.8)	−19.6 (−42.9; 3.8)	−2.2 (−11.3; 6.9)	−0.2 (−7.9; 7.6)	1.7 (−6.8; 10.1)
Topic 12	−1.5 (−4.3; 1.4)	−3.2 (−7.3; 1.0)	−3.1 (−9.2; 3.1)	−0.6 (−3.0; 1.8)	−1.1 (−3.1; 1.0)	−0.8 (−3.0; 1.4)
Topic 13	−4.9 (−13.2; 3.3)	−7.6 (−19.6; 4.4)	−4.4 (−22.4; 13.7)	0.8 (−6.2; 7.8)	2.9 (−3.1; 8.9)	2.1 (−4.4; 8.6)
Topic 14	1.7 (−7.4; 10.8)	−2.5 (−15.7; 10.8)	−3 (−22.8; 16.9)	−1 (−8.8; 6.7)	−2.9 (−9.5; 3.7)	−1 (−8.2; 6.1)
Topic 15	16.6 (6.5; 26.7) *	19.9 (5.2; 34.6) *	34.8 (12.8; 56.8) *	−20.8 (−29.3; −12.2) *	−18.9 (−26.2; −11.6) *	−17 (−24.9; −9) *

* $p < 0.05$; [1] Compared to Low-income countries. The model was adjusted to natural logarithm of GDP per capita, number of cases, number of deaths, and WHO COVID-19 transmission classification; [2] Compared to Pending classification. The model was adjusted to natural logarithm of GDP per capita, number of cases, number of deaths, and World Bank Income Classification.

Regarding transmission classifications, comorbidities in patients with COVID-19 (Topic 8) were found to receive less attention among countries with sporadic cases in comparison with countries having "pending" transmission classification. Treatment interventions had less attention in countries having sporadic cases, a cluster of cases, and community transmission compared with those with "pending" transmission classification.

4. Discussion

By using LDA as the natural language processing approach, this study was able to capture the foci of COVID-19 related publications in different settings. This paper informed the rapid growth of research publications, and the global variation in research productivity and research interests. Moreover, findings of this study indicated that global scholars are paying attention to clinical management, viral pathogenesis, and public health responses, while other issues, such as psycho-social problems or impacts of COVID-19 on different vulnerable populations, are not-well investigated.

In this study, we found a greater number of publications regarding COVID-19 and SARS-CoV-2 in comparison with previous bibliometric studies [21–23]. For example, Lou et al. used the Medline database and only found 183 publications through February 29, 2020 [22]. This disparity could be justified that our search was far more comprehensive than these studies by using three major databases including the Medline, Scopus, and WOS. In addition, we included other document types such as letters, commentaries, or notes rather than concentrating only on original articles. As original papers require a long period for peer-review [30], scientists tended to publish their ideas in those document types first for receiving rapid feedbacks from others [31]. Therefore, we believed that our approach was appropriate given that these documents might partly reflect the research focus in each country.

The thematic maps of authors' keywords and terms reveal that major research themes included virological and molecular analysis of the virus; clinical, laboratory and radiology examinations;

and global and public health responses. Our findings are in line with a previous bibliometric study, which showed that virology, clinical characteristics, and epidemiology of COVID-19 were found to be the major research foci with the highest volume of papers [22]. Indeed, it has been a short period of time since the onset of the pandemic, and these research areas are essential components for preventing and controlling the pandemic. Understanding the biology of SARS-CoV-2 is critical for the development of effective and safe screening tests, drugs, and vaccines, while investigations into clinical and paraclinical characteristics of COVID-19 could inform a fundamental method for appropriate patient management. Research on public health responses could illustrate the effectiveness of different policies and strategies to mitigate the consequences of the COVID-19 pandemic [32–34]. Notably, we believed that much research is ongoing as well as numerous papers are under reviewed, which will remarkably contribute to the global knowledge about COVID-19 in the short coming.

Results of topic modeling offer more penetrating insights into the emerging research themes. Of all identified topics, clinical aspects, particularly guidelines for emergency care and surgical management during the COVID-19 pandemic, were most frequent. Along with the rapid increase in the number of confirmed cases, the heavy demand for health facilities and health workers, along with the lack of effective treatment regimens, place a heavy burden and prevent the healthcare systems from operating efficiently. Without guidelines for prompt responses in emergency care, the burden caused by COVID-19 would go beyond the capacity of most health systems, especially for ICU care [35]. In addition, a number of SARS-CoV-2 infections emerged from operations were reported in China, suggesting the risk of virus exposure despite strict hygienic requirements and aseptic techniques during the surgical process [36]. Research for clinical guidelines, therefore, plays a critical role in mitigating the impact of COVID-19 on the healthcare system.

The origin and pathophysiology of the virus have attracted a great deal of attention since the beginning of the outbreak [37–39]. The interest in this topic has continued to rise as the virus has gone beyond China, where the first infection was reported, and positive cases have been found in most countries and territories [40]. On the other hand, the information that SARS-CoV-2 is a laboratory derived virus, albeit that this has been confirmed to be a false claim, gave rise to considerable controversy and also facilitated research on the nature of the virus [41]. Another topic that should be mentioned is national public health responses and actions against COVID-19, especially at the beginning of the pandemic when there was a wide difference in policies introduced by different governments. In particular, some countries advocated achieving herd immunity, whereas low- and middle-income countries (LMICs) implemented strict actions, including quarantine, isolation, social distancing, and community containment as soon as the outbreak occurred [42–45]. Although such measures have demonstrated their effectiveness, for optimal public health as well as economic outcomes, further investigations into their implementation within specific contextual factors should be prioritized [46]. Moreover, continued medical training for healthcare workers [47] and preventive measures for the workforce [48], along with frequent transparent communication and educational interventions for the public, is essential to strengthen the preventive capacity of each individual and thus, contribute to the global fight against COVID-19. Meanwhile, since COVID-19 has been reported to have no noticeable effect on pregnancy, research on COVID-19 among pregnant women received relatively slight interest [49].

Regarding the research foci in different country groups, it appeared that the share of publications regarding psychological health and related interventions was negatively associated with income level. This finding might imply that this topic might not be the priority of the countries, or in other words, developed nations show even less interest than the ones having lower-income [50]. However, COVID-19 caused a significant psychiatric impact [51], and this impact was maintained when the total number of COVID-19 cases continued to rise [52]. Developed nations are not immune from mental health issues and mental health services have often been disrupted during the COVID-19 pandemic [53]. Another reason which might play a role in this phenomenon is that most of the studies about this topic were cross-sectional surveys in the community, which were more affordable for low-income countries to perform compared to other topics. Therefore, the share of publications in this topic in low-income countries might be higher than that in high-income countries.

In terms of treatment interventions, although all countries are making efforts to develop effective treatment regimens, high-income countries, with their vast financial resources, greater expertise, and infrastructure, demonstrated their bold attempt in this research area [54,55]. Meanwhile, compared to low-income nations, we observed a lower share of SARS-CoV-2 test-related publications among low-middle income countries, which might imply that these countries prioritized to other research fields such as treatment interventions given their resource-constraint [56]. In addition, while rapid transmission of COVID-19 has been triggering a strong need for the development of an effective vaccine, our results show minimal research on this topic. However, we do believe that the amount of research on vaccine development is possibly abundant according to the number of studies about COVID-19 vaccination registered in clinicaltrials.gov and the WHO Trial Registry Network. Because it requires remarkable amount of time to obtain results, the small amount of publications compared with other topics is understandable.

Findings also suggested that research on comorbidities associated with COVID-19 is relatively underdeveloped in countries with sporadic cases, in contrast with the extensive understanding and research on the effects of comorbidities on COVID-19 in those countries with a high number of infections [57,58]. On the other hand, the increase of transmission level was negatively correlated with the interest in treatment interventions. Although some high-income countries such as the United States, Canada, or the United Kingdom were classified as "community transmission" and greatly contributed to the progress of finding treatment interventions, most of the nations in this category were low-middle income countries (e.g., South American and African countries) and the governments tends to focus on preventive methods to prevent the pandemic from getting worse [2].

This study has several implications. To begin with, since there has been anecdotal evidence that promising drugs for COVID-19 such as Lopinavir/ritonavir (LPV/RTV), Chloroquine (CQ), and hydroxychloroquine (H0) have shown no significant benefits to health outcomes of patients, developing effective and safe medications specific for the treatment of COVID-19 is of utmost importance [59–61]. Furthermore, the findings show a lack of behavioral psychosocial research on how people react with COVID-19 emergency [32]. Future research should consider the risk factors of psychosocial distress at interpersonal or cultural aspect, impact of mass media and social media on behaviors of population to COVID-19, as well as behavior-change interventions to each research subject. Additionally, we found a lack of research on the social stigma caused by COVID-19. Due to the rapid contagion of the virus, fear and anxiety about being infected can give rise to stigma and discrimination toward people, places, or things. For instance, people associated with the disease, such as being in a neighborhood of high risk or being a civilian of a nation with a high rate of COVID-19 infection, are often stigmatized [62,63]. Stigma can also arise when people are released from quarantine, even though they have been confirmed to be negative and are no longer risk. Although there have been several published guidelines for reducing social stigma related to COVID-19, further investigations into the detrimental effects of social stigma and development of interventions for this problem should be considered [62,63]. Finally, due to the rapid spread of this disease, the vulnerable population, such as the elderly living in nursing homes, workers in industrial zones, refugees, migrants, or persons with disabilities are at higher risk of getting an infection, will need extra precautions [64]. However, these high-risk clusters have not received enough concern from the researchers, even on commentary or local government. More research and preventive actions should be done so as to not leave these people behind [64].

To our knowledge, this is the first analysis using text mining and text modeling to investigate the research foci of the worldwide COVID-19 publications. However, some limitations should be noted. The restriction of the search strategy to the English language might not reflect globalized practices and the research priority of a country. Analyses of keywords, titles, and abstracts may not fully reflect the content of articles. However, with the combination of three large datasets and various techniques of text mining, this study is useful for an overview of the research direction. Moreover, our correlation analysis was based on population data, which might not reflect the causes of the research tendency in each country. Since the publications on COVID-19 will rapidly grow in the coming time, further studies should be performed with more advanced techniques to elucidate our findings.

5. Conclusions

This study showed that COVID-19 related publications were primarily contributed by major research hubs such as the United States, China, and European countries. Global researchers have been currently focused on clinical management, viral pathogenesis, and public health responses in combating against COVID-19. Meanwhile, little attention has been paid to psycho-social problems or of the impacts of COVID-19 on different vulnerable populations. Findings of this study suggest the need for global research collaboration among high- and low/middle-income countries in the different stages of the pandemic prevention and control. This paper can serve as a reference for governments and research institutions to identify the research priority in their settings and allocate appropriate resources for research on COVID-19.

Author Contributions: Conceptualization, B.X.T., G.T.V., C.A.L., and R.C.M.H.; data curation, G.H.H., M.T.H., H.T.L., and C.S.H.H.; formal analysis, B.X.T., L.H.N., G.T.V., M.T.H., and C.A.L.; funding acquisition, C.S.H.H. and R.C.M.H.; investigation, B.X.T., L.H.N., and C.S.H.H.; methodology, G.H.H., L.H.N., G.T.V., M.T.H., H.T.L., C.A.L., and R.C.M.H.; resources, B.X.T., G.H.H., L.H.N., G.T.V., and C.S.H.H.; software, G.H.H., H.T.L., C.A.L., and R.C.M.H.; supervision, B.X.T., G.T.V., H.T.L., C.S.H.H., and R.C.M.H.; validation, B.X.T., M.T.H., and C.A.L.; visualization, L.H.N., and G.T.V.; writing—original draft, B.X.T., G.H.H., L.H.N., G.T.V., M.T.H., H.T.L., C.A.L., C.S.H.H., and R.C.M.H.; and writing—review and editing, B.X.T., G.H.H., L.H.N., G.T.V., M.T.H., H.T.L., C.A.L., C.S.H.H., and R.C.M.H. All authors have read and agreed to the published version of the manuscript.

Funding: This research is supported by Vingroup Innovation Foundation (VINIF) in project code VINIF.2020.COVID-19.DA03.

Acknowledgments: This research is supported by Vingroup Innovation Foundation (VINIF) in project code VINIF.2020.COVID-19.DA03.

Conflicts of Interest: The authors declare no conflict of interest.

Appendix A

Table A1. Search query (Web of Science).

No	Search Query	Result
1	TS = ("COVID-19")	998
2	TS = ("2019 novel coronavirus")	151
3	TS = ("2019-nCoV")	255
4	TS = ("severe acute respiratory syndrome coronavirus 2")	84
5	TS = ("SARS-CoV-2")	286
6	#5 OR #4 OR #3 OR #2 OR #1	1304
7	#5 OR #4 OR #3 OR #2 OR #1 Refined by: [excluding] PUBLICATION YEARS: (2011 OR 2003)	1302
8	#5 OR #4 OR #3 OR #2 OR #1 Refined by: [excluding] PUBLICATION YEARS: (2011 OR 2003) AND [excluding] DOCUMENT TYPES: (CORRECTION OR DATA PAPER OR REPRINT)	1281
9	#5 OR #4 OR #3 OR #2 OR #1 Refined by: [excluding] PUBLICATION YEARS: (2011 OR 2003) AND [excluding] DOCUMENT TYPES: (CORRECTION OR DATA PAPER OR REPRINT) AND [excluding] AUTHORS: (ANONYMOUS)	1247
10	#5 OR #4 OR #3 OR #2 OR #1 Refined by: [excluding] PUBLICATION YEARS: (2011 OR 2003) AND [excluding] DOCUMENT TYPES: (CORRECTION OR DATA PAPER OR REPRINT) AND [excluding] AUTHORS: (ANONYMOUS) AND [excluding] LANGUAGES: (GERMAN OR HUNGARIAN OR FRENCH OR PORTUGUESE OR ITALIAN OR SPANISH OR TURKISH OR CZECH OR NORWEGIAN)	1207

Table A2. Search query (MEDLINE/PubMed).

No	Search Query	Result
1	Search (((("COVID-19"[Title/Abstract]) OR "2019 novel coronavirus"[Title/Abstract]) OR "2019-nCoV"[Title/Abstract]) OR "severe acute respiratory syndrome coronavirus 2"[Title/Abstract]) OR "SARS-CoV-2"[Title/Abstract]	5779

Table A3. Search query (Scopus).

No	Search Query	Result
1	(TITLE-ABS-KEY ("COVID-19")) OR (TITLE-ABS-KEY ("2019 novel coronavirus")) OR (TITLE-ABS-KEY ("2019-nCoV")) OR (TITLE-ABS-KEY ("severe acute respiratory syndrome coronavirus 2")) OR (TITLE-ABS-KEY ("SARS-CoV-2"))	3348
2	(TITLE-ABS-KEY ("COVID-19")) OR (TITLE-ABS-KEY ("2019 novel coronavirus")) OR (TITLE-ABS-KEY ("2019-nCoV")) OR (TITLE-ABS-KEY ("severe acute respiratory syndrome coronavirus 2")) OR (TITLE-ABS-KEY ("SARS-CoV-2")) AND (EXCLUDE (PUBYEAR , 2011) OR EXCLUDE (PUBYEAR , 2006) OR EXCLUDE (PUBYEAR , 2004) OR EXCLUDE (PUBYEAR , 2003))	3309
3	(TITLE-ABS-KEY ("COVID-19")) OR (TITLE-ABS-KEY ("2019 novel coronavirus")) OR (TITLE-ABS-KEY ("2019-nCoV")) OR (TITLE-ABS-KEY ("severe acute respiratory syndrome coronavirus 2")) OR (TITLE-ABS-KEY ("SARS-CoV-2")) AND (EXCLUDE (PUBYEAR , 2011) OR EXCLUDE (PUBYEAR , 2006) OR EXCLUDE (PUBYEAR , 2004) OR EXCLUDE (PUBYEAR , 2003)) AND (EXCLUDE (DOCTYPE , "er") OR EXCLUDE (DOCTYPE , "cp") OR EXCLUDE (DOCTYPE , "dp"))	3309
4	(TITLE-ABS-KEY ("COVID-19")) OR (TITLE-ABS-KEY ("2019 novel coronavirus")) OR (TITLE-ABS-KEY ("2019-nCoV")) OR (TITLE-ABS-KEY ("severe acute respiratory syndrome coronavirus 2")) OR (TITLE-ABS-KEY ("SARS-CoV-2")) AND (EXCLUDE (PUBYEAR , 2011) OR EXCLUDE (PUBYEAR , 2006) OR EXCLUDE (PUBYEAR , 2004) OR EXCLUDE (PUBYEAR , 2003)) AND (EXCLUDE (DOCTYPE , "er") OR EXCLUDE (DOCTYPE , "cp") OR EXCLUDE (DOCTYPE , "dp")) AND (EXCLUDE (PREFNAMEAUID , "Undefined#Undefined"))	3295
5	(TITLE-ABS-KEY ("COVID-19")) OR (TITLE-ABS-KEY ("2019 novel coronavirus")) OR (TITLE-ABS-KEY ("2019-nCoV")) OR (TITLE-ABS-KEY ("severe acute respiratory syndrome coronavirus 2")) OR (TITLE-ABS-KEY ("SARS-CoV-2")) AND (EXCLUDE (PUBYEAR , 2011) OR EXCLUDE (PUBYEAR , 2006) OR EXCLUDE (PUBYEAR , 2004) OR EXCLUDE (PUBYEAR , 2003)) AND (EXCLUDE (DOCTYPE , "er") OR EXCLUDE (DOCTYPE , "cp") OR EXCLUDE (DOCTYPE , "dp")) AND (EXCLUDE (PREFNAMEAUID , "Undefined#Undefined")) AND (EXCLUDE (SUBJAREA , "Undefined")) AND (EXCLUDE (LANGUAGE , "Chinese") OR EXCLUDE (LANGUAGE , "German") OR EXCLUDE (LANGUAGE , "Spanish") OR EXCLUDE (LANGUAGE , "French") OR EXCLUDE (LANGUAGE , "Norwegian") OR EXCLUDE (LANGUAGE , "Portuguese") OR EXCLUDE (LANGUAGE , "Italian") OR EXCLUDE (LANGUAGE , "Dutch") OR EXCLUDE (LANGUAGE , "Icelandic") OR EXCLUDE (LANGUAGE , "Korean") OR EXCLUDE (LANGUAGE , "Swedish") OR EXCLUDE (LANGUAGE , "Turkish"))	3032

References

1. Cucinotta, D.; Vanelli, M. WHO Declares COVID-19 a Pandemic. *Acta Biomed.* **2020**, *91*, 157–160. [CrossRef] [PubMed]
2. John Hopkins University and Medicine. Covid-19 Dashbroad by the Center for Systems Science and Engineering at John Hopskin University. Available online: https://coronavirus.jhu.edu/map.html (accessed on 26 April 2020).
3. World Health Organization. *WHO Director-General's Opening Remarks at the Media Briefing on COVID-19, 11 March 2020*; World Health Organization: Geneva, Switzerland, 2020.
4. Rajgor, D.D.; Lee, M.H.; Archuleta, S.; Bagdasarian, N.; Quek, S.C. The many estimates of the COVID-19 case fatality rate. [published online ahead of print, 2020 Mar 27]. *Lancet Infect. Dis.* **2020**. [CrossRef]
5. Nikolich-Zugich, J.; Knox, K.S.; Rios, C.T.; Natt, B.; Bhattacharya, D.; Fain, M.J. SARS-CoV-2 and COVID-19 in older adults: What we may expect regarding pathogenesis, immune responses, and outcomes. *Geroscience* **2020**, *42*, 505–514. [CrossRef] [PubMed]
6. Congressional Research Service. *Global Economic Effects of COVID-19*; Congressional Research Service: New York, NY, USA, 2020.
7. International Monetary Fund. Chapter 1 The Great Lockdown. 2020. In *World Economic Outlook*; International Monetary Fund: Washington, DC, USA, 2020.
8. The Lancet. Redefining vulnerability in the era of COVID-19. *Lancet* **2020**, *395*, 1089. [CrossRef]
9. Kandel, N.; Chungong, S.; Omaar, A.; Xing, J. Health security capacities in the context of COVID-19 outbreak: An analysis of International Health Regulations annual report data from 182 countries. *Lancet* **2020**, *395*, 1047–1053. [CrossRef]
10. World Health Organization. Country & Technical Guidance-Coronavirus Disease (COVID-19). Available online: https://www.who.int/emergencies/diseases/novel-coronavirus-2019/technical-guidance (accessed on 26 April 2020).
11. World Health Organization. *Coronavirus Disease 2019 (COVID-19)-Situation Report–65*; World Health Organization: Geneva, Switzerland, 2020.
12. Thorlund, K.; Dron, L.; Park, J.; Hsu, G.; Forrest, J.I.; Mills, E.J. A Real-Time Dashboard of Clinical Trials for COVID-19. *Lancet Digit. Health* **2020**, *2*, 286–287. [CrossRef]

13. World Health Organization. Global Research on Coronavirus Disease (COVID-19). Available online: https://www.who.int/emergencies/diseases/novel-coronavirus-2019/global-research-on-novel-coronavirus-2019-ncov (accessed on 28 April 2020).
14. Commission on a Global Health Risk Framework for the Future. *The Neglected Dimension of Global Security: A Framework to Counter Infectious Disease Crises*; National Academies Press: Washington, DC, USA, 2016.
15. World Health Organization. Statement on the Meeting of the International Health Regulations (2005) Emergency Committee Regarding the Outbreak of Novel Coronavirus (2019-nCoV). Available online: https://www.who.int/news-room/detail/23-01-2020-statement-on-the-meeting-of-the-international-health-regulations-(2005)-emergency-committee-regarding-the-outbreak-of-novel-coronavirus-(2019-ncov) (accessed on 29 April 2020).
16. Fu, L.; Wang, B.; Yuan, T.; Chen, X.; Ao, Y.; Fitzpatrick, T.; Li, P.; Zhou, Y.; Lin, Y.; Duan, Q. Clinical characteristics of coronavirus disease 2019 (COVID-19) in China: A systematic review and meta-analysis. *J. Infect.* **2020**. [CrossRef]
17. Lovato, A.; de Filippis, C. Clinical Presentation of COVID-19: A Systematic Review Focusing on Upper Airway Symptoms. [published online ahead of print, 2020 Apr 13]. *Ear. Nose Throat. J.* **2020**. [CrossRef]
18. Cortegiani, A.; Ingoglia, G.; Ippolito, M.; Giarratano, A.; Einav, S. A systematic review on the efficacy and safety of chloroquine for the treatment of COVID-19. *J. Crit. Care* **2020**. [CrossRef]
19. Shamshirian, A.; Hessami, A.; Heydari, K.; Alizadeh-Navaei, R.; Ebrahimzadeh, M.A.; Ghasemian, R.; Aboufazeli, E.; Baradaran, H.; Karimifar, K.; Eftekhari, A. Hydroxychloroquine Versus COVID-19: A Rapid Systematic Review and Meta-Analysis. Available online: https://www.medrxiv.org/ (accessed on 29 April 2020). [CrossRef]
20. Viner, R.M.; Russell, S.J.; Croker, H.; Packer, J.; Ward, J.; Stansfield, C.; Mytton, O.; Bonell, C.; Booy, R. School closure and management practices during coronavirus outbreaks including COVID-19: A rapid systematic review. *Lancet Child Adolesc. Health* **2020**, *4*, 397–404. [CrossRef]
21. Nasab, F.R. Bibliometric Analysis of Global Scientific Research on SARSCoV-2 (COVID-19). Available online: https://www.medrxiv.org/ (accessed on 29 April 2020). [CrossRef]
22. Lou, J.; Tian, S.; Niu, S.; Kang, X.; Lian, H.; Zhang, L.; Zhang, J. Coronavirus disease 2019: A bibliometric analysis and review. *Eur. Rev. Med. Pharmacol. Sci.* **2020**, *24*, 3411–3421.
23. Chahrour, M.; Assi, S.; Bejjani, M.; Nasrallah, A.A.; Salhab, H.; Fares, M.Y.; Khachfe, H.H. A bibliometric analysis of Covid-19 research activity: A call for increased output. *Cureus* **2020**, *12*, e7357. [CrossRef]
24. World Health Organization. Naming the Coronavirus Disease (COVID-19) and the Virus That Causes It. Available online: https://www.who.int/emergencies/diseases/novel-coronavirus-2019/technical-guidance/naming-the-coronavirus-disease-(covid-2019)-and-the-virus-that-causes-it (accessed on 25 April 2020).
25. Van Eck, N.J.; Waltman, L. Text mining and visualization using VOSviewer. *arXiv* **2011**, arXiv:1109.2058.
26. Van Eck, N.J.; Waltman, L. Visualizing bibliometric networks. In *Measuring Scholarly Impact*; Springer: Berlin, Germany, 2014; pp. 285–320.
27. Blei, D.M.; Ng, A.Y.; Jordan, M.I. Latent dirichlet allocation. *J. Mach. Learn. Res.* **2003**, *3*, 993–1022.
28. The World Bank. World Bank Country and Lending Groups. Available online: https://datahelpdesk.worldbank.org/knowledgebase/articles/906519-world-bank-country-and-lending-groups (accessed on 26 April 2020).
29. World Health Organization. *Critical Preparedness, Readiness and Response Actions for COVID-19*; World Health Organization: Geneva, Switzerland, 2020.
30. Voight, M.L.; Hoogenboom, B.J. Publishing your work in a journal: Understanding the peer review process. *Int. J. Sports Phys. Ther.* **2012**, *7*, 452–460. [PubMed]
31. Berterö, C. Guidelines for writing a commentary. *Int. J. Qual. Stud. Health Well-Being* **2016**, *11*, 31390. [CrossRef] [PubMed]
32. World Health Organization. Clinical Management of Severe Acute Respiratory Infection When Novel Coronavirus (2019 nCoV) Infection Is Suspected: Interim Guidance, 28 January 2020. Available online: https://apps.who.int/iris/handle/10665/330893 (accessed on 26 April 2020).
33. Jiang, S. Don't rush to deploy COVID-19 vaccines and drugs without sufficient safety guarantees. *Nature* **2020**, *579*, 321. [CrossRef]
34. Andersen, K.G.; Rambaut, A.; Lipkin, W.I.; Holmes, E.C.; Garry, R.F. The proximal origin of SARS-CoV-2. *Nat. Med.* **2020**, *26*, 450–452. [CrossRef]

35. Murray, C.J. Forecasting COVID-19 Impact on Hospital Bed-Days, ICU-Days, Ventilator-Days and Deaths by US State in the Next 4 Months. Available online: https://www.medrxiv.org/ (accessed on 28 April 2020). [CrossRef]
36. Novel Coronavirus Pneumonia Emergency Response Epidemiology T. [The epidemiological characteristics of an outbreak of 2019 novel coronavirus diseases (COVID-19) in China]. *Zhonghua Liu Xing Bing Xue Za Zhi* **2020**, *41*, 145–151. [CrossRef]
37. Chan, J.F.; Yuan, S.; Kok, K.H.; To, K.K.; Chu, H.; Yang, J.; Xing, F.; Liu, J.; Yip, C.C.; Poon, R.W.; et al. A familial cluster of pneumonia associated with the 2019 novel coronavirus indicating person-to-person transmission: A study of a family cluster. *Lancet* **2020**, *395*, 514–523. [CrossRef]
38. Chen, Y.; Liu, Q.; Guo, D. Emerging coronaviruses: Genome structure, replication, and pathogenesis. *J. Med. Virol.* **2020**, *92*, 418–423. [CrossRef] [PubMed]
39. Chan, J.F.; Kok, K.H.; Zhu, Z.; Chu, H.; To, K.K.; Yuan, S.; Yuen, K.Y. Genomic characterization of the 2019 novel human-pathogenic coronavirus isolated from a patient with atypical pneumonia after visiting Wuhan. *Emerg. Microbes. Infect.* **2020**, *9*, 221–236. [CrossRef] [PubMed]
40. Center for Infectious Disease Research and Policy. U.o.M. Global COVID-19 Deaths Pass 70,000; More Nations Emerge as Hot Spots. Available online: https://www.cidrap.umn.edu/news-perspective/2020/04/europe-urged-ease-pandemic-distancing-slowly-brazil-notes-hot-spot (accessed on 26 April 2020).
41. Shmerling, R.H. Be Careful Where You Get Your News about Coronavirus. Available online: https://www.health.harvard.edu/blog/be-careful-where-you-get-your-news-about-coronavirus2020020118801 (accessed on 27 April 2020).
42. Pen, C.L. The Theory of Herd Immunity, or the Ayatollahs of Public Health. Available online: https://www.institutmontaigne.org/en/blog/theory-herd-immunity-or-ayatollahs-public-health (accessed on 28 April 2020).
43. Ellyatt, H. Sweden Resisted A Lockdown, and Its Capital Stockholm Is Expected to Reach 'Herd Immunity' in Weeks. Available online: https://www.cnbc.com/2020/04/22/no-lockdown-in-sweden-but-stockholm-could-see-herd-immunity-in-weeks.html (accessed on 28 April 2020).
44. Adam, D. Special report: The simulations driving the world's response to COVID-19. *Nature* **2020**, *580*, 316–318. [CrossRef] [PubMed]
45. Hopman, J.; Allegranzi, B.; Mehtar, S. Managing COVID-19 in Low-and Middle-Income Countries. *JAMA* **2020**. [CrossRef] [PubMed]
46. Wilder-Smith, A.; Freedman, D.O. Isolation, quarantine, social distancing and community containment: Pivotal role for old-style public health measures in the novel coronavirus (2019-nCoV) outbreak. *J. Travel Med.* **2020**, *27*. [CrossRef]
47. Chew, N.W.; Lee, G.K.; Tan, B.Y.; Jing, M.; Goh, Y.; Ngiam, N.J.; Yeo, L.L.; Ahmad, A.; Khan, F.A.; Shanmugam, G.N. A Multinational, Multicentre Study on the Psychological Outcomes and Associated Physical Symptoms Amongst Healthcare Workers During COVID-19 Outbreak. *Brain Behav. Immun.* **2020**, S0889-1591(20)30523-7. [CrossRef]
48. Tan, W.; Hao, F.; McIntyre, R.S.; Jiang, L.; Jiang, X.; Zhang, L.; Zhao, X.; Zou, Y.; Hu, Y.; Luo, X. Is Returning to Work during the COVID-19 Pandemic Stressful? A Study on Immediate Mental Health Status and Psychoneuroimmunity Prevention Measures of Chinese Workforce. *Brain Behav. Immun.* **2020**, S0889-1591(20)30603-6. [CrossRef]
49. Chen, H.; Guo, J.; Wang, C.; Luo, F.; Yu, X.; Zhang, W.; Li, J.; Zhao, D.; Xu, D.; Gong, Q.; et al. Clinical characteristics and intrauterine vertical transmission potential of COVID-19 infection in nine pregnant women: A retrospective review of medical records. *Lancet* **2020**, *395*, 809–815. [CrossRef]
50. Rajkumar, R.P. COVID-19 and mental health: A review of the existing literature. *Asian J. Psychiatry* **2020**, *52*, 102066. [CrossRef]
51. Wang, C.; Pan, R.; Wan, X.; Tan, Y.; Xu, L.; Ho, C.S.; Ho, R.C. Immediate psychological responses and associated factors during the initial stage of the 2019 coronavirus disease (COVID-19) epidemic among the general population in China. *Int. J. Environ. Res. Public Health* **2020**, *17*, 1729. [CrossRef]
52. Wang, C.; Pan, R.; Wan, X.; Tan, Y.; Xu, L.; McIntyre, R.S.; Choo, F.N.; Tran, B.; Ho, R.; Sharma, V.K. A longitudinal study on the mental health of general population during the COVID-19 epidemic in China. *Brain Behav. Immun.* **2020**, S0889-1591(20)30511-0. [CrossRef]

53. Hao, F.; Tan, W.; Jiang, L.; Ling, Z.; Zhao, X.; Zoua, Y.; Hua, Y.; Luoa, X.; Jiang, X.; McIntyree, R.S.; et al. Do Psychiatric Patients Experience More Psychiatric Symptoms during COVID-19 Pandemic and Lockdown? A Case-Control Study with Service and Research Implications for Immunopsychiatry. *Brain Behav. Immun.* 2020. Available online: https://doi.org/10.1016/j.bbi.2020.04.069 (accessed on 27 April 2020).
54. Dean, S. Covid-19 Vaccine Trial on Humans Starts as UK Warns Restrictions Could Stay in Place Until Next Year. Available online: https://edition.cnn.com/2020/04/23/health/coronavirus-vaccine-trial-uk-gbr-intl/index.html (accessed on 28 April 2020).
55. Reuters. Germany Approves Trials of COVID-19 Vaccine Candidate. Available online: https://www.nytimes.com/reuters/2020/04/22/world/europe/22reuters-health-coronavirus-vaccine-biontech.html (accessed on 28 April 2020).
56. World Economic Forum. 80 Countries are Hoarding Medical Supplies—Here's Why It Damages the Global Response to COVID-19. Available online: https://www.weforum.org/agenda/2020/04/wto-report-80-countries-limiting-exports-medical-supplies/ (accessed on 26 April 2020).
57. Guan, W.J.; Liang, W.H.; Zhao, Y.; Liang, H.R.; Chen, Z.S.; Li, Y.M.; Liu, X.Q.; Chen, R.C.; Tang, C.L.; Wang, T.; et al. Comorbidity and its impact on 1590 patients with Covid-19 in China: A Nationwide Analysis. *Eur. Respir. J.* **2020**. [CrossRef] [PubMed]
58. Yang, J.; Zheng, Y.; Gou, X.; Pu, K.; Chen, Z.; Guo, Q.; Ji, R.; Wang, H.; Wang, Y.; Zhou, Y. Prevalence of comorbidities in the novel Wuhan coronavirus (COVID-19) infection: A systematic review and meta-analysis. *Int. J. Infect. Dis.* **2020**, *94*, 91–95. [CrossRef] [PubMed]
59. Lu, C.C.; Chen, M.Y.; Chang, Y.L. Potential therapeutic agents against COVID-19: What we know so far. *J. Chin. Med. Assoc.* **2020**. [CrossRef]
60. Ledford, H. Chloroquine hype is derailing the search for coronavirus treatments. *Nature* **2020**, *580*, 7805. [CrossRef]
61. Ferner, R.E.; Aronson, J.K. Chloroquine and Hydroxychloroquine in COVID-19. *BMJ* **2020**, *369*, m1432. [CrossRef]
62. United Nations International Children's Emergency Fund (UNICEF). Social Stigma Associated with the Coronavirus Disease (COVID-19). Available online: https://www.unicef.org/documents/social-stigma-associated-coronavirus-disease-covid-19 (accessed on 29 April 2020).
63. Center for Disease Control and Prevention. Reducing Stigma. Available online: https://www.cdc.gov/coronavirus/2019-ncov/daily-life-coping/reducing-stigma.html (accessed on 29 April 2020).
64. United Nations. COVID-19 Response. Available online: https://www.un.org/en/un-coronavirus-communications-team/un-working-ensure-vulnerable-groups-not-left-behind-covid-19 (accessed on 26 April 2020).

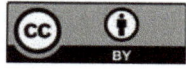

© 2020 by the authors. Licensee MDPI, Basel, Switzerland. This article is an open access article distributed under the terms and conditions of the Creative Commons Attribution (CC BY) license (http://creativecommons.org/licenses/by/4.0/).

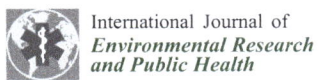 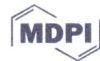

Article

Global Mapping of Research Trends on Interventions to Improve Health-Related Quality of Life in Asthma Patients

Hai Thanh Phan [1], Giap Van Vu [2,3], Giang Thu Vu [4], Giang Hai Ha [5,6,*], Hai Quang Pham [5,7], Carl A. Latkin [8], Bach Xuan Tran [1,8], Cyrus S.H. Ho [9] and Roger C.M. Ho [10,11,12]

[1] Institute for Preventive Medicine and Public Health, Hanoi Medical University, Hanoi 100000, Vietnam; 020101190574@daihocyhanoi.edu.vn (H.T.P.); bach.ipmph@gmail.com (B.X.T.)
[2] Department of Internal Medicine, Hanoi Medical University, Hanoi 100000, Vietnam; vuvangiap@hmu.edu.vn
[3] Respiratory Center, Bach Mai Hospital, Hanoi 100000, Vietnam
[4] Center of Excellence in Evidence-based Medicine, Nguyen Tat Thanh University, Ho Chi Minh City 700000, Vietnam; giang.coentt@gmail.com
[5] Institute for Global Health Innovations, Duy Tan University, Da Nang 550000, Vietnam; phamquanghai@duytan.edu.vn
[6] Faculty of Pharmacy, Duy Tan University, Da Nang 550000, Vietnam
[7] Faculty of Medicine, Duy Tan University, Da Nang 550000, Vietnam
[8] Bloomberg School of Public Health, Johns Hopkins University, Baltimore, MD 21205, USA; carl.latkin@jhu.edu
[9] Department of Psychological Medicine, National University Hospital, Singapore 119074, Singapore; cyrushosh@gmail.com
[10] Institute for Health Innovation and Technology (iHealthtech), National University of Singapore, Singapore 119077, Singapore; pcmrhcm@nus.edu.sg
[11] Department of Psychological Medicine, Yong Loo Lin School of Medicine, National University of Singapore, Singapore 119228, Singapore
[12] Center of Excellence in Behavioral Medicine, Nguyen Tat Thanh University, Ho Chi Minh City 700000, Vietnam
* Correspondence: hahaigiang@duytan.edu.vn; Tel.: +84-6954-8561

Received: 30 March 2020; Accepted: 12 May 2020; Published: 19 May 2020

Abstract: Globally, approximately 335 million people are being affected by asthma. Given that asthma is a chronic airway condition that cannot be cured, the disease negatively impacts physical health and results in losses of productivity of people experiencing asthma, leading to decrease in quality of life. This study aims at demonstrating the research trends worldwide and identifying the research gaps in interventions for improving quality of life of patients with asthma. Bibliometric approach and content analysis, which can objectively evaluate the productivity and research landscapes in this field, were utilized. In this study, we systematically quantified the development of research landscapes associated with interventions for improving quality of life of people experiencing asthma. Along with the gradual growth in the number of publications, these research topics have relatively expanded in recent years. While the understanding of the pathophysiology, diagnosis and treatment of asthma has been well-established, recent research has showed high interest in the control and management of asthma. Findings of this study suggest the need for more empirical studies in developing countries and further investigation into the effects of environment factors on asthma outcomes, as well as the economic burden of asthma.

Keywords: scientometrics; content analysis; text mining; interventions; asthma; quality of life; HRQoL

1. Introduction

According to the Global Initiative for Asthma (GINA), asthma is a heterogeneous disease characterized by chronic airway inflammation [1]. The hallmark features of asthma include reversible airflow obstruction, airway eosinophilia, and history of recurrent wheeze along with cough and breathlessness [1,2]. The pathophysiology of asthma involves various cells and cellular elements, such as mast cells, eosinophils, T lymphocytes, macrophages, neutrophils, and epithelial cells. The inflammation not only causes recurrent episodes of cough, wheezing, shortness of breath, and chest tightness, but also results in an associated increase in the existing bronchial hyperresponsiveness to various stimuli [3].

Globally, approximately 335 million people are being affected by asthma, and in 2015 only, about 383,000 deaths were attributed to asthma [4,5]. Asthma is ranked 14th among the most serious disorders due to its negative impacts on the people experiencing the disease, and its economic burden on healthcare facilities and governments [6]. Asthma has been observed in both children and adults. The incidence and prevalence of pediatric asthma appear to be higher, while morbidity and mortality are more common among adults. Children with asthma may have impaired airway development as well as reduced maximally attained lung function, which may persist into adulthood without further progressive loss. Meanwhile, in adults, asthma usually facilitates a decline in lung function and enhances the risk of fixed airflow obstructions, especially for asthmatics who smoke [7]. Asthma is also associated with a number of respiratory comorbidities, namely rhinosinusitis, allergen rhinitis, sleep-disordered breathing in children, and chronic obstructive pulmonary disease (COPD) and chronic sinusitis for adults. Such comorbidities may not only somewhat enhance the asthma symptoms but also complicate clinical care in various ways [8–10].

Since traditional measures of asthma outcome, such as pulmonary functions and respiratory symptoms, are insufficient to demonstrate the limitations that asthma causes to patients, subjective experience of health-related quality of life of patients plays a critical role in the evaluation of interventions' effectiveness [11–13]. A number of factors have been reported to have an association with poor quality of life among people suffering from asthma, including sociodemographic characteristics (higher age, female gender, lower education level and unemployment), clinical conditions (severity, hospitalization, high levels of immune markers), poor control and management, and associated comorbidities [14,15]. Therefore, conceptualized healthcare beyond medical treatment is crucial for individuals living with asthma, who need to be able to deal with and manage the symptoms themselves. The evaluation of health-related quality of life among patients with asthma is beyond a mere measurement of their situation and healthcare needs, as it also makes a great contribution to the assessment of the effectiveness of clinical interventions.

In addition to pharmacological treatment, including the use of bronchodilator and inhaled corticosteroids (ICS), or biological therapy, such as omalizumab, mepolizumab, and reslizumab, interventions to improve quality of life of asthmatics involve a personalized and comprehensive approach [1–3]. Self-management, namely training in proper use of inhaler for children as well as caregivers, family members, and teachers, and writing asthma action plans are among common interventions [1]. Since incorrect practice of using inhaler is highly common and usually results in an increased risk of asthma attacks, inhaler training with physical demonstration does play a crucial role. Regularly repeated inhaler training has been proved to improve the level of asthma control in adult patients [16]. Along with self-monitoring, the importance of a written asthma action plan that guides the patients and their caregivers on how to promptly recognize and make correct responses to asthma exacerbations is undeniable. Such education has helped to reduce up to two-thirds of urgent healthcare, work and school absenteeism, and even night waking [17,18]. Other approaches target comorbidities and/or modifiable risk factors, such as reducing the use of aspirin or other non-steroidal anti-inflammatory drugs (NSAIDs) in patients with aspirin-exacerbated respiratory disease, and avoidance of exposure to tobacco smokes, occupational pollution, and mold or damp [1].

This study aims at demonstrating the research trends worldwide and identifying the research gaps in interventions for improving quality of life of patients with asthma. In order to report the trend in available articles over time and measure the global research growth based on the existing literature, we applied a bibliometric approach and content analysis, which can objectively evaluate the productivity and research landscapes generated by researchers, health professionals and institutions in this field. By pointing out the current research patterns, we are able to examine the development as well as productivity, and identify research gaps of the literature on quality of life among people suffering from asthma, and thus better inform health professionals worldwide.

2. Materials and Methods

2.1. Search Strategy

The data were retrieved from the Web of Science (WoS) Core Collection, which covers a large number of scientific domains and technology fields. WoS provides publications from high-quality scientific journals, which have been accessed by the experts of literature review committees. WoS is also among the databases with widest coverage, with citation and bibliographic data going back until the 1900s [19].

The search strategy can be described as follows:

- Step 1: With the use of Boolean operators "OR", the search query was developed to identify the number of published items included "quality of life" OR "QoL" OR "HRQoL" OR "well-being". We downloaded papers in text format (txt.) and imported to STATA for further extraction.
- Step 2: Among papers found in Step 1, we used STATA syntax to filter the papers with the following terms in titles or abstracts: ("asthma" OR "asthmatic*") AND ("intervention*" OR "trial*"). Papers that did not mention "asthma" in their titles and abstracts were removed at this step.
- Step 3: We screened the abstracts of the papers from Step 2 to figure out the papers with asthmatics as study participants and which mentioned quality of life as an outcome. The process was performed by two independent researchers. Any arisen disagreement was solved by discussing with the research team and senior researchers.

2.2. Data Download and Extraction

In addition to titles and abstracts, metadata of each paper and reports generated by WoS database were downloaded in text format and imported in Excel for analyzing, including:

1. Total number of publications
2. Authors' names, their affiliations and the number of total papers, and total citations for each author
3. Most prolific countries and collaborations
4. Institutional affiliations and frequency of citation
5. The top cited articles with titles, authors, journal details, year of publication, total citations and citation per year.
6. Titles, abstracts and keywords

Selected papers were research articles written in English. Grey literature, conference proceedings, reviews and books/book chapters were excluded. As the search was performed in the middle of 2019, only papers published before and in the year 2018 were included in the analysis.

2.3. Data Analysis

We used STATA version 15.0 (STATACorp., College Station, TX, USA) to analyze the final data in step 4 using the following information on the articles: authors' affiliations, titles, journals' names, keywords, total number of citations, and abstracts.

Publications' general characteristics, namely year of publication, the number of papers per year of each country, accumulative citations from published year to 2018, yearly mean citation rate, total usage in the last six months and the last five years, and mean use rate in the last six months and the last five years, were described. We used STATA to calculate the number of papers by country in abstracts.

A network graph showing the co-occurrence of terms in title and abstracts was established by VOSviewer (version 1.6.11, Center for Science and Technology, Leiden University, Leiden, The Netherlands). A co-occurrence network can be described as the collective interconnection of terms and is generated by connecting pairs of terms based on a set of criteria that defines co-occurrence. In this study, when term A and term B both appear in title and/or abstract of a particular publication, they are said to "co-occur". Additionally, another paper may contain terms B and C, and so on. By linking the co-occurrence of the identified terms, we created a co-occurrence network of terms.

Latent Dirichlet Allocation (LDA) was applied to classify papers into corresponding topics. LDA is a common topic modeling algorithm for text mining to determine the relationships of text documents. In LDA, each term is regarded as a random vector with the probability of drawing the words/texts associated with that term, in other words, that vector. The probability of a paper is calculated based on the probability of the terms, and papers with similar probability will be classified into one group [20–25]. Thus, by applying LDA, we would be able to recognize the interdisciplinary structure of research development as well as obtain an in-depth view of hidden themes of research on interventions in asthma [26]. We reviewed and read through the most cited papers of each group and assign the labels for each topic manually. In addition, to analyze the relationship of the research area, we utilized coincidence analysis using the STATA command 'precoin' and presented the results in the form of a dendrogram. Dendrograms graphically illustrate the information concerning which observations are grouped together at various levels of similarity.

Analytical techniques for each data types are summarized below (Table 1):

Table 1. Summary of techniques used for each type of data.

Type of Data	Unit of Analysis	Analytical Methods	Presentations of Results
Keywords, Countries	Words	Frequency of co-occurrence	Map of keywords clusters
Abstracts	Papers	Latent Dirichlet Allocation	10 classifications of research topics
WoS classification of research areas	WoS research areas	Frequency of co-occurrence	Dendrogram of research disciplines (WoS classification)

3. Results

3.1. Number of Published Items and Publication Trend

The process of screening and selecting papers is presented in Figure 1. Among 326,405 articles about quality of life, a total of 1624 publications met the eligible criteria and was selected for further analysis.

General characteristics of the selected publications are presented in Table 2. Since 1991, when the first studies on quality of life of people suffering from asthma were published, the number of papers considering this research interest has grown gradually. The total citations of articles published during the 2000s were relatively high compared to publications in recent years. Meanwhile, the total usage, defined by the total downloads, and mean use rate during the last six months were considerable for the research in 2017 and 2018, suggesting the continuous update and rising interest in the topic recently.

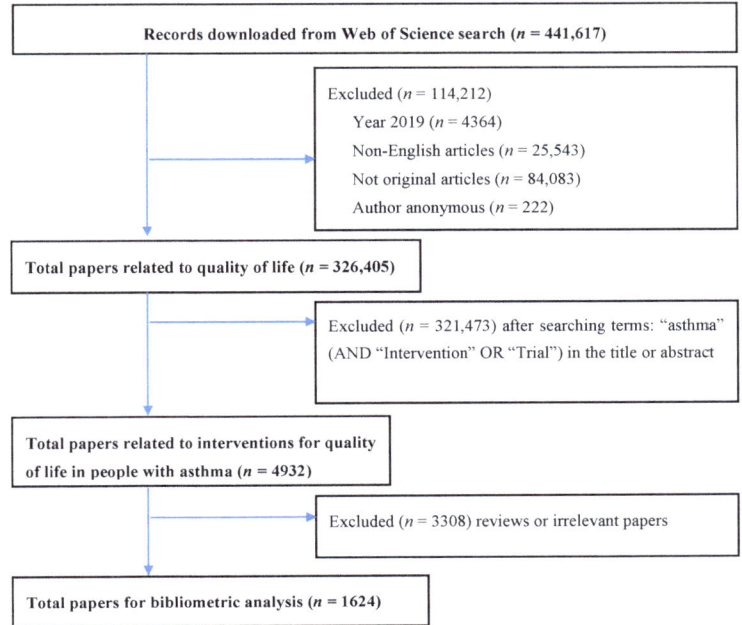

Figure 1. Selection of papers.

Table 2. General characteristics of publications.

Year Published	Total Number of Papers	Total Citations	Mean Cite Rate Per Year [1]	Total Usage [2] Last 6 Months	Total Usage [2] Last 5 Years	Mean Use rate Last 6 Months [3]	Mean Use Rate Last 5 Years [4]
2018	129	229	1.78	228.00	364.00	1.77	0.56
2017	143	640	2.24	171.00	725.00	1.20	1.01
2016	109	888	2.72	70.00	718.00	0.64	1.32
2015	95	1056	2.78	49.00	677.00	0.52	1.43
2014	93	1185	2.55	37.00	785.00	0.40	1.69
2013	85	1710	3.35	43.00	996.00	0.51	2.34
2012	73	1467	2.87	24.00	664.00	0.33	1.82
2011	72	1880	3.26	23.00	475.00	0.32	1.32
2010	82	2259	3.06	44.00	509.00	0.54	1.24
2009	76	3302	4.34	33.00	464.00	0.43	1.22
2008	67	1833	2.49	11.00	280.00	0.16	0.84
2007	74	3357	3.78	29.00	359.00	0.39	0.97
2006	60	2601	3.33	22.00	271.00	0.37	0.90
2005	69	3399	3.52	18.00	274.00	0.26	0.79
2004	65	2539	2.60	13.00	203.00	0.20	0.62
2003	47	2009	2.67	12.00	161.00	0.26	0.69
2002	48	2528	3.10	11.00	191.00	0.23	0.80
2001	47	2559	3.02	6.00	160.00	0.13	0.68
2000	49	2366	2.54	8.00	187.00	0.16	0.76
1999	32	3088	4.83	9.00	96.00	0.28	0.60
1998	32	1764	2.63	1.00	53.00	0.03	0.33
1997	26	2001	3.50	4.00	84.00	0.15	0.65
1996	16	2268	6.16	5.00	57.00	0.31	0.71
1995	12	865	3.00	1.00	41.00	0.08	0.68
1994	10	1908	7.63	2.00	36.00	0.20	0.72
1993	8	1132	5.44	4.00	27.00	0.50	0.68
1992	2	1094	20.26	0.00	22.00	0.00	2.20
1991	3	469	5.58	0.00	7.00	0.00	0.47

[1] mean cite rate per year = total citations/[total citations × (2018 − that year)]; [2] total usage: total downloads; [3] mean use rate last 6 months = total usage last 6 months/total number of papers; [4] mean use rate last 5 years = total usage last 5 years/(total number of papers × 5).

3.2. Number of Study Settings by Countries

Table 3 show the number of papers categorized by the countries of the study settings as mentioned in abstracts. There was a total of 407 articles describing locations of settings, and 14.3% of these were set up in the United States, making this country the top of the list. Over half of the study settings (55.6%) belonged to the top 10 countries, which are all classified as developed countries.

Table 3. Number of papers by countries as study settings.

	Country Settings	Frequency	%		Country Settings	Frequency	%
1	United States	58	14.3%	36	Cuba	2	0.5%
2	Australia	37	9.1%	37	Finland	2	0.5%
3	United Kingdom	32	7.9%	38	Georgia	2	0.5%
4	Sweden	18	4.4%	39	Greece	2	0.5%
5	Spain	17	4.2%	40	Hungary	2	0.5%
6	Netherlands	15	3.7%	41	Kuwait	2	0.5%
7	Canada	13	3.2%	42	Norway	2	0.5%
8	Japan	13	3.2%	43	South Africa	2	0.5%
9	Taiwan	12	2.9%	44	Sri Lanka	2	0.5%
10	Brazil	11	2.7%	45	Tunisia	2	0.5%
11	India	11	2.7%	46	United Arab Emirates	2	0.5%
12	Italy	11	2.7%	47	Wallis and Futuna	2	0.5%
13	China	10	2.5%	48	Argentina	1	0.2%
14	Germany	10	2.5%	49	Barbados	1	0.2%
15	France	9	2.2%	50	Benin	1	0.2%
16	Ireland	9	2.2%	51	Chile	1	0.2%
17	Saudi Arabia	7	1.7%	52	Czech	1	0.2%
18	Switzerland	7	1.7%	53	Dominica	1	0.2%
19	Egypt	6	1.5%	54	Dominican Republic	1	0.2%
20	Jordan	5	1.2%	55	Iceland	1	0.2%
21	Singapore	5	1.2%	56	Indonesia	1	0.2%
22	Belgium	4	1.0%	57	Iran	1	0.2%
23	Hong Kong	4	1.0%	58	Israel	1	0.2%
24	Mexico	4	1.0%	59	Jamaica	1	0.2%
25	Turkey	4	1.0%	60	Jersey	1	0.2%
26	Denmark	3	0.7%	61	Lebanon	1	0.2%
27	Malaysia	3	0.7%	62	Lithuania	1	0.2%
28	New Zealand	3	0.7%	63	Malta	1	0.2%
29	Niger	3	0.7%	64	Oman	1	0.2%
30	Nigeria	3	0.7%	65	Peru	1	0.2%
31	Pakistan	3	0.7%	66	Puerto Rico	1	0.2%
32	Poland	3	0.7%	67	Qatar	1	0.2%
33	Portugal	3	0.7%	68	Serbia	1	0.2%
34	Thailand	3	0.7%	69	Uruguay	1	0.2%
35	Austria	2	0.5%				

3.3. Thematic Analysis of Literature and Research Interests Over Time

Figure 2, which was generated by the analysis of content of abstracts and titles, provides an illustration of the most frequently co-occurred groups of terms. There were four clusters emerging from 458 terms with co-occurrence at least 30 times. Red cluster points out indicators of pulmonary function tests, such as forced vital capacity (FVC), forced expiratory volume in one second (FEV1), peak expiratory flow (PEF), and treatment for different asthma conditions, including inhaled corticosteroids (ICS), mometasone furoate dry powder inhaler (MF-DPI), salmeterol, etc. Yellow cluster focuses on common questionnaires for measuring asthma-related quality of life, namely Asthma Quality of Life Questionnaire (AQLQ), Pediatric Quality of Life Inventory (PedsQL) and Living with Asthma Questionnaire (LWAQ). Blue nodes reveal various approaches of intervention for asthma, while green cluster refers to comorbidity of asthma and factors associated with quality of life among asthmatics.

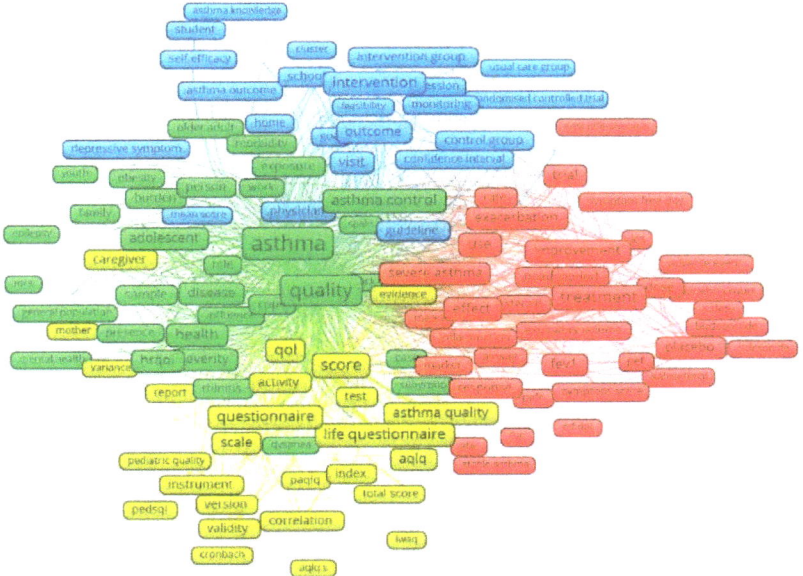

Figure 2. Co-occurrence of most frequent terms in titles and abstracts. Note: the colors of the nodes indicate principle components of the data structure; the node size was scaled to the keywords' occurrences. Abbreviations: (red cluster) fvc—forced vital capacity, fev1—forced expiratory volume in one second, pef—peak expiratory flow, pefr—peak expiratory flow rate, ahr—airway hyperresponsiveness, ics—inhaled corticosteroids, mf dpi—mometasone furoate dry powder inhaler; (yellow cluster) qol—quality of life, aqlq—Asthma Quality of Life Questionnaire, aqlq s—Asthma Quality of Life Questionnaire (Standardized), paqlq—Pediatric Asthma Quality of Life Questionnaire, pedsql—Pediatric Quality of Life Inventory, lwaq—Living with Asthma Questionnaire; (green cluster) mcs—multiple chemical sensitivity.

By applying Latent Dirichlet Allocation for the abstracts, we constructed research articles into ten major topics (Table 4, Figure 3). We extracted a list of papers most likely to be associated with each topic identified, then reviewed the titles and abstracts of the most cited papers within each group to determine the name for each topic. The topic number was assigned by the number of papers belonging to the topic in the last five years. The n (%) is the total number and percentage of papers classified into the topic over the research period. We also rank the topics by highest literature volume produced in the last five years. According to the results of the LDA analysis, asthma control and self-management education interventions was the topic of most interest over time as well as in the last five years, accounting for over one-fifth of the literature volume. Meanwhile, the total number of studies on application and impact of non-medical treatment og asthma have received relatively little attention.

In addition, Figure 3 provides an evident illustration of the trend in the interest in each topic throughout the research period. Despite being ignored in the first years, research on asthma control and education interventions for asthmatics (Topic 1) has increased rapidly and become the research topic that covers a large body of the literature, with a robust rise, especially in recent years. Studies into specific types of asthma (Topic 2 and Topic 7), and the association between diet and exercise and quality of life of people with asthma (Topic 3), albeit having a modest start, have been significantly increasing in recent years. By contrast, as the instruments for measuring asthma-related quality of life, to a certain extent, have become well-established and proved their validity, there has been a slight decline of research volume for Topic 4.

Table 4. Ten research topics classified by LDA.

Topic (Ranked by the Highest Volume in the Last 5 Years)	Research Topics	n (%)
middleic 1	Asthma control and education interventions for asthmatics	355 (21.8)
middleic 2	Development of medication for persistent asthma and allergic asthma	238 (14.6)
middleic 3	Association between diet and exercises and quality of life of people with asthma	167 (10.3)
middleic 4	Validation of questionnaires and evaluation of instruments	308 (18.9)
middleic 5	Impact of psychological and environmental factors on asthma-related quality of life	232 (14.3)
middleic 6	Asthma care and intervention for children and adolescents	160 (9.8)
middleic 7	Drugs for refractory asthma, eosinophilic asthma and non-eosinophilic asthma	71 (4.4)
middleic 8	Quality of life of asthmatics' caregiversAsthma-related quality of life among the elderly	36 (2.2)
middleic 9	Relationship between allergens, allergic rhinitis and asthma status	52 (3.2)
middleic 10	Impact of non-medical treatment on health outcomes	7 (0.5)

LDA: Latent Dirichlet Allocation.

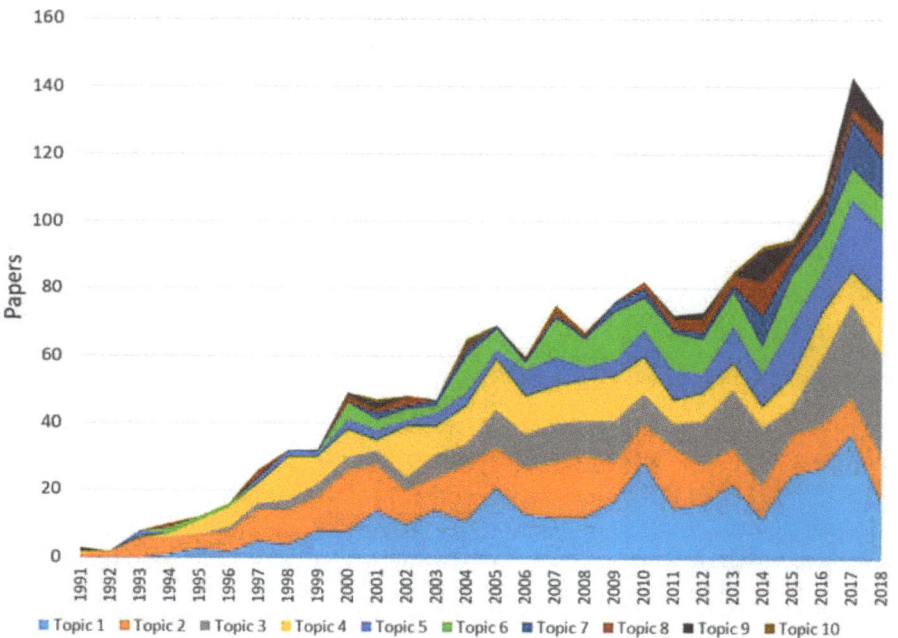

Figure 3. Changes in research topics development.

Figure 4 presents the dendrogram, in other words, the hierarchical clustering of research disciplines in quality of life of patients with asthma. The distance or dissimilarity between clusters is indicated in the horizontal axis, while the vertical axis shows the research disciplines. The red lines show the depth for the cut-off of the analysis [27]. According to Figure 4, the research landscapes in quality of life among patients with asthma are rooted in the following disciplines: (a) Health policy and services, (b) Health care sciences and services and (c) Public, Environmental and Occupational health, as the first chunk in the bottom the dendrogram. In the top part, we found the integration of: (a) Respiratory system, (b) Critical care medicine, and (c) Cardiac and Cardiovascular system.

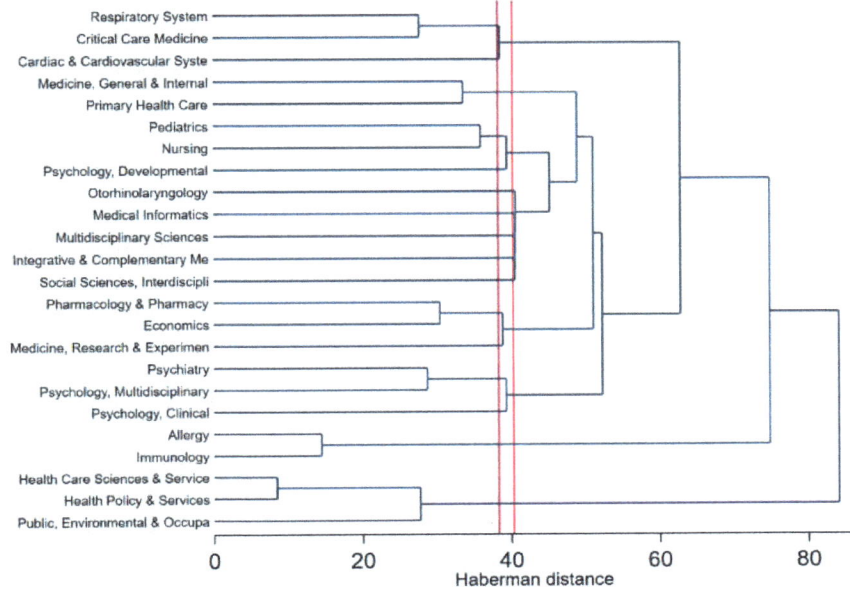

Figure 4. Dendrogram of coincidence of research areas using the Web of Science (WoS) lassifications.

4. Discussion

4.1. Summary of Findings

This study provides a quantitative as well as qualitative overview of interdisciplinary research landscapes of quality of life among individuals with asthma. In this study, we have systematically quantified the development of research landscapes associated with interventions for improving quality of life of asthmatics in the past 28 years. While the number of publications showed an insignificant change over years, the substantial total usage and mean use rate in the last six months of studies published in 2017 and 2018 implies an increasing interest and the need for a continuous update of understandings of this topic. Along with the growth in the number of publications, the research topics have also been expanded in recent years. Besides the conventional research areas such as development of instruments and treatment, asthma control and education interventions for people living with asthma, research into specific types of asthma have also emerged and attracted a great deal of attention.

4.2. Current Research on Asthma in Different Countries

In terms of the countries involved in the research area, the top nine countries with the highest number of study settings belonged to the high-income group [28]. In addition to the United States, which led in research on interventions to improve quality of life of asthmatics, a large number of study settings on quality of life of people living with asthma took place in Australia, the United Kingdom and Europe (Table 2). These efforts have resulted in the stabilized or decreasing prevalence of asthma in such developed countries, as opposed to developing countries, which have been facing a steep increase in the burden of asthma [4,29,30]. It is also noteworthy that low- and lower-middle income countries accounted for more than 80% of asthma-related deaths worldwide, which calls for more empirical studies to be conducted in developing countries [5].

4.3. Emerging Research Interests

Realizing the growing importance of asthma control in improving quality of life of people with asthma at a population level, one of the emerging research domains that has attracted much attention from researchers in recent years is asthma control and education interventions for asthmatics (Topic 1—Table 3, Figure 3). Aside from clinical history and manifestations, namely experience of near-fatal asthma, sensitivity to mold and other allergens, and comorbidities with other respiratory diseases and infections, poor management and control of asthma has been reported to be responsible for a large number of asthma exacerbation and asthma-related preventable deaths [4,31–39]. Whilst understanding of the pathophysiology, diagnosis and treatment of asthma has been well-established (Figure 2), research on controlling the distribution of asthmatics and how to increase their access to appropriate and high-quality interventions for better quality of life remains relatively scarce. Despite the development of various medications and interventions to improve the quality of life of asthmatics, asthma management and control, especially in developing countries, has been facing such barriers as unaffordability of inhaled corticosteroids, inadequate education on asthma for the general population and poor infrastructure, which frequently leads to lack of adherence to treatment as well as lack of appropriate and prompt actions in case of asthma attack [4,38,40,41]. Self-management, including the use of healthy diet and physical exercises (Topic 3), is also an important component of asthma management [42–45]. Although studies have demonstrated the association between food allergy and pathogenesis of asthma, and dietary factors are reported to directly influence asthma outcomes regardless of level of allergy, a number of people suffering from asthma and their caregivers have not yet been made aware of the importance of a healthy and appropriate diet [31,44,46–48]. Meanwhile, exercise showed positive effects on asthma control and can be recommended for children and young adults [43,49]. Given that a person best understands his or her allergy and physical status, self-management, considering diet and exercise, therefore plays an important role in alleviating asthma symptoms and improving quality of life.

4.4. Identified Research Gaps

Based on the results obtained, we have identified certain research gaps. Even though understanding of the pathogenesis of asthma has been extensively studied, the association between asthma and environmental factors deserves more attention from researchers. Asthma has been long recognized as a chronic condition and with the proper treatment and management, the symptoms can be well controlled and asthma patients are able to live a full and rewarding life [5]. Nevertheless, under the influence of continuously worsening air quality, it is undeniable that asthmatics have become more and more vulnerable [50–53]. Increased levels of ambient ozone, nitrogen dioxide (NO_2), sulfur dioxide (SO_2) and particulates ($PM_{2.5}$, PM_{10}) were proved to be associated with higher prevalence of asthma and symptoms onset, as well as increased hospital admission due to asthma attack [54]. Children and adolescents with asthma are particular susceptible to these pollutants due to their underdeveloped lung function and immature metabolic pathways [51,55–57]. The current environmental situation has showed little sign of improvement and has continued to bring about detrimental effects on health-related quality of life of asthma patients, suggesting the need for further update research on this topic.

In the meanwhile, notwithstanding the fact that asthma is a chronic condition with both direct and indirect cost, the financial burden of asthma is not among the emerging research domains identified in this study. According to the Global Asthma Report 2018, annual direct cost per patient ranged from under USD 150 in United Arab Emirates to more than USD 3000 in USA and, at national level, total annual costs for asthma in the USA witnessed an increase of 3 billion USD from 2002 to 2011. Total costs for asthma patients aged 15 to 64 in Europe were USD 24.7 billion during 1999–2002, in which the United Kingdom itself accounted for USD 9.8 billion [4]. The data indicates that asthma is an economic burden even for high-income countries. While indirect costs are regularly ignored by cost estimates, studies have consistently indicated that indirect costs constitute a significant part of the economic burden of asthma [58–60]. On the other hand, high cost of treatment can be regarded as an important limiting factor for improving quality of life of asthma patients in developing countries. While access to inhaled corticosteroids has been recognized as one of the keys to improve quality of life among asthmatics, for many asthma patients in developing countries, such as India, Malaysia and Thailand, inhaled corticosteroids are either inaccessible or unaffordable [4,61,62]. In Indonesia, although inhaled corticosteroid is available and covered by health insurance, many people are unable to afford a spacer, which is the best delivery system for the drug [4]. Therefore, there presents a call for more research on the economic aspects of asthma.

4.5. Limitations

In this study, we introduced an efficient approach to analyzing the extant literature about quality of life among asthmatics. Nonetheless, there exist some limitations. Even though a fairly large proportion of publications relating to quality of life is available on WoS, the choice of WoS as the only data source would leave out relevant studies. Another limitation that should be acknowledged is that the language of selected papers was restricted to English, potentially causing a bias toward English-speaking countries. Besides, instead of analyzing full texts, the content analysis and text mining involved solely titles and abstracts. Nevertheless, provided that the major content of a study is normally included in the title and abstract, this bibliometric analysis is able to provide meaningful findings and offer a comprehensive overview of current research trends.

5. Conclusions

In conclusion, by conducting a bibliometric analysis and applying a scientometric approach, we have presented the global research patterns and current interests and identified the research gaps in the literature relevant to quality of life among people suffering from asthma. Recent research has showed high interest in the control and management of asthma. Findings of this study suggest the need for more empirical studies in developing countries and further investigation into the effects of environment factors on asthma outcomes as well as the economic burden of asthma.

Author Contributions: Conceptualization, H.T.P., G.V.V., C.A.L., B.X.T., C.S.H.H. and R.C.M.H.; data curation, G.H.H. and H.Q.P.; formal analysis, H.T.P., G.H.H. and C.S.H.H.; funding acquisition, R.C.M.H.; investigation, H.T.P. and G.T.V.; methodology, H.T.P.; project administration, G.T.V., G.H.H. and B.X.T.; software, G.H.H. and H.Q.P.; supervision, G.T.V. and B.X.T.; validation, G.V.V., C.A.L. and C.S.H.H.; visualization, H.Q.P.; writing—original draft, H.T.P.; writing—review & editing, H.T.P., G.V.V., G.T.V., C.A.L. and R.C.M.H. All authors have read and agreed to the published version of the manuscript.

Funding: The article processing charge is funded by the National University of Singapore Healthtech Other Operating Expense (R-722-000-004-731).

Conflicts of Interest: The authors declare no conflict of interest.

References

1. Global Initiative for Asthma. Global Strategy for Asthma Management and Prevention. 2017. Available online: www.ginasthma.org (accessed on 20 June 2019).
2. Poddighe, D.; Brambilla, I.; Licari, A.; Marseglia, G.L. Omalizumab in the Therapy of Pediatric Asthma. *Recent Pat. Inflamm. Allergy Drug Discov.* **2018**, *12*, 103–109. [CrossRef] [PubMed]
3. Busse, W.W. *Expert Panel Report 3: Guidelines for the Diagnosis and Management of Asthma*; National Institutes of Health: Bethesda, MD, USA, 2007.
4. *The Global Asthma Report 2018*; Global Asthma Network: Auckland, New Zealand, 2018.
5. World Health Organization (WHO). Asthma. Available online: https://www.who.int/news-room/fact-sheets/detail/asthma (accessed on 30 September 2019).
6. *The Global Asthma Report*; Global Asthma Network: Auckland, New Zealand, 2014.
7. Dharmage, S.C.; Perret, J.L.; Custovic, A. Epidemiology of Asthma in Children and Adults. *Front. Pediatr.* **2019**, *7*, 246. [CrossRef]

8. Poddighe, D.; Brambilla, I.; Licari, A.; Marseglia, G.L. Pediatric rhinosinusitis and asthma. *Respir Med.* **2018**, *141*, 94–99. [CrossRef] [PubMed]
9. Kercsmar, C.M.; Shipp, C. Management/Comorbidities of School-Aged Children with Asthma. *Immunol. Allergy Clin. N. Am.* **2019**, *39*, 191–204. [CrossRef] [PubMed]
10. Weatherburn, C.J.; Guthrie, B.; Mercer, S.W.; Morales, D.R. Comorbidities in adults with asthma: Population-based cross-sectional analysis of 1.4 million adults in Scotland. *Clin. Exp. Allergy* **2017**, *47*, 1246–1252. [CrossRef] [PubMed]
11. Juniper, E.F.; Guyatt, G.H.; Ferrie, P.J.; Griffith, L.E. Measuring quality of life in asthma. *Am. Rev. Respir Dis.* **1993**, *147*, 832–838. [CrossRef] [PubMed]
12. Krishnan, J.A.; Lemanske, R.F., Jr.; Canino, G.J.; Elward, K.S.; Kattan, M.; Matsui, E.C.; Mitchell, H.; Sutherland, E.R.; Minnicozzi, M. Asthma outcomes: Symptoms. *J. Allergy Clin. Immunol.* **2012**, *129*, S124–S135. [CrossRef]
13. Tepper, R.S.; Wise, R.S.; Covar, R.; Irvin, C.G.; Kercsmar, C.M.; Kraft, M.; Liu, M.C.; O'Connor, G.T.; Peters, S.P.; Sorkness, R.; et al. Asthma outcomes: Pulmonary physiology. *J. Allergy Clin. Immunol.* **2012**, *129*, S65–S87. [CrossRef]
14. Kalyva, E.; Eiser, C.; Papathanasiou, A. Health-Related Quality of Life of Children with Asthma: Self and Parental Perceptions. *Int. J. Behav. Med.* **2016**, *23*, 730–737. [CrossRef]
15. Stern, J.; Pier, J.; Litonjua, A.A. Asthma epidemiology and risk factors. *Semin. Immunopathol.* **2020**, *42*, 5–15. [CrossRef]
16. Melani, A.S.; Bonavia, M.; Cilenti, V.; Cinti, C.; Lodi, M.; Martucci, P.; Serra, M.; Scichilone, N.; Sestini, P.; Aliani, M.; et al. Inhaler mishandling remains common in real life and is associated with reduced disease control. *Respir. Med.* **2011**, *105*, 930–938. [CrossRef] [PubMed]
17. Boyd, M.; Lasserson, T.J.; McKean, M.C.; Gibson, P.G.; Ducharme, F.M.; Haby, M. Interventions for educating children who are at risk of asthma-related emergency department attendance. *Cochrane Database Syst. Rev.* **2009**, CD001290. [CrossRef] [PubMed]
18. Pinnock, H.; Parke, H.L.; Panagioti, M.; Daines, L.; Pearce, G.; Epiphaniou, E.; Bower, P.; Sheikh, A.; Griffiths, C.J.; Taylor, S.J.; et al. Systematic meta-review of supported self-management for asthma: A healthcare perspective. *BMC Med.* **2017**, *15*, 64. [CrossRef]
19. Aghaei chadegani, A.; Salehi, H.; Yunus, M.; Farhadi, H.; Fooladi, M.; Farhadi, M.; Ale Ebrahim, N. A Comparison between Two Main Academic Literature Collections: Web of Science and Scopus Databases. *Asian Soc. Sci.* **2013**, *9*, 18–26. [CrossRef]
20. Ding, Y.; Rousseau, R.; Wolfram, D. *Measuring Scholarly Impact: Methods and Practice*; Springer: Berlin, Germany, 2014.
21. Li, Y.; Rapkin, B.; Atkinson, T.M.; Schofield, E.; Bochner, B.H. Leveraging Latent Dirichlet Allocation in processing free-text personal goals among patients undergoing bladder cancer surgery. *Qual. Life Res.* **2019**, *28*, 1441–1455. [CrossRef] [PubMed]
22. Valle, D.; Albuquerque, P.; Zhao, Q.; Barberan, A.; Fletcher, R.J., Jr. Extending the Latent Dirichlet Allocation model to presence/absence data: A case study on North American breeding birds and biogeographical shifts expected from climate change. *Glob. Chang. Biol.* **2018**, *24*, 5560–5572. [CrossRef] [PubMed]
23. Chen, C.; Zare, A.; Trinh, H.N.; Omotara, G.O.; Cobb, J.T.; Lagaunne, T.A. Partial Membership Latent Dirichlet Allocation for Soft Image Segmentation. *IEEE Trans. Image Process. Publ. IEEE Signal. Process. Soc.* **2017**, *26*, 5590–5602. [CrossRef]
24. Lu, H.M.; Wei, C.P.; Hsiao, F.Y. Modeling healthcare data using multiple-channel latent Dirichlet allocation. *J. Biomed. Inform.* **2016**, *60*, 210–223. [CrossRef]
25. Gross, A.; Murthy, D. Modeling virtual organizations with Latent Dirichlet Allocation: A case for natural language processing. *Neural Netw. Off. J. Int. Neural Netw. Soc.* **2014**, *58*, 38–49. [CrossRef]
26. Tong, Z.; Zhang, H. A document exploring system on LDA topic model for Wikipedia articles. *Int. J. Multimed. Its Appl.* **2016**, *8*. [CrossRef]
27. Moffat, D.; Ronan, D.; Reiss, J.D. Unsupervised taxonomy of sound effects. *Context* **2017**, *6*, 7.
28. Bank, T.W. High Income. Available online: https://data.worldbank.org/income-level/high-income (accessed on 1 February 2020).

29. Asher, M.I.; Montefort, S.; Bjorksten, B.; Lai, C.K.; Strachan, D.P.; Weiland, S.K.; Williams, H.; Group, I.P.T.S. Worldwide time trends in the prevalence of symptoms of asthma, allergic rhinoconjunctivitis, and eczema in childhood: ISAAC Phases One and Three repeat multicountry cross-sectional surveys. *Lancet* **2006**, *368*, 733–743. [CrossRef]
30. Mallol, J.; Crane, J.; von Mutius, E.; Odhiambo, J.; Keil, U.; Stewart, A.; Group, I.P.T.S. The International Study of Asthma and Allergies in Childhood (ISAAC) Phase Three: A global synthesis. *Allergol. Immunopathol. (Madr.)* **2013**, *41*, 73–85. [CrossRef] [PubMed]
31. Pumphrey, R.S.; Gowland, M.H. Further fatal allergic reactions to food in the United Kingdom, 1999–2006. *J. Allergy Clin. Immunol.* **2007**, *119*, 1018–1019. [CrossRef] [PubMed]
32. Black, P.N.; Udy, A.A.; Brodie, S.M. Sensitivity to fungal allergens is a risk factor for life-threatening asthma. *Allergy* **2000**, *55*, 501–504. [CrossRef]
33. Kodadhala, V.; Obi, J.; Wessly, P.; Mehari, A.; Gillum, R.F. Asthma-related mortality in the United States, 1999 to 2015: A multiple causes of death analysis. *Ann. Allergy Asthma Immunol.* **2018**, *120*, 614–619. [CrossRef]
34. Levy, M.L. The national review of asthma deaths: What did we learn and what needs to change? *Breathe (Sheff)* **2015**, *11*, 14–24. [CrossRef]
35. Fu, L.S.; Tsai, M.C. Asthma exacerbation in children: A practical review. *Pediatr. Neonatol.* **2014**, *55*, 83–91. [CrossRef]
36. Castillo, J.R.; Peters, S.P.; Busse, W.W. Asthma Exacerbations: Pathogenesis, Prevention, and Treatment. *J. Allergy Clin. Immunol.* **2017**, *5*, 918–927. [CrossRef]
37. Bloom, C.I.; Nissen, F.; Douglas, I.J.; Smeeth, L.; Cullinan, P.; Quint, J.K. Exacerbation risk and characterisation of the UK's asthma population from infants to old age. *Thorax* **2018**, *73*, 313–320. [CrossRef]
38. Royal College of Physicians. *Why Asthma Still Kills: The National Review of Asthma Deaths (NRAD) Confidential Enquiry Report*; Royal College of Physicians: London, UK, 2014.
39. Fy, O.K.R. Why Asthma Still Kills. *Ulst. Med. J.* **2017**, *86*, 44.
40. Lenney, W.; Bush, A.; Fitzgerald, D.A.; Fletcher, M.; Ostrem, A.; Pedersen, S.; Szefler, S.J.; Zar, H.J. Improving the global diagnosis and management of asthma in children. *Thorax* **2018**, *73*, 662–669. [CrossRef]
41. Tan, W.C. Asthma management in the developing world: Achievements and challenges. *Expert Rev. Respir Med.* **2008**, *2*, 323–328. [CrossRef] [PubMed]
42. McDonald, V.M.; Gibson, P.G. Asthma self-management education. *Chron. Respir. Dis.* **2006**, *3*, 29–37. [CrossRef] [PubMed]
43. Heikkinen, S.A.M.; Makikyro, E.M.S.; Hugg, T.T.; Jaakkola, M.S.; Jaakkola, J.J.K. Effects of regular exercise on asthma control in young adults. *J. Asthma* **2018**, *55*, 726–733. [CrossRef] [PubMed]
44. Hakami, R.; Gillis, D.E.; Poureslami, I.; FitzGerald, J.M. Patient and Professional Perspectives on Nutrition in Chronic Respiratory Disease Self-Management: Reflections on Nutrition and Food Literacies. *Health Lit. Res. Pract.* **2018**, *2*, e166–e174. [CrossRef] [PubMed]
45. Kouba, J.; Velsor-Friedrich, B.; Militello, L.; Harrison, P.R.; Becklenberg, A.; White, B.; Surya, S.; Ahmed, A. Efficacy of the I Can Control Asthma and Nutrition Now (ICAN) pilot program on health outcomes in high school students with asthma. *J. Sch. Nurs.* **2013**, *29*, 235–247. [CrossRef]
46. Julia, V.; Macia, L.; Dombrowicz, D. The impact of diet on asthma and allergic diseases. *Nat. Rev. Immunol.* **2015**, *15*, 308–322. [CrossRef]
47. Guo, C.H.; Liu, P.J.; Lin, K.P.; Chen, P.C. Nutritional supplement therapy improves oxidative stress, immune response, pulmonary function, and quality of life in allergic asthma patients: An open-label pilot study. *Altern Med. Rev.* **2012**, *17*, 42–56.
48. Roberts, G.; Patel, N.; Levi-Schaffer, F.; Habibi, P.; Lack, G. Food allergy as a risk factor for life-threatening asthma in childhood: A case-controlled study. *J. Allergy Clin. Immunol.* **2003**, *112*, 168–174. [CrossRef]
49. Wanrooij, V.H.; Willeboordse, M.; Dompeling, E.; van de Kant, K.D. Exercise training in children with asthma: A systematic review. *Br. J. Sports Med.* **2014**, *48*, 1024–1031. [CrossRef] [PubMed]
50. Orru, H.; Ebi, K.L.; Forsberg, B. The Interplay of Climate Change and Air Pollution on Health. *Curr. Environ. Health Rep.* **2017**, *4*, 504–513. [CrossRef]
51. Khreis, H.; Kelly, C.; Tate, J.; Parslow, R.; Lucas, K.; Nieuwenhuijsen, M. Exposure to traffic-related air pollution and risk of development of childhood asthma: A systematic review and meta-analysis. *Environ. Int.* **2017**, *100*, 1–31. [CrossRef] [PubMed]
52. Vardoulakis, S.; Osborne, N. Air pollution and asthma. *Arch. Dis. Child.* **2018**, *103*, 813–814. [CrossRef]

53. Cai, Y.; Zijlema, W.L.; Doiron, D.; Blangiardo, M.; Burton, P.R.; Fortier, I.; Gaye, A.; Gulliver, J.; de Hoogh, K.; Hveem, K.; et al. Ambient air pollution, traffic noise and adult asthma prevalence: A BioSHaRE approach. *Eur. Respir. J.* **2017**, *49*. [CrossRef]
54. Guan, W.J.; Zheng, X.Y.; Chung, K.F.; Zhong, N.S. Impact of air pollution on the burden of chronic respiratory diseases in China: Time for urgent action. *Lancet* **2016**, *388*, 1939–1951. [CrossRef]
55. Orellano, P.; Quaranta, N.; Reynoso, J.; Balbi, B.; Vasquez, J. Effect of outdoor air pollution on asthma exacerbations in children and adults: Systematic review and multilevel meta-analysis. *PLoS ONE* **2017**, *12*, e0174050. [CrossRef]
56. Romeo, E.; De Sario, M.; Forastiere, F.; Compagnucci, P.; Stafoggia, M.; Bergamaschi, A.; Perucci, C.A. PM 10 exposure and asthma exacerbations in pediatric age: A meta-analysis of panel and time-series studies. *Epidemiol. Prev.* **2006**, *30*, 245–254.
57. Weinmayr, G.; Romeo, E.; De Sario, M.; Weiland, S.K.; Forastiere, F. Short-term effects of PM10 and NO_2 on respiratory health among children with asthma or asthma-like symptoms: A systematic review and meta-analysis. *Environ. Health Perspect* **2010**, *118*, 449–457. [CrossRef]
58. Barbosa, J.P.; Ferreira-Magalhaes, M.; Sa-Sousa, A.; Azevedo, L.F.; Fonseca, J.A. Cost of asthma in Portuguese adults: A population-based, cost-of-illness study. *Rev. Port. Pneumol.* **2017**, *23*, 323–330. [CrossRef]
59. Ehteshami-Afshar, S.; FitzGerald, J.M.; Doyle-Waters, M.M.; Sadatsafavi, M. The global economic burden of asthma and chronic obstructive pulmonary disease. *Int. J. Tuberc. Lung Dis.* **2016**, *20*, 11–23. [CrossRef] [PubMed]
60. Sharifi, L.; Dashti, R.; Pourpak, Z.; Fazlollahi, M.R.; Movahedi, M.; Chavoshzadeh, Z.; Soheili, H.; Bokaie, S.; Kazemnejad, A.; Moin, M. Economic Burden of Pediatric Asthma: Annual Cost of Disease in Iran. *Iran. J. Public Health* **2018**, *47*, 256–263. [PubMed]
61. Ait-Khaled, N.; Enarson, D.A.; Bissell, K.; Billo, N.E. Access to inhaled corticosteroids is key to improving quality of care for asthma in developing countries. *Allergy* **2007**, *62*, 230–236. [CrossRef] [PubMed]
62. Rodriguez-Martinez, C.E.; Nino, G.; Castro-Rodriguez, J.A. Cost-utility analysis of daily versus intermittent inhaled corticosteroids in mild-persistent asthma. *Pediatr. Pulmonol.* **2015**, *50*, 735–746. [CrossRef]

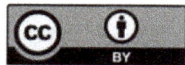 © 2020 by the authors. Licensee MDPI, Basel, Switzerland. This article is an open access article distributed under the terms and conditions of the Creative Commons Attribution (CC BY) license (http://creativecommons.org/licenses/by/4.0/).

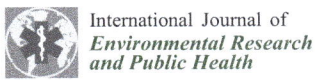 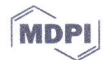

Article

Interventions to Improve the Quality of Life of Patients with Chronic Obstructive Pulmonary Disease: A Global Mapping during 1990–2018

Giap Van Vu [1,2], Giang Hai Ha [3,4,*], Cuong Tat Nguyen [3,5], Giang Thu Vu [6], Hai Quang Pham [7], Carl A. Latkin [8], Bach Xuan Tran [7,8], Roger C.M. Ho [9,10,11] and Cyrus S.H. Ho [12]

1. Department of Internal Medicine, Hanoi Medical University, Hanoi 100000, Vietnam; vuvangiap@hmu.edu.vn
2. Respiratory Center, Bach Mai Hospital, Hanoi 100000, Vietnam
3. Institute for Global Health Innovations, Duy Tan University, Da Nang 550000, Vietnam; nguyentatcuong@duytan.edu.vn
4. Faculty of Pharmacy, Duy Tan University, Da Nang 550000, Vietnam
5. Faculty of Medicine, Duy Tan University, Da Nang 550000, Vietnam
6. Center of Excellence in Evidence-based Medicine, Nguyen Tat Thanh University, Ho Chi Minh City 700000, Vietnam; giang.coentt@gmail.com
7. Institute for Preventive Medicine and Public Health, Hanoi Medical University, Hanoi 100000, Vietnam; quanghai23hmu@gmail.com (H.Q.P.); bach.ipmph@gmail.com (B.X.T.)
8. Bloomberg School of Public Health, Johns Hopkins University, Baltimore, MD 21205, USA; carl.latkin@jhu.edu
9. Institute for Health Innovation and Technology (iHealthtech), National University of Singapore, Singapore 119077, Singapore; pcmrhcm@nus.edu.sg
10. Department of Psychological Medicine, Yong Loo Lin School of Medicine, National University of Singapore, Singapore 119228, Singapore
11. Center of Excellence in Behavioral Medicine, Nguyen Tat Thanh University, Ho Chi Minh City 700000, Vietnam
12. Department of Psychological Medicine, National University Hospital, Singapore 119074, Singapore; cyrushosh@gmail.com
* Correspondence: hahaigiang@duytan.edu.vn; Tel.: +84-869-548-561

Received: 31 March 2020; Accepted: 24 April 2020; Published: 29 April 2020

Abstract: Chronic obstructive pulmonary disease (COPD) has been considered a significant health challenge globally in recent years, which affects different aspects of the quality-of-life (QoL). A review was conducted of research output, research topics, and landscape to have a global view of the papers mentioning the interventions to increase QoL of patients with COPD. A total of 3242 research items from Web of Science during the period 1990–2018 were downloaded and analyzed. Analyses based on the different levels of data and methods using using VOSviewer software tool (version 1.16.15, Centre for Science and Technology Studies (CWTS), Leiden University, Leiden, The Netherlands) and Latent Dirichlet allocation. By exploring the trends in research productivity and topics, an increase was found in the number of papers mentioning non-pharmacological interventions as well as mental health illness and QoL among patients with COPD. In conclusion, the research on the interventions to increase the QoL of patients with COPD has attracted scientists globally. It is suggested that more research should be conducted on the effectiveness of non-pharmacological therapies to increase QoL of patients with COPD that can be applied broadly in the community. The collaboration and support from developed countries to developing countries are needed to increase the QoL of people living with COPD.

Keywords: scientometrics; content analysis; text mining; interventions; COPD; QoL

1. Introduction

Chronic obstructive pulmonary disease (COPD) is one of the chronic airway diseases, which characterized by the limitation in airflow and not fully reversible [1]. The reported prevalence of COPD is different among regions: 4% in Europe [2], 6.3% in the Asia Pacific region [3], from less than 4% to over 9% [4] in the US and predicted, with limited epidemiological evidence, to be at about 11% in 2010 in the African region [5,6].

This chronic disease has significant adverse effects on physical and mental conditions of those patients [7–9], as other systems and organs other than the lungs suffered the negative impacts, leading to pneumonia [10], pulmonary hypertension [11], and cardiovascular disease (CVD) [12]. A worsening mental status has been found in patients with COPD compared to non-COPD subjects, with higher rates of anxiety and depression [13,14], and the severity of fatigue [15]. Patients with COPD less frequently report a partner compared to others, and, when having a partner, they were less likely to be 'very satisfied' with the daily support and less often perceived emotional support from the partner [16]. They suffer worse quality of life with early-morning and nighttime symptoms compared to those without COPD [17,18]. COPD often results in a reduction in quality of life.

Quality of life (QoL) is defined by World Health Organization as a broad and complex concept of an individual about their physical health, mental health, social relationships and beliefs in the context of their living enviroment [19]. It is a "multidimensional measure" which focus on at least three domains: physics, psychology and society. Thus, several studies applied dimensions of QoL to to: (1) evaluate the efficiency of clinical therapies [20–22] or alternative therapies [23,24]; (2) identify factors associated with QoL [25] and increase health service quality [24]. In the case of COPD, improving QoL of patients with COPD becomes critical due to the incurables [26]. Medical methods have been used mainly to control COPD and strengthen prevention efforts, such as: (1) smoking cessation [27,28], (2) pharmacotherapy [29], and (3) Non-pharmacological therapy [30]. Therefore, measuring QoL could be useful in applying suitable interventions and preventing risk factors affected COPD.

Systematic reviews of interventions and treatments are considered as a reliable source of evidence to inform clinical practice and policy development [31]. Several systematic reviews and meta-analyses mentioning interventions to patients with COPD have been conducted. Gregersen et al. confirmed that telehealth showed promise for improving QoL of patients living with COPD, yet, this method call for more research to prove its effectiveness [32]. According to Coronini-Cronberg et al., psychosocial and pharmacological support is an effective intervention for smoking cessation [33], which raises the QoL in some health domains [34]. Moreover, breathing exercises can be used to improve the QoL of patients living with COPD, yet, the use of this method as a complementary therapy needs more research [35]. These literature review studies answer specific questions by gathering available empirical research evidence. However, a limitation of this approach is that it could review one method, which makes it difficult to compare the effects of all methods during a long period of study.

In addition, several researchers have used indicators of scientometric to review literature [36]. Prvevious studies used bibliometrics to explore research output, country collaboration, journal ranking or fundings of all papers mentioning COPD in European countries [37] or in Arab countries [38]. However, scientometric analyses may not have a deep understanding of the context of research or the landscape of research areas. Therefore, by combining scientometric and Latent Direcht allocation, topic modeling (in titles and abstracts), this study aims to describe the global trend in research outputs, countries collaboration, interdisciplinary research areas, as well as ten common topics among papers mentioning interventions to improve QoL of patients with COPD. The findings will emphasize research gaps, and make it possible to recommend some implications for future studies and policy.

2. Materials and Methods

2.1. Database and Search Strategy

The data were retrieved in the middle of 2019 from the Web of Science (WoS) Core Collection. It was decided to choose WoS because WoS (1) allows to download a large number of papers and (2) provides necessary information for scientometrics analysis, such as authors' affiliations, authors' keywords, the title of papers, publication year, research areas, as well as the number of citations and download times for each paper [39,40].

The search strategy was described as follow:

- Step 1: With the use of Boolean operators "OR", the search query was developed to identify the number of published items related to "Quality of life" OR "well-being". Only English research articles and research reviews were included, while grey literature, conference proceedings, or books/book chapters in any other language were excluded. Papers having anonymous authors and publications in 2019 were also limited. This research began in the middle of 2019; thus, this data could not reflect the research trend for the whole year. Data in WoS databases under text format was downloaded and imported to STATA version 15.0 (STATACorp., Texas, TX, USA) for further extraction. (See Table A1)
- Step 2: STATA syntax was applied to filter the papers in step 1 with the terms "Intervention" OR "Interventions" OR "trial" OR "trials" in titles or abstracts.
- Step 3: The COPD keywords were formed by COPD specialists and reviewing some papers and MeSH term library of PubMed. These terms were used to search in the title and keyword fields among papers in step 2 (see Table A1), and there were 5784 papers for further screening.
- Step 4: Two researchers separately screened the titles and abstracts of 5784 papers to exclude papers not related to COPD. A group discussion with a senior researcher was conducted if there were any contradictions. A total of 3242 papers were imported to STATA for further analysis. (See Figure A1).

2.2. Data Analysis

The corrected data after the screening was imported to STATA for further analysis using the following information of the articles: authors' affiliations, the title of papers, the journals' name, authors' keywords, the number of citations, research areas, and abstracts.

Several basic characteristics of the data sets were included publication year, the number of papers /per year, total citations up to 2018, average citation rate per year, total number of downloads in the last six months/five years, and average number of downloads (mean use rate) the last six months/five years. Two network graphs showing the countries collaboration and co-occurrence terms in title and abstracts were established by VOSviewer (version 1.16.15, Centre for Science and Technology Studies (CWTS), Leiden University, Leiden, The Netherlands). Latent dirichlet allocation (LDA) was used for classifying papers into topics [41–45]. The titles and abstracts of most cited papers within each group were reviewed. After discussing with COPD specialists, the labels for each topic were named. In addition to the number and percentage of publications of each topic, these topics were ranked based on the total number of publications in the past five years to explore the research interests. Table 1 shows the methods and results for each kind of data.

Table 1. Summary of analytical techniques for each data types.

Type of Data	Unit of Analysis	Analytical Methods	Presentations of Results
Terms, Countries	Words	Frequency of co-occurrence	Map of terms co-occurrence clusters
Abstracts	Papers	Latent Dirichlet Allocation	Ten classifications of research topics
WoS classification of research areas	WoS research areas	Frequency of co-occurrence	Dendrogram of research disciplines (WoS classification)

3. Results

Overall Growth and Essential Characteristics of Research

Table 2 described the basic characteristics of publications. The first seven papers related to this health issues in dataset were published in 1991. There has been a gradual raise in the annual number of papers on intervention to improve the QoL of patients with COPD within the period 1991–2018, contributing to a total of 3242 papers. The papers in 2018 showed the reading interests of readers in last six month with the average times of download (mean use rate) was 1.8; meanwhile, the papers in 2013 received the highest concern in last five years with average times of download (the mean use rate) was 2.1. The papers in the year 2000 had the highest average citation with 6.9 citations per paper.

Table 2. General characteristics of publications.

Year Published	Total Number of Papers	Total Citations	Mean Cite Rate per Year	Total Usage Last 6 Month	Total Usage Last 5 Years	Mean Use Rate Last 6 Month	Mean Use Rate Last 5 Year
2018	314	197	0.6	562	822	1.8	0.5
2017	295	1763	3.0	356	1756	1.2	1.2
2016	306	1946	2.1	254	2055	0.8	1.3
2015	270	3311	3.1	219	2198	0.8	1.6
2014	284	5101	3.6	177	2753	0.6	1.9
2013	234	3970	2.8	128	2451	0.5	2.1
2012	199	4653	3.3	78	1825	0.4	1.8
2011	189	6880	4.6	90	1424	0.5	1.5
2010	144	5733	4.4	75	1146	0.5	1.6
2009	128	5719	4.5	61	823	0.5	1.3
2008	127	6549	4.7	36	819	0.3	1.3
2007	109	5158	3.9	33	492	0.3	0.9
2006	107	6800	4.9	28	514	0.3	1.0
2005	86	4625	3.8	37	422	0.4	1.0
2004	75	5445	4.8	30	448	0.4	1.2
2003	62	6317	6.4	20	385	0.3	1.2
2002	56	5847	6.1	15	257	0.3	0.9
2001	40	2757	3.8	3	157	0.1	0.8
2000	43	5670	6.9	28	324	0.7	1.5
1999	28	1612	2.9	6	112	0.2	0.8
1998	32	3324	4.9	14	196	0.4	1.2
1997	29	2223	3.5	8	146	0.3	1.0
1996	18	2275	5.5	3	91	0.2	1.0
1995	16	1681	4.4	9	80	0.6	1.0
1994	10	1060	4.2	0	40	0.0	0.8
1993	12	559	1.8	4	20	0.3	0.3
1992	9	420	1.7	2	14	0.2	0.3
1991	7	426	2.2	0	11	0.0	0.3

The paper having the highest influence was the second report entitled Global Strategy for the Diagnosis, Management, and Prevention of COPD published in 2007 with 3456 citations [46].

Figure 1 shows countries collaboration network. In total, there were 89 countries contributing for the research field (automatically calculated by VOSviewer). In figure there were 64 countries with minimum of 5 papers. Of those, the United States of America led in the number of studies with 786 papers (24.2%), followed by England (452 papers, 13.9%), the Netherlands (322 papers, 9.9%), and Canada (268 papers, 8.3%). Although people living in low-and middle-income countries (LMICs) are more vulnerable to developing COPD [47], there was only China in the list of top 10 countries having the highest volume. As can ben seen, there were four main clusters in this countries network (1) Asia with the leadership of China in collaboration with two East European countries (Czech and Romania) (red cluster); (2) the U.S and South American countries (yellow cluster); (3) Canada, South Africa, New Zealandm and European countries (turquoise cluster); (4) European countries with three subgroups with the lead of France, the Netherlands, and England (the rest).

By analyzing abstracts and titles, the most co-occurrence terms were found to discover the scope of COPD research (Figure 2). Three major clusters were formed by 279 most common terms in title and abstract with the minimum appearance of 95 times. The three significant clusters are: Cluster 1 (red) refers to comorbidity and COPD, among which mental health illness (depression and anxiety) was most frequently mentioned. Cluster 2 (blue) focuses on interventions and treatment to increase QoL of people with COPD. Cluster 3 (yellow) points out the risk and mortality of exacerbation of COPD.

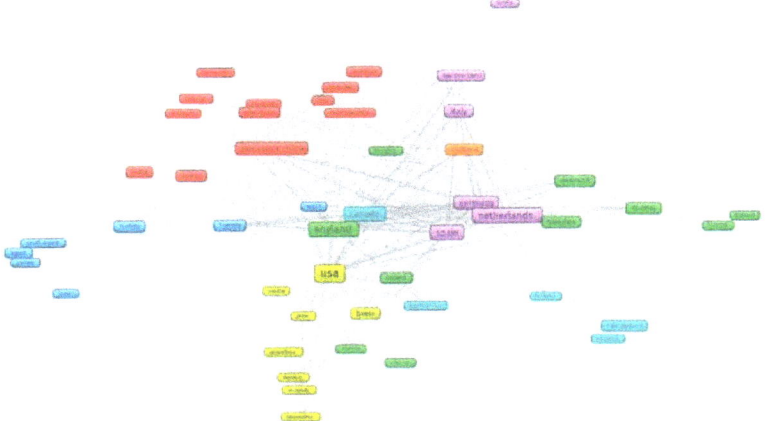

Figure 1. Countries collaboration network. Note: four main clusters, including (1) red cluster: Asia countries and two East European countries (Czech and Romania); (2) yellow cluster: the U.S and South American countries; (3) turquoise cluster Canada and South Africa, New Zealand and European countries; (4) the rest: European countries with three subgroups with the lead of France, the Netherlands and England.

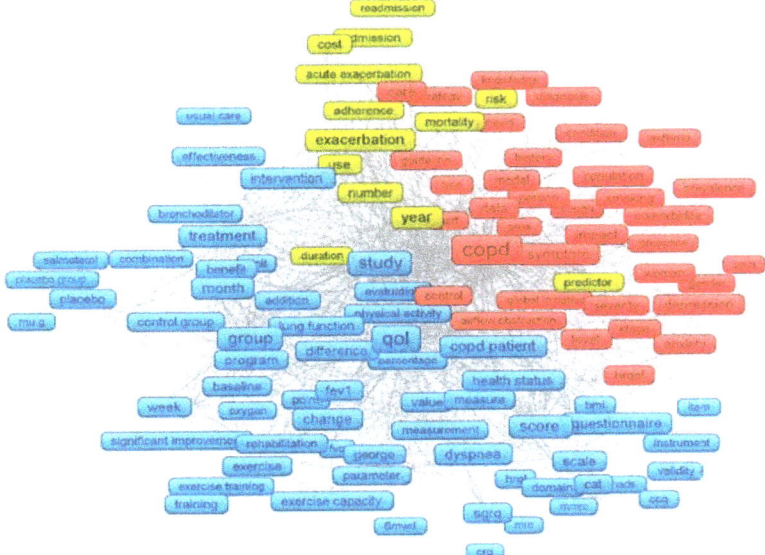

Figure 2. Text mining using VOSviewer (titles and abstracts). Note: the colors of each node were automatically assigned by VOSviewer based on its score; the node size was based on the frequency of each term; the length and thickness of the lines reflected the association between two terms. Cluster 1 (red) refers to comorbidity and COPD; cluster 2 (blue) focuses on interventions and treatment to increase QoL of people with COPD, cluster 3 (yellow) points out the risk and mortality of exacerbation of COPD.

Table 3 shows the most cited papers. Each had more than 100 citations during the study period. Based on the list, three main topics which have been recently attracted the attention of researchers were: (1) The Global Initiative for chronic obstructive lung disease (GOLD) reports and other national reports. GOLD was a consensus report published periodically since 2001. It included the latest evidence for diagnosis and prevention from experts, which were as "strategy documents" for adequate care for COPD at a global level [48] (paper 1, paper 7, paper 4, paper 9, paper 28, paper 36); (2) Exacerbations in patients with COPD (paper 2, paper 3, paper 12, paper 25, paper 29, paper 32); (3) Treatments and interventions of COPD (paper 5, paper 6, paper 11, paper 14, paper 15, paper 17, paper 19, paper 20, paper 23, paper 24, paper 27, paper 33, paper 34, paper 35, paper 39, paper 40), (4) QoL, health-related QoL and COPD (paper 26, paper 30, paper 31, and paper 41), others topic (rehabilitation—paper 8; COPD and comorbidity—paper 10; COPD and its effects to patient health and life—paper 22 and paper 37).

Applying latent dirichlet allocation in title and abstracts, ten major research topics were formed (Table 4). Topic 2 (n = 468 papers), Topic 1 (n = 436 papers), and topic 3 (n = 355 papers) were three topics with the highest volume of publications. Pulmonary rehabilitation has been a rapidly developed field in the last decades [49]. Further, improving QoL of patients living with COPD by pharmacological therapies (topic 6) or non-pharmacological therapies (topic 3, topic 10) has been a major area of focus. Notably, the domain of mental health received frequent attention from the scientific community with 436 papers. The reason for it could be that about 85% of people living with COPD were at high risk of developing anxiety disorders compared with healthy people [50].

Figure 3 shows the changes in the development of topics. Topic 1 in the last five years (2014–2018) had the highest number of published papers (n = 237), followed by topic 2 (n = 186) and topic 3 (n = 141).

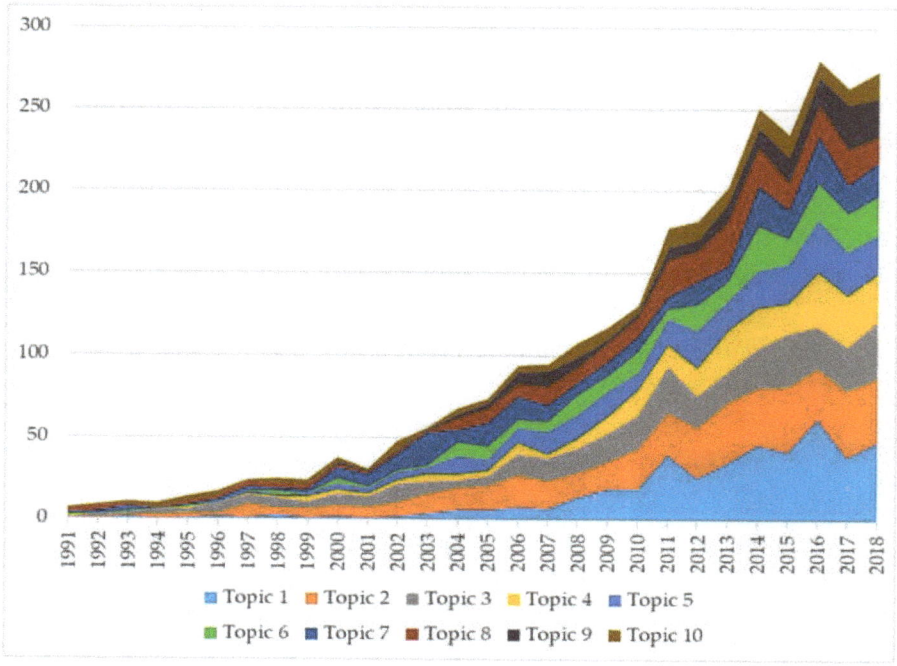

Figure 3. Changes in research topics development.

Table 3. Most cited papers.

No	Title	Total Citation	Published Year	Cite Rate
1	The body-mass index, airflow obstruction, dyspnea, and exercise capacity index in chronic obstructive pulmonary disease	2046	2004	136.4
2	A 4-year trial of tiotropium in chronic obstructive pulmonary disease	1390	2008	126.4
3	Susceptibility to Exacerbation in Chronic Obstructive Pulmonary Disease.	1298	2010	144.2
4	Effect of exacerbation on quality of life in patients with chronic obstructive pulmonary disease	1223	1998	58.2
5	Randomised, double blind, placebo-controlled study of fluticasone propionate in patients with moderate to severe chronic obstructive pulmonary disease: the ISOLDE trial*	964	2000	50.7
6	Development and first validation of the COPD Assessment Test	933	2009	93.3
7	Severe acute exacerbations and mortality in patients with chronic obstructive pulmonary disease	868	2005	62.0
8	Outcomes following acute exacerbation of severe chronic obstructive lung disease	863	1996	37.5
9	Combined salmeterol and fluticasone in the treatment of chronic obstructive pulmonary disease: a randomised controlled trial	749	2003	46.8
10	Chronic obstructive pulmonary disease: current burden and future projections	698	2006	53.7
11	Time course and recovery of exacerbations in patients with chronic obstructive pulmonary disease	655	2000	34.5
12	A long-term evaluation of once-daily inhaled tiotropium in chronic obstructive pulmonary disease	609	2002	35.8
13	Azithromycin for Prevention of Exacerbations of COPD	578	2011	72.3
14	Reduction of hospital utilization in patients with chronic obstructive pulmonary disease—A disease-specific self-management intervention	576	2003	36.0
15	Effects of pulmonary rehabilitation on physiological and psychosocial outcomes in patients with chronic obstructive pulmonary disease	568	1995	23.7
16	Efficacy and safety of budesonide/formoterol in the management of chronic obstructive pulmonary disease	550	2003	34.4
17	Results at 1 year of outpatient multidisciplinary pulmonary rehabilitation: a randomised controlled trial	536	2000	28.2
18	Dyspnea is a better predictor of 5-year survival than airway obstruction in patients with COPD	500	2002	29.4
19	Improved health outcomes in patients with COPD during 1 year's treatment with tiotropium	492	2002	28.9
20	Maintenance therapy with budesonide and formoterol in chronic obstructive pulmonary disease	472	2003	29.5
21	Global Strategy for the Diagnosis, Management, and Prevention of Chronic Obstructive Lung Disease 2017 Report	467	2017	233.5
22	Relation of sputum inflammatory markers to symptoms and lung function changes in COPD exacerbations	458	2000	24.1
23	Tiotropium in combination with placebo, salmeterol, or fluticasone-salmeterol for treatment of chronic obstructive pulmonary disease—A randomized trial	448	2007	37.3
24	Meta-analysis of respiratory rehabilitation in chronic obstructive pulmonary disease	443	1996	19.3
25	Risk factors of readmission to hospital for a COPD exacerbation: a prospective study	421	2003	26.3
26	Mortality after hospitalization for COPD	380	2002	22.4
27	Depressive symptoms and chronic obstructive pulmonary disease—Effect on mortality, hospital readmission, symptom burden, functional status, and quality of life	369	2007	30.8
28	How well do we care for patients with end stage chronic obstructive pulmonary disease (COPD)? A comparison of palliative care and quality of life in COPD and lung cancer	338	2000	17.8
29	Randomized controlled trial of respiratory rehabilitation	337	1994	13.5
30	Early therapy improves the chronic obstructive outcomes of exacerbations pulmonary disease	335	2004	22.3
31	Quality of life changes in COPD patients treated with salmeterol	331	1997	15.0
32	Prevalence of COPD in Spain: impact of undiagnosed COPD on quality of life and daily life activities	323	2009	32.3
33	A 6-month, placebo-controlled study comparing lung function and health status changes in COPD patients treated with tiotropium or salmeterol	323	2002	19.0
34	Health outcomes following treatment for six months with once daily tiotropium compared with twice daily salmeterol in patients with COPD	317	2003	19.8
35	Roflumilast—an oral anti-inflammatory treatment for chronic obstructive pulmonary disease: a randomised controlled trial	315	2005	22.5
36	Analysis of the factors related to mortality in chronic obstructive pulmonary disease—Role of exercise capacity and health status	314	2003	19.6
37	Interpreting thresholds for a clinically significant change in health status in asthma and COPD	313	2002	18.4
38	Short- and long-term effects of outpatient rehabilitation in patients with chronic obstructive pulmonary disease: A randomized trial	308	2000	16.2
39	Effect of exacerbations on quality of life in patients with chronic obstructive pulmonary disease: a 2 year follow up study	299	2004	19.9
40	Phosphodiesterase-4 inhibitors for asthma and chronic obstructive pulmonary disease	298	2005	21.3

Note: * The inhaled steroids in obstructive lung disease in Europe (ISOLDE).

Table 4. Research topics classified by LDA.

Rank by the Highest Volume	Research Topics	N	Percent
Topic 2	Pulmonary rehabilitation for COPD	468	16.30%
Topic 1	Comorbidities, mental health and QoL in COPD patients	436	15.20%
Topic 3	QoL of patients with COPD: validity of questionnaire	355	12.40%
Topic 5	Predictors for mortality due to acute exacerbation of COPD	287	10.00%
Topic 7	Pharmacological Therapy and COPD	272	9.50%
Topic 8	Management of COPD	257	9.00%
Topic 4	Multicomponent interventions: home care, rehabilitation, self-care education, integrated care, and pharmacy-led management	255	8.90%
Topic 6	Perception and QoL of patients living with COPD and their caregivers	217	7.60%
Topic 10	Noninvasive Ventilation and Oxygen Therapy in patient with COPD	160	5.60%
Topic 9	COPD Phenotype and quality of life	157	5.50%

Figure 4 shows the cluster of research areas in QoL of patients with COPD. The horizontal axis represents the distance between clusters, while the vertical axis displays the research areas [51]. The red lines show the depth for the cut-off of the analysis [52]. Research landscapes were divided into three main parts. The root (first group) in the top of the dendrogram included (a) respiratory system and (b) critical care medicine. This cluster had a close relationship with (1) intervention and health care such as general & internal medicine, pharmacy, nursing, and cardiovascular system (second group); (2) comorbidities, for instance, psychiatry, clinical psychology, clinical neurology (third group). However, the first group did not have a strong relatedness to the cluster in the bottom, such as rehabiliation or the integration of public health, environmental and occupational health (health care science & services; health policy & services, occupational &public, environment, interdiscriplinary social sciences).

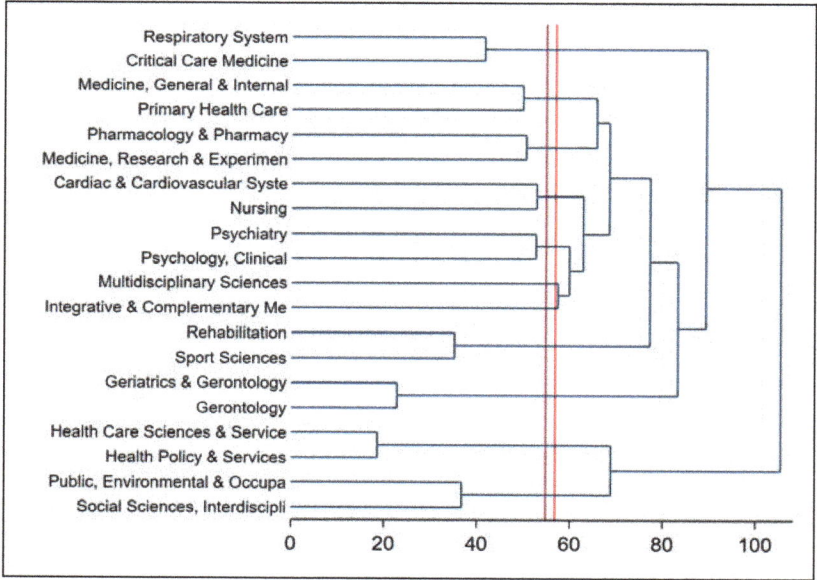

Figure 4. Dendrogram of coincidence of research areas.

4. Discussion

This study investigated the global trend of 3242 research publications regarding interventions to increase QoL of patients with COPD. It was found that the publications of research related to in topic increased annually and gradually, and most of the contribution came from high income countries

(HICs). Mental health issues and non-pharmacological therapy, including exercise, home care, self-care education, noninvasive ventilation, and oxygen therapy were common approaches. Current findings emphasize the importance of research that focuses on the effects of non-pharmacological therapy, which should be considered to increase QoL of people living with COPD. Additionally, mental health problems among people living with COPD have received more focus, especially in the last five years.

Notably, but unsurprisingly, a high number of research were conducted by authors from HICs than that of LMICs although more than 90% of COPD-related deaths occur in LMICs [53]. This work supports the conclusion of previous studies, which confirmed the main contribution of HICs in diabetes research [54] or HIV/AIDS research [55]. This phenomenon may be explained by the fact that risk factor prevention has not been fully recognized by the LMICs' governments and populations, including using biomass fuels indoors for cooking [56] or occupational exposure [57]. Moreover, many LMICs faced the barriers in research and implication planning, such as information and communication technology limitations [58], lack of human resources and finance, and scientific findings [59]. Therefore, the support of HICs and actively joining in collaboration network with HICs are critical to LMICs [60].

Chronic obstructive pulmonary disease is a chronic disorder, which requires a long-term treatment with complementary and alternative therapy to reduce exacerbation and improve patients' QoL [61]. Our finding were in line with the results of previous studies, which emphasized that pharmacological therapy [62], exercise [63], non-invasive ventilation [64], and oxygen therapy [65] increase the QoL of people living with COPD. In our study, the number of papers mentioning pharmacological treatment was in the top five of highest volume of work by LDA. It showed the concern of researchers and physicians on this therapy to control the symptoms in stable COPD as well as improve QoL of people suffered COPD. It confirmed the results of some papers which emphasize the effectiveness of pharmacotherapy in controlling symptoms to decrease recurrence and seriousness of exacerbations and improve QoL [66,67]. However, this topic rose at a lower level in the last five years compared with non-pharmacy therapies, such as mental health, or rehabilita. The results might be explained by the efficiency of the alternative therapies in improving the quality of life, controlling symptoms in daily life and when exacerbations occur [68], and reducing the frequency of hospitalization [69].

Furthermore, the topics receiving the most attention in the last five years were comorbidities and mental health issues in patients with COPD. A previous study showed that about one-third of patients living with COPD with depression or anxiety did not received appropriate treatment [50]. The comorbid condition of mental illness can increase the risk of exacerbations, reduce QoL, and raise the chance of mortality [70,71]. Thus, mental health illness should receive further piority, which may help to increase QoL among patients living with COPD [72].

The results provide some evidence to enhance designing interventions, health research, and policy. Most of the death cases related to COPD happened in LMICs, yet, most of the studies were conducted in HICs. The health research capacity in LMICs is lower than that of HICs could be explained by (1) the limitation of infrastructure and capacity [73], (2) a lack of investment funding in universities and research institutions, low wages for researchers [74], and (3) a lack of clear national research priorities [74]. Therefore, LMICs need to (1) actively create collaboration research networks with HICs and (2) prepare the national research priorities under the circumstance of understanding the local context. Moreover, the LMICs' national health research priorities should be considered when international organizations or donors from HICs invest in LMICs. Secondly, we call for multidisciplinary collaboration of researchers and physicians among research areas, especially between psychological and respiratory physiologists since the complexity of this disease and negatives effects of depression and anxiety to patients with COPD.

Several limitations of this study should be mentioned. Firstly, WOS was the only database used in the analysis. However, for a large number of papers for analysis, there was a high possibility that these articles were in other databases, including PubMed and Scopus. Secondly, only English publications were included. Thus, it was more likely that our study did not reflect the trend in COPD research where English is not used. Finally, only titles and abstracts were used for topic modeling. However, by applying a different level of data and alternative method, the trends and hidden themes of the research studies could be discovered [74].

5. Conclusions

The findings of the study show that the interventions to increase QoL of patients with COPD has attracted increasing research interest in the last two decades. Non-pharmacological therapy and mental health problems were two common approaches. In addition, increasing support from HICs to LMICs in research together with the multidisciplinary collaboration of research areas are needed to improve the QoL of people living with COPD in LMICs.

Author Contributions: Conceptualization, G.V.V., G.H.H., H.Q.P., C.A.L. and R.C.M.H.; Data curation, G.H.H., C.T.N. and H.Q.P.; Formal analysis, G.H.H., C.T.N., G.T.V., H.Q.P. and B.X.T.; Investigation, G.V.V., B.X.T. and C.S.H.H.; Methodology, G.H.H., C.T.N. and B.X.T.; Project administration, G.T.V. and C.S.H.H.; Software, C.T.N.; Supervision, G.V.V., C.A.L. and B.X.T.; Validation, G.V.V., C.A.L., R.C.M.H. and C.S.H.H.; Writing—original draft, G.H.H., G.V.V.and H.Q.P.; Writing—review & editing, G.V.V., C.A.L. and R.C.M.H. All authors have read and agreed to the published version of the manuscript.

Funding: This research received no external funding.

Conflicts of Interest: The authors declare no conflict of interest.

Appendix A

Table A1. Search query for "Quality of life" and "well-being".

No	Search Query	Search Result
# 1	TS = ("quality of life")	355,541
# 2	TS = ("well-being")	104,048
# 3	#2 OR #1	441,617
# 4	#2 OR #1 Refined by: [excluding] Publication Years: (2019)	437,253
# 5	#2 OR #1 Refined by: [excluding] Publication Years: (2019) AND [excluding] Document Types: (Meeting Abstract Or Proceedings Paper Or Editorial Material Or Book Chapter Or Letter Or Book Review Or Correction Or Note Or News Item Or Book Or Reprint Or Early Access Or Retracted Publication Or Biographical Item Or Correction Addition Or Discussion Or Data Paper Or Retraction Or Bibliography Or Fiction Creative Prose Or Item About An Individual Or Poetry Or Software Review)	353,171
# 6	#2 OR #1 Refined by: [excluding] Publication Years: (2019) AND [excluding] Document Types: (Meeting Abstract Or Proceedings Paper Or Editorial Material Or Book Chapter Or Letter Or Book Review Or Correction Or Note Or News Item Or Book Or Reprint Or Early Access Or Retracted Publication Or Biographical Item Or Correction Addition Or Discussion Or Data Paper Or Retraction Or Bibliography Or Fiction Creative Prose Or Item About An Individual Or Poetry Or Software Review) AND [excluding] Document Types: (Tv Review Radio Review)	353,170
# 7	#2 OR #1 Refined by: [excluding] Publication Years: (2019) AND [excluding] Document Types: (Meeting Abstract Or Proceedings Paper Or Editorial Material Or Book Chapter Or Letter Or Book Review Or Correction Or Note Or News Item Or Book Or Reprint Or Early Access Or Retracted Publication Or Biographical Item Or Correction Addition Or Discussion Or Data Paper Or Retraction Or Bibliography Or Fiction Creative Prose Or Item About An Individual Or Poetry Or Software Review) AND [excluding] Document Types: (Tv Review Radio Review) AND [excluding]Languages: (German Or Spanish Or French Or Portuguese Or Russian Or Turkish Or Polish Or Italian Or Korean Or Czech Or Hungarian Or Croatian Or Greek Or Dutch Or Japanese Or Slovenian Or Slovak Or Lithuanian Or Serbian Or Persian Or Malay Or Romanian Or Chinese Or Icelandic Or Arabic Or Afrikaans Or Norwegian Or Ukrainian Or Danish Or Catalan Or Swedish Or Estonian Or Bulgarian Or Serbo Croatian Or Galician Or Georgian Or Esperanto Or Finnish Or Hebrew Or Indonesian Or Welsh)	327,627
# 8	AU = ("Anonymous" OR "anonymous")	1,406,800
# 9	#7 NOT #8	327,405

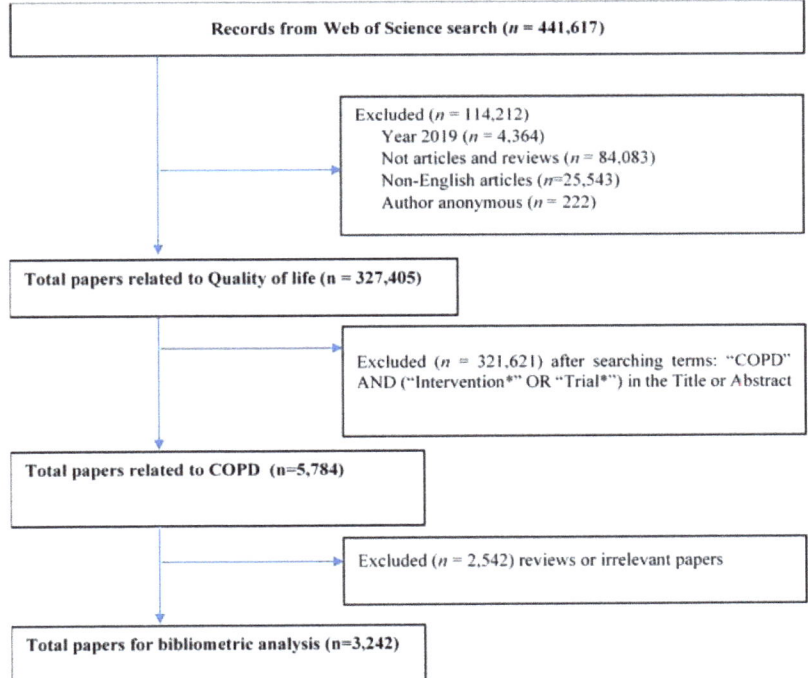

Figure A1. Selection of papers.

References

1. World Health Organization. Chronic obstructive pulmonary disease: Definition. Available online: https://www.who.int/respiratory/copd/definition/en/ (accessed on 12 July 2019).
2. OECD/EUROPEAN UNION 2016. Asthma and COPD prevalence. In *Health at a Glance: Europe 2016–State of Health in the EU Cycle*; OECD Publishing: Paris, France, 2016. [CrossRef]
3. Group, R.C.W. COPD prevalence in 12 Asia–Pacific countries and regions: Projections based on the COPD prevalence estimation model. *Respirology* **2003**, *8*, 192–198.
4. National Center for Chronic Disease Prevention and Health Promotion. COPD Prevalence in the United States. Available online: https://www.cdc.gov/copd/data.html (accessed on 12 July 2019).
5. Mehrotra, A.; Akanbi, M.O.; Gordon, S.B. The burden of COPD in Africa: A literature review and prospective survey of the availability of spirometry for COPD diagnosis in Africa. *Trop. Med. Int. Health TM IH* **2009**, *14*, 840–848. [CrossRef] [PubMed]
6. Adeloye, D.; Basquill, C.; Papana, A.; Chan, K.Y.; Rudan, I.; Campbell, H. An estimate of the prevalence of COPD in Africa: A systematic analysis. *Copd J. Chronic Obstr. Pulm. Dis.* **2015**, *12*, 71–81. [CrossRef] [PubMed]
7. Peruzza, S.; Sergi, G.; Vianello, A.; Pisent, C.; Tiozzo, F.; Manzan, A.; Coin, A.; Inelmen, E.; Enzi, G. Chronic obstructive pulmonary disease (COPD) in elderly subjects: Impact on functional status and quality of life. *Respir. Med.* **2003**, *97*, 612–617. [CrossRef] [PubMed]
8. Agusti, À.; Soriano, J.B. COPD as a systemic disease. *Copd J. Chronic Obstr. Pulm. Dis.* **2008**, *5*, 133–138. [CrossRef] [PubMed]
9. Agusti, A.; Calverley, P.M.; Celli, B.; Coxson, H.O.; Edwards, L.D.; Lomas, D.A.; MacNee, W.; Miller, B.E.; Rennard, S.; Silverman, E.K. Characterisation of COPD heterogeneity in the ECLIPSE cohort. *Respir. Res.* **2010**, *11*, 122. [CrossRef]

10. Restrepo, M.I.; Sibila, O.; Anzueto, A. Pneumonia in patients with chronic obstructive pulmonary disease. *Tuberc. Respir. Dis. (Seoul)* **2018**, *81*, 187–197. [CrossRef]
11. Chaouat, A.; Naeije, R.; Weitzenblum, E. Pulmonary hypertension in COPD. *Eur. Respir. J.* **2008**, *32*, 1371–1385. [CrossRef]
12. Quint, J. The Relationship between COPD and Cardiovascular Disease. *Tanaffos* **2017**, *16*, S16–S17.
13. Maurer, J.; Rebbapragada, V.; Borson, S.; Goldstein, R.; Kunik, M.E.; Yohannes, A.M.; Hanania, N.A.; Anxiety, A.W.P.O.; Depression, C. Anxiety and depression in COPD: Current understanding, unanswered questions, and research needs. *Chest* **2008**, *134*, 43S–56S. [CrossRef]
14. Kim, H.F.S.; Kunik, M.E.; Molinari, V.A.; Hillman, S.L.; Lalani, S.; Orengo, C.A.; Petersen, N.J.; Nahas, Z.; Goodnight-White, S. Functional impairment in COPD patients: The impact of anxiety and depression. *Psychosomatics* **2000**, *41*, 465–471. [CrossRef] [PubMed]
15. Spruit, M.A.; Vercoulen, J.H.; Sprangers, M.A.G.; Wouters, E.F.M. Fatigue in COPD: An important yet ignored symptom. *Lancet Respir. Med.* **2017**, *5*, 542–544. [CrossRef]
16. Franssen, F.M.E.; Smid, D.E.; Deeg, D.J.H.; Huisman, M.; Poppelaars, J.; Wouters, E.F.M.; Spruit, M.A. The physical, mental, and social impact of COPD in a population-based sample: Results from the Longitudinal Aging Study Amsterdam. *NPJ Prim. Care Respir. Med.* **2018**, *28*, 30. [CrossRef]
17. Price, D.; Small, M.; Milligan, G.; Higgins, V.; Gil, E.G.; Estruch, J. Impact of night-time symptoms in COPD: A real-world study in five European countries. *Int. J. Chron. Obs. Pulmon. Dis.* **2013**, *8*, 595. [CrossRef] [PubMed]
18. Stephenson, J.J.; Cai, Q.; Mocarski, M.; Tan, H.; Doshi, J.A.; Sullivan, S.D. Impact and factors associated with nighttime and early morning symptoms among patients with chronic obstructive pulmonary disease. *Int. J. Chron. Obs. Pulmon. Dis.* **2015**, *10*, 577. [CrossRef]
19. World Health Organization. WHOQOL: Measuring Quality of Life. Available online: https://www.who.int/healthinfo/survey/whoqol-qualityoflife/en/ (accessed on 21 April 2020).
20. Gandhi, S.K.; Kong, S.X. Quality-of-life measures in the evaluation of antihypertensive drug therapy: Reliability, validity, and quality-of-life domains. *Clin. Ther.* **1996**, *18*, 1276–1295. [CrossRef]
21. Taylor, S.H. Drug therapy and quality of life in angina pectoris. *Am. Heart J.* **1987**, *114*, 234–240. [CrossRef]
22. Wright, E.K.; Kamm, M.A. Impact of drug therapy and surgery on quality of life in Crohn's disease: A systematic review. *Inflamm. Bowel Dis.* **2015**, *21*, 1187–1194. [CrossRef]
23. Benzo, R.P.; Abascal-Bolado, B.; Dulohery, M.M. Self-management and quality of life in chronic obstructive pulmonary disease (COPD): The mediating effects of positive affect. *Patient Educ. Couns.* **2016**, *99*, 617–623. [CrossRef]
24. Tran, B.X.; Harijanto, C.; Vu, G.T.; Ho, R.C. Global Mapping of Interventions to improve Quality of Life using Mind-body therapies during 1990–2018. *Complementary Ther. Med.* **2020**, *49*, 102350. [CrossRef]
25. Hawthorne, G.; Richardson, J.; Osborne, R. The Assessment of Quality of Life (AQoL) instrument: A psychometric measure of health-related quality of life. *Qual. Life Res. Int. J. Qual. Life Asp. Treat. Care Rehabil.* **1999**, *8*, 209–224. [CrossRef] [PubMed]
26. Feldman, G.J. Improving the quality of life in patients with chronic obstructive pulmonary disease: Focus on indacaterol. *Int. J. Chron. Obs. Pulmon. Dis.* **2013**, *8*, 89. [CrossRef] [PubMed]
27. Godtfredsen, N.S.; Lam, T.H.; Hansel, T.T.; Leon, M.; Gray, N.; Dresler, C.; Burns, D.; Prescott, E.; Vestbo, J. COPD-related morbidity and mortality after smoking cessation: Status of the evidence. *Eur. Respir. J.* **2008**, *32*, 844–853. [CrossRef] [PubMed]
28. Zamarro, C.G.; Bernabé, M.B.; Santamaría, B.R.; Rodríguez, J.H. Smoking in COPD. *Arch. De Bronconeumol.* **2011**, *47*, 3–9.
29. Antus, B. Pharmacotherapy of Chronic Obstructive Pulmonary Disease: A Clinical Review. *ISRN Pulmonol.* **2013**, *2013*, 11. [CrossRef]
30. Safka, K.A.; McIvor, R.A. Non-pharmacological management of chronic obstructive pulmonary disease. *Ulst. Med. J.* **2015**, *84*, 13–21.
31. Ahn, E.; Kang, H. Introduction to systematic review and meta-analysis. *Korean J. Anesth.* **2018**, *71*, 103–112. [CrossRef]
32. Gregersen, T.L.; Green, A.; Frausing, E.; Ringbæk, T.; Brøndum, E.; Suppli Ulrik, C. Do telemedical interventions improve quality of life in patients with COPD? A systematic review. *Int. J. Chron. Obs. Pulmon. Dis.* **2016**, *11*, 809–822. [CrossRef]

33. Coronini-Cronberg, S.; Heffernan, C.; Robinson, M. Effective smoking cessation interventions for COPD patients: A review of the evidence. *JRSM Short Rep.* **2011**, *2*, 1–12. [CrossRef]
34. Papadopoulos, G.; Vardavas, C.I.; Limperi, M.; Linardis, A.; Georgoudis, G.; Behrakis, P. Smoking cessation can improve quality of life among COPD patients: Validation of the clinical COPD questionnaire into Greek. *BMC Pulm. Med.* **2011**, *11*, 13. [CrossRef]
35. Ubolnuar, N.; Tantisuwat, A.; Thaveeratitham, P.; Lertmaharit, S.; Kruapanich, C.; Mathiyakom, W. Effects of Breathing Exercises in Patients With Chronic Obstructive Pulmonary Disease: Systematic Review and Meta-Analysis. *Ann. Rehabil. Med.* **2019**, *43*, 509–523. [CrossRef] [PubMed]
36. Alvarez, G.R.; Vanz, S.A.S.; Barbosa, M.C. Scientometric indicators for Brazilian research on High Energy Physics, 1983–2013. *An. Da Acad. Bras. De Ciências* **2017**, *89*, 2525–2543. [CrossRef] [PubMed]
37. Begum, M.; Lewison, G.; Wright, J.S.; Pallari, E.; Sullivan, R. European non-communicable respiratory disease research, 2002–2013: Bibliometric study of outputs and funding. *PLoS ONE* **2016**, *11*. [CrossRef] [PubMed]
38. Sweileh, W.M.; Al-Jabi, S.W.; Sa'ed, H.Z.; Sawalha, A.F. Bronchial asthma and chronic obstructive pulmonary disease: Research activity in Arab countries. *Multidiscip. Respir. Med.* **2014**, *9*, 38. [CrossRef] [PubMed]
39. Martín-Martín, A.; Orduna-Malea, E.; Delgado López-Cózar, E. Coverage of highly-cited documents in Google Scholar, Web of Science, and Scopus: A multidisciplinary comparison. *Scientometrics* **2018**, *116*, 2175–2188. [CrossRef]
40. Clarivate Analytics. Web of Science databases. Available online: https://clarivate.com/products/web-of-science/databases/ (accessed on 26 June 2019).
41. Li, Y.; Rapkin, B.; Atkinson, T.M.; Schofield, E.; Bochner, B.H. Leveraging Latent Dirichlet Allocation in processing free-text personal goals among patients undergoing bladder cancer surgery. *Qual. Life Res. Int. J. Qual. Life Asp. Treat. Care Rehabil.* **2019**. [CrossRef]
42. Valle, D.; Albuquerque, P.; Zhao, Q.; Barberan, A.; Fletcher, R.J., Jr. Extending the Latent Dirichlet Allocation model to presence/absence data: A case study on North American breeding birds and biogeographical shifts expected from climate change. *Glob. Chang. Biol.* **2018**, *24*, 5560–5572. [CrossRef]
43. Chen, C.; Zare, A.; Trinh, H.N.; Omotara, G.O.; Cobb, J.T.; Lagaunne, T.A. Partial Membership Latent Dirichlet Allocation for Soft Image Segmentation. *IEEE Trans. Image Process. A Publ. IEEE Signal. Process. Soc.* **2017**, *26*, 5590–5602. [CrossRef]
44. Lu, H.M.; Wei, C.P.; Hsiao, F.Y. Modeling healthcare data using multiple-channel latent Dirichlet allocation. *J. Biomed. Inform.* **2016**, *60*, 210–223. [CrossRef]
45. Gross, A.; Murthy, D. Modeling virtual organizations with Latent Dirichlet Allocation: A case for natural language processing. *Neural Netw. Off. J. Int. Neural Netw. Soc.* **2014**, *58*, 38–49. [CrossRef]
46. Rabe, K.F.; Hurd, S.; Anzueto, A.; Barnes, P.J.; Buist, S.A.; Calverley, P.; Fukuchi, Y.; Jenkins, C.; Rodriguez-Roisin, R.; van Weel, C.; et al. Global strategy for the diagnosis, management, and prevention of chronic obstructive pulmonary disease: GOLD executive summary. *Am. J. Respir. Crit. Care Med.* **2007**, *176*, 532–555. [CrossRef] [PubMed]
47. World Health Organization. *Global Status Report on Noncommunicable Diseases 2014*; World Health Organization: Geneva, Switzerland, 2014.
48. Global Initiative for Chronic Obstructive Lung Disease. *Global Strategy for the Diagnosis, Management, and Prevention of COPD*; Global Initiative for Chronic Obstructive Lung Disease, Inc.: Fontana, WI, USA, 2019.
49. Troosters, T.; Gosselink, R.; Janssens, W.; Decramer, M. Exercise training and pulmonary rehabilitation: New insights and remaining challenges. *Eur. Respir. Rev.* **2010**, *19*, 24–29. [CrossRef] [PubMed]
50. Yohannes, A.M.; Alexopoulos, G.S. Depression and anxiety in patients with COPD. *Eur. Respir. Rev.* **2014**, *23*, 345–349. [CrossRef] [PubMed]
51. STATA. Cluster Dendrogram—Dendrograms for Hierarchical Cluster Analysis. Available online: https://www.stata.com/manuals13/mvclusterdendrogram.pdf (accessed on 22 April 2020).
52. Moffat, D.; Ronan, D.; Reiss, J.D. Unsupervised taxonomy of sound effects. *Context* **2017**. *6*, 7.
53. Laniado-Laborin, R. Smoking and chronic obstructive pulmonary disease (COPD). Parallel epidemics of the 21 century. *Int. J. Environ. Res. Public Health* **2009**, *6*, 209–224. [CrossRef] [PubMed]
54. Tran, B.X.; Nguyen, L.H.; Pham, N.M.; Vu, H.T.T.; Nguyen, H.T.; Phan, D.H.; Ha, G.H.; Pham, H.Q.; Nguyen, T.P.; Latkin, C.A. Global Mapping of Interventions to Improve Quality of Life of People with Diabetes in 1990–2018. *Int. J. Environ. Res. Public Health* **2020**, *17*, 1597. [CrossRef]

55. Vu, G.T.; Tran, B.X. Global Research on Quality of Life of Patients with HIV/AIDS: Is It Socio-Culturally Addressed? (GAP(RESEARCH)). *Int. J. Environ. Res. Public Health* **2020**, *17*, 2127. [CrossRef]
56. Torres-Duque, C.; Maldonado, D.; Perez-Padilla, R.; Ezzati, M.; Viegi, G. Biomass fuels and respiratory diseases: A review of the evidence. *Proc. Am. Thorac. Soc.* **2008**, *5*, 577–590. [CrossRef]
57. Pleasants, R.A.; Riley, I.L.; Mannino, D.M. Defining and targeting health disparities in chronic obstructive pulmonary disease. *Int. J. Chron. Obs. Pulmon. Dis.* **2016**, *11*, 2475–2496. [CrossRef]
58. Bezuidenhout, L.; Chakauya, E. Hidden concerns of sharing research data by low/middle-income country scientists. *Glob. Bioeth. Probl. Di Bioet.* **2018**, *29*, 39–54. [CrossRef]
59. Ritchie, L.M.P.; Khan, S.; Moore, J.E.; Timmings, C.; van Lettow, M.; Vogel, J.P.; Khan, D.N.; Mbaruku, G.; Mrisho, M.; Mugerwa, K. Low-and middle-income countries face many common barriers to implementation of maternal health evidence products. *J. Clin. Epidemiol.* **2016**, *76*, 229–237. [CrossRef] [PubMed]
60. Nuwayhid, I.A. Occupational health research in developing countries: A partner for social justice. *Am. J. Public Health* **2004**, *94*, 1916–1921. [CrossRef] [PubMed]
61. Viniol, C.; Vogelmeier, C.F. Exacerbations of COPD. *Eur. Respir. Rev.* **2018**, *27*, 170103. [CrossRef] [PubMed]
62. Montuschi, P. Pharmacological treatment of chronic obstructive pulmonary disease. *Int. J. Chron. Obs. Pulmon. Dis.* **2006**, *1*, 409. [CrossRef] [PubMed]
63. Xu, Y.; Wang, J.; Li, H.; Zhu, X.; Wang, G. Efficacy of integrative respiratory rehabilitation training in exercise ability and quality of life of patients with chronic obstructive pulmonary disease in stable phase: A randomized controlled trial. *Zhong Xi Yi Jie He Xue Bao J. Chin. Integr. Med.* **2010**, *8*, 432–437. [CrossRef] [PubMed]
64. Díaz-Lobato, S.; Alises, S.M.; Rodríguez, E.P. Current status of noninvasive ventilation in stable COPD patients. *Int. J. Chron. Obs. Pulmon. Dis.* **2006**, *1*, 129–135. [CrossRef]
65. Murphy, P.B.; Rehal, S.; Arbane, G.; Bourke, S.; Calverley, P.M.A.; Crook, A.M.; Dowson, L.; Duffy, N.; Gibson, G.J.; Hughes, P.D.; et al. Effect of Home Noninvasive Ventilation With Oxygen Therapy vs Oxygen Therapy Alone on Hospital Readmission or Death After an Acute COPD Exacerbation: A Randomized Clinical Trial. *JAMA* **2017**, *317*, 2177–2186. [CrossRef]
66. National Institute for Health and Care Excellence. *Chronic Obstructive Pulmonary Disease in over 16s: Diagnosis and Management Evidence Reviews for Self Management, Education and Telehealth*; National Institute for Health and Care Excellence: London, UK, 2018.
67. Zwerink, M.; Brusse-Keizer, M.; van der Valk, P.D.; Zielhuis, G.A.; Monninkhof, E.M.; van der Palen, J.; Frith, P.A.; Effing, T. Self management for patients with chronic obstructive pulmonary disease. *Cochrane Database Syst. Rev.* **2014**. [CrossRef]
68. Smith, M.C.; Wrobel, J.P. Epidemiology and clinical impact of major comorbidities in patients with COPD. *Int. J. Chron. Obs. Pulmon. Dis.* **2014**, *9*, 871. [CrossRef]
69. Cavaillès, A.; Brinchault-Rabin, G.; Dixmier, A.; Goupil, F.; Gut-Gobert, C.; Marchand-Adam, S.; Meurice, J.-C.; Morel, H.; Person-Tacnet, C.; Leroyer, C. Comorbidities of COPD. *Eur. Respir. Rev.* **2013**, *22*, 454–475. [CrossRef]
70. Australian Institute of Health and Welfare. COPD, associated Comorbidities and Risk Factors. Available online: https://www.aihw.gov.au/reports/chronic-respiratory-conditions/copd-associated-comorbidities-risk-factors/contents/about-copd-and-associated-comorbidities (accessed on 17 June 2019).
71. Khanal, P. Bringing all together for research capacity building in LMICs. *Lancet Glob. Health* **2017**, *5*, e868. [CrossRef]
72. ESSENCE on Health Research. *Seven Principle for Strengthening Research Capacity in Low-and-middle-income Countries: Simple Ideas in a Complex World*; TDR/World Health Organization: Geneva, Switzerland, 2014.
73. Ali, N.; Hill, C.; Kennedy, A.; IJsselmuiden, C.C. COHRED Record Paper 5. In *What Factors Influence National Health Research Agendas in Low and Middle Income Countries?* Council on Health Research for Development (COHRED): Geneva, Switzerland, 2006.
74. Wang, H.; Wu, F.; Lu, W.; Yang, Y.; Li, X.; Li, X.; Zhuang, Y. Identifying Objective and Subjective Words via Topic Modeling. *IEEE Trans. Neural Netw. Learn. Syst.* **2018**, *29*, 718–730. [CrossRef] [PubMed]

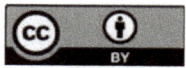

© 2020 by the authors. Licensee MDPI, Basel, Switzerland. This article is an open access article distributed under the terms and conditions of the Creative Commons Attribution (CC BY) license (http://creativecommons.org/licenses/by/4.0/).

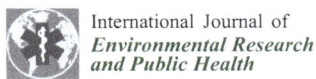
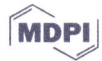

Article

Global Research on Quality of Life of Patients with HIV/AIDS: Is It Socio-Culturally Addressed? (GAP_{RESEARCH})

Giang Thu Vu [1], Bach Xuan Tran [2,3], Chi Linh Hoang [4], Brian J. Hall [3,5], Hai Thanh Phan [6], Giang Hai Ha [6,*], Carl A. Latkin [3], Cyrus S.H. Ho [7] and Roger C.M. Ho [4,8,9]

1. Center of Excellence in Evidence-Based Medicine, Nguyen Tat Thanh University, Ho Chi Minh City 700000, Vietnam; giang.coentt@gmail.com
2. Institute for Preventive Medicine and Public Health, Hanoi Medical University, Hanoi 100000, Vietnam; bach.ipmph@gmail.com
3. Bloomberg School of Public Health, Johns Hopkins University, Baltimore, MD 21205, USA; brianhall@umac.mo (B.J.H.); carl.latkin@jhu.edu (C.A.L.)
4. Center of Excellence in Behavioral Medicine, Nguyen Tat Thanh University, Ho Chi Minh City 700000, Vietnam; chi.coentt@gmail.com (C.L.H.); pcmrhcm@nus.edu.sg (R.C.M.H.)
5. Global and Community Mental Health Research Group, University of Macau, Macau 999078, China
6. Institute for Global Health Innovations, Duy Tan University, Da Nang 550000, Vietnam; haipt.ighi@gmail.com
7. Department of Psychological Medicine, National University Hospital, Singapore 119074, Singapore; cyrushosh@gmail.com
8. Department of Psychological Medicine, Yong Loo Lin School of Medicine, National University of Singapore, Singapore 119228, Singapore
9. Institute for Health Innovation and Technology (iHealthtech), National University of Singapore, Singapore 119077, Singapore
* Correspondence: giang.ighi@gmail.com; Tel.: +84-8-6954-8561

Received: 21 December 2019; Accepted: 19 March 2020; Published: 23 March 2020

Abstract: Quality of life (QOL) has been considered as an important outcome indicator in holistic care for HIV-infected people, especially as HIV/AIDS transforms from a fatal illness to a chronic condition. This study aimed to identify trends and emerging topics among research concerning the QOL of people living with HIV/AIDS (PLWHA). The analyzed data were English papers published from 1996 to 2017, searched and extracted from the Web of Science Core Collection. Collaborations between countries and the correlation between the keywords were visualized by VOSviewer while the abstracts' content was analyzed using exploratory factor analysis and Jaccard's' similarity index. There has been an increase in both the number of publications and citations. The United Nations of America leads in terms of paper volume. The cross-nation collaborations are mainly regional. Despite a rather comprehensive coverage of topics relating to QOL in PLWHA, there has evidently been a lack of studies focusing on socio-cultural factors and their impacts on the QOL of those who are HIV-infected. Further studies should consider investigating the role of socio-cultural factors, especially where long-term treatment is involved. Policy-level decisions are recommended to be made based on the consideration of cultural factors, while collaborations between developed and developing nations, in particular in HIV/AIDS-ridden countries, are strongly recommended.

Keywords: scientometrics; HIV/AIDS; bibliometric; quality of life

1. Introduction

Human immunodeficiency viruses (HIV) is one of the leading causes of disability and mortality worldwide, with more than 76.1 infected people and 35.0 million deaths [1–3]. In 2017, there were

1.8 million people newly infected with HIV and Acquired immunodeficiency syndrome (AIDS), 36.9 million people living with HIV and AIDS (PLWHA), and 940,000 deaths related to life-threatening infections and cancers [4]. Hence, ensuring sufficient care and treatment, as well as treatment provision, has become a challenge for global public health systems.

Quality of life (QOL), as noted by the existing literature, has been described as an umbrella term for a variety of human needs, including the position in life, goals, standards, expectations, and concerns in the context of the culture and value systems. It manifests within patients as symptomatic, social functioning, and spirituality [5]. In terms of health promotion, health-related quality of life (HRQOL) is also considered as a priority health indicator. Since 1996, optimizing adherence to Antiretroviral Therapy (ART) has brought the chance to transform HIV—an incurable disease—into a chronic health condition [6], which in turn prolongs the life of PLWHA and improves their QOL [6]. In many settings, poor QOL is associated with a lower immune response, non-adherence, poor mental health, and greater disease severity [7–9]. Therefore, QOL attracted great attention from regulatory authorities and health providers as an important outcome to evaluate the effectiveness of HIV treatment [10–13]. People who were effectively treated with HAART, however, have been found to have a lower QOL compared with other long-term chronic illnesses [14]. Over time, the expansion of HAART coverage not only prolonged the life expectancy of PLWHA, but also boosted the innovation of new QOL instruments to adapt to the complexity of care. The previous literature has reported a high burden of comorbidities suffered by PLWHA, as well as adverse side impacts of long-term treatment on their health [15,16], while a complex combination of psychological and social factors which also influence their physical, mental and social conditions, directly and indirectly, affect their QOL [17–22]. On the other hand, in recent years, the availability of early HIV diagnosis, antiretroviral (ARV) treatments and enhanced healthcare services have been found to support the improvement in the QOL of PLWHA [23].

Thus, in order to improve the quality and effectiveness of HIV/AIDS treatment and prevention programs, qualitative as well as quantitative analyses on the QOL of PLWHA are needed. In 2017, Cooper, et al. conducted a systematic review on the finding of existing reviews on QOL of the HIV/AIDS-infected population in various aspects, including the development, validation, and effectiveness of the most commonly used instruments [12]. Though informative, reviews of such kind suffer from the limitation of a narrow focus on specific questions or issues. In order to broaden the scope of research, a new approach is needed that has the ability to cover a large volume of global data on QOL in PWLHA research and allows for complex analysis to identify the research trend [12,18,24,25].

Our study adopts the scientometrics approach that gathers and analyze publications on a global level, coupled with more a technical analysis approach applied to the content of papers' title and abstract to identify emerging research topics as well as the current level of international collaboration in research on the QOL of PLWHA. This study aims to supplement the current literature while uncovering research gaps, suggest directions for future studies, and act as a reference point for priority settings and strategies initiating in HIV/AIDS management.

2. Materials and Methods

2.1. Study Design

Serving as the best approach to evaluate evidence, the increase in the number of systematic reviews of QOL regarding HIV/AIDS could provide an insightful view of various aspects, including evaluating the effectiveness of instruments, clinical intervention, and HIV/AIDS programs in vulnerable populations. In addition to having a limited scope of research; such reviews also remain lack of the comparison of findings over time and overlap with information. Several researchers use bibliometrics with the expectation that it could fill the gap in the literature and provide the research trend using quantitative analysis. It can be seen that the bibliometric approach sometimes could not draw a full picture because the majority only present the number without a comprehensive reading of the literature [26]. In order to provide a comprehensive view of the current status of the quality of life in terms of the HIV/AIDS literature, we conducted the scientometric approach combined with content analysis.

The current study is a part of a larger project, Global Analysis for Policy in Research (GAPRESEARCH), that aims to set priorities in global health evolution and provide empirical evidence for designing effective interventions and policies [27–32]. The findings of this study, therefore, can be used as a reference point for directing investments, allocating resources, and crafting policies.

2.2. Search Strategy

A search for HIV/AIDS publications was performed on the Web of Science (WoS) Core Collection. This database was prioritized because it has covered all scientific publications with full cited reference indexing since 1900 and allowed downloading information with a diversity of research disciplines that far outweigh other databases such as Scopus or MEDLINE [32].

We applied a search query containing the search terms of "HIV" OR "human-immunodeficiency-virus" OR "AIDS" OR "Acquired-Immune-Deficiency-Syndrome". Data were extracted in a unit of 500 publications from the first publication in the dataset end up in 2017. As the process was conducted in July 2018, we excluded all papers published in 2018 as the partial coverage of publications published in 2018 would not fully reflect the publication trend of the year. The selection criteria for study subjects were English peer-review articles, including original articles and reviews (see Figure A1). Any paper with anonymous or no authors would be excluded. In the next step, we continue refined relevant research by using the research term "quality of life", articles could be removed if they did not include "quality of life" in titles and abstracts. Any disagreement during the screening process could be discussed with a senior researcher.

2.3. Summary Measures

The retrieved data consisting mainly of publication indexes were contained the following information: Title; years of publication; the total number of papers; citations up to 2017; usages/number of downloads; keywords (authors' keywords); authors' affiliations; most prolific countries and collaborations. In order to describe the change of publication over time, we calculated several fundamental domains including the speed of publication (total number of papers), the level of reader attention (mean cited rate per year), the level of short-term and long-term interest (mean usage rate last 6 months/5 years). We also illustrated the major topic clusters and landscapes of QOL in the field of HIV/AIDS by calculating the frequency of co-occurrence of keywords and synthesized from abstract's content.

2.4. Data Analysis

The extracted data were sorted by Macro in Microsoft Excel to calculate the indexes. The connection among countries by sharing co-authorships' data (we applied full counting for papers sharing by more than one country), networks of co-occurrence authors' keywords, and clusters of topic groups were visualized by VOSviewer (version 1.6.11, Center for Science and Technology, Leiden University, the Netherlands). The cluster topics of QO were then identified from the frequency of keywords and named by expert opinions.

The exploratory factor analysis (EFA) and Jaccard's similarity index were performed using STATA software version 15.0. This index was defined as the magnitude of the intersection divided by the magnitude of the union of two sets of co-occurring terms; thus, multi-dimensional scaling could be used to adjust a point for a topic category, the distance between items and color presented the partnership of certain key terms. To measure the likelihood of research trends (e.g., emerging research domains and landscapes), we utilized exploratory factor analysis (EFA), which allows us to test the variance in the domains and landscape appearing from the abstract's contents. The summary of the technique used for analyzing is described in Table A1.

3. Results

Table 1 shows an expansion in the volume of publications on QOL among HIV/AIDS populations. The period between 2007 and 2017 saw the number of papers grow from 114 to 234. In particular, the total citation (from the year published up to 2017) has also risen remarkably in 2005 and 2013.

Table 1. General indicators of publications

Year Published	Total Number of Papers	Total Citations	Mean Cite Rate per Year [1]	Total Usage* Last 6 Months	Total Usage* Last 5 Years	Mean Use Rate Last 6 Months [2]	Mean Use Rate Last 5 Years [3]
2017	234	11,965	51.1	356	1,151	1.5	1.0
2016	215	11,221	26.1	211	1,619	1.0	1.5
2015	218	10,985	16.8	174	1,972	0.8	1.8
2014	211	9,638	11.4	107	1,891	0.5	1.8
2013	213	9,866	9.3	96	2,286	0.5	2.1
2012	185	8,773	7.9	52	1,692	0.3	1.8
2011	169	8,476	7.2	65	1,315	0.4	1.6
2010	167	7,462	5.6	46	1,160	0.3	1.4
2009	140	6,445	5.1	62	908	0.4	1.3
2008	122	5,468	4.5	53	818	0.4	1.3
2007	114	5,639	4.5	33	622	0.3	1.1
2006	96	4,588	4.0	41	606	0.4	1.3
2005	112	5,265	3.6	61	767	0.5	1.4
2004	80	3,746	3.3	36	414	0.4	1.0
2003	73	3,012	2.8	25	374	0.3	1.0
2002	58	2,579	2.8	10	226	0.2	0.8
2001	51	2,163	2.5	11	264	0.2	1.0
2000	66	2,759	2.3	11	309	0.2	0.9
1999	49	2,291	2.5	13	212	0.3	0.9
1998	56	2,385	2.1	16	214	0.3	0.8
1997	39	1,708	2.1	7	128	0.2	0.7
1996	44	1,455	1.5	11	169	0.3	0.8

* Usage: downloaded time; [1] Mean cited rate per year = Total citations/(Total citations × (2018-that year)); [2] Mean usage rate last 6 months = Total usage last 6 months/Total number of papers; [3] Mean use rate last 5 years = total usage last 5 years/(total number of papers × 5).

Table 2 indicates the frequency of countries by counting such study settings in the mentioned abstracts. In the top 10, except countries with the highest HIV prevalence, such as South Africa, the number of studies were mostly produced in upper-middle-income and high-income countries (United States, Brazil, China, Canada, Thailand, England, Australia) [33]. The low and middle-income countries such as Botswana, Zambia, Lesotho, Swaziland had below 10 papers, even though these countries have been reported as having the highest rate of HIV/AIDS [34].

Figure 1 displays the global network between 102 countries having co-authorships of selected papers. These countries have been classified into 10 clusters of at least five countries, depending on their level of international collaboration.

Cluster 1 (red) refers to the network of countries in the two regions: South-East Asia and the Western Pacific. Cluster 2 (purple) indicates the link of the USA with European countries and Saudi Arabia. Cluster 3 (blue) illustrates international collaborations between the Americas, South Africa, and some countries in Asia. Cluster 4 (brown and green) demonstrates the co-authorship between countries within Southeast Africa. In addition, they have an additional link with England. The European countries tend to associate with each other by geographical areas, such as orange, pink, light blue, and yellow (French West Africa).

Table 2. A number of papers by countries as study settings.

No.	Country Settings	Frequency	%	No.	Country Settings	Frequency	%
1	United States	271	21.1%	31	Sweden	8	0.6%
2	South Africa	108	8.4%	32	Zambia	8	0.6%
3	India	74	5.8%	33	Cambodia	7	0.5%
4	Brazil	60	4.7%	34	Ghana	7	0.5%
5	China	60	4.7%	35	Lesotho	7	0.5%
6	Uganda	52	4.0%	36	Netherlands	7	0.5%
7	Canada	42	3.3%	37	Swaziland	7	0.5%
8	Thailand	32	2.5%	38	Switzerland	7	0.5%
9	United Kingdom	30	2.3%	39	Hong Kong	6	0.5%
10	Australia	29	2.3%	40	Jamaica	6	0.5%
11	Ethiopia	27	2.1%	41	Japan	6	0.5%
12	Niger	25	1.9%	42	Nepal	6	0.5%
13	Nigeria	25	1.9%	43	Germany	5	0.4%
14	Malawi	21	1.6%	44	Mexico	5	0.4%
15	Viet Nam	20	1.6%	45	Peru	5	0.4%
16	Ireland	19	1.5%	46	Wallis and Futuna	5	0.4%
17	Taiwan	18	1.4%	47	Colombia	4	0.3%
18	Rwanda	17	1.3%	48	Georgia	4	0.3%
19	Kenya	15	1.2%	49	Haiti	4	0.3%
20	Iran	14	1.1%	50	Jersey	4	0.3%
21	Spain	14	1.1%	51	Portugal	4	0.3%
22	Tanzania	14	1.1%	52	Romania	4	0.3%
23	Zimbabwe	14	1.1%	53	Singapore	4	0.3%
24	Malaysia	13	1.0%	54	Burkina Faso	3	0.2%
25	Cameroon	12	0.9%	55	Democratic Republic of the Congo	3	0.2%
26	Italy	12	0.9%	56	Republic of the Congo	3	0.2%
27	France	11	0.9%	57	Finland	3	0.2%
28	Botswana	9	0.7%	58	Guinea	3	0.2%
29	Indonesia	9	0.7%	59	Lebanon	3	0.2%
30	Puerto Rico	8	0.6%	60	Mali	3	0.2%

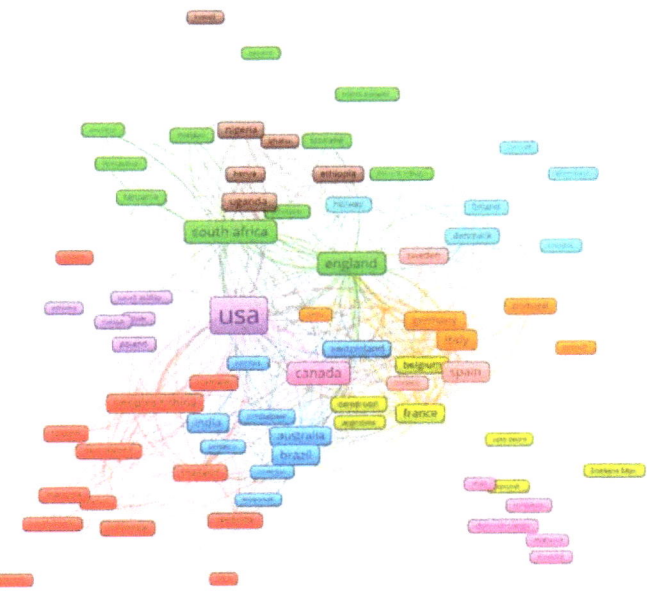

Figure 1. The network of 102 countries having international co-authorships in quality of life research in HIV/AIDS.

Figure 2 describes the core components of the keywords with the most common groups of terms. There were four major clusters that emerged from 205 most frequent co-occurrence keywords with a minimum frequency of 20 times. Three major clusters (red, blue, and green) indicate three topics of quality of life.

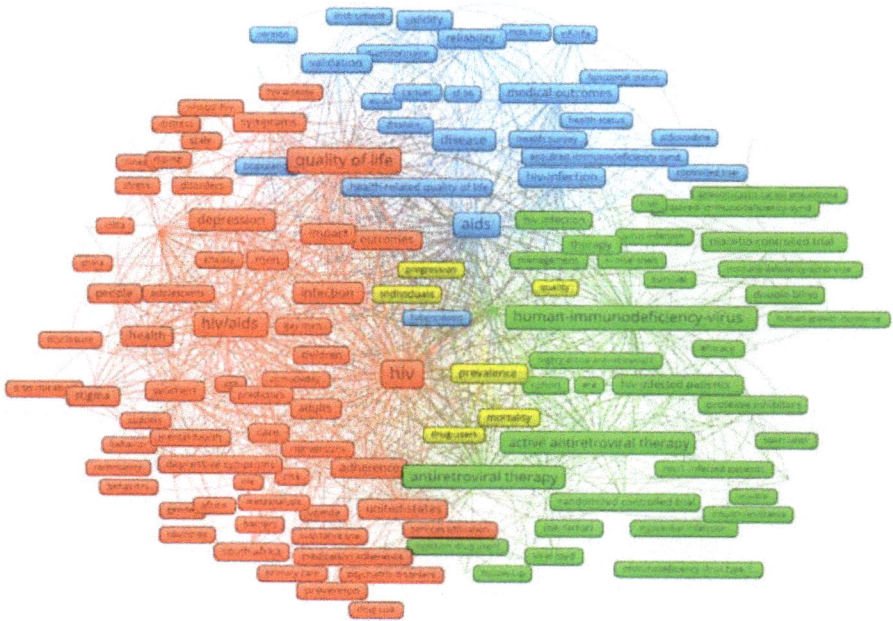

Figure 2. The most common author keywords. Note: the principal components of the data structure were visualized regarding the colors of the nodes; the node size was identified by the keywords' occurrences; the closer the nodes are, the stronger the association between two keywords are.

Cluster 1 (red) covers mental health, social, and associated factors. It includes psychological disorders (depression, anxiety, stress); social behavior (stigma, discrimination); specific HIV groups (such as gay, children, women, and men), and regions (India, South Africa, Uganda). Cluster 2 (blue) presents physical health-related aspects: treatment, outcome, mortality, and disability. Cluster 3 (green) indicates ART adherence studies: study design and laboratory results.

The top 50 emerging research domains have been discovered from the content analysis of abstracts using exploratory factor analysis (Table 3). Mental health (62.6% of papers containing mental health-related keywords) appears to receive more attention from researchers compared to other health problems (e.g., chronic conditions 23.4%, or cost-effectiveness 37.5%). Other major domains cover coping strategies and social support. Nearly half of the articles have keywords related to the randomized and controlled trial. Meanwhile, the keywords concern comorbidities account for less than 10%.

Figure 3 illustrates the similarity between QOL and the top 50 co-occurrence terms. In particular, physical, social, and health were the most common terms that co-occurred with QOL in all abstracts. The term related to women was more common than that of men in the literature. Antiretroviral, treatment, and infection were also co-occurrence terms with a high frequency of appearance.

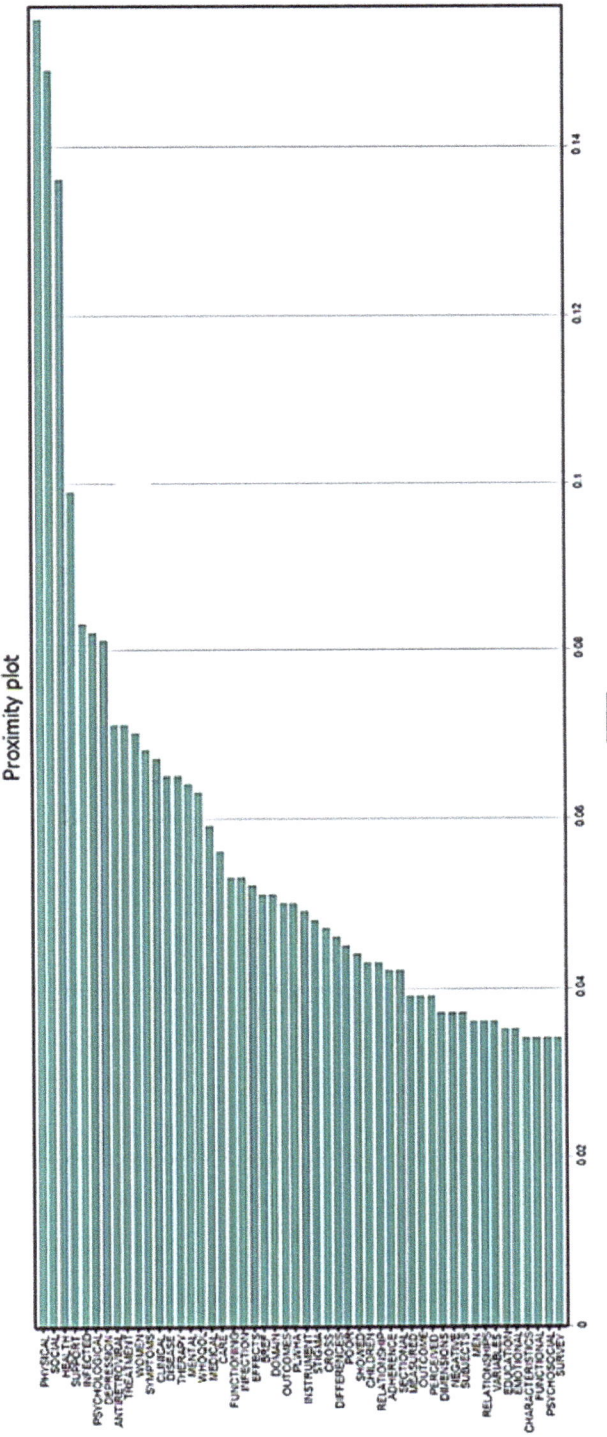

Figure 3. Proximity Plots of "quality of life" with the top 50 most frequent concurrence terms in abstracts.

Table 3. Top 50 research domains emerged from exploratory factor analysis of all abstracts' contents.

Name	Keywords	Eigen Value	FREQ	% Cases
Mental health summary	Medical Outcomes Study (MOS); summary; mental; survey; physical; scores; medical; score; health related quality of life (HRQOL); outcomes; short form (SF)	26.1	4123	62.60%
Criteria; controlled trials	Criteria; trials; objectives; controlled; main; evidence; performed; review; evaluate	1.9	2357	48.90%
The World Health Organization Quality of Life brief (WHOQOL-BREF); Domain	WHOQOL; BREF; Domain; domains; world; version; QOL; psychological; social	3.3	2335	44.20%
Randomized; Controlled trial	Randomized; trial; placebo; controlled; weeks; week; groups; primary; intervention	7.2	2312	39.30%
Cost-effectiveness; costs	Cost; costs; effectiveness; effective; economic; model; year	1.9	1643	37.50%
Coping strategies; social support	Coping; strategies; support; social	1.3	1522	37.10%
Depressive; anxiety and depression	Depressive; depression; symptoms; anxiety; psychiatric; psychological	2.7	1722	36.10%
Reliability and validity; item scale	Validity; reliability; item; items; instrument; factor; scales; measure; good; scale	2.2	1923	36.10%
Care access	Access; services; care	1.3	1220	33.40%
Role functioning	Role; function; cognitive; functioning	1.5	1025	27.30%
Viral load; count	Load; viral; count; counts; cells	1.8	1384	27.00%
Literature; review	Literature; review; evidence	5	919	24.10%
Sex; men and women	Sexual; men; sex; women	1.8	1002	23.90%
Chronic conditions	Conditions; chronic; diseases	1.6	840	23.40%
Stigma; disclosure	Stigma; disclosure; perceived; negative	3.7	837	23.20%
Cross-sectional	Sectional; cross; prevalence	2.5	1128	23.00%
Side effects	Side; effects	1.5	815	22.80%
Follow-up period	Period; follow; month; year	2.3	852	22.50%
Body mass; fat loss	Mass; body; fat; weight; kg; loss; nutritional; exercise; testosterone; index	3.3	1169	21.40%
Drug users	Users; methadone; drug; substance	2.3	766	21.00%
Outcome measures	Outcome; measures	1.3	718	20.60%
Control	Controls; control; intervention	1.7	712	20.10%
Anti; development	Anti; development; resistance; therapeutic	1.2	712	19.70%
Palliative; cancer pain	Palliative; cancer; advanced; pain	1.9	620	18.20%
Adherence to medication	Medication; adherence	1.6	639	18.10%
Developed countries	Countries; developed; settings	1.2	600	18.00%
Screening; early	Screening; early; settings	1.2	500	15.50%
Combination	Combination; response	1.3	416	13.50%
Demographic	Demographic; characteristics	1.5	456	13.40%
Children	Children; adoslescents; caregivers; family	1.7	499	13.30%
EuroQOL (EQ); HRQOL demension	EQ; HRQOL; Dimensions	1.6	445	13.30%
Reduction	Reduction; improvement	1.4	407	13.10%
Morbidity and mortality	Mortality; morbidity	1.7	497	12.60%
Inhibitor; protease inhibitor (PI) regimens	Inhibitor; PI; regimen; regimens	3.1	498	12.20%
Death	Death; hospital	1.3	357	12.00%
Emotional	Emotional; functional	1.3	358	11.80%
Exercise	Exercise; activity; week	1.3	374	11.70%

Table 3. *Cont.*

Name	Keywords	Eigen Value	FREQ	% Cases
Moderate to severe	Severe; moderate; haemophilia	1.5	390	11.70%
Long-term	Term; long	2.1	522	11.20%
Adverse effect	Events; adverse	1.4	426	11.20%
Cytomegalovirus (CMV); Prophylaxis	CMV; prophylaxis; infections	1.4	348	10.80%
South Africa	South; Africa	2	344	8.60%
Food	Food; people living with HIV (PLHIV); nutritional	1.3	225	6.90%
Facial	Facial; satisfaction	1.3	177	5.90%
Hepatitis	Hepatitis; hepatitis C virus (HCV)	1.9	215	5.60%
Sleep	Sleep; fatigue	1.4	155	4.80%
Failure	Failure	1.4	120	4.30%
Anemia	Anemia	1.4	49	1.70%
Diarrhea	Diarrhea	1.5	44	1.60%
Tuberculosis (TB)	TB	1.4	38	1.40%

4. Discussion

By analyzing the volume and abstract contents of global publications on the QOL of PLWHA during 1996–2017, our research captured and visualized the level of attention, current research trends, and the global networking of researches. The results show rather extensive coverage of topics in the existing literature, ranging from physical-related aspects to mental health, from issues concerning clinical trials to social support. Nonetheless, the current bibliography shows the lack of socio-cultural factors involved in the development and measurement of QOL.

Our study reports an increase in the number of papers using QOL as an important instrument for evaluating HIV/AIDS interventions since 1996, when highly active antiretroviral therapy (HAART) was first introduced [6]. This result is in line with a study conducted by Eltony et al., which confirmed an increasing trend in the volume of publications on QOL of PLWHA [35]. On the other hand, our findings draw a troubling picture regarding the degree of inequality in contributions and collaborative partnerships across settings. While most HIV incidence is located in LMICs, for instance, nearly 70% of individuals infected with HIV live in Sub-Saharan Africa [36], the highest amount of relevant studies belonged to high-income countries. It is widely acknowledged that the combination of low socioeconomic conditions and limited access to health services result in increasing HIV prevalence in sub-Saharan Africa, the Caribbean, and Central Asia [37]. Therefore, these countries may be more focused on the prevention of HIV transmission rather than investing interventions to improve mental health or social situation, for instance, to reduce stigma against HIV patients when accessing general health facilities. The reduction in global funds for HIV—the major source of financing for HIV/AIDS management in LMICs—would also lead to a lack of funding for the crucial activities of collecting empirical data, planning essential investigations, and HIV/AIDS management strategies [38]. Meanwhile, cross-regional collaborations, and especially research partnerships between high-income countries and their low-middle-income counterparts, have been found to still be rather limited (Figure 1). These findings call for more collaboration efforts between developed and developing nations, in which support both in terms of finance and knowledge/ technology should be transferred from advanced to disadvantaged regions. In addition, further research in favor of economic evaluation should be conducted to identify the appropriate interventions in the context of limited funding for HIV/AIDS management.

Knowing the association between the QOL of PLWHA and the effectiveness of HIV programs, QOL has been used as a criteria in assessing HIV/AIDS prevention programs, clinical treatment, and harm reduction strategies [39–41]. This is reflected in the finding of our study, as terms relating to QOL measurements like MOS-HIV, EQ-5D, SF-36, and WHOQOL-HIV are found to frequently co-occur with QOL in analyzed publications (Figure 2), while the EFA of abstract content identifies QOL measurements to be an emerging research domain (Table 3). EQ-5D and SF-36 have been broadly used thanks to their ability to be adopted for economic analyses. Meanwhile, MOS-HIV and WHOQOL-HIV have been developed and validated as QOL measurements specifically for the HIV/AIDS-infected population [42–46].

Even with the advancement of health services as well as the high ART coverage, the HIV/AIDS programs remain complex, contextual, and are often referred to as complicated because appropriate recommendations vary according to subpopulation and epidemiological context [23]. Previous studies have reported that in LMIC, a combination of factors, instead only one or two major ones, have major impacts on optimal adherence and rates of virological suppression when a patient is lost to follow-up [23]. The combined language and ethnicity profile of a country has been found to significantly influence culturally sensitive healthcare services—those at risk of HIV infection may face delayed treatment initiation and access to prevention services in regions where stigma against infectious diseases is common, for instance [47]. Some of the most HIV/AIDS-ridden nations in North-Central Africa, such as Cameroon, Nigeria, and the Democratic Republic of the Congo, have been found to also be the most culturally diverse countries [48]. The absence of culture-related terms like language, belief and religion in the keywords and abstract content of our analyzed publications suggest a gap in the research concerning the QoL of PLWHA. Further studies thus may consider assessing the role of cultural factors on QoL of PLWHA, as well as the impacts of diverse beliefs, for instance, on the effectiveness of the programs initiated to improve the QoL of those infected with HIV. Similarly, those involved in developing HIV/AIDS management programs, including policy-makers and non-governmental organizations, should take into account the impact of cultural factors.

The analysis of a principal component of terms in titles and abstracts reveals that QOL tends to co-occur with terms relating to mental disorders and high-risk populations, including adolescents, children, women, and gay. Disclosure, discrimination, and stigma have also been found to appear together with the aforementioned terms, along with keywords like barriers and primary care (Figure 2). This finding suggests that topics on the mental health consequences of HIV infection and its treatments, barriers to treatment due to stigmatization and social-related issues like reluctance to disclose have been covered in the existing literature. The focus on single domains of QOL, such as physical [14,49,50], psychological [49,51–53], social [50,52–54], and environmental [55,56] can be said to be common in research concerning QOL among PLWHA. However, given the complex, multi-dimensional nature of the QOL construct, the lack of contextualized factors (sociological perspective, culture, religion for instance) in the titles and abstracts of published papers, as our results reveal, can undermine the power and scope of impact of QOL on PLWHA and the effectiveness of treatments. Therefore, further studies are encouraged to address more contextualized factors and consider adopting multiple QOL measures when attempting to evaluate the association and influence of QOL on PLWHA.

Despite the positive findings of the study, several limitations should be mentioned. As our search strategy was conducted via Web of Science Core Collection solely and only English reviews and articles were included, despite the extensive coverage of WoS and the dominance of English publications, there is a chance that relevant publications not recorded in such a database and/or in other languages would be missed. Our decision to use only the term "quality of life" when conducting a publication search would also filter out possibly related papers where variations of the construct such as "satisfaction with life", "well-being"; "satisfaction" or "value of life" were used instead. Thus, further researches are strongly encouraged to consider investigating deviations of "quality of life" both as a term and a concept, especially research with a sociological focus. In addition, future studies may also be conducted in the form of systematic reviews and meta-analyses, for instance, on how QOL can or has been used as a measurement for assessing the effectiveness of HIV/AIDS treatments or interventions.

5. Conclusions

Using bibliometrics analysis, we illustrate the development and current global trends of research on the QOL of PLWHA. Meanwhile, the results of the text mining techniques adopted provide a picture of current emerging research trends and topics and highlight research gaps. Despite a rather comprehensive coverage of topics relating to QOL in PLWHA, there has evidently been a lack of studies focusing on socio-cultural factors and their impacts on the QOL of those that are HIV-infected. Further studies should consider investigating the role of socio-cultural factors, especially where long-term treatment is involved. Policy-level decisions are recommended to be made based on the consideration of cultural factors, while collaborations between developed and developing nations, in particular with HIV/AIDS-ridden countries, are strongly recommended.

Author Contributions: Conceptualization, G.T.V., C.L.H., H.T.P., G.H.H. and R.C.M.H.; Data curation, B.J.H., H.T.P. and C.A.L.; Formal analysis, B.X.T., C.L.H., B.J.H. and H.T.P.; Funding acquisition, C.S.H.H. and G.H.H.; Investigation, B.X.T., B.J.H. and C.A.L.; Methodology, B.X.T., C.L.H., C.S.H.H. and G.H.H.; Project administration, G.T.V. and R.C.M.H.; Software, C.A.L. and G.H.H.; Supervision, G.T.V. and R.C.M.H.; Validation, C.S.H.H. and R.C.M.H.; Visualization, C.S.H.H.; Writing—original draft, G.T.V.; Writing—review and editing, G.T.V., B.X.T., C.L.H., B.J.H., H.T.P., C.A.L., C.S.H.H., G.H.H. and R.C.M.H. All authors have read and agreed to the published version of the manuscript.

Funding: This research received no external funding

Acknowledgments: Not applicable.

Conflicts of Interest: The authors declare no conflict of interest.

Appendix A

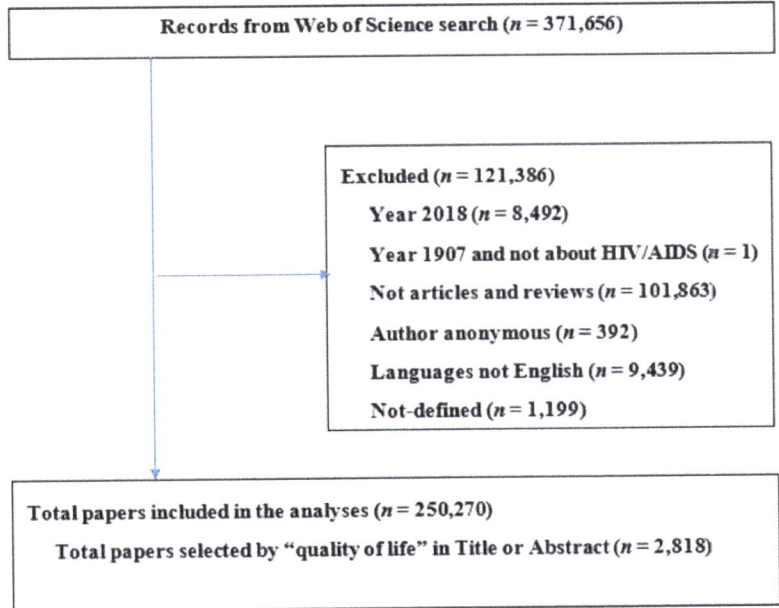

Figure A1. Selection of papers. The searching and paper selection process identified 250,270 related to HIV/AIDS. Among those, 2818 papers included the terms "quality of life".

Table A1. Summary of the techniques and methods.

Type of Data	Unit of Analysis	Analytical Methods	Presentations of Results
Abstracts Keywords	Words	Frequency of co-occurrence	1. The number of articles by countries mentioned in the abstract 2. Networks of co-occurrence authors' keywords 3. Networks of countries by sharing co-authorships data
Abstracts	WoS research domains	Exploratory factor analysis	1. Top 50 research domains
Abstracts	Words	Jaccard's similarity index	1. Top 50 most frequent co-occurrence terms

References

1. Fauci, A.S. The AIDS epidemic–considerations for the 21st century. *N. Engl. J. Med.* **1999**, *341*, 1046–1050. [CrossRef]
2. World Health Organization. Data on the size of the HIV/AIDS epidemic. Available online: http://apps.who.int/gho/data/view.main.22100WHO?lang=en (accessed on 26 January 2019).
3. GBD 2015 HIV Collaborators. Estimates of Global, Regional, and National Incidence, Prevalence, and Mortality of HIV, 1980–2015: The Global Burden of Disease Study 2015. *Lancet HIV* **2016**, *3*, e361–e387. [CrossRef]
4. UNAIDS. Global HIV & AIDS statistics—2018 fact sheet. Available online: Aidsinfo.unaids.org (accessed on 12 December 2019).
5. Dennison, C.R. The role of patient-reported outcomes in evaluating the quality of oncology care. *Am. J. Manag. Care* **2002**, *8*, S580–S586.
6. Hudelson, C.; Cluver, L. Factors associated with adherence to antiretroviral therapy among adolescents living with HIV/AIDS in low- and middle-income countries: A systematic review. *AIDS Care* **2015**, *27*, 805–816. [CrossRef] [PubMed]
7. Safren, S.A.; Hendriksen, E.S.; Smeaton, L.; Celentano, D.D.; Hosseinipour, M.C.; Barnett, R.; Guanira, J.; Flanigan, T.; Kumarasamy, N.; Klingman, K.; et al. Quality of life among individuals with HIV starting antiretroviral therapy in diverse resource-limited areas of the world. *AIDS Behav.* **2012**, *16*, 266–277. [CrossRef] [PubMed]
8. Nojomi, M.; Anbary, K.; Ranjbar, M. Health-related quality of life in patients with HIV/AIDS. *Arch. Iran. Med.* **2008**, *11*, 608–612.
9. Pereira, M.; Canavarro, M.C. Gender and age differences in quality of life and the impact of psychopathological symptoms among HIV-infected patients. *AIDS Behav.* **2011**, *15*, 1857–1869. [CrossRef]
10. Wu, A.W.; Mathews, W.C.; Brysk, L.T.; Atkinson, J.H.; Grant, I.; Abramson, I.; Kennedy, C.J.; McCutchan, J.A.; Spector, S.A.; Richman, D.D. Quality of life in a placebo-controlled trial of zidovudine in patients with AIDS and AIDS-related complex. *J. Acquir. Immune Defic. Syndr.* **1990**, *3*, 683–690.
11. Freedberg, K.A.; Losina, E.; Weinstein, M.C.; Paltiel, A.D.; Cohen, C.J.; Seage, G.R.; Craven, D.E.; Zhang, H.; Kimmel, A.D.; Goldie, S.J. The cost effectiveness of combination antiretroviral therapy for HIV disease. *N. Engl. J. Med.* **2001**, *344*, 824–831. [CrossRef]
12. Cooper, V.; Clatworthy, J.; Harding, R.; Whetham, J.; Emerge, C. Measuring quality of life among people living with HIV: A systematic review of reviews. *Health Qual. Life Outcomes* **2017**, *15*, 220. [CrossRef]
13. Ragsdale, D.; Morrow, J.R.J.N.R. Quality of life as a function of HIV classification. *Nurs. Res.* **1990**, *39*, 355–359. [CrossRef] [PubMed]
14. Miners, A.; Phillips, A.; Kreif, N.; Rodger, A.; Speakman, A.; Fisher, M.; Anderson, J.; Collins, S.; Hart, G.; Sherr, L.J.T.l.H. Health-related quality-of-life of people with HIV in the era of combination antiretroviral treatment: A cross-sectional comparison with the general population. *Lancet HIV* **2014**, *1*, e32–e40. [CrossRef]
15. Hasan, S.S.; Keong, S.C.; Choong, C.L.; Ahmed, S.I.; Ching, T.W.; Anwar, M.; Ahmadi, K.; Babar, M.G. Patient-reported adverse drug reactions and drug-drug interactions: A cross-sectional study on Malaysian HIV/AIDS patients. *Med. Princ. Pract.* **2011**, *20*, 265–270. [CrossRef] [PubMed]
16. Boyer, S.; Protopopescu, C.; Marcellin, F.; Carrieri, M.P.; Koulla-Shiro, S.; Moatti, J.P.; Spire, B.; Group, E.S. Performance of HIV care decentralization from the patient's perspective: Health-related quality of life and perceived quality of services in Cameroon. *Health Policy Plan.* **2012**, *27*, 301–315. [CrossRef] [PubMed]

17. Liu, C.; Johnson, L.; Ostrow, D.; Silvestre, A.; Visscher, B.; Jacobson, L.P. Predictors for lower quality of life in the HAART era among HIV-infected men. *J. Acquir. Immune Defic. Syndr.* **2006**, *42*, 470–477. [CrossRef]
18. Drewes, J.; Gusy, B.; Ruden, U. More than 20 years of research into the quality of life of people with HIV and AIDS–a descriptive review of study characteristics and methodological approaches of published empirical studies. *J. Int. Assoc. Provid. AIDS Care* **2013**, *12*, 18–22. [CrossRef]
19. Mafirakureva, N.; Dzingirai, B.; Postma, M.J.; van Hulst, M.; Khoza, S. Health-related quality of life in HIV/AIDS patients on antiretroviral therapy at a tertiary care facility in Zimbabwe. *AIDS Care* **2016**, *28*, 904–912. [CrossRef]
20. Aranda-Naranjo, B. Quality of life in the HIV-positive patient: Implications and consequences. *J. Assoc. Nurses AIDS Care* **2004**, *15*, 20S–27S. [CrossRef]
21. Davis, S. Clinical sequelae affecting quality of life in the HIV-infected patient. *J. Assoc. Nurses AIDS Care* **2004**, *15*, 28S–33S. [CrossRef]
22. Tran, B.X.; Hwang, J.; Nguyen, L.H.; Nguyen, A.T.; Latkin, N.R.; Tran, N.K.; Minh Thuc, V.T.; Nguyen, H.L.; Phan, H.T.; Le, H.T.; et al. Impact of Socioeconomic Inequality on Access, Adherence, and Outcomes of Antiretroviral Treatment Services for People Living with HIV/AIDS in Vietnam. *PLoS ONE* **2016**, *11*, e0168687. [CrossRef]
23. Jin, Y.; Liu, Z.; Wang, X.; Liu, H.; Ding, G.; Su, Y.; Zhu, L.; Wang, N. A systematic review of cohort studies of the quality of life in HIV/AIDS patients after antiretroviral therapy. *Int. J. STD AIDS* **2014**, *25*, 771–777. [CrossRef] [PubMed]
24. Gakhar, H.; Kamali, A.; Holodniy, M. Health-related quality of life assessment after antiretroviral therapy: A review of the literature. *Drugs* **2013**, *73*, 651–672. [CrossRef] [PubMed]
25. Wu, A.W.; Hanson, K.A.; Harding, G.; Haider, S.; Tawadrous, M.; Khachatryan, A.; Pashos, C.L.; Simpson, K.N. Responsiveness of the MOS-HIV and EQ-5D in HIV-infected adults receiving antiretroviral therapies. *Health Qual. Life Outcomes* **2013**, *11*, 42. [CrossRef] [PubMed]
26. Jeavons, S.; Greenwood, K.M.; Horne, D.J. Accident cognitions and subsequent psychological trauma. *J. Trauma. Stress* **2000**, *13*, 359–365. [CrossRef]
27. Tran, B.X.; Vu, G.T.; Ha, G.H.; Vuong, Q.H.; Ho, M.T.; Vuong, T.T.; La, V.P.; Ho, M.T.; Nghiem, K.P.; Nguyen, H.L.T.; et al. Global Evolution of Research in Artificial Intelligence in Health and Medicine: A Bibliometric Study. *J. Clin. Med.* **2019**, *8*, 360. [CrossRef]
28. Tran, B.X.; Moir, M.; Latkin, C.A.; Hall, B.J.; Nguyen, C.T.; Ha, G.H.; Nguyen, N.B.; Ho, C.S.H.; Ho, R.C.M. Global research mapping of substance use disorder and treatment 1971–2017: Implications for priority setting. *Subst. Abus. Treat. Prev. Policy* **2019**, *14*, 21. [CrossRef]
29. Tran, B.X.; Ho, R.C.M.; Ho, C.S.H.; Latkin, C.A.; Phan, H.T.; Ha, G.H.; Vu, G.T.; Ying, J.; Zhang, M.W.B. Depression among Patients with HIV/AIDS: Research Development and Effective Interventions (GAPRESEARCH). *Int. J. Environ. Res. Public Health* **2019**, *16*, 1772. [CrossRef]
30. Tran, B.X.; Dang, K.A.; Le, H.T.; Ha, G.H.; Nguyen, L.H.; Nguyen, T.H.; Tran, T.H.; Latkin, C.A.; Ho, C.S.H.; Ho, R.C.M. Global Evolution of Obesity Research in Children and Youths: Setting Priorities for Interventions and Policies. *Obes. Facts* **2019**, *12*, 137–149. [CrossRef]
31. Hoang, C.L.; Ha, G.H.; Kiet, P.H.T.; Tran, B.X.; Latkin, C.A.; Ho, C.S.H.; Ho, R.C.M. Global Mapping of Interventions to Improve Quality of Life of Patients with Alzheimer's Disease during 1990–2018. *Dement. Geriatr. Cogn. Disord.* **2020**, 1–3. [CrossRef]
32. Analytics, C. Web of Science platform: Web of Science: Summary of Coverage. Available online: https://clarivate.libguides.com/webofscienceplatform/coverage (accessed on 18 March 2020).
33. Katz, D.I.; Cohen, S.I.; Alexander, M.P. Mild traumatic brain injury. *Handb. Clin. Neurol.* **2015**, *127*, 131–156. [CrossRef]
34. Kessler, R.C.; Barker, P.R.; Colpe, L.J.; Epstein, J.F.; Gfroerer, J.C.; Hiripi, E.; Howes, M.J.; Normand, S.L.; Manderscheid, R.W.; Walters, E.E.; et al. Screening for serious mental illness in the general population. *Arch. Gen. Psychiatry* **2003**, *60*, 184–189. [CrossRef] [PubMed]
35. Diwakar, P. *O16. 1 Quality of Life and HIV—A Bibliometric Analysis of Publication Trends between 1995 to 2013*; BMJ Publishing Group Ltd.: London, UK, 2017.
36. Kharsany, A.B.; Karim, Q.A. HIV Infection and AIDS in Sub-Saharan Africa: Current Status, Challenges and Opportunities. *Open AIDS J.* **2016**, *10*, 34–48. [CrossRef] [PubMed]

37. Shao, Y.; Williamson, C. The HIV-1 epidemic: Low- to middle-income countries. *Cold Spring Harb. Perspect. Med.* **2012**, *2*, a007187. [CrossRef] [PubMed]
38. UNAIDS. *The Collapse of Global AIDS Funding*; UNAIDS: Geneva, Switzerland, 2016.
39. Rueda, S.; Mitra, S.; Chen, S.; Gogolishvili, D.; Globerman, J.; Chambers, L.; Wilson, M.; Logie, C.H.; Shi, Q.; Morassaei, S.; et al. Examining the associations between HIV-related stigma and health outcomes in people living with HIV/AIDS: A series of meta-analyses. *BMJ Open* **2016**, *6*, e011453. [CrossRef] [PubMed]
40. Swindells, S.; Mohr, J.; Justis, J.C.; Berman, S.; Squier, C.; Wagener, M.M.; Singh, N. Quality of life in patients with human immunodeficiency virus infection: Impact of social support, coping style and hopelessness. *Int. J. STD AIDS* **1999**, *10*, 383–391. [CrossRef]
41. Pozniak, A. Quality of life in chronic HIV infection. *Lancet HIV* **2014**, *1*, e6–e7. [CrossRef]
42. Canavarro, M.C.; Pereira, M. Factor structure and psychometric properties of the European Portuguese version of a questionnaire to assess quality of life in HIV-infected adults: The WHOQOL-HIV-Bref. *AIDS Care* **2012**, *24*, 799–807. [CrossRef]
43. Pereira, M.; Martins, A.; Alves, S.; Canavarro, M.C. Assessing quality of life in middle-aged and older adults with HIV: Psychometric testing of the WHOQOL-HIV-Bref. *Qual. Life Res.* **2014**, *23*, 2473–2479. [CrossRef]
44. Hsiung, P.C.; Fang, C.T.; Wu, C.H.; Sheng, W.H.; Chen, S.C.; Wang, J.D.; Yao, G. Validation of the WHOQOL-HIV BREF among HIV-infected patients in Taiwan. *AIDS Care* **2011**, *23*, 1035–1042. [CrossRef]
45. Saddki, N.; Noor, M.M.; Norbanee, T.H.; Rusli, M.A.; Norzila, Z.; Zaharah, S.; Sarimah, A.; Norsarwany, M.; Asrenee, A.R.; Zarina, Z.A. Validity and reliability of the Malay version of WHOQOL-HIV BREF in patients with HIV infection. *AIDS Care* **2009**, *21*, 1271–1278. [CrossRef]
46. Tran, B.X. Quality of life outcomes of antiretroviral treatment for HIV/AIDS patients in Vietnam. *PLoS ONE* **2012**, *7*, e41062. [CrossRef] [PubMed]
47. Tucker, C.M.; Marsiske, M.; Rice, K.G.; Nielson, J.J.; Herman, K. Patient-centered culturally sensitive health care: Model testing and refinement. *Health Psychol.* **2011**, *30*, 342–350. [CrossRef] [PubMed]
48. Nota, S.P.; Bot, A.G.; Ring, D.; Kloen, P.J.I. Disability and depression after orthopaedic trauma. *Injury* **2015**, *46*, 207–212. [CrossRef]
49. Larios, S.E.; Davis, J.N.; Gallo, L.C.; Heinrich, J.; Talavera, G. Concerns about stigma, social support and quality of life in low-income HIV-positive Hispanics. *Ethn. Dis.* **2009**, *19*, 65–70. [PubMed]
50. Medeiros, R.; Medeiros, J.A.; Silva, T.; Andrade, R.D.; Medeiros, D.C.; Araujo, J.S.; Oliveira, A.M.G.; Costa, M.A.A.; Dantas, P.M.S. Quality of life, socioeconomic and clinical factors, and physical exercise in persons living with HIV/AIDS. *Rev. Saude Publica* **2017**, *51*, 66. [CrossRef] [PubMed]
51. Calvetti, P.Ü.; Giovelli, G.R.M.; Gauer, G.J.C.; Moraes, J.F.D.d. Psychosocial factors associated with adherence to treatment and quality of life in people living with HIV/AIDS in Brazil %J Jornal Brasileiro de Psiquiatria. *J. Brasileiro De Psiquiatria* **2014**, *63*, 8–15. [CrossRef]
52. Ruiz Perez, I.; Rodriguez Bano, J.; Lopez Ruz, M.A.; del Arco Jimenez, A.; Causse Prados, M.; Pasquau Liano, J.; Martin Rico, P.; de la Torre Lima, J.; Prada Pardal, J.L.; Lopez Gomez, M.; et al. Health-related quality of life of patients with HIV: Impact of sociodemographic, clinical and psychosocial factors. *Qual. Life Res.* **2005**, *14*, 1301–1310. [CrossRef]
53. Lutgendorf, S.; Antoni, M.H.; Schneiderman, N.; Fletcher, M.A. Psychosocial counseling to improve quality of life in HIV infection. *Patient Educ. Couns.* **1994**, *24*, 217–235. [CrossRef]
54. Bastardo, Y.M.; Kimberlin, C.L. Relationship between quality of life, social support and disease-related factors in HIV-infected persons in Venezuela. *AIDS Care* **2000**, *12*, 673–684. [CrossRef]
55. Sowell, R.L.; Seals, B.F.; Moneyham, L.; Demi, A.; Cohen, L.; Brake, S. Quality of life in HIV-infected women in the south-eastern United States. *AIDS Care* **1997**, *9*, 501–512. [CrossRef]
56. Bachmann, M.O.; Louwagie, G.; Fairall, L.R. *Quality of life and financial measures in HIV/AIDS in Southern Africa*; Springer: New York, NY, USA, 2010; pp. 3223–3243.

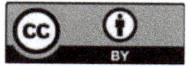

© 2020 by the authors. Licensee MDPI, Basel, Switzerland. This article is an open access article distributed under the terms and conditions of the Creative Commons Attribution (CC BY) license (http://creativecommons.org/licenses/by/4.0/).

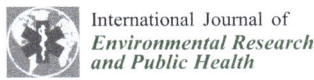 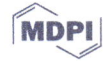

Article

Modeling the Research Landscapes of Artificial Intelligence Applications in Diabetes (GAP_{RESEARCH})

Giang Thu Vu [1], Bach Xuan Tran [2,3], Roger S. McIntyre [4,5,6,7], Hai Quang Pham [8], Hai Thanh Phan [8], Giang Hai Ha [8,*], Kenneth K. Gwee [9], Carl A. Latkin [3], Roger C.M. Ho [9,10,11] and Cyrus S.H. Ho [12]

[1] Center of Excellence in Evidence-based Medicine, Nguyen Tat Thanh University, Ho Chi Minh City 700000, Vietnam; giang.coentt@gmail.com
[2] Institute for Preventive Medicine and Public Health, Hanoi Medical University, Hanoi 100000, Vietnam; bach.ipmph@gmail.com
[3] Bloomberg School of Public Health, Johns Hopkins University, Baltimore, MD 21205, USA; carl.latkin@jhu.edu
[4] Institute of Medical Science, University of Toronto, Toronto, ON M5S 1A8, Canada; roger.mcintyre@uhn.ca
[5] Mood Disorders Psychopharmacology Unit, University Health Network, Toronto, ON M5G 2C4, Canada
[6] Department of Psychiatry, University of Toronto, Toronto, ON M5T 1R8, Canada
[7] Department of Toxicology and Pharmacology, University of Toronto, Toronto, ON M5S 1A8, Canada
[8] Institute for Global Health Innovations, Duy Tan University, Da Nang 550000, Vietnam; qhai.ighi@gmail.com (H.Q.P.); haipt.ighi@gmail.com (H.T.P.)
[9] Department of Psychological Medicine, Yong Loo Lin School of Medicine, National University of Singapore, Singapore 119228, Singapore; e0012499@u.nus.edu (K.K.G.); pcmrhcm@nus.edu.sg (R.C.M.H.)
[10] Center of Excellence in Behavioral Medicine, Nguyen Tat Thanh University, Ho Chi Minh City 700000, Vietnam
[11] Institute for Health Innovation and Technology (iHealthtech), National University of Singapore, Singapore 117599, Singapore
[12] Department of Psychological Medicine, National University Hospital, Singapore 119074, Singapore; cyrushosh@gmail.com
* Correspondence: giang.ighi@gmail.com; Tel.: +84-869548561

Received: 18 December 2019; Accepted: 9 March 2020; Published: 17 March 2020

Abstract: The rising prevalence and global burden of diabetes fortify the need for more comprehensive and effective management to prevent, monitor, and treat diabetes and its complications. Applying artificial intelligence in complimenting the diagnosis, management, and prediction of the diabetes trajectory has been increasingly common over the years. This study aims to illustrate an inclusive landscape of application of artificial intelligence in diabetes through a bibliographic analysis and offers future direction for research. Bibliometrics analysis was combined with exploratory factor analysis and latent Dirichlet allocation to uncover emergent research domains and topics related to artificial intelligence and diabetes. Data were extracted from the Web of Science Core Collection database. The results showed a rising trend in the number of papers and citations concerning AI applications in diabetes, especially since 2010. The nucleus driving the research and development of AI in diabetes is centered around developed countries, mainly consisting of the United States, which contributed 44.1% of the publications. Our analyses uncovered the top five emerging research domains to be: (i) use of artificial intelligence in diagnosis of diabetes, (ii) risk assessment of diabetes and its complications, (iii) role of artificial intelligence in novel treatments and monitoring in diabetes, (iv) application of telehealth and wearable technology in the daily management of diabetes, and (v) robotic surgical outcomes with diabetes as a comorbid. Despite the benefits of artificial intelligence, challenges with system accuracy, validity, and confidentiality breach will need to be tackled before being widely applied for patients' benefits.

Keywords: artificial intelligence; machine learning; diabetes; bibliometric; LDA

1. Introduction

Diabetes is a chronic medical disease that is characterized by increased levels of blood glucose, which causes microvascular and macrovascular complications with time. This chronic condition is concerning because the prevalence of diabetes has been steadily increasing for the past three decades. In 2014, the worldwide prevalence of diabetes was 8.5% among those aged 18 years and older, a escalation from 4.7% in 1980 [1]. In 2016, an estimated 1.6 million deaths were directly attributable to diabetes alone with World Health Organization (WHO) estimating that diabetes was the seventh leading cause of death in 2016. This figure is expected to rise even further in the future [1].

The global health expenditure on diabetes among people of ages 20 and 79 is expected to rise from USD 376 billion in 2010 to an estimated USD 490 billion in 2030 [2]. All these alarming statistics justify the need for ongoing research and active management to prevent and treat diabetes and its complications to optimize quality of life as well as to reduce the economic healthcare burden.

One of the promising research areas that are ongoing in the field of diabetes, is the use of artificial intelligence (AI). Artificial intelligence is a domain in computer science which accentuates the creation and use of intelligent machines that are able to function and respond like humans. According to a recent 2019 bibliometric study, there has been a tripled fold increase in the number of studies on the applications of AI in the past three years alone, with Diabetes being among the top ten areas of interest [3].

The techniques applied in the research of AI and diabetes include machine learning, artificial neural networks, and natural language processing. These techniques have allowed several applications of AI into the diagnosis and management of diabetes such as the diagnosis of microalbuminuria in type II diabetes patients without the need to measure urinary albumin levels. Microalbuminuria (MA) is a known complication of diabetes and is one of the measures of the renal function in diabetic patients The gold standard of such a diagnosis is to collect 24-hour urine albumin excretion, but with artificial intelligence on the rise, the detection of MA can be done with clinical parameters usually monitored in type II diabetes patients such as age, duration of diabetes, body mass index, and HbA1c (which is the average of blood glucose over the past three months, commonly used to assess diabetic control) [4].

Another promising application of artificial intelligence in diabetes is the development of a model that helps to generate a risk score with the ability to predict future glycemic control in individuals with type II diabetes. Machine learning models have been established and used to forecast the trajectories using clinical parameters such as body mass index, glycated hemoglobin, and triglycerides. This developed model can be used to estimate the patient's journey with diabetes and determine the follow-up period based on their risk score. Patients with higher risk scores should be followed up more closely compared to those who have lower risk scores to optimize their health outcomes, particularly in diabetes [5].

The evidently increasing interest of academics and practitioners in applications of AI in diabetes management sparked a need for having a comprehensive and up-to-date picture of what has been done in terms of research on this topic, highlighting areas that have been investigated, the emerging research domains, and potential research gaps that need further investigation. Informed readers may, in turn, be able to decide on a better direction for their future researches on the topic. To the best of our knowledge, there has not been a publication looking into AI application in diabetes on a comprehensive, global scale. This study is conducted to fill such gap in literature by adopting a combination of bibliometric approach and more complex analysis of title and abstracts of publications.

2. Materials and Methods

2.1. Search Strategy

We did a search on the Web of Science (WOS) Core Collection, an online database covering the bibliographic data of various research areas since 1900 [6], and retrieved all papers related to artificial intelligence in diabetes [7]. The full search strategy has been presented in another paper [3]. In this analysis, we selected and retrieved the data on AIs that were related to diabetes in two steps:

(a) Step 1: the publications related to AI in medicine and healthcare were extracted [3];
(b) Step 2: among the papers in step 1, we used terms related to diabetes for identifying studies related to diabetes in AI in health and medicine.

2.2. Data Extraction

All data in .txt format were downloaded from the WOS including title, authors' names, journal, year of publication, affiliations, a total of citation, keywords, and abstracts. All of these data were converted to xls. file (Microsoft Excel) for checking data error. After this, we filtered all downloaded data by sieving out papers that were: (1) not original articles and reviews, (2) unrelated to diabetes and AIs, and (3) not in English. Two researchers worked independently to guarantee the quality of data download and extraction. Any conflict in terms of paper selection was resolved by discussion. The collective dataset was eventually transferred into Stata 14.0 to be further analyzed (STATACorp., College Station, Texas, USA).

2.3. Data Analysis

We analyzed the dataset based on the following information: general characteristic (number of papers per year, citations, the total and average number of download publications), keywords (most common keywords and co-occurrence keywords), and text mining (abstract). After we have downloaded and extracted the data, descriptive statistical analysis using Stata was applied to calculate the number of papers by countries mentioned in abstracts. A network graph that illustrated the connection among authors' keyword co-occurrence network was created by the VOSviewer (version 1.6.8, Center for Science and Technology, Leiden University, Leiden, the Netherlands). For analyzing the contents of the abstracts, exploratory factor analysis (EFA) was employed to identify and visualize the research domains that stem from all content of the abstracts; to highlight research topics or terms most commonly co-occurring with each other, we used the 0.4. Jaccard's similarity index. Latent Dirichlet Allocation (LDA) was used for classifying papers into corresponding topics [8–12]. Principal component analysis (PCA) was used to create the keyword map as the technique is able to reduce the number of variables, and thus, cluster them into more manageable groups [13]. EFA, LDA, and PCA were conducted using Stata. The analytical techniques for each data type are shown in Table 1.

Table 1. Overview of analytical techniques utilized for each data type. WOS, Web of Science.

Type of Data	Unit of Analysis	Analytical Methods	Presentations of Results
Keywords, Countries	Words	Frequency of co-occurrence	Map of keywords clusters
Abstracts	Words	Exploratory factors analyses	Top 50 constructed research domains Clustering map of the landscapes constructed by these domains.
Abstracts	Papers	Latent Dirichlet Allocation	10 classifications of research topics
WOS [1] classification of research areas	WOS research areas	Frequency of co-occurrence	Dendrogram of research disciplines

[1] WOS: Web of Science.

2.4. Ethical Statement

This study used statistics on papers and citations retrieved from the Web of Sciences databases. No human subjects involved, so that this is not subject to ethical review requirements for biomedical research.

3. Results

Table 2 gives the basic characteristic of the research papers. There has been an increased interest in studies applying AI to diabetes during 1991–2018. The number of papers has been growing gradually, with two-thirds of the total of 372 papers being published in the 2014–2018 period. Notably, the papers being published in 2009 have the highest total citations, mean cite rate and mean use rate in the last five years (2014–2018).

Table 2. General characteristics of publications.

Year Published	Total Number of Papers	Total Citations	Mean Cite Rate per Year	Total Usage Last 6 Months [1]	Total Usage Last 5 Years [1]	Mean Use Rate Last 6 Months [2]	Mean Use Rate Last 5 Years [2]
2018	74	60	0.8	405	739	5.5	2.0
2017	56	243	2.2	157	788	2.8	2.8
2016	57	400	2.3	61	656	1.1	2.3
2015	33	288	2.2	39	462	1.2	2.8
2014	22	196	1.8	29	403	1.3	3.7
2013	27	380	2.3	28	400	1.0	3.0
2012	17	135	1.1	9	117	0.5	1.4
2011	14	300	2.7	8	206	0.6	2.9
2010	12	343	3.2	8	107	0.7	1.8
2009	8	435	5.4	7	197	0.9	4.9
2008	8	291	3.3	8	75	1.0	1.9
2007	8	323	3.4	4	98	0.5	2.5
2006	8	213	2.0	9	130	1.1	3.3
2005	2	30	1.1	0	4	0.0	0.4
2004	5	321	4.3	3	56	0.6	2.2
2003	2	134	4.2	1	16	0.5	1.6
2002	5	177	2.1	0	21	0.0	0.8
2001	1	23	1.3	0	0	0.0	0.0
2000	4	44	0.6	0	10	0.0	0.5
1999	1	18	0.9	0	2	0.0	0.4
1998	2	48	1.1	0	5	0.0	0.5
1997	2	14	0.3	0	3	0.0	0.3
1996	1	22	1.0	0	4	0.0	0.8
1994	1	8	0.3	0	0	0.0	0.0
1993	1	2	0.1	0	0	0.0	0.0
1991	1	2	0.1	0	2	0.0	0.4

[1] Total usage: Total number of download; [2] Use rate: Total number of downloads/Total number of papers.

In terms of study settings (i.e., the country where the study was conducted), there were a total of 36 countries being mentioned in the abstracts of 372 publications (see Table 3). Of those, the United States of America was mentioned 44.1%, followed by Ireland (10.2%) and Italy (6.1%). The top 10 countries accounted for over 80% of the total study settings. Noticeably, in some countries where the prevalence of diabetes is higher than others [14] such as Saudi Arabia ($n = 3$, 1.2%), Egypt ($n = 1$, 0.4%), and United Arab of Emirates ($n = 2$, 0.8%), the number of papers was small compared to others with less prevalence of diabetes like Ireland, Italy, and Japan.

Table 3. Number of papers by countries as study settings.

No.	Country Settings	Frequency	%	No.	Country	Frequency	%
1	United States	108	44.1%	19	Czech	2	0.8%
2	Ireland	25	10.2%	20	France	2	0.8%
3	Italy	15	6.1%	21	Netherlands	2	0.8%
4	India	14	5.7%	22	Singapore	2	0.8%
5	Australia	9	3.7%	23	United Arab Emirates	2	0.8%
6	Japan	8	3.3%	24	Antarctica	1	0.4%
7	Taiwan	6	2.4%	25	Brazil	1	0.4%
8	Spain	5	2.0%	26	Bulgaria	1	0.4%
9	United Kingdom	5	2.0%	27	Egypt	1	0.4%
10	Germany	4	1.6%	28	Greece	1	0.4%
11	Israel	4	1.6%	29	Jordan	1	0.4%
12	Switzerland	4	1.6%	30	Malaysia	1	0.4%
13	Iran	3	1.2%	31	Mexico	1	0.4%
14	Poland	3	1.2%	32	New Zealand	1	0.4%
15	Saudi Arabia	3	1.2%	33	Pakistan	1	0.4%
16	Austria	2	0.8%	34	Sweden	1	0.4%
17	Canada	2	0.8%	35	Tunisia	1	0.4%
18	China	2	0.8%	36	Turkey	1	0.4%

By analyzing the keywords and abstracts' contents, it provided us with a clearer comprehension of the scopes of studies and development of research landscapes. Figure 1 describes the co-occurrence of keywords with the most common groups of terms. There were 17 major clusters that emerged from 165 most common keywords with co-occurrence of 5 times and higher. Of which, we could arrange into three major clusters: (1) AI types and its application in diabetes such as red cluster (machine learning, deep learning and clinical predictions), turquoise cluster (data mining and type II diabetes diagnosis), and green cluster (artificial neural network, big data and gene expression in diabetes diagnosis); (2) diabetes types: light yellow cluster and blue cluster (type II diabetes) and orange cluster (type 1 diabetes); (3) robotics in surgery, risk factor (obesity) and epidemiology of diabetes.

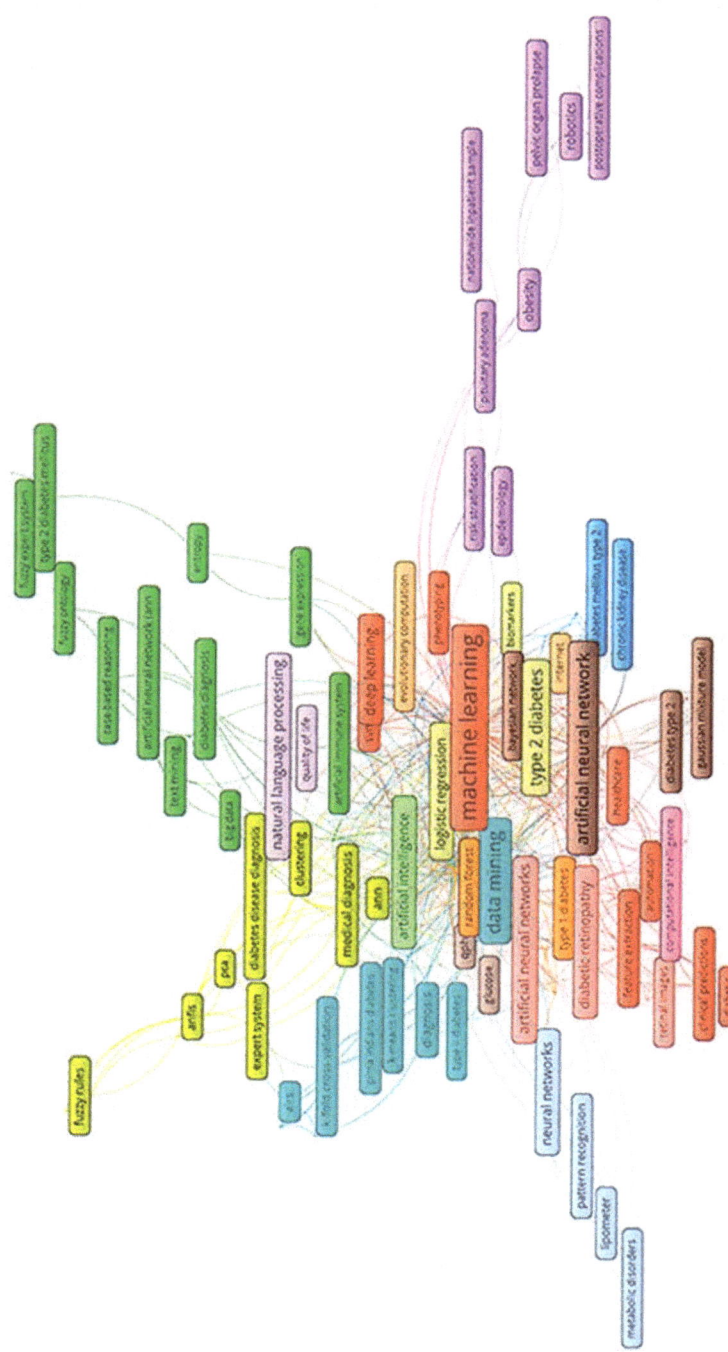

Figure 1. Co-occurrence of most frequent authors' keywords. The colors of the nodes indicate principal components of the data structure; the size of the node was scaled to the keywords' occurrences; the thickness of the lines was drawn based on the strength of the association between two keywords.

As for the content analysis of abstracts, the top 20 emerging research domains that were highlighted via the exploratory factor analysis of abstracts are listed in Table 4. Some AI techniques have been most used in this dataset including fuzzy expert system, support vector machine, artificial neural network, and machine learning. Those branches were applied in the following fields of diabetes: (1) clinical prediction (health records collecting or support vector machine modeling for prediction); (2) diabetes management (monitor blood sugar levels); (3) robot-assisted surgery with complication (hypertension, or obesity); (4) the cost of diabetes care.

Table 4. Top 20 research domains emerged from exploratory factor analysis of all abstracts' contents.

No.	Name	Keywords	Eigenvalue	Frequency	% Cases
1	Predict; Predictors	Prediction; Predictors; Predict; Random; Models; Learning; Machine; Records	2.89	173	74.39%
2	Events; Lead	Events; Lead; Developing; Detection; Potential; Treatment; Drug; Optimal; Medical; Work	2.2	114	71.95%
3	UCI [1]; Fuzzy	UCI; Fuzzy; Heart; Disease; Proposed; Obtained; Problems	2.36	117	69.51%
4	Early; Rate	Early; Rate; Complications; Medical; Detection; Work	1.88	89	65.85%
5	Technique; Cross	Technique; Cross; Applied; Validation; Machine; Metabolic; Learning	2	132	64.63%
6	Support Vector Machine (SVM)	Vector; Support; SVM; Machine	3.04	101	59.76%
7	Development; Present	Development; Present; Show; Conditions; Mellitus; Real	2.33	75	58.54%
8	Classification	Classification; Predictive; Achieved	2.1	57	54.88%
9	Monitoring; Blood Glucose	Monitoring; Glucose; Short; Insulin; Blood; Long; Treatment	3.29	96	54.88%
10	Artificial Neural Network	Neural; Artificial; Network; Ann; Values; Parameters; DM [2]; Obtained	3.58	121	53.66%
11	Large; Physicians	Large; Physicians; Screening; Processing; Performance; Long; Set; AUC	2.58	84	50.00%
12	Cost; Healthcare	Cost; Healthcare; Records; Predicting; Common; Risk	2.68	71	48.78%
13	Body Mass; Index	Mass; Body; Index; Testing; Surgery; Rate; Complications; Robotic	2.62	86	45.12%
14	Information; Develop	Information; Develop; Heart; Features; Long	2.47	60	43.90%
15	Clinical Decision	Decision; Tree; Clinical; Major	1.95	58	42.68%
16	Test; Neuropathy	Test; Neuropathy; Parameters; Component; Classifier; Accurate	2.23	59	41.46%
17	Feature Selection; Features	Feature; Selection; Features; Proposed; Paper	2.95	68	41.46%
18	Cohort; Hypertension	Cohort; Hypertension; Outcomes; Stage; Robotic; Surgery; Similar; Database; Complications	15.05	73	41.46%
19	Area; Curve (AUC) [3]	Area; Curve; AUC; Identifying; Set; Evaluated	3.82	79	39.02%
20	Sensitivity, Specificity	Specificity; Sensitivity; Develop	1.85	42	26.83%

[1] UCI: Machine Learning Repository; [2] DM: Diabetes mellitus; [3] AUC: Area Under the Curve.

The co-occurrence of the most frequent landscape was shown in Figure 2 by using exploratory factor analysis. In particular, we have the following major landscapes: (1) AI techniques in diabetes diagnosis (machine learning, Support Vector Machine (SVM), Fuzzy) (red); (2) diabetes prediction using model (green); (3) risk factors prediction (yellow and orange); and (4) diabetes treatments.

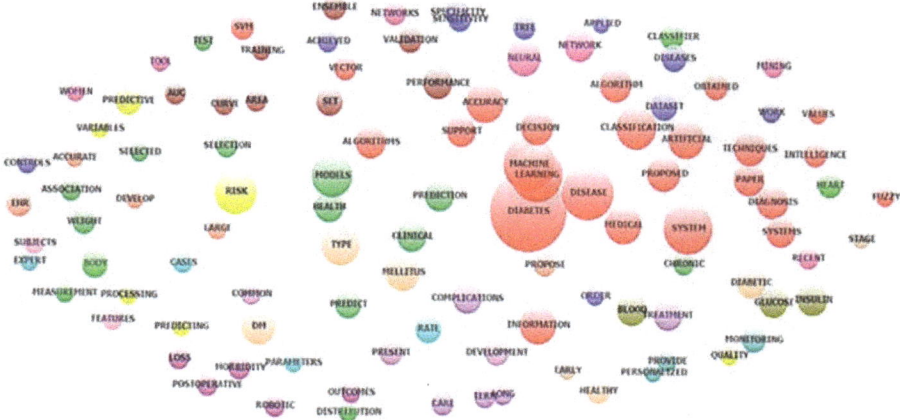

Figure 2. Co-occurrence of most frequent topics emerged from exploratory factor analysis of abstracts contents.

In Table 5, we showcased the research topics that were constructed via the use of latent Dirichlet allocation where we scrutinized the most frequent words and titles for each topic and manually annotated the labels of the topics. The topics found to have the highest volumes of publications included: (1) AI application in diabetes prediction and diagnosis; (2) complications of diabetes prediction; (3) biomedicine and molecular biology in diabetes; (4) e-health for diabetes care, and (5) robot-assisted surgery for patients with diabetes.

Table 5. 10 research topics classified by Latent Dirichlet Allocation

Year	Research areas	Frequency	%
Topic 1	AI application in diabetes prediction and diagnosis	100	31.1%
Topic 2	Complications of diabetes prediction	83	25.8%
Topic 3	Biomedicine and molecular biology in diabetes	43	13.4%
Topic 4	E-health for diabetes care	56	17.4%
Topic 5	Robot-assisted surgery for patients with diabetes	40	12.4%

In Figure 3, we illustrate the changes in research productivity over time. It shows that the number of publications related to AI in diabetes increased during the research period, especially from the beginning of the 21st century, especially in Topic 1 and Topic 2.

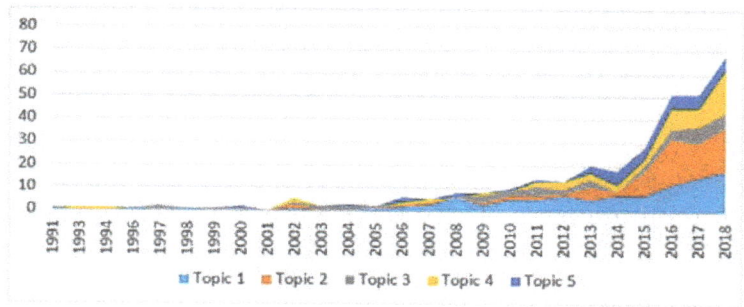

Figure 3. Changes in applications of Artificial Intelligence to diabetes research during 1991–2018.

Based on WOS categories, we identified the dendrogram for those (Figure 4). The horizontal axis shows the dissimilarity between research areas. The vertical position of the split, shown by a short bar indicates the dissimilarity between research areas. AI in diabetes focused on the following research areas: (1) computer Application in health care and biomedicine for diabetes; (2) biotechnological investigation and physiological mechanisms of diabetes; (3) AI application in biomedicine and comorbidities of diabetes; (4) health policy and diabetes, and (5) technology and diabetes.

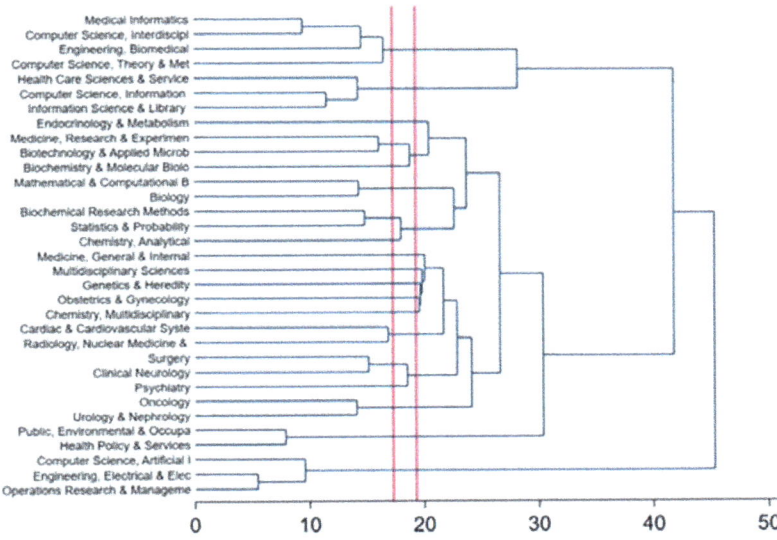

Figure 4. The clustering of research disciplines (WOS classification) used in Artificial Intelligence and Diabetes.

4. Discussion

The study clearly demonstrates a strong and increasing interest in the field of AI in the diagnosis and management of diabetes. This is evident by the increasing number of studies and a considerably higher extent of articles being published and applied. The gain in traction of such studies started from 2010 and has been steadily increasing to 2018, where a record number of 74 papers were published (Table 2). The nucleus driving the research and development of AI in diabetes is centered around developed countries mainly consisting of the United States, which contributed 44.1% of the publications with Ireland and Italy following behind (Table 3).

The study has found the top five emerging research domains (Table 5) pertaining to the application of AI in the diagnosis and management of diabetes: (1) uses of AI in the diagnosis of diabetes, (2) risk Assessment diabetes and its complications, (3) role of AI in novel treatments and monitoring in diabetes, (4) applications of telehealth and wearable technology in the daily management of diabetes, (5) robotic surgical outcomes with diabetes as a comorbid.

4.1. Uses of AI in the Diagnosis of Diabetes

Under this area of interest, the papers published in this category center around the diagnosis of diabetes using branches of AI. The intention of such research is not to replace the diagnosis work done by the doctors in healthcare, but to complement their efforts as such to optimize the patient's diagnosis timings as well as to cut down on the workload burden.

There are many methods published under this category, examples include the diagnosis of type II diabetes via the analysis of parameters such as heart rate variability and arterial blood glucose alterations. They are performed using non-linear methods such as detrended fluctuation analysis (DFA) and Poincare plot to produce two metrics termed standard deviation ratio (SDR) and alpha-ratio. These two metrics are then fed into a machine-learning algorithm to dichotomize the subjects as diabetic or non-diabetic. The paper reports an accuracy of 94.7% in the correct categorization of subjects, which offers the possibility that it could be further developed as a non-invasive screening tool for predicting whether an individual has type II diabetes [15].

Using AI to diagnose different conditions such as diabetes is interesting, but it comes with drawbacks as well. The main problem with AI is that firstly, it needs to be well-trained, which would require a large number of patients in the training set. This is a problem because personal details protection and privacy is a concern. Another problem with AI diagnostics is that it needs to be consistent, replicable, and reliable, but so far many of the studies have not been applying the evidence-based approaches that are seen in established fields [16].

There have been questions about whether the use of AI can improve diagnostic ability in terms of efficacy and time reduction. For instance, a study found the AI model can detect breast cancer in whole slide images better than 11 pathologists, with the pathologists being limited by the allowed assessment time of one minute per image, while the AI is not limited by any factors. However, when the pathologists were given unlimited time, they performed similarly to the AI and detected more difficult cases more frequently than the computers [17]. This raised the possibility that AI may better be employed in the diagnosis of clear-cut simple cases, whereas more complex cases that require detailed assessment may be more worthwhile to be tackled by humans.

4.2. Risk Assessment of Diabetes and its Complications

A crucial principle in the management of type II diabetes is to retard the progression of the chronic disease as well as to prevent the onset of complications resulting from the condition. Many barriers to the optimal detection of the progression include patients defaulting appointments, non-compliance to medical advice, and financial barriers that include treatment costs and costs of a healthy diet [18]. Therefore, the development of AI in such a setting is beneficial to both doctors and patients as doctors will be able to foretell the course of the disease to individualize and cater to the proper management of the patient based on their risk.

A novel method of achieving the above objective is noted in a paper that studies the application of an artificial neural network model that aims to diagnose type II diabetes mellitus and establishes the relative importance of risk factors. The study was conducted on a cohort of 234 people who were diagnosed with type II diabetes mellitus using glycated hemoglobin levels. A multilayer perceptron artificial neural network that was utilized to highlight the demographic risk factors revealed that risk factors such as age, hypertension, waist circumference, body mass index, sedentary lifestyle, etc. were predictors of type II diabetes. However, the final analysis showed that the most important predictors and risk assessment of diabetes type II were waist circumference, age, BMI, hypertension, stress, smoking, and positive family history of type II diabetes [19].

These risk assessment models developed with the assistance of AI help to improve the detection/screening of diabetes type II by enabling the optimization of health resources for people who are known to be high risk, compared to screening the entire population at large. This not only improves the cost at a population level, but also the landscape of screening for chronic diseases such as diabetes.

4.3. Role of AI in Novel Treatments and Monitoring of Diabetes

Monitoring blood glucose levels is a crucial tool to prevent complications such as hypoglycemia, which may lead to coma, seizures, or even death. AI has been applied to analyze breath samples taken from different subjects to determine hypoglycemic states. This was inspired by diabetes alert dogs which could detect hypoglycemia based on their owner's breath [20]. This presents a new way of monitoring glucose control and may help in the future to increase the uptake of self-glucose monitoring, that is currently mostly done with a glucometer, which is still quite troublesome for the patient and involves the pricking of the fingers, which some might not be comfortable with.

4.4. Applications of Telehealth and Wearable Technology in the Daily Management of Diabetes

In today's day and age, telehealth and wearable technology is catching up and may soon be one of the revolutionary tools used in clinical healthcare. The benefits of such technology are not only convenience, but it also allows the patients to take up more responsibility for their own healthcare. Some of the applications include monitoring of the patient's vitals through wearable technology such as a watch. In the future, it is possible for AI to be introduced to analyze biological information such as ultrasound scans or electrocardiography (ECG) obtained via the patient's phone, and provide real-time analysis for the patient. These results can also be shared with the primary doctor or a hospital for further evaluation and action.

A mobile application for managing diabetic patients' nutrition is currently being developed with the help of AI. This application combines AI techniques with a knowledge base constructed from the guidelines of the American Diabetes Association. This application recommends snacks based on the patient's favorites as well as current diabetic condition, which may help to improve glycemic control and prevent episodes of hypoglycemia [21].

Promoting beneficial behavior change in people with or at risk of diabetes is also a promising area of application for AI [22]. Studies have shown that the use of fitness tracking applications in smartphones and/or wearable health devices such as smart watch have been found to be associated with increased physical activities and fitness level in diabetic patients [22,23]. The incorporation of behavior change strategies, for instance environmental restructuring, attitude adjusting, or identifying barriers to changes that are specific to each individual, which, argued Sullivan and Lachman to be possibly the most change influencing factors, but have had limited appearance in fitness and health applications [24], yet application in fitness/health applications would supposedly be easy and effective, given the power of AI to record and process a large amount information.

4.5. Robotic Surgery with Diabetes as a Co-Morbid

AI has also been able to assist surgeons in the form of robotic surgery known to come with greater precision, lesser complication rates, as well as quicker healing times. However, that is not all that AI can do in the field of surgery. Machine learning techniques have been known to be applied to the field of surgery, where it concluded that new-onset diabetes and preexisting diabetes are correlated with a decrease in long term survival after liver transplants. Using AI, this has enabled the comparison of different surgical techniques, their complication rates as well as to identify different factors that may affect the outcomes during and after the surgery [25].

4.6. Challenges in the Use of AI

The increasingly deeper integration of AI applications in the diagnosis, management, and prediction of diabetes has also come with challenges. Ethical issues, in particular the privacy and confidentiality of patient data, have been a topic of debate in existing literature [26]. It is noted that most of the AI technology is still under development and not yet utilized in clinical practice. For this to happen, AI needs to be more developed so that it can be as sensitive and specific as possible. This requires large datasets to train the AI or computer models. These datasets may consist of sensitive and confidential patient biodata such as their age, body mass index, etc. The use of wearable technology that constantly records data on behavior of diabetic users while also encouraging users to input their sensitive health data for it to provide more accurate, tailor-made suggestions would inherently expose users to the risk of having personal data leaked or being used for other purposes without their consent. Furthermore, with large datasets, massive amounts of data may lead to difficulty in human efforts to design intricate and perfectly logical models for specific clinical tasks or to provide appropriate, effective treatment, or behavior suggestions for users. Other common limitations of mathematical models such as the lack of model validations, especially for model of novel approach, data/measurement bias, issues in sample representations, and the occurrence of outliers, would also potentially be found with AI models. Therefore, further research and development would be needed to tackle these problems before AI may be reliably used in clinical practice as well as in diabetic care.

This bibliometric analysis has put forward several key developments in the field of AI in diabetes and has included large quantities of literature on the topic of interest. However, since the study has only included papers written in the English language, a bias towards Western countries may be present. In addition, another limitation of the study was that of a restriction to purely peer-reviewed research publications, which possibly could have affected the extensiveness of the analyzed results. Future studies may also benefit from applying sensitivity analysis for type I and type II diabetes when conducting research using the method applied in this study.

5. Conclusions

The application of AI in diabetes has evidently become more common in recent years, with AI-related technologies being found to assist from diagnosis and clinical treatment to daily management of diabetes. As a condition with severity depending heavily on the lifestyle and behavior of patients and those at risk, continuous monitoring and initiating specific treatments based on data of individual's conditions and behavior as well as their specific surrounding would likely be effective, and is an area that AI applications can be seen as a promising solution. With such opportunities to enhance diabetes management also come challenges associated with the use of AI, of which privacy and confidentiality remain the major ones. These issues must be tackled and resolved before clinical use of AI-related technology is approved and available for the patient's benefit.

Author Contributions: Conceptualization, G.T.V., B.X.T, R.S.M., K.K.G and R.C.M.H; Data curation, G.T.V., R.S.M, H.Q.P, H.T.P. and G.H.H.; Formal analysis, G.T.V., B.X.T., H.Q.P. and H.T.P.; Investigation, G.T.V., K.K.G. and R.C.M.H.; Methodology, G.T.V., B.X.T. and H.T.P.; Software, R.S.M., H.Q.P. and G.H.H.; Supervision, B.X.T., C.A.L. and C.S.H.H.; Validation, C.A.L., R.C.M.H. and C.S.H.H; Visualization, G.H.H.; Writing – original draft, G.T.V. and K.K.G.; Writing – review & editing, C.A.L., R.C.M.H. and C.S.H.H. All authors have read and agreed to the published version of the manuscript.

Funding: This research received no external funding.

Conflicts of Interest: The authors declare no conflicts of interest.

References

1. WHO.int. Diabetes. Available online: https://www.who.int/news-room/fact-sheets/detail/diabetes (accessed on 6 December 2019).
2. Zhang, P.; Zhang, X.; Brown, J.; Vistisen, D.; Sicree, R.; Shaw, J.; Nichols, G. Global healthcare expenditure on diabetes for 2010 and 2030. *Diabetes Res. Clin. Pract.* **2010**, *87*, 293–301. [CrossRef]
3. Tran, B.X.; Vu, G.T.; Ha, G.H.; Vuong, Q.-H.; Ho, M.-T.; Vuong, T.-T.; La, V.-P.; Ho, M.-T.; Nghiem, K.-C.P.; Nguyen, H.L.T.; et al. Global Evolution of Research in Artificial Intelligence in Health and Medicine: A Bibliometric Study. *J. Clin. Med.* **2019**, *8*, 360. [CrossRef]
4. Marateb, H.R.; Mansourian, M.; Faghihimani, E.; Amini, M.; Farina, D. A hybrid intelligent system for diagnosing microalbuminuria in Type II diabetes patients without having to measure urinary albumin. *Comput. Biol. Med.* **2014**, *45*, 34–42. [CrossRef]
5. Hertroijs, D.F.L.; Elissen, A.M.J.; Brouwers, M.C.G.J.; Schaper, N.C.; Köhler, S.; Popa, M.C.; Asteriadis, S.; Hendriks, S.H.; Bilo, H.J.; Ruwaard, D. A risk score including body mass index, glycated haemoglobin and triglycerides predicts future glycaemic control in people with Type II diabetes. *Diabetes Obes. Metab.* **2018**, *20*, 681–688. [CrossRef]
6. Web of Science Group. Web of Science Core Collection. Available online: https://clarivate.com/webofsciencegroup/solutions/web-of-science-core-collection/?fbclid=IwAR1YnyjGtbiE3cOizWZvlblrBhr86xZCOrbzDmFJ1pAFIDGBm5xdw5PU5qM (accessed on 25 January 2020).

7. Chadegani, A.A.; Salehi, H.; Yunus, M.M.; Farhadi, H.; Fooladi, M.; Farhadi, M.; Ebrahim, N.A. A Comparison between Two Main Academic Literature Collections: Web of Science and Scopus Databases. *ASS* **2013**, *9*, 18. [CrossRef]
8. Chen, C.; Zare, A.; Trinh, H.N.; Omotara, G.O.; Cobb, J.T.; Lagaunne, T.A. Partial Membership Latent Dirichlet Allocation for Soft Image Segmentation. *IEEE Trans. Image Process. Publ. IEEE Signal Process. Soc.* **2017**, *26*, 5590–5602. [CrossRef]
9. Gross, A.; Murthy, D. Modeling virtual organizations with Latent Dirichlet Allocation: A case for natural language processing. *Neural Netw. Off. J. Int. Neural Netw. Soc.* **2014**, *58*, 38–49. [CrossRef]
10. Li, Y.; Rapkin, B.; Atkinson, T.M.; Schofield, E.; Bochner, B.H. Leveraging Latent Dirichlet Allocation in processing free-text personal goals among patients undergoing bladder cancer surgery. *Qual. Life Res. Int. J. Qual. Life Asp. Treat. Care Rehabil.* **2019**, *28*, 1441–1455. [CrossRef]
11. Lu, H.M.; Wei, C.P.; Hsiao, F.Y. Modeling healthcare data using multiple-channel latent Dirichlet allocation. *J. Biomed. Inform.* **2016**, *60*, 210–223. [CrossRef]
12. Valle, D.; Albuquerque, P.; Zhao, Q.; Barberan, A.; Fletcher, R.J., Jr. Extending the Latent Dirichlet Allocation model to presence/absence data: A case study on North American breeding birds and biogeographical shifts expected from climate change. *Glob. Chang. Biol.* **2018**, *24*, 5560–5572. [CrossRef]
13. Cobo, M.J.; López-Herrera, A.G.; Herrera-Viedma, E.; Herrera, F. Science mapping software tools: Review, analysis, and cooperative study among tools. *J. Am. Soc. Inf. Sci. Technol.* **2011**, *62*, 1382–1402. [CrossRef]
14. Worldbank.org. Diabetes Prevalence (% of Population Ages 20 to 79) | Data. Available online: https://data.worldbank.org/indicator/SH.STA.DIAB.ZS?view=map&year_low_desc=false (accessed on 1 December 2019).
15. Jong, G.-J.; Huang, C.-S.; Yu, G.-J.; Horng, G.-J. Artificial Neural Network Expert System for Integrated Heart Rate Variability. *Wirel. Pers. Commun.* **2014**, *75*, 483–509. [CrossRef]
16. Liu, W.; Huang, C.; Cai, J.; Wang, X.; Zou, Z.; Sun, C. Household environmental exposures during gestation and birth outcomes: A cross-sectional study in Shanghai, China. *Sci. Total Environ.* **2018**, *615*, 1110–1118. [CrossRef]
17. Ehteshami Bejnordi, B.; Veta, M.; Johannes van Diest, P.; van Ginneken, B.; Karssemeijer, N.; Litjens, G.; van der Laak, J.A.W.M.; The CAMELYON16 Consortium; Hermsen, M.; Manson, Q.F.; et al. Diagnostic Assessment of Deep Learning Algorithms for Detection of Lymph Node Metastases in Women With Breast CancerMachine Learning Detection of Breast Cancer Lymph Node MetastasesMachine Learning Detection of Breast Cancer Lymph Node Metastases. *JAMA* **2017**, *318*, 2199–2210. [CrossRef]
18. McBrien, K.A.; Naugler, C.; Ivers, N.; Weaver, R.G.; Campbell, D.; Desveaux, L.; Hemmelgarn, B.R.; Edwards, A.L.; Saad, N.; Nicholas, D.; et al. Barriers to care in patients with diabetes and poor glycemic control—A cross-sectional survey. *PLoS ONE* **2017**, *12*, e0176135. [CrossRef]
19. Borzouei, S.; Soltanian, A.R. Application of an artificial neural network model for diagnosing Type II diabetes mellitus and determining the relative importance of risk factors. *Epidemiol. Health* **2018**, *40*, e2018007. [CrossRef]
20. Siegel, A.P.; Daneshkhah, A.; Hardin, D.S.; Shrestha, S.; Varahramyan, K.; Agarwal, M. Analyzing breath samples of hypoglycemic events in type 1 diabetes patients: Towards developing an alternative to diabetes alert dogs. *J. Breath Res.* **2017**, *11*, 026007. [CrossRef]
21. Norouzi, S.; Kamel Ghalibaf, A.; Sistani, S.; Banazadeh, V.; Keykhaei, F.; Zareishargh, P.; Amiri, F.; Nematy, M.; Etminani, K. A Mobile Application for Managing Diabetic Patients' Nutrition: A Food Recommender System. *Arch. Iran. Med.* **2018**, *21*, 466–472.
22. Cvetkovic, B.; Janko, V.; Romero, A.E.; Kafali, O.; Stathis, K.; Lustrek, M. Activity Recognition for Diabetic Patients Using a Smartphone. *J. Med. Syst.* **2016**, *40*, 256. [CrossRef]
23. Plotnikoff, R.C.; Wilczynska, M.; Cohen, K.E.; Smith, J.J.; Lubans, D.R. Integrating smartphone technology, social support and the outdoor physical environment to improve fitness among adults at risk of, or diagnosed with, Type II Diabetes: Findings from the 'eCoFit' randomized controlled trial. *Prev. Med.* **2017**, *105*, 404–411. [CrossRef]
24. Sullivan, A.N.; Lachman, M.E. Behavior Change with Fitness Technology in Sedentary Adults: A Review of the Evidence for Increasing Physical Activity. *Front. Public Health* **2016**, *4*, 289. [CrossRef]

25. Bhat, V.; Tazari, M.; Watt, K.D.; Bhat, M. New-Onset Diabetes and Preexisting Diabetes Are Associated With Comparable Reduction in Long-Term Survival After Liver Transplant: A Machine Learning Approach. *Mayo Clin. Proc.* **2018**, *93*, 1794–1802. [CrossRef]
26. Rigby, M.J. Ethical Dimensions of Using Artificial Intelligence in Health Care. *AMA J. Ethics* **2019**, *21*, 121–124. [CrossRef]

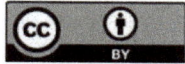

© 2020 by the authors. Licensee MDPI, Basel, Switzerland. This article is an open access article distributed under the terms and conditions of the Creative Commons Attribution (CC BY) license (http://creativecommons.org/licenses/by/4.0/).

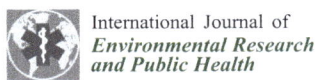 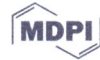

Article

Global Mapping of Interventions to Improve Quality of Life of People with Diabetes in 1990–2018

Bach Xuan Tran [1,2,*,†], Long Hoang Nguyen [3,†], Ngoc Minh Pham [4,5], Huyen Thanh Thi Vu [6,7], Hung Trong Nguyen [8], Duong Huong Phan [9], Giang Hai Ha [10,11], Hai Quang Pham [10,12], Thao Phuong Nguyen [13], Carl A. Latkin [2], Cyrus S.H. Ho [14] and Roger C.M. Ho [15,16,17]

1. Institute for Preventive Medicine and Public Health, Hanoi Medical University, Hanoi 100000, Vietnam
2. Bloomberg School of Public Health, Johns Hopkins University, Baltimore, MD 21205, USA; carl.latkin@jhu.edu
3. Department of Public Health Sciences, Karolinska Institutet, 17177 Stockholm, Sweden; hoang.nguyen@ki.se
4. School of Public Health, Faculty of Health Sciences, Curtin University, Perth, WA 2605, Australia; minh.pn@tnu.edu.vn
5. Thai Nguyen University of Medicine and Pharmacy, Thai Nguyen 250000, Vietnam
6. Department of Gerontology and Geriatrics, Hanoi Medical University, Hanoi 100000, Vietnam; vuthanhhuyen11@hmu.edu.vn
7. Scientific Research Department, National Geriatric Hospital, Hanoi 100000, Vietnam
8. Clinical Nutrition and Dietetics Department, National Institute of Nutrition, Hanoi 100000, Vietnam; nguyentronghung9602@yahoo.com
9. National Hospital of Endocrinology, Hanoi 100000, Vietnam; phanhuongduong@gmail.com
10. Institute for Global Health Innovations, Duy Tan University, Da Nang 550000, Vietnam; hahaigiang@duytan.edu.vn (G.H.H.); phamquanghai@duytan.edu.vn (H.Q.P.)
11. Faculty of Pharmacy, Duy Tan University, Danang 550000, Vietnam
12. Faculty of Medicine, Duy Tan University, Danang 550000, Vietnam
13. Center of Excellence in Evidence-based Medicine, Nguyen Tat Thanh University, Ho Chi Minh City 700000, Vietnam; thao.coentt@gmail.com
14. Department of Psychological Medicine, National University Hospital, Singapore 119074, Singapore; cyrushosh@gmail.com
15. Center of Excellence in Behavioral Medicine, Nguyen Tat Thanh University, Ho Chi Minh City 700000, Vietnam; pcmrhcm@nus.edu.sg
16. Department of Psychological Medicine, Yong Loo Lin School of Medicine, National University of Singapore, Singapore 119228, Singapore
17. Institute for Health Innovation and Technology (iHealthtech), National University of Singapore, Singapore 119077, Singapore

* Correspondence: bach.ipmph@gmail.com; Tel.: +84-98222-8662
† These authors contributed equally to the paper.

Received: 21 January 2020; Accepted: 21 February 2020; Published: 2 March 2020

Abstract: Improving the quality of life (QOL) of people living with diabetes is the ultimate goal of diabetes care. This study provides a quantitative overview of global research on interventions aiming to improve QOL among people with diabetes. A total of 700 English peer-reviewed papers published during 1990–2018 were collected and extracted from the Web of Science databases. Latent Dirichlet Allocation (LDA) analysis was undertaken to categorize papers by topic or theme. Results showed an increase in interventions to improve the QOL of patients with diabetes across the time period, with major contributions from high-income countries. Community- and family-based interventions, including those focused on lifestyle and utilizing digital technologies, were common approaches. Interventions that addressed comorbidities in people with diabetes also increased. Our findings emphasize the necessity of translating the evidence from clinical interventions to community interventions. In addition, they underline the importance of developing collaborative research between developed and developing countries.

Keywords: scientometrics; content analysis; text mining; interventions; diabetes; QOL

1. Introduction

Diabetes mellitus is well recognized as a global public health crisis. It is a chronic metabolic disorder characterized by elevated blood glucose levels due to the body's impaired insulin secretion and/or insulin resistance [1]. Persistent diabetes devastates vascular and nerve systems, causing many severe life-threatening complications (e.g., cardiovascular diseases, neuropathy, diabetic foot complications, diabetic retinopathies, or renal failure) and increasing the risk of hospitalization and mortality [2–4]. This disease has now been among the leading causes of disease burden worldwide [5]. According to global estimates, in 2017, over 451 million people were reported to be living with diabetes, with more than 5 million diabetes-related deaths [1].

Like other chronic diseases, diabetes cannot be completely cured [6]. Therefore, ensuring that people living with diabetes have a good quality of life (QOL) and can function adequately has become the ultimate goal of diabetic care [7]. Research increasingly looks to QOL as a favorable outcome of interventions focused on diabetes [2,6]. QOL is a multidimensional concept that does not have a unified definition [8–11]. The World Health Organization defines QOL as "an individual's perceptions of their position in life, in the context of the culture and value systems in which they live, and in relation to their goals, expectations, standards, and concerns" [11]. When two treatments have similar clinical outcomes, measuring QOL can reflect patients' different experiences or perceptions of treatments and symptoms, helping clinicians to identify which intervention's benefits outweigh its drawbacks [12]. In the case of diabetes, evaluating QOL is critically important as its enhancement is associated with good self-care management, including adherence to prescribed medication and suggested lifestyle modifications, which are significant protective factors for diabetes care [2,6,13,14].

A growing body of literature (including trials, systematic reviews, and meta-analyses) examines the effectiveness of various approaches (from health education to behavioral modification, pharmacotherapy, and surgery [12,15–18]) in enhancing treatment outcomes and QOL among people with diabetes. However, few publications feature updated quantitative data (i.e, bibliometric or scientometric analysis) focusing on interventions aimed at improving QOL in people living with diabetes. Recently, most of the published bibliometric studies have concentrated on diabetes in general [19–21], diabetic complications [22] or comorbidities [23], and the use of specific therapy in diabetes treatment [24]. Looking at these offers a comprehensive picture of the current approaches utilized for improving QOL, the status of international collaboration, and the gap between high- and low-income nations, which is vital in developing a roadmap for a global research agenda that will help optimize diabetes treatment outcomes. The aim of this study is thus to assess the outcomes of recent interventions to improve QOL of people with diabetes.

2. Materials and Methods

2.1. Searching Strategy

We performed a combined bibliometric and content analysis of publications covering the interventions to improve QOL among people with diabetes. The Web of Science (WOS) Core Collection was selected for the retrieval of data from 1900 to 31 December, 2018. The reasons for selecting the WOS include the availability of necessary information for analyzing contents of papers such as names and addresses of authors, titles/abstracts of articles, keywords, total citations and downloads, and research area coverage, which is far more than other accessible databases. Moreover, this database has a high citation report coverage and supports various analysis measures that facilitate bibliometric analysis of the existing literature [25,26].

Articles were included if they (1) involved interventions (randomized controlled trials [RCTs], pre-post or quasi-experiments); (2) focused on people with diabetes as the targeted population; (3) had QOL or health-related QOL as primary or secondary outcomes; (4) were original articles; (5) were published in English scientific journals indexed in the WOS; and (6) had comprehensive information on the authors.

We excluded gray literature (e.g., reports, dissertations, theses, letters, news, etc.), book and book chapters, and conference abstracts/proceedings because some of these might have been published as scientific papers in peer-reviewed journals which could cause duplications. Papers without author information were also excluded because they could not be used to analyze the affiliation and collaboration networks across countries. Additionally, papers about narrative reviews/systematic reviews/meta-analysis studies were excluded because they were not original studies, which might not reflect the tendency of research development. Study protocols of interventions or papers reporting only baseline characteristics were not eligible because they did not assess the effect of specific interventions on the QOL.

To identify relevant articles, we performed the search strategy as follows:

- First, we produced a QOL dataset by employing topic search terms such as "quality of life" and "well-being" on the WOS. Among 441,617 records after searching, we excluded 114,212 documents (including: 4364 papers that were published in 2019; 25,543 documents that were non-English articles; 84,083 documents that were not articles/reviews; and 222 documents that had insufficient author information). A total of 327,405 quality of life-related papers were used for the next step.
- Second, we filtered the papers regarding interventions in diabetes populations by using a set of title/abstract terms related to "diabetes" (AND "intervention" OR "trial") and saved it as the final dataset. A total of 323,079 papers were excluded, resulting in 4326 papers that were included in the next phase.
- Finally, we screened 4326 papers by reading their titles and abstracts and excluded 3626 papers that were not eligible according to the inclusion and exclusion criteria.

Full records of articles were exported and downloaded independently by two members in the research team. The third researcher performed a cross-check between two datasets to ensure their consistency.

2.2. Data Analysis

STATA version 15.0 (STATA Corp., TX, USA) was utilized for data analysis. We performed a descriptive analysis using the following indicators: publication year, the number of papers per country/per year, total citations up to 2018, mean citation rate per year, total usage in the last six months/five years, and mean use rate in the last six months/five years. The VOSviewer (version 1.6.8, Center for Science and Technology, Leiden University, the Netherlands) was employed to illustrate the co-occurrence of the most frequent terms in titles and abstracts. Country collaboration networks were illustrated by using the Circos platform [27]. As for content analysis, we analyzed the hierarchical clustering of major research disciplines in the interventions and visualized it in a Dendrogram. Thematic analysis was performed using the Latent Dirichlet Allocation (LDA) technique, which supports classified papers in ten major themes/topics [18,28–31]. Titles and abstracts of papers in every topic/theme were then reviewed by two researchers. Any disagreements were addressed by discussing it with a senior researcher. We then calculated the number of papers per topic and determined any change in research interests by ranking the total number of publications per topic in the past five years (from 2013–2018).

3. Results

Figure 1 illustrates the searching process. Among the 327,405 papers on QOL, 700 papers on interventions to improve QOL of people with diabetes were selected as eligible.

Table 1 shows that in the period 1990–2018, there were a total of 700 papers published about interventions to improve the QOL among people with diabetes. From the first paper counted in 1990, the volume of annual articles increased significantly over time to reach a peak of 67 papers in 2015, before falling to 63 papers by the end of 2018. Papers published in 2005 and 1998 had the highest mean citation rate per year (9.7 and 9.0, respectively). Articles published in 2015 and 2005 had the highest total usage (i.e., the total number of downloads) and mean use rate in the last five years, respectively. In the last six months, the total usage and the mean use rate of papers published in 2018 were higher than those published in other years.

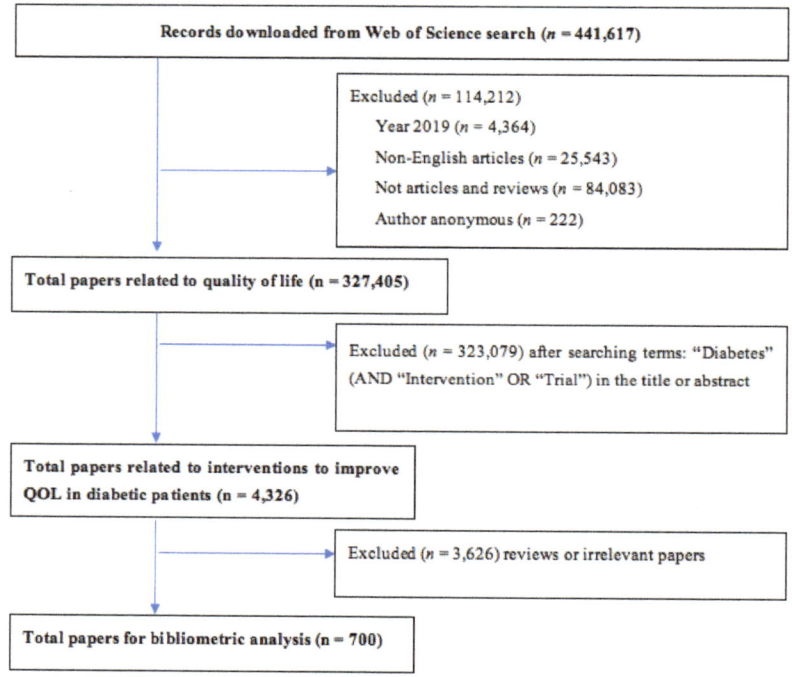

Figure 1. Selection of papers.

Overall, 700 papers were published by authors in 61 countries. The United States (U.S.) and the United Kingdom (U.K.) contributed the most publications (322 and 160 papers, respectively), followed by Germany (101 papers), Australia (87 papers), and the Netherlands (85 papers). Only China was the only middle-income country in the top ten nations with the greatest number of publications, while the others were high-income nations. Meanwhile, among the top 20 countries, only China, India, Malaysia, and Iran were middle-income countries.

Table 1. General characteristics of publications analyzed.

Year Published	Total Number of Papers	Total Citations	Mean Cite Rate Per Year	Total Usage Last 6 Months [1]	Total Usage Last 5 Years [2]	Mean Use Rate Last 6 Months	Mean Use Rate Last 5 Years
2018	63	158	2.5	218	405	3.5	1.3
2017	56	556	5.0	95	494	1.7	1.8
2016	57	455	2.7	51	601	0.9	2.1
2015	67	1009	3.8	77	1,135	1.1	3.4
2014	59	1845	6.3	67	927	1.1	3.1
2013	46	1205	4.4	25	808	0.5	3.5
2012	53	1342	3.6	28	871	0.5	3.3
2011	41	1127	3.4	16	501	0.4	2.4
2010	33	1020	3.4	24	380	0.7	2.2
2009	34	1590	4.7	23	370	0.7	2.2
2008	24	1372	5.2	10	297	0.4	2.5
2007	27	1244	3.8	18	308	0.7	2.3
2006	20	1038	4.0	8	156	0.4	1.6
2005	18	2438	9.7	18	335	1.0	3.7
2004	17	930	3.6	3	94	0.2	1.1
2003	9	870	6.0	3	79	0.3	1.8
2002	13	1233	5.6	1	79	0.1	1.2
2001	12	978	4.5	0	65	0.0	1.1
2000	13	1355	5.5	8	140	0.6	2.2
1999	3	202	3.4	1	9	0.3	0.6
1998	12	2265	9.0	1	98	0.1	1.6
1997	4	208	2.4	2	14	0.5	0.7
1996	8	1177	6.4	4	60	0.5	1.5
1995	2	202	4.2	2	13	1.0	1.3
1994	3	220	2.9	2	10	0.7	0.7
1993	2	13	0.3	0	0	0.0	0.0
1992	2	171	3.2	0	12	0.0	1.2
1990	1	37	1.3	0	0	0.0	0.0

[1] Total usage: Total number of downloads. [2] Use rate: Total number of downloads/total number of papers.

Figure 2 depicts networks of collaboration among the top 20 countries having the highest volume of publications. The U.K. and the U.S. had the highest amount of collaborations, with 28 and 25 countries, correspondingly. In the U.S., among 322 published papers, there were more than 610 affiliations mentioned. Approximately 80% of them were from U.S. authors (~490 affiliations), 4% were from the U.K. (~23 affiliations), and 2% were from Denmark (~10 affiliations). Similarly, in the U.K., 160 papers were products of authors from 290 affiliations (or organizations), with ~58% from the U.K., 8% from the U.S. and 6% from Australia. These countries were followed by Germany (22 countries), Denmark (18 countries), and the Netherlands (18 countries).

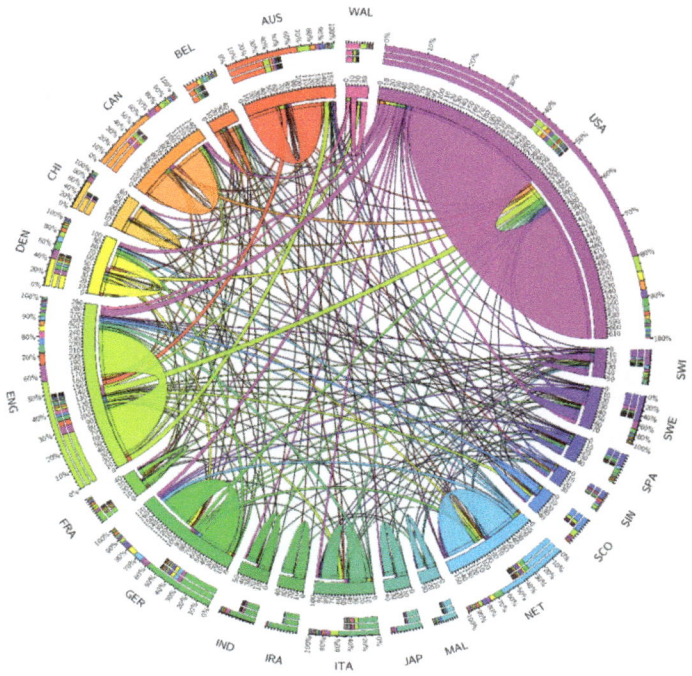

Figure 2. Collaboration network between the top 20 countries by the number of publications. The outer rim reflects the volume of collaborations between each country and the other countries in the top 20, showing collaboration among countries. Abbreviation: USA, the United States of America; ENG, England; GER, Germany; AUS, Australia; NET, the Netherlands; CAN, Canada; DEN, Denmark; ITA, Italy; SWE, Sweden; CHI, China; IND, India; SWI, Switzerland; BEL, Belgium; SPA, Spain; MAL, Malaysia; FRA, France; JAP, Japan; SCO, Scotland; IRA, Iran; SIN, Singapore.

To illustrate the scope of the selected studies, we performed a content analysis to evaluate the co-occurrence of the most frequent terms in the abstracts and titles. Figure 3 shows four major clusters emerging from the 271 most common keywords with a co-occurrence rate of at least 15: (1) the yellow cluster refers to clinical trials to test the efficacy and safety of drugs, as well as to control pain and overweight/obesity among people with diabetes (e.g., placebo, efficacy, safety, dose, pain, body weight, obesity, weight loss); (2) the blue cluster indicates trials focusing on diabetes prevention such as lifestyle- or behavior-related interventions (e.g., physical activity, exercise training, diet, etc.); (3) the green cluster covers the interventions using insulin-related therapies to control blood glucose level, particularly among patients with type 1 diabetes (e.g., insulin treatment, insulin glargine, etc.); and (4) the red cluster refers to interventions in the community to promote self-care capability (e.g., self-care, practice, self-efficacy, caregivers, etc.), as well as reduce the risk of psychological problems (e.g., depression or distress) among people with diabetes, especially in adolescents and children (e.g., adolescent, child, parent).

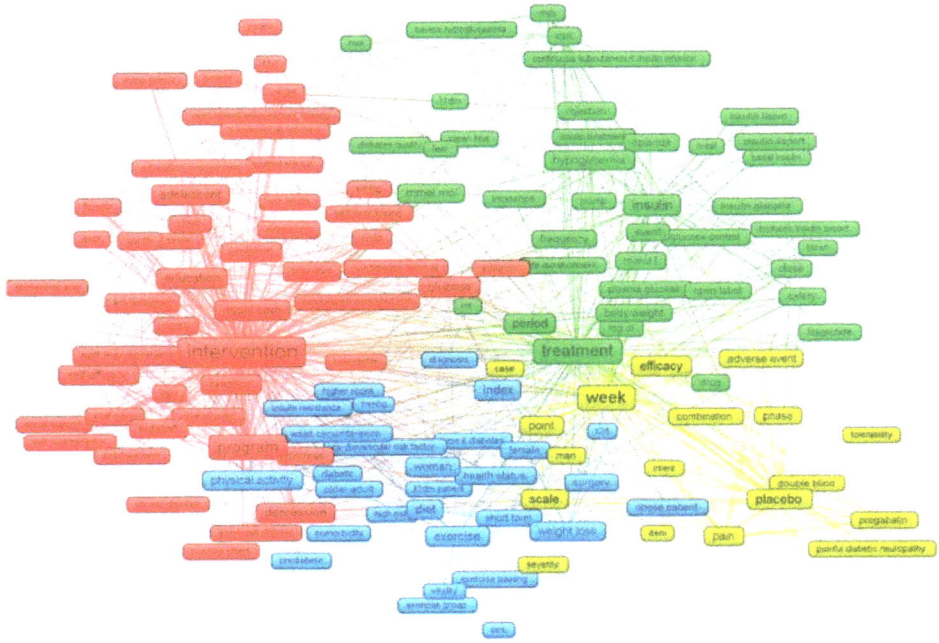

Figure 3. Co-occurrence of most frequent terms in titles and abstracts. The colors of the nodes indicate principal components of the data structure; the node size was scaled to the keywords' occurrences; the thickness of the lines was drawn based on the strength of the association between two keywords.

The top 10 clinical trials having the highest number of citations are presented in Table 2. All of them were RCTs, which focused mainly on the effectiveness of different medications, surgery, or behavioral therapies in controlling blood glucose; reducing the negative effects of diabetic complications (such as diabetic neuropathy, obesity, limb ischemia, or perinatal complications); and improving QOL in people with diabetes, especially pregnant women, children, and adolescents. Among the top three papers, the first paper, by Crowther et al., titled "Effect of treatment of gestational diabetes mellitus on pregnancy outcomes," published in 2005 in the *New England Journal of Medicine*, had the highest number of citations and evaluated the efficacy of dietary advice, blood glucose monitoring, and insulin therapy (by comparing the intervention group to a control group receiving only routine care) in treating gestational diabetes in pregnant women to prevent perinatal complications [32]. By using the Short-form 36 (SF-36) instrument, the results of this study showed a significant increase in QOL among participants [32]. The second paper, titled "Gabapentin for the symptomatic treatment of painful neuropathy in patients with diabetes mellitus—A randomized controlled trial," also used SF-36 and showed that gabapentin use significantly improved the QOL of patients with diabetic neuropathy compared to the placebo group [33]. The SF-36 was also used in the third-most cited paper, entitled "Bariatric Surgery versus Intensive Medical Therapy for Diabetes-3-Year Outcomes" [34]. The authors of this study indicated that bariatric surgery significantly enhanced health-related QOL among obese patients with type 2 diabetes compared to those receiving intensive medical therapy only [34].

Table 2. Top 10 most cited clinical trials.

Title	Journal	Total Citations	Publication Year	Cite Rate	Study Design	Type of Diabetes	Type of Interventions	QOL Tool
Effect of treatment of gestational diabetes mellitus on pregnancy outcomes [32]	New England Journal of Medicine	1,516	2005	108.3	RCT	gestational diabetes mellitus	dietary advice, blood glucose monitoring, and insulin therapy	SF-36
Gabapentin for the symptomatic treatment of painful neuropathy in patients with diabetes mellitus - A randomized controlled trial [33]	Journal of the American Medical Association	981	1998	46.7	RCT	Type 1 and type 2	Gabapentin	SF-36
Bariatric surgery versus intensive medical therapy for diabetes – 3-year outcomes [34]	New England Journal of Medicine	798	2014	159.6	RCT	Type 2	Bariatric Surgery, Intensive Medical Therapy	RAND-36
Does increased access to primary care reduce hospital readmissions?	New England Journal of Medicine	504	1996	21.9	RCT	General	Access to Primary Care	SF-36
Effectiveness of the diabetes education and self-management for ongoing and newly diagnosed (DESMOND) programme for people with newly diagnosed type 2 diabetes: Cluster randomized controlled trial [35]	British Medical Journal	356	2008	32.4	RCT	Type 2	Group education programme	WHOQOL-BREF
Double-blind randomized trial of tramadol for the treatment of the pain of diabetic neuropathy [36]	Neurology	351	1998	16.7	RCT	Type 1 and type 2	Tramadol	MOS
Controlled-release oxycodone relieves neuropathic pain: A randomized controlled trial in painful diabetic neuropathy [37]	Pain	324	2003	20.3	RCT	Type 1 and type 2	Controlled-release oxycodone	SF-36
Randomized placebo-controlled clinical trial of Lorcaserin for weight loss in Type 2 diabetes mellitus: The BLOOM-DM study [38]	Obesity	294	2012	42.0	RCT	Type 2	Lorcaserin	IWQOL-LITE
Bariatric surgery versus intensive medical therapy for diabetes – 5-year outcomes [39]	New England Journal of Medicine	293	2017	146.5	RCT	Type 2	Bariatric Surgery, Intensive Medical Therapy	RAND-36
Bariatric-metabolic surgery versus conventional medical treatment in obese patients with type 2 diabetes: 5-year follow-up of an open-label, single-centre, randomized controlled trial [40]	Lancet	289	2015	72.3	RCT	Type 2	Bariatric-metabolic Surgery	RAND-36

RCT: Randomized controlled trials, SF-36 = Short-form 36, WHOQOL-BREF = WHO Quality of Life-BREF; MOS = Medical Outcomes Studies; IWQOL-LITE = Impact of Weight on Quality of Life-LITE.

Figure 4 presents the hierarchical clustering of major research disciplines in interventions aiming to improve the QOL of people with type 2 diabetes. The horizontal axis reflects the dissimilarity between clusters, while the vertical axis reveals disciplines of pooled papers. This figure shows that interventions were separated into five major clusters. In the first cluster, the "Pediatrics" grouping is connected to "Endocrinology and Metabolism," suggesting that the majority of interventions for children with diabetes and adolescents were concentrated on using medications to enhance metabolic pathways such as insulin infusion or an insulin pump.

Meanwhile, the second cluster indicated clinical and lifestyle interventions to improve QOL in people with diabetes in general or with multiple comorbidities (such as cardiac disease and mental problems). For example, the "Pharmacology and Pharmacy" grouping was joined with "Medicine, Research and Experiment," which indicated that interventions using a pharmacological approach such as fenofibrate, ranolazine, or other drugs in glycemic control, reduced the damage done by diabetes and its complications and improved QOL. In addition, the "Sport Sciences" discipline was combined with the "Geriatrics and Gerontology" disciplines, showing that the common intervention approaches in older people with diabetes were facilitating physical activity. Similarly, for people with diabetes suffering cardiac illnesses ("Cardiac and Cardiovascular System"), "Surgery" and "Nutrition and Dietetics" were the two most common interventions.

The third cluster reveals clinical interventions to improve the QOL of people with diabetes in primary care settings. These included home- or community-based interventions.

Meanwhile, the fourth cluster indicated clinical interventions to enhance the QOL of people with diabetes suffering from neurological pain.

Finally, the fifth cluster showed public health, health service, health policy, and medical-information-technology-related interventions aiming to improve the QOL of people with diabetes. Notably, this cluster is not close to other groupings in the figure.

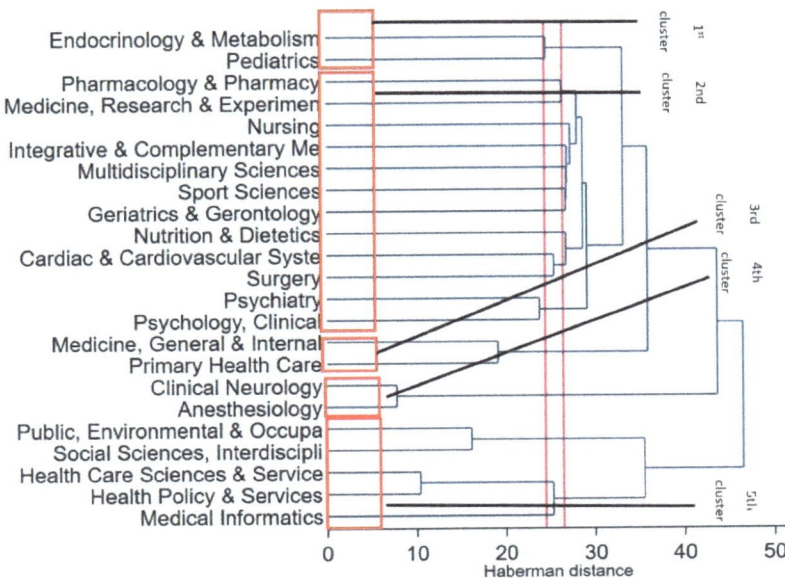

Figure 4. Dendrogram of coincidence of research areas using WOS classifications.

By using LDA, we categorized the selected interventions under ten major topic headings. The three topics with the highest number of publications included: (1) community-, family-, and eHealth-based interventions to improve self-management and self-efficacy; (2) lifestyle (e.g., physical activity and dietary) interventions in people with diabetes; (3) interventions focused on comorbidities in people with diabetes (Table 3). The first topic was investigated in 187 papers, accounting for 26.7% of total papers. Meanwhile, the second and third topics accounted for 17.7% and 15.3%, respectively.

Table 3. Ten research topics classified by Latent Dirichlet Allocation.

Rank	Research Topics	n	Percent
Topic 1	Community-, family-, and telehealth-based interventions to improve self-management and self-efficacy	187	26.7%
Topic 2	Lifestyle (e.g., physical activity and dietary) interventions in people with diabetes	124	17.7%
Topic 3	Interventions address comorbidities in people with diabetes	107	15.3%
Topic 4	Education-based interventions on different aspects of the disease	74	10.6%
Topic 5	Pharmacological treatment to control blood glucose levels	66	9.4%
Topic 6	Pharmacological treatment for diabetic neuropathic pain	52	7.4%
Topic 7	Functional complication interventions	29	4.1%
Topic 8	Interventions addressing mental disorders in people with diabetes	27	3.9%
Topic 9	Surgery and dietary interventions to promote weight loss	18	2.6%
Topic 10	Pharmacological and surgical interventions to address cardiovascular complications	16	2.3%

Figure 5 shows the correlation of publications to the ten topics. Recently, topics 1 and 2 received the greatest attention, with the largest number of publications every year in the three years 2015–2018. In the same period, the number of publications on topics 3 and 4 also increased, while the volume of publications on other topics decreased.

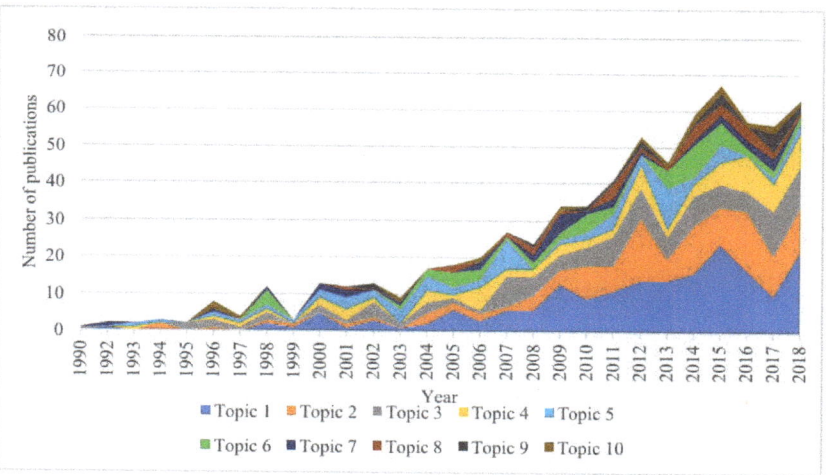

Figure 5. Changes in research topic development.

4. Discussion

Our study presents an overview of global research on interventions supporting QOL among people with diabetes during the period 1990–2018. The findings of this study indicated a general increase in the overall number of articles about this issue over time, and a significant disparity in the contributing countries based on income level. Community- and family-based interventions, including those focused on lifestyle and those utilizing digital technologies, were common approaches. Interventions that addressed comorbidities in people with diabetes also increased over the period.

Our findings emphasize the necessity of translating the evidence from clinical interventions to community interventions. In addition, they underline the importance of developing collaborative research between high-income countries (HICs) and low- and middle-income countries (LMICs). It is particularly true since LMICs are predicted to experience a substantially greater diabetes burden in the coming years [41].

Diabetes is a chronic condition and requires good self-management and long-term metabolic control for patients' QOL to improve [42]. Our analysis confirmed the findings of previous reviews [43] regarding approaches seen to increase the QOL of people with diabetes, including pharmacotherapy, surgery, and educational or lifestyle interventions to control blood glucose or diabetic complications, in both online (e.g., Internet or telephone) and offline settings (e.g., hospital, community, family, or school). Amid the increase in the diabetes burden as well as its pervasiveness in communities around the world, there is no doubt that community-, family-, or even online-based interventions are important to consider. This is confirmed by the high and growing number of publications on them, relative to other topics in the healthcare sector. We found that most studies focused on improving the self-management and self-efficacy of patients with diabetes, helping them monitor and control their blood glucose levels, as well as prevent the onset of diabetic complications [44]. This topic is followed by the application of lifestyle interventions (including diet with active physical activity), which plays a major role in enhancing diabetes outcomes and improving QOL. An earlier review of this type of intervention showed that it was more effective than pharmacotherapy in alleviating diabetic symptoms and complications, as well as in preventing the onset of diabetes [45]. The remaining topics included interventions to control and treat comorbidities and other complications such as neuropathic pain, mental disorders, cardiac diseases, and functional impairment such as foot ulcers or sexual disfunction. It has been confirmed in prior reviews that these problems significantly affect the QOL of people with diabetes [42,46]; therefore, medical approaches to solving these issues are critical to improving QOL not only in hospital settings but also in primary care and community settings.

Notably, this study revealed a skewed geographical distribution of the selected publications toward HICs such as the United States, England, Germany, Australia, and the Netherlands. China was the only middle-income country among the top 10 active nations. However, it should be noted that the burden of diabetes has been much greater for LMICs than for HICs. In 2016, a global report showed that among the 425 million people living with diabetes, approximately 80% of them resided in LMICs, and this figure is expected to increase significantly in the coming decades [1]. This disparity was in line with a previous bibliometric study about diabetes, depression, and suicide, though these same countries had the highest volume of publications on this topic [23]. Other scientometric studies also underlined the insufficient contribution of LMICs to research, which does not help diminish the diabetes burden in these nations [19,20,47,48]. The concept of QOL refers to the individual's perception of physical, psychological, and social conditions in a specific context and culture [11]. Thus, more contextualized evidence about the effects of interventions on the QOL of people with diabetes in LMICs is required to increase the applicability of these interventions. Insufficient evidence from LMICs might be due to a lack of funding sources, human resources, and infrastructure for research institutions [47–49]. This gap may not be fulfilled in the short term, but these countries might benefit from using evidence from neighboring nations having similar cultural, socioeconomic, and value systems. Regional collaborative networks may be developed such that LMICs with high research productivity (such as China and India) play a central role, with support from HICs. Such initiatives could strengthen the research capacity of member countries as well as increase the quality of evidence, which would serve as a foundation for further strategies to increase QOL of people with diabetes.

This study has several limitations. First, our sample was limited to English-language publications indexed in the WOS database. This may not reflect the development of publications on interventions improving QOL among people with diabetes in countries where English is not a native language. Therefore, publications from these countries, many of them LMICs, might be underestimated. Additionally, we did not use the full text of publications for our content analysis. That said, we analyzed various levels of data, including keywords, the text of the title and abstract, and research discipline categories, and also employed advanced analytical methods such as LDA [50].

5. Conclusions

Global research on interventions to improve the QOL of people with diabetes gradually increased in recent decades, with major contributions from HICs. Community- and family-based interventions, including those focused on lifestyle and utilizing digital technologies, have been common. Interventions to address comorbidities in people with diabetes have also been on the rise. More contextualized interventions in LMICs, as well as regional initiatives to support LMICs in translating worldwide evidence, should be facilitated to alleviate the diabetes burden in these countries.

Author Contributions: Conceptualization, B.X.T., L.H.N., H.T.T.V., G.H.H., C.A.L., C.S.H.H. and R.C.M.H.; Data curation, B.X.T., N.M.P., H.T.N., D.H.P., G.H.H. and H.Q.P.; Formal analysis, B.X.T., L.H.N. and H.T.N.; Funding acquisition, H.T.T.V. and D.H.P.; Investigation, L.H.N., N.M.P. and T.P.N.; Methodology, B.X.T., L.H.N. and H.T.T.V.; Resources, R.C.M.H.; Software, N.M.P., D.H.P., H.Q.P. and T.P.N.; Supervision, C.A.L.; Validation, H.T.N. and C.S.H.H.; Writing—original draft, L.H.N. and G.H.H.; Writing—review & editing, B.X.T., H.Q.P., C.A.L., C.S.H.H. and R.C.M.H. All authors have read and agreed to the published version of the manuscript.

Funding: This research received no external funding.

Acknowledgments: We would like to express our gratitude to the Stanford Asia Health Policy Program for the support in reviewing and editing this paper.

Conflicts of Interest: The authors declare no conflict of interest.

References

1. Cho, N.H.; Shaw, J.E.; Karuranga, S.; Huang, Y.; da Rocha Fernandes, J.D.; Ohlrogge, A.W.; Malanda, B. IDF Diabetes Atlas: Global estimates of diabetes prevalence for 2017 and projections for 2045. *Diabetes Res. Clin. Pract.* **2018**, *138*, 271–281. [CrossRef]
2. Smith-Palmer, J.; Bae, J.P.; Boye, K.S.; Norrbacka, K.; Hunt, B.; Valentine, W.J. Evaluating health-related quality of life in type 1 diabetes: A systematic literature review of utilities for adults with type 1 diabetes. *Clin. Outcomes Res. Ceor* **2016**, *8*, 559–571. [CrossRef]
3. World Health Organization. Diabetes: Fact Sheet. Available online: https://www.who.int/news-room/fact-sheets/detail/diabetes (accessed on 29 July 2019).
4. Baena-Diez, J.M.; Penafiel, J.; Subirana, I.; Ramos, R.; Elosua, R.; Marin-Ibanez, A.; Guembe, M.J.; Rigo, F.; Tormo-Diaz, M.J.; Moreno-Iribas, C.; et al. Risk of Cause-Specific Death in Individuals With Diabetes: A Competing Risks Analysis. *Diabetes Care* **2016**, *39*, 1987–1995. [CrossRef]
5. Global, regional, and national disability-adjusted life-years (DALYs) for 359 diseases and injuries and healthy life expectancy (HALE) for 195 countries and territories, 1990–2017: A systematic analysis for the Global Burden of Disease Study 2017. *Lancet* **2018**, *392*, 1859–1922. [CrossRef]
6. Jing, X.; Chen, J.; Dong, Y.; Han, D.; Zhao, H.; Wang, X.; Gao, F.; Li, C.; Cui, Z.; Liu, Y.; et al. Related factors of quality of life of type 2 diabetes patients: A systematic review and meta-analysis. *Health Qual. Life Outcomes* **2018**, *16*, 189. [CrossRef]
7. Saleh, F.; Ara, F.; Mumu, S.J.; Hafez, M.A. Assessment of health-related quality of life of Bangladeshi patients with type 2 diabetes using the EQ-5D: A cross-sectional study. *BMC Res. Notes* **2015**, *8*, 497. [CrossRef]
8. Costanza, R.; Fisher, B.; Ali, S.; Beer, C.; Bond, L.; Boumans, R.; Danigelis, N.L.; Dickinson, J.; Elliott, C.; Farley, J.; et al. Quality of life: An approach integrating opportunities, human needs, and subjective well-being. *Ecol. Econ.* **2007**, *61*, 267–276. [CrossRef]
9. Galloway, S.; Bell, D.; Hamilton, C.; Scullion, A. *Quality of Life and Well-Being: Measuring the Benefits of Culture and Sport: Literature Review and Thinkpiece*; 0755929071; Analytical Services Division, Scottish Executive Education Department: Edinburgh, UK, 2006.
10. Cummins, R.A. *Quality of Life Definition and Terminology: A Discussion Document from the International Society for Quality of Life Studies*; International Society for Quality-of-Life Studies: Gilbert, AZ, UAS, 1998.
11. WHOQoL Group. Study protocol for the World Health Organization project to develop a Quality of Life assessment instrument (WHOQOL). *Qual. Life Res.* **1993**, *2*, 153–159. [CrossRef]

12. Zhang, X.; Norris, S.L.; Chowdhury, F.M.; Gregg, E.W.; Zhang, P. The effects of interventions on health-related quality of life among persons with diabetes: A systematic review. *Med. Care* **2007**, *45*, 820–834. [CrossRef]
13. Luscombe, F.A. Health-related quality of life measurement in type 2 diabetes. *Value Health J. Int. Soc. Pharm. Outcomes Res.* **2000**, *3* (Suppl. 1), 15–28. [CrossRef]
14. Watkins, K.; Connell, C.M. Measurement of health-related QOL in diabetes mellitus. *Pharmacoeconomics* **2004**, *22*, 1109–1126. [CrossRef] [PubMed]
15. Cai, H.; Li, G.; Zhang, P.; Xu, D.; Chen, L. Effect of exercise on the quality of life in type 2 diabetes mellitus: A systematic review. *Qual. Life Res.* **2017**, *26*, 515–530. [CrossRef] [PubMed]
16. Magwood, G.S.; Zapka, J.; Jenkins, C. A Review of Systematic Reviews Evaluating Diabetes Interventions. *Diabetes Educ.* **2008**, *34*, 242–265. [CrossRef] [PubMed]
17. Ayadurai, S.; Hattingh, H.L.; Tee, L.B.G.; Md Said, S.N. A Narrative Review of Diabetes Intervention Studies to Explore Diabetes Care Opportunities for Pharmacists. *J. Diabetes Res.* **2016**, *2016*, 11. [CrossRef]
18. Massey, C.N.; Feig, E.H.; Duque-Serrano, L.; Wexler, D.; Moskowitz, J.T.; Huffman, J.C. Well-being interventions for individuals with diabetes: A systematic review. *Diabetes Res. Clin. Pract.* **2019**, *147*, 118–133. [CrossRef]
19. Emami, Z.; Hariri, N.; Khamseh, M.E.; Nooshinfard, F. Mapping diabetes research in Middle Eastern countries during 2007–2013: A scientometric analysis. *Med. J. Islamic Repub. Iran* **2018**, *32*, 84. [CrossRef]
20. Rasolabadi, M.; Khaledi, S.; Ardalan, M.; Kalhor, M.M.; Penjvini, S.; Gharib, A. Diabetes Research in Iran: A Scientometric Analysis of Publications Output. *Acta Inform. Med.* **2015**, *23*, 160–164. [CrossRef]
21. Bruggmann, D.; Richter, T.; Klingelhofer, D.; Gerber, A.; Bundschuh, M.; Jaque, J.; Groneberg, D.A. Global architecture of gestational diabetes research: Density-equalizing mapping studies and gender analysis. *Nutr. J.* **2016**, *15*, 36. [CrossRef]
22. Ramin, S.; Gharebaghi, R.; Heidary, F. Scientometric Analysis and Mapping of Scientific Articles on Diabetic Retinopathy. *Med. Hypothesisdiscov. Innov. Ophthalmol. J.* **2015**, *4*, 81–100.
23. Sweileh, W.M. Analysis of global research output on diabetes depression and suicide. *Ann. Gen. Psychiatry* **2018**, *17*, 44. [CrossRef]
24. Tabatabaei-Malazy, O.; Ramezani, A.; Atlasi, R.; Larijani, B.; Abdollahi, M. Scientometric study of academic publications on antioxidative herbal medicines in type 2 diabetes mellitus. *J. Diabetes Metab. Disord.* **2016**, *15*, 48. [CrossRef] [PubMed]
25. Martín-Martín, A.; Orduna-Malea, E.; Delgado López-Cózar, E. Coverage of highly-cited documents in Google Scholar, Web of Science, and Scopus: A multidisciplinary comparison. *Scientometrics* **2018**, *116*, 2175–2188. [CrossRef]
26. Clarivate Analytics. Web of Science databases. Available online: https://clarivate.com/products/web-of-science/databases/ (accessed on 26 June 2019).
27. Krzywinski, M.; Schein, J.; Birol, I.; Connors, J.; Gascoyne, R.; Horsman, D.; Jones, S.J.; Marra, M.A. Circos: An information aesthetic for comparative genomics. *Genome Res.* **2009**, *19*, 1639–1645. [CrossRef] [PubMed]
28. Valle, D.; Albuquerque, P.; Zhao, Q.; Barberan, A.; Fletcher, R.J., Jr. Extending the Latent Dirichlet Allocation model to presence/absence data: A case study on North American breeding birds and biogeographical shifts expected from climate change. *Glob. Chang. Biol.* **2018**, *24*, 5560–5572. [CrossRef] [PubMed]
29. Chen, C.; Zare, A.; Trinh, H.N.; Omotara, G.O.; Cobb, J.T.; Lagaunne, T.A. Partial Membership Latent Dirichlet Allocation for Soft Image Segmentation. *IEEE Trans. Image Process.* **2017**, *26*, 5590–5602. [CrossRef] [PubMed]
30. Lu, H.M.; Wei, C.P.; Hsiao, F.Y. Modeling healthcare data using multiple-channel latent Dirichlet allocation. *J. Biomed. Inf.* **2016**, *60*, 210–223. [CrossRef]
31. Gross, A.; Murthy, D. Modeling virtual organizations with Latent Dirichlet Allocation: A case for natural language processing. *Neural. Netw.* **2014**, *58*, 38–49. [CrossRef]
32. Crowther, C.A.; Hiller, J.E.; Moss, J.R.; McPhee, A.J.; Jeffries, W.S.; Robinson, J.S. Effect of Treatment of Gestational Diabetes Mellitus on Pregnancy Outcomes. *N. Engl. J. Med.* **2005**, *352*, 2477–2486. [CrossRef]
33. Backonja, M.; Beydoun, A.; Edwards, K.R.; Schwartz, S.L.; Fonseca, V.; Hes, M.; LaMoreaux, L.; Garofalo, E. Gabapentin for the symptomatic treatment of painful neuropathy in patients with diabetes mellitus: A randomized controlled trial. *JAMA* **1998**, *280*, 1831–1836. [CrossRef]

34. Schauer, P.R.; Bhatt, D.L.; Kirwan, J.P.; Wolski, K.; Brethauer, S.A.; Navaneethan, S.D.; Aminian, A.; Pothier, C.E.; Kim, E.S.H.; Nissen, S.E.; et al. Bariatric Surgery versus Intensive Medical Therapy for Diabetes—3-Year Outcomes. *N. Engl. J. Med.* **2014**, *370*, 2002–2013. [CrossRef]
35. Weinberger, M.; Oddone, E.Z.; Henderson, W.G. Does increased access to primary care reduce hospital readmissions? Veterans Affairs Cooperative Study Group on Primary Care and Hospital Readmission. *N. Engl. J. Med.* **1996**, *334*, 1441–1447. [CrossRef]
36. Davies, M.J.; Heller, S.; Skinner, T.C.; Campbell, M.J.; Carey, M.E.; Cradock, S.; Dallosso, H.M.; Daly, H.; Doherty, Y.; Eaton, S.; et al. Effectiveness of the diabetes education and self management for ongoing and newly diagnosed (DESMOND) programme for people with newly diagnosed type 2 diabetes: Cluster randomised controlled trial. *BMJ* **2008**, *336*, 491–495. [CrossRef] [PubMed]
37. Harati, Y.; Gooch, C.; Swenson, M.; Edelman, S.; Greene, D.; Raskin, P.; Donofrio, P.; Cornblath, D.; Sachdeo, R.; Siu, C.O.; et al. Double-blind randomized trial of tramadol for the treatment of the pain of diabetic neuropathy. *Neurology* **1998**, *50*, 1842–1846. [CrossRef] [PubMed]
38. Watson, C.P.N.; Moulin, D.; Watt-Watson, J.; Gordon, A.; Eisenhoffer, J. Controlled-release oxycodone relieves neuropathic pain: A randomized controlled trial in painful diabetic neuropathy. *Pain* **2003**, *105*, 71–78. [CrossRef]
39. O'Neil, P.M.; Smith, S.R.; Weissman, N.J.; Fidler, M.C.; Sanchez, M.; Zhang, J.; Raether, B.; Anderson, C.M.; Shanahan, W.R. Randomized Placebo-Controlled Clinical Trial of Lorcaserin for Weight Loss in Type 2 Diabetes Mellitus: The BLOOM-DM Study. *Obesity* **2012**, *20*, 1426–1436. [CrossRef]
40. Schauer, P.R.; Bhatt, D.L.; Kirwan, J.P.; Wolski, K.; Aminian, A.; Brethauer, S.A.; Navaneethan, S.D.; Singh, R.P.; Pothier, C.E.; Nissen, S.E.; et al. Bariatric Surgery versus Intensive Medical Therapy for Diabetes—5-Year Outcomes. *N. Engl. J. Med.* **2017**, *376*, 641–651. [CrossRef]
41. Mingrone, G.; Panunzi, S.; De Gaetano, A.; Guidone, C.; Iaconelli, A.; Nanni, G.; Castagneto, M.; Bornstein, S.; Rubino, F. Bariatric-metabolic surgery versus conventional medical treatment in obese patients with type 2 diabetes: 5 year follow-up of an open-label, single-centre, randomised controlled trial. *Lancet* **2015**, *386*, 964–973. [CrossRef]
42. Satterfield, D.W.; Volansky, M.; Caspersen, C.J.; Engelgau, M.M.; Bowman, B.A.; Gregg, E.W.; Geiss, L.S.; Hosey, G.M.; May, J.; Vinicor, F. Community-Based Lifestyle Interventions to Prevent Type 2 Diabetes. *Diabetes Care* **2003**, *26*, 2643–2652. [CrossRef] [PubMed]
43. Shrestha, P.; Ghimire, L. A review about the effect of life style modification on diabetes and quality of life. *Glob. J. Health Sci.* **2012**, *4*, 185–190. [CrossRef] [PubMed]
44. Trikkalinou, A.; Papazafiropoulou, A.K.; Melidonis, A. Type 2 diabetes and quality of life. *World J. Diabetes* **2017**, *8*, 120–129. [CrossRef]
45. Liu, L.; Jiao, J.H.; Chen, L. Bibliometric study of diabetic retinopathy during 2000–2010 by ISI. *Int. J. Ophthalmol.* **2011**, *4*, 333–336. [CrossRef] [PubMed]
46. Somogyi, A.; Schubert, A.J.S. Correlation between national bibliometric and health indicators: The case of diabetes. *Scientometrics* **2005**, *62*, 285–292. [CrossRef]
47. Khanal, P. Bringing all together for research capacity building in LMICs. *Lancet Glob. Health* **2017**, *5*, e868. [CrossRef]
48. ESSENCE on Health Research. *Seven Principle for Strengthening Research Capacity in Low-and-Middle-Income Countries: Simple Ideas in a Complex World*; TDR/World Health Organization: Geneva, Switzerland, 2014.
49. Ali, N.; Hill, C.; Kennedy, A.; IJsselmuiden, C. *What Factors Influence National Health Research Agendas in Low and Middle Income Countries*; Council on Health Research for Development (COHRED): Geneva, Switzerland, 2006.
50. Baghaei Lakeh, A.; Ghaffarzadegan, N. Global Trends and Regional Variations in Studies of HIV/AIDS. *Sci. Rep.* **2017**, *7*, 4170. [CrossRef] [PubMed]

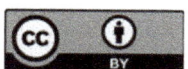

© 2020 by the authors. Licensee MDPI, Basel, Switzerland. This article is an open access article distributed under the terms and conditions of the Creative Commons Attribution (CC BY) license (http://creativecommons.org/licenses/by/4.0/).

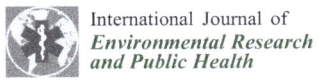

Article

Worldwide Research Trends on Medicinal Plants

Esther Salmerón-Manzano [1], Jose Antonio Garrido-Cardenas [2] and Francisco Manzano-Agugliaro [3],*

1. Faculty of Law, Universidad Internacional de La Rioja (UNIR), 26006 Logroño, Spain; esther.salmeron@unir.net
2. Department of Biology and Geology, University of Almeria, ceiA3, 04120 Almeria, Spain; jcardena@ual.es
3. Department of Engineering, University of Almeria, ceiA3, 04120 Almeria, Spain
* Correspondence: fmanzano@ual.es; Tel.: +34-950-015-396; Fax: +34-950-015-491

Received: 22 March 2020; Accepted: 11 May 2020; Published: 12 May 2020

Abstract: The use of medicinal plants has been done since ancient times and may even be considered the origin of modern medicine. Compounds of plant origin have been and still are an important source of compounds for drugs. In this study a bibliometric study of all the works indexed in the Scopus database until 2019 has been carried out, analyzing more than 100,000 publications. On the one hand, the main countries, institutions and authors researching this topic have been identified, as well as their evolution over time. On the other hand, the links between the authors, the countries and the topics under research have been analyzed through the detection of communities. The last two periods, from 2009 to 2014 and from 2015 to 2019, have been examined in terms of research topics. It has been observed that the areas of study or clusters have been reduced, those of the last period being those engaged in unclassified drug, traditional medicine, cancer, in vivo study—antidiabetic activity, and animals—anti-inflammatory activity. In summary, it has been observed that the trend in global research is focused more on the search for new medicines or active compounds rather than on the cultivation or domestication of plant species with this demonstrated potential.

Keywords: medicinal plants; drugs; worldwide research; bibliometrics; traditional medicine

---

1. Introduction

Ten percent of all vascular plants are used as medicinal plants [1], and there are estimated to be between 350,000 [2] and almost half a million [3] species of them. Since ancient times, plants have been used in medicine and are still used today [4]. In the beginning, the trial and error method was used to treat illnesses or even simply to feel better, and in this way, to distinguish useful plants with beneficial effects [5]. The use of these plants has been gradually refined over the generations, and this has become known in many contexts as traditional medicine. The official definition of traditional medicine can be considered as "the sum total of the knowledge, skills and practices based on the theories, beliefs and experiences indigenous to different cultures, whether explicable or not, used in the maintenance of health, as well as in the prevention, diagnosis, improvement or treatment of physical and mental illnesses" [6].

It is a fact that all civilizations have developed this form of medicine [7] based on the plants in their own habitat [8]. There are even authors who claim that this transmitted knowledge is the origin of medicine and pharmacy. Even today, hundreds of higher plants are cultivated worldwide to obtain useful substances in medicine and pharmacy [9]. The therapeutic properties of plants gave rise to medicinal drugs made from certain plants with these benefits [10].

Until the 18th century, the therapeutic properties of many plants, their effect on the human organism and their method of treatment were known, but the active compound was unknown [11].

As an example, the Canon of Medicine written by the Persian physician and scientist Avicenna (Ibn Sina) was used until the 18th century [12].

The origin of modern science, especially in the Renaissance, in particular chemical analysis, and the associated instrumentation such as the microscope, was what made it possible to isolate the active principles of medical plants [13]. Since then, these active principles have been obtained synthetically in the laboratory to produce the medicines later [14]. The use of medicines was gradually expanded. Until today, the direct use of medicinal plants is apparently displaced in modern medicine [15]. Today's medicine needs the industry producing pharmaceutical medicines, which are largely based on the active principles of plants, and therefore, these are used as raw materials in many cases [16]. Yet, today, the underdeveloped world does not have access to this modern medicine of synthetic origin, and therefore, large areas of the world continue to use traditional medicine based on the direct use of medicinal plants due to their low cost [17].

However, it should be noted that the possible trend to return to this type of traditional medicine may have two major drawbacks. The first is the use of medicinal plants without sanitary control, without thinking about the possible harmful aspects for health [18]. Although many plants do not have side effects like the aromatic plants used in infusions: chamomile, rosemary, mint, or thyme; however, others may have dangerous active principles. To cite an example, Bitter melon (*Momordica charantia L.*) used to cure fever and in cases of malaria [19], its green seeds are very toxic as they can cause a sharp drop in blood sugar and induce a patient's coma (hypoglycemic coma) [20]; this is due to the fact that the components of bitter melon extract appear to have structural similarities to animal insulin [21]. Secondly, there has been a proliferation of products giving rise to false perspectives, as they are not sufficiently researched [22].

Examining the specialized literature of reviews and bibliometric studies on medicinal plants, three types of studies are found: those focused on a geographical area, those focused on a specific plant or family, and those focused on some type of medical interest activity. Regarding the studies of geographical areas, for example, there are the studies of Africa. Specifically, in South Africa, the plants that are marketed [23], as these plants of medical interest have been promoted [24], or for the treatment of specific diseases such as Alzheimer's [25]. In Central Africa, the studies of Cameroon are remarkable, where for general bibliometric studies of its scientific output, the topic of medicinal plants stands out as one of the most important in this country [26]. Or those of Ghana, regarding frequent diseases in this country such as malaria, HIV/AIDS, hypertension, tuberculosis, or bleeding disorders [27]. Other countries that have conducted a bibliometric study of their medicinal plants have been Cuba [28] and China [29].

The other direction of the bibliometric studies mentioned, those that focus on specific plants, are those of: *Artemisia annua L.* [30], *Aloe vera* [31], *Panax ginseng* [32], *Punica grantum L.* [33], *Apocynum cannabinum* [34], or *Andrographis paniculata* [35]. The third line of the bibliometric research on medicinal plants deals with some kind of specific activity; there are studies for example for the activities of: antibacterial or antifungal [36], antioxidant [37], and anticancer [38–40].

As a common feature of the bibliometric studies published so far, none of them has a worldwide perspective. Furthermore, they are generally based on Web of Science and some of them on other more specific databases such as CAB Abstracts or PlantMedCUBA, but no work based on Scopus has been observed. Therefore, this paper aims to study what types of scientific advances are being developed around medicinal plants, what research trends are being carried out, and by which countries and research institutions. To this purpose, it is proposed to carry out a bibliometric analysis of all the scientific publications on this topic.

2. Materials and Methods

The data analyzed in this work have been obtained through a query in the Scopus database, which has been successfully used in a large number of bibliometric studies [41]. Due to the large amount of results, it was necessary to use the Scopus API to download the data, whose methodology has been developed in previous works [42,43]. In this study, the query used was: (TITLE-ABS-KEY("medic* plant*")). An outline of the methodology used is shown in Figure 1. The analysis of the scientific communities, both in terms of keywords and the relationship between authors or between countries was done with the SW VosViewer [44].

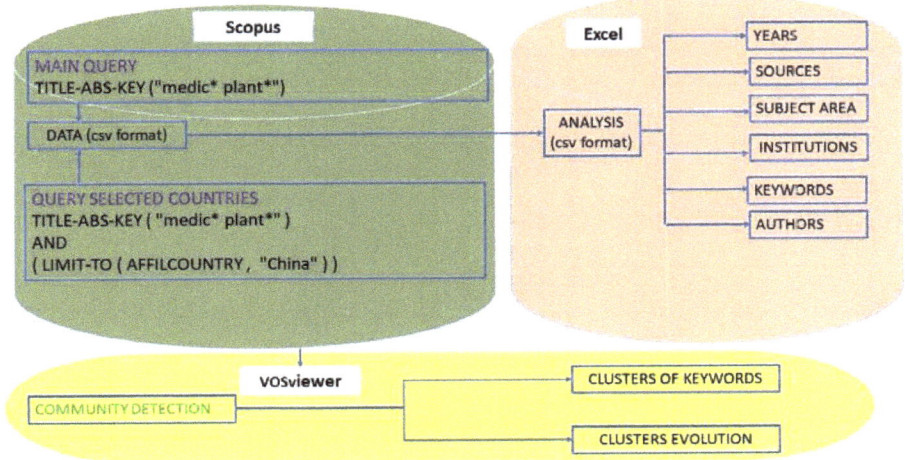

Figure 1. Methodology.

3. Results

3.1. Global Evolution Trend

From 1960 to 2019, more than 110,000 studies related to medicinal plants have been published. Figure 2 shows the trend in research in this field. Overall, it can be said that there was a continuous increase from 1960 to 2001, with just over 1300 published studies. From here, the trend increases faster until 2011, when it reaches a maximum of just over 6200 publications. After this period, publications stabilize at just over 5000 per year. These three periods identified are highlighted in Figure 2.

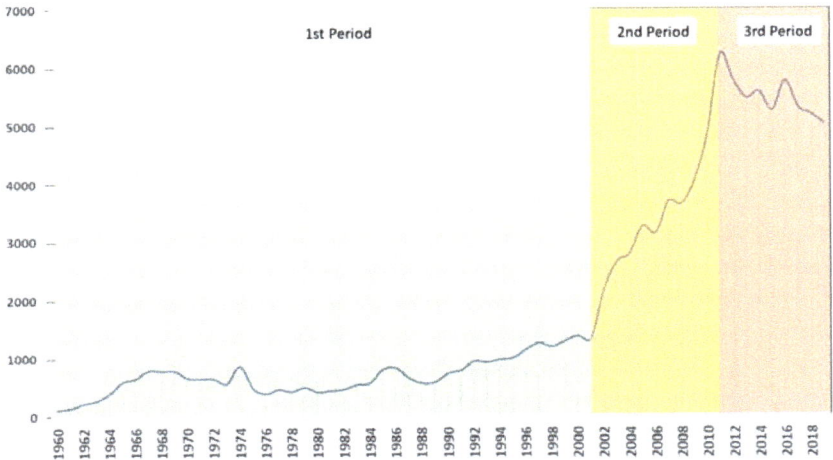

Figure 2. Worldwide temporal evolution of medical plants publications.

3.2. Global Subject Category

If the results are analyzed according to the categories in which they have been published (see Figure 3), according to the Scopus database, it can be seen that most of them have been carried out in the Pharmacology, Toxicology and Pharmaceutics category with 27.1 % of the total. Other categories with significant relative relevance have been: Medicine (23.8%), Biochemistry, Genetics and Molecular Biology (16.7%), Agricultural and Biological Sciences (11%), Chemistry (8.7%), Immunology and Microbiology (2.5%), Environmental Science (2.1%), and Chemical Engineering (1.5%). All other categories are below 1%, such as: Nursing, Multidisciplinary, or Engineering.

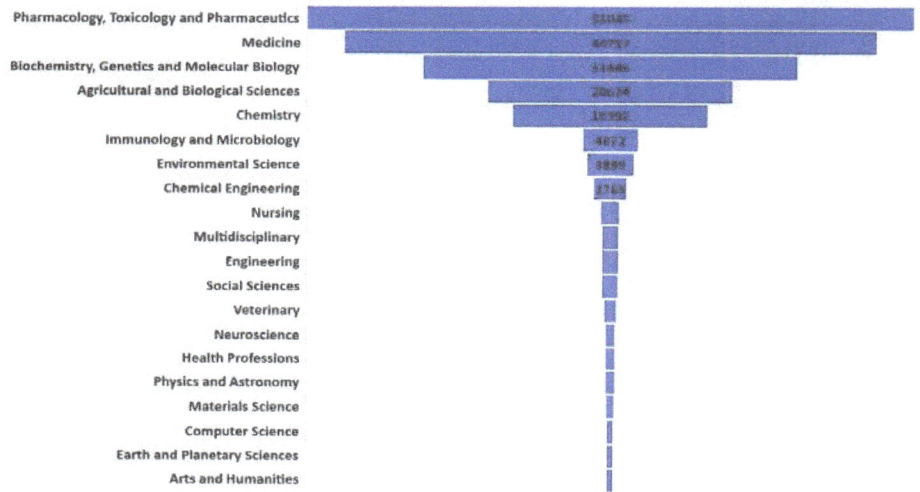

Figure 3. Medicinal plants publications by scientific categories indexed in Scopus.

3.3. Distribution of Publications by Countries

If the results obtained are analyzed by country, a total of 159 countries have published on this topic. Figure 4 shows the countries that have published on the subject and the intensity with which they published has been shown. It is observed that China and India stand out over the rest of the countries with more than 10,000 publications, perhaps influenced by traditional medicine, although their most cited works are related to antioxidant activity, both for China [45], and for India [46,47], and in this last country also antidiabetic potential [4]. The third place is the USA followed by Brazil, both with more than 5000 publications. The most frequently cited publications from these countries focus on antioxidant activity [48], and antimicrobial activity [49] for the USA and anti-inflammatory activity for Brazil [50,51].

As mentioned, the list of countries is very long, but those with more than 2000 publications are included: Japan, South Korea, Germany, Iran, United Kingdom, Pakistan, Italy, and France. If the overall results obtained are analyzed in their evolution by years, for this list of countries with more than 2000 publications, Figure 5 is obtained. From this point onwards, three groups of countries can be identified.

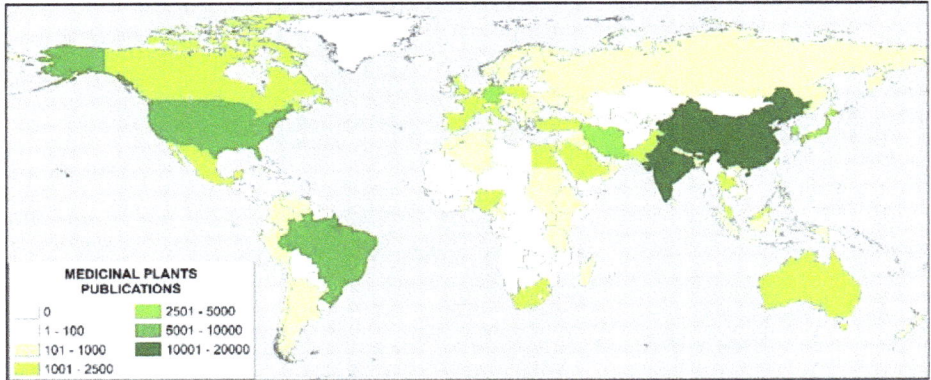

Figure 4. Worldwide research on medical plants.

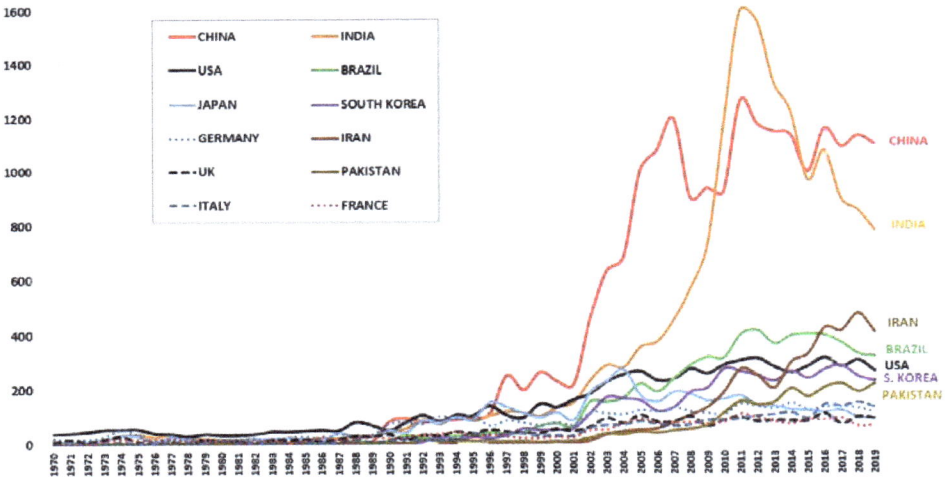

Figure 5. Temporal evolution on medical plants publications for Top 12 countries.

The first group is the leaders of this research, China and India, with between 800 and 1100 publications per year. China led the research from 1996 to 2010, and from this year to 2016, the leader was India, after which it returned to China. The second group of five countries is formed in order in the last year of the study: Iran, Brazil, USA, South Korea and Pakistan. This group of countries has a sustained growth over time, with a rate of publications between 200 and 400 per year. It should be noted that Brazil led the third place for a decade, from 2007 to 2016, since then that position is for Iran. The third group of five countries is made up of: Japan, Germany, United Kingdom, Italy, and France. They are keeping the publications around 100 a year, with an upward trend, but at a very slight rate.

If the analysis of the publications by country is made according to the categories in which they publish, Figure 6 is obtained, which shows the relative effort between the different themes or categories is shown. At first look, it might seem that they have a similar distribution. However, in relative terms the category of Pharmacology, Toxicology and Pharmaceutics is led by Brazil with 35% of its own publications followed by India with 33%. For the Medicine category, in relative terms it is led by China with 29 %, followed by Germany with 27 %. The category of Biochemistry, Genetics and Molecular

Biology always takes second or third place for this ranking of countries, standing out especially for Japan and South Korea with 23% and for France with 22%. The fourth category for many countries is Agricultural and Biological Sciences, with Pakistan standing out with 20%, followed by Italy with 16%. The category of Chemistry occupies the fourth category for countries such as Japan with 20% or Iran with 14%. The other categories: Chemical Engineering, Immunology and Microbiology, Environmental Science, Multidisciplinary, or Engineering, are below 5 % in all countries.

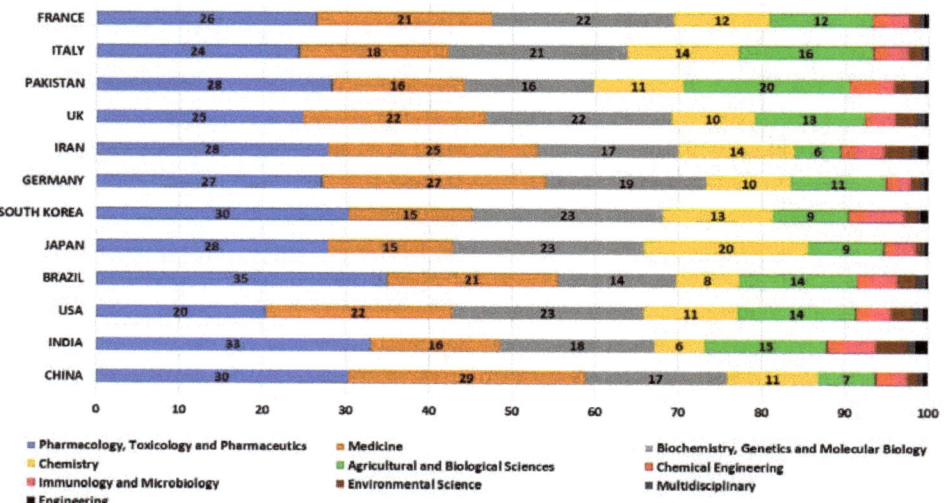

Figure 6. Distribution by scientific categories according to countries.

According to these results, it can be seen the relative lack of relevance of the category of Agricultural and Biological Sciences for medicinal plants, compared to the categories of Pharmacology, Toxicology and Pharmaceutics, Medicine, or Biochemistry, Genetics and Molecular Biology.

3.4. Institutions (Affiliations)

So far, the distribution by country has been seen, but the research is done in specific research centers (institution or affiliations as are indexed in Scopus) and therefore, it is important to study them. Table 1 shows the 25 institutions with more than 400 publications, of which 13 are from China (including the first 7), 3 from Brazil, 2 from South Korea, and now with 1: Saudi Arabia, Pakistan, Iran, Mexico, Cameroon, France, and Malaysia.

If the three main keywords of these affiliations are analyzed, it can be seen that there are no great differences, and in fact, they are often the same: Unclassified Drug, Drug Isolation, Drug Structure, Chemistry, Controlled Study, Isolation And Purification, Chemistry, and Plant Extract. They only call attention to "Drugs, Chinese Herbal" which appears in two affiliations: China Academy of Chinese Medical Sciences, and Beijing University of Chinese Medicine, which of course is a very specific issue in this country.

Table 1. Top 25 affiliations and main keywords.

Institution	Country	N	Keyword 1	Keyword 2	Keyword 3
Chinese Academy of Sciences	China	2322	Unclassified Drug	Drug Isolation	Drug Structure
Chinese Academy of Medical Sciences	China	1432	Chemistry	Unclassified Drug	Isolation And Purification
Peking Union Medical College Hospital	China	1200	Chemistry	Unclassified Drug	Isolation And Purification
Ministry of Education China	China	1192	Unclassified Drug	Controlled Study	Chemistry
China Pharmaceutical University	China	851	Unclassified Drug	Chemistry	Plant Extract
Kunming Institute of Botany Chinese Academy of Sciences	China	694	Unclassified Drug	Drug Isolation	Drug Structure
China Academy of Chinese Medical Sciences	China	650	Unclassified Drug	Chemistry	Drugs, Chinese Herbal
Universidade de Sao Paulo—USP	Brazil	626	Unclassified Drug	Plant Extract	Controlled Study
Shenyang Pharmaceutical University	China	598	Unclassified Drug	Chemistry	Drug Isolation
University of Chinese Academy of Sciences	China	549	Unclassified Drug	Controlled Study	Drug Isolation
UNESP-Universidade Estadual Paulista	Brazil	534	Unclassified Drug	Plant Extract	Controlled Study
Kyung Hee University	South Korea	533	Unclassified Drug	Controlled Study	Plant Extract
King Saud University	Saudi Arabia	533	Unclassified Drug	Plant Extract	Controlled Study
Beijing University of Chinese Medicine	China	533	Chemistry	Drugs, Chinese Herbal	Herbaceous Agent
University of Karachi	Pakistan	520	Unclassified Drug	Plant Extract	Drug Isolation
Zhejiang University	China	497	Unclassified Drug	Chemistry	Controlled Study
Seoul National University	South Korea	496	Unclassified Drug	Controlled Study	Plant Extract
Tehran University of Medical Sciences	Iran	461	Unclassified Drug	Plant Extract	Controlled Study
Universidad Nacional Autónoma de México	Mexico	453	Unclassified Drug	Plant Extract	Controlled Study
Université de Yaoundé I	Cameroon	451	Unclassified Drug	Plant Extract	Controlled Study
Peking University	China	434	Unclassified Drug	Chemistry	Isolation And Purification
Second Military Medical University	China	425	Unclassified Drug	Plant Extract	Controlled Study
Universidade Federal do Rio de Janeiro	Brazil	414	Unclassified Drug	Plant Extract	Controlled Study
CNRS Centre National de la Recherche Scientifique	France	410	Unclassified Drug	Plant Extract	Controlled Study
Universiti Putra Malaysia	Malaysia	406	Unclassified Drug	Plant Extract	Controlled Study

3.5. Authors

The main authors researching this topic are shown in Table 2, which are those with more than 100 publications on this topic. It is observed that they are authors with a significantly high h-index. On the other hand, it is noteworthy that the first two are not from China or India, which as we have seen were the most productive countries, and also had the most relevant institutions in this area. The lead author is from South Africa, J. Van Staden, and the second from Bangladesh, M. Rahmatullah. The author with the highest h-index is from Germany, T. Efferth.

Table 2. Main authors in medicinal plants.

	Author	Scopus Author ID	N	Affiliation, Country	h-Index
1	Van Staden, J.	7201832631	238	University of KwaZulu-Natal, South Africa	69
2	Rahmatullah, M.	6701489271	175	University of Dhaka, Bangladesh	38
3	Huang, L.Q.	56156528000	150	China Academy of Chinese Medical Sciences, China	36
4	Choudhary, M.I.	35228815600	142	University of Karachi, Pakistan	53
5	Afolayan, A.J.	7003478648	137	University of Fort Hare, South Africa	41
6	Heinrich, M.	16156235300	124	UCL, London, United Kingdom	54
7	Khan, I.A.	26643155300	124	University of Mississippi, United States	54
8	Efferth, T.	7005243974	122	Johannes Gutenberg Universität Mainz, Germany	70
9	Farnsworth, N.R.	35392089500	118	University of Illinois at Chicago, United States	63
10	Rafieian-Kopaei, M.	6506929448	115	Shahrekord University of Medical Sciences, Iran	60
11	Kuete, V.	15757756200	114	University of Dschang, Cameroon	38
12	Xiao, P.G.	7103088959	113	Ministry of Education China, China	37
13	Vilegas, W.	7004140097	107	UNESP-Universidade Estadual Paulista, Brazil	36
14	Hao, X.J.	7202000647	105	Chinese Academy of Sciences, China	38
15	Sun, H.D.	7404828012	105	Kunming Institute of Botany Chinese Academy of Sciences, China	47
16	Li, P.	56381767900	101	China Pharmaceutical University, China	51

If the network of collaboration between authors with more than 40 documents is established, Figure 7 is obtained. Here, there are 33 clusters, where the most important is the red one with 195 authors, where the central author is Huang, L.Q. The second more abundant cluster is the green one, composed of 69 authors. In this cluster, there is no central author, but instead, a collaboration between prominent authors such as Kim, J.S., Lee, K.R. or Park, J.S. The third cluster, in blue, is composed of 64 authors, led by the authors M.I. Choudhary and M. Ahmad.

The fourth cluster, of yellow color is composed of 63 authors, the central authors are Y. Li and H-D. Sun. The fifth cluster, in purple, is also composed of 51 authors, the central author is W. Villegas. It should be noted that this cluster is not linked to the whole network, so they must research very specific topics in their field. The sixth cluster is composed of 48 authors and is cyan colored, the central author is Rahmatullah, M. The cluster of the main author of Table 2, Van Staden, J., is composed of 23 authors, and would be number 17 in order of importance by number of authors, is light brown, and is located next to that of W. Vilegas but without any apparent connection.

3.6. Keywords

3.6.1. Global Perspective

The central aspect of bibliometric studies is to study the keywords in the publications and, through the relationships between them, to establish the clusters or scientific communities in which the different topics associated with a field of study can be grouped together. If keywords are extracted from the total number of publications, an overview can be made of the most used keywords in relation to the subject of medicinal plants (see Figure 8). As expected, the search terms are the main ones, but then, there are two indexing terms, Human and Nonhuman, and then Unclassified Drug and Plant Extract.

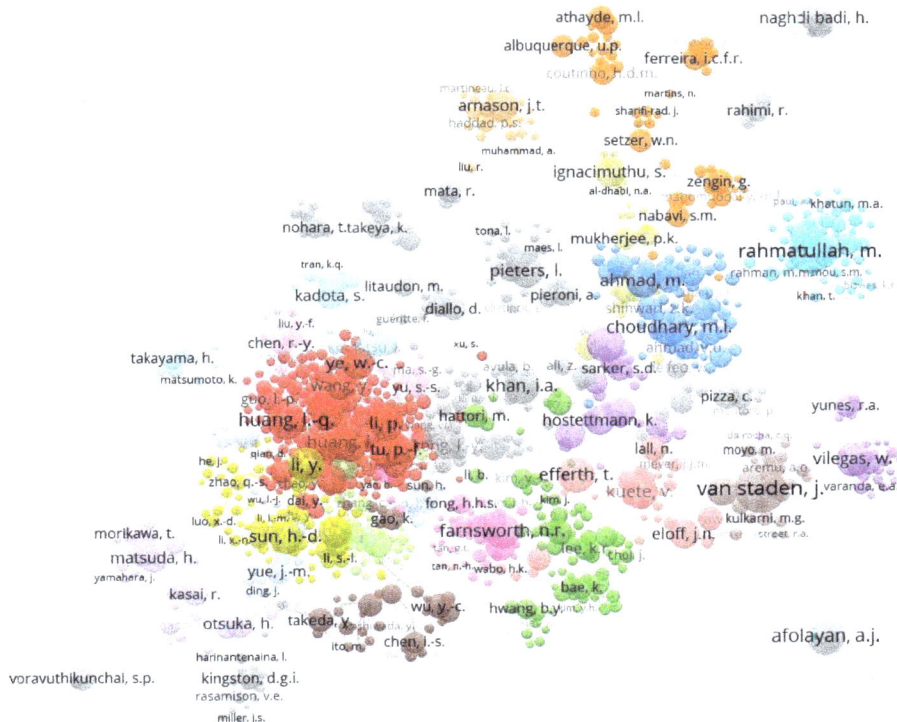

Figure 7. A collaborative network of authors with more than 40 publications on medicinal plants.

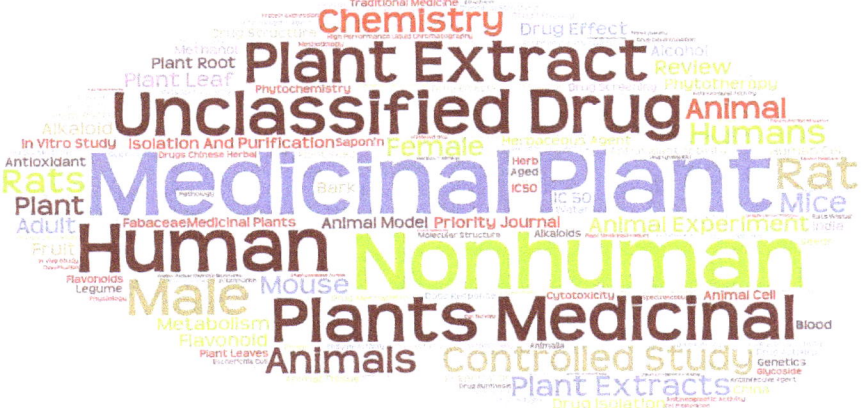

Figure 8. Cloudword of keywords in medical plants publications.

If the keywords are analyzed by country, and we do not take into account the search terms, the results are obtained in Table 3, where the four main keywords of the main countries that research this topic are shown. It can be seen that the terms: Unclassified Drug, Plant Extract, and Controlled Study, are the ones that dominate without a doubt.

Table 3. Main keywords by country.

Rank	Country	N	1	2	3	4
1	China	19,846	Unclassified Drug	Chemistry	Controlled Study	Plant Extract
2	India	16,372	Unclassified Drug	Plant Extract	Controlled Study	Animal Experiment
3	USA	7339	Unclassified Drug	Plant Extract	Controlled Study	Chemistry
4	Brazil	5993	Unclassified Drug	Plant Extract	Controlled Study	Animal Experiment
5	Japan	4557	Unclassified Drug	Plant Extract	Drug Isolation	Controlled Study
6	South Korea	4131	Unclassified Drug	Controlled Study	Plant Extract	Animals
7	Germany	3867	Unclassified Drug	Plant Extract	Controlled Study	Chemistry
8	Iran	3771	Unclassified Drug	Plant Extract	Controlled Study	Essential Oil
9	United Kingdom	2377	Unclassified Drug	Plant Extract	Controlled Study	Chemistry
10	Pakistan	2220	Unclassified Drug	Plant Extract	Controlled Study	Chemistry
11	Italy	2135	Unclassified Drug	Plant Extract	Controlled Study	Chemistry
12	France	2031	Unclassified Drug	Plant Extract	Controlled Study	Drug Isolation

3.6.2. Keywords Related to Plants

If this keyword analysis is done by parts of the plant (see Table 4), which shows which parts of the plant have been most investigated. It should be noted that the number of documents is less than the sum of the individual keywords, since a publication contains more than one keyword. It has been obtained that the parts of the plant most studied in order of importance have been the value expressed in relative terms: Leaf-Leaves (33%), Root-Roots (22%), Seed (12%), Stem (10%), Fruit (10%), Bark (7%), and Flower (6%). The table also shows which plant families have been most used for the study of that part of the plant.

Table 4. Main keywords related to plant parts and plant families studied.

Part of the Plant	Documents	Main Family Studied	Keyword	N
Leaf-Leaves	14652	Asteraceae, Fabaceae, Lamiaceae	Plant Leaf	12,009
			Plant Leaves	4664
Root-Roots	9581	Asteraceae, Fabaceae	Plant Root	7695
			Plant Roots	3920
Seed	5204	Fabaceae, Asteraceae	Plant Seed	3789
			Seeds	2149
Stem	4480	Fabaceae, Asteraceae, Apocynaceae	Plant Stem	3561
			Plant Stems	1462
Fruit	4357	Fabaceae, Asteraceae,	Fruit	3423
			Fruits	259
Bark	3358	Fabaceae, Meliaceae, Euphorbiaceae, Apocynaceae, Asteraceae	Bark	3146
			Plant Bark	1171
Flower	2615	Asteraceae, Lamiaceae, Fabaceae	Flower	2081
			Flowers	804
Rhizome	2519	Zingiberaceae, Asteraceae	Rhizome	1969

To give an idea of the most studied plant families, see Table 5. Although the first two are the same family, it has been left separately to indicate the indexing preferences of the two main affiliations that study them. This is also the situation with Compositae that correspond to the family of Asteraceae. This table lists for each plant family the main institution working on its study. However, it is curious that even if a country is a leader in certain studies related to plant families, most often it is found that the institution leading the issue is not from the country leading the study on that plant family. This helps to establish a certain amount of global leadership on the side of the institutions.

Table 5. Plant families and Institutions.

Rank	Plant Family	Documents	Main Country	Main Affiliation (Country)
1	Fabaceae	4492	USA	Universidade de Sao Paulo – USP (Brazil)
2	Leguminosae	3255	USA	Wageningen University and Research Centre (Netherlands)
3	Asteraceae	2743	China	Chinese Academy of Sciences (China)
4	Lamiaceae	1825	China	Chinese Academy of Sciences (China)
5	Apocynaceae	962	India	Chinese Academy of Sciences (China)
6	Angiosperm	914	China	Chinese Academy of Medical Sciences & Peking Union Medical College (China)
7	Euphorbiaceae	898	India	Chinese Academy of Sciences (China)
8	Apiaceae (Umbelliferae)	884(135)	China	Tehran University of Medical Sciences (Iran)
9	Rubiaceae	814	India	Chinese Academy of Sciences (China)
10	Rutaceae	732	India	CNRS Centre National de la Recherche Scientifique (France)
11	Solanaceae	539	India	University of Development Alternative (Bangladesh)
12	Rosaceae	582	China	Chinese Academy of Sciences (China)
13	Compositae	352	China	Lanzhou University (China)

3.7. Clusters

The analysis of the clusters formed by the keywords allows the classification of the different groups into which the research trends are grouped. A first analysis has been made with the documents published between 2009 and 2019 and in two periods, from 2009 to 2014 and from 2015 to 2019. Figure 9 shows the clusters obtained for the period 2009 to 2014, showing seven clusters, which can be distinguished by color, and in Table 6 its main keywords have been collected.

The first of these clusters, in red (1-1), is linked to traditional medicine. This is reflected in the main keywords associated with this cluster: phytotherapy, herbaceous agent, traditional medicine, ethnobotany. Within this cluster, the most cited publications are related to the antioxidant function of plants. This includes the prevention of hyperglycemia hypertension [52], and the prevention of cancer. Of the latter, studies suggest that a reduced risk of cancer is associated with high consumption of vegetables and fruits [53]. Another topic frequently addressed is the antidiabetic properties, as some plants have hypoglycemic properties [34]. It should be remembered that diabetes mellitus is one of the common metabolic disorders, acquiring around 2.8% of the world's population and is expected to double by 2025 [54].

The second cluster, in green (1-2), appears to be the central cluster, and is related to drugs—chemistry. The main keywords are: drug isolation, drug structure, chemistry, drug determination, and molecular structure. Here, the most cited publications are the search for new drugs [55] or in natural antimicrobials for food preservation [56].

The third cluster, in purple (1-3), is focused on in vivo study through studies with laboratory animals, as shown by keywords such as mouse and mice. As it is known that in vivo drug trials are initiated in laboratory animals such as mice, in general studies focused on anti-inflammatory effect [57,58].

The fourth cluster, in yellow (1-4), is engaged in the search for drugs. The main keywords in this regard are unclassified drug and drug screening. Within this cluster, the studies of flavonoids stand out [59]. Flavonoids have been shown to be antioxidant, free radical scavenger, coronary heart disease prevention, hepatoprotective, anti-inflammatory and anticancer, while some flavonoids show possible antiviral activities [60].

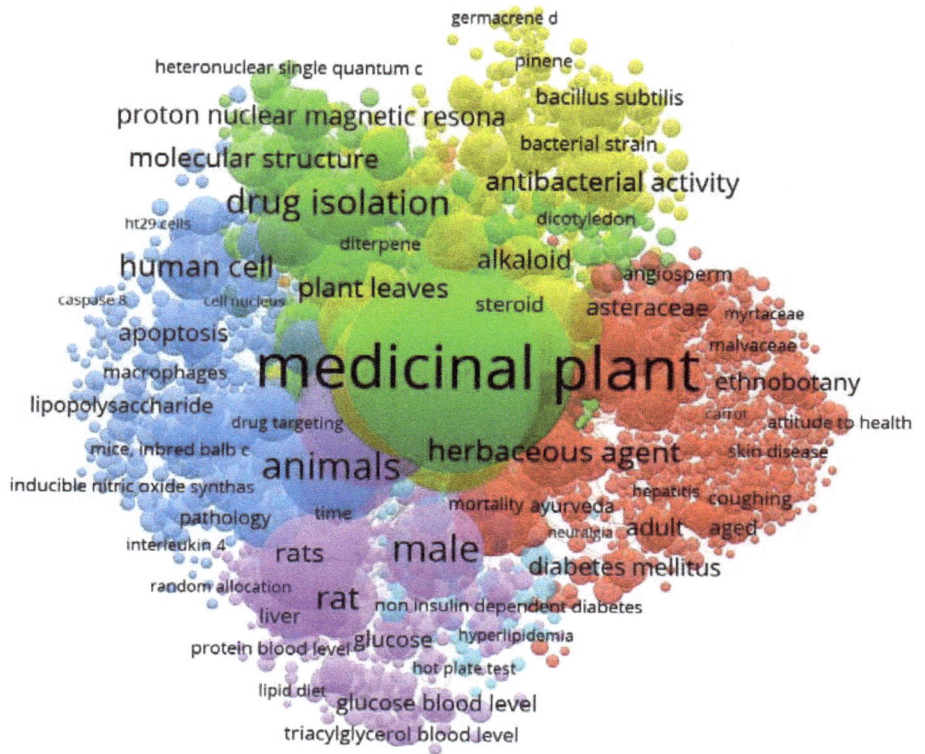

Figure 9. Network of keywords in medical plants publications: Clusters between 2009–2014.

Table 6. Main keywords used by the communities detected in the topic in the period 2009–2014.

Cluster	Color	Main Keywords	Topic
1-1	Red	Human, Phytotherapy, herbaceous agent, traditional medicine, ethnobotany, diabetes mellitus	Traditional medicine
1-2	Green	Drug isolation, drug structure, chemistry, drug determination, molecular structure	Drug determination
1-3	Purple	Animal, mouse, mice, animal cell, apoptosis, anti-inflammatory effect, protein expression	Animals-in vivo study
1-4	Yellow	Unclassified drug, drug screening, flavonoid, phytochemistry, plant leaf	Unclassified drug
1-5	Blue	Drug efficacy, animal experiment, dose response, oxidative stress, histopathology	Drug efficacy
1-6	Cian	Solvent, ethanol, neuroprotection, acetic acid, sodium chloride	Effect of extraction solvent
1-7	Orange	antimalarial activity, antimalarials, *Plasmodium berghei*, *Plasmodium falciparum*	Malaria

The fifth cluster, in blue (1-5), is focused on the effectiveness of some drugs, and their experimentation on animals. Some of the most cited publications of this cluster over this period are those focused on genus *Scutellaria* [61], Epimedium (*Berberidaceae*) [62] and Vernonia (*Asteraceae*) [63].

The sixth cluster, in cyan (1-6), is aimed at the effect of extraction solvent/technique on the antioxidant activity. One of the most cited publications in this regard studies the effects on barks of *Azadirachta indica*, *Acacia nilotica*, *Eugenia jambolana*, *Terminalia arjuna*, leaves and roots of *Moringa oleifera*, fruit of *Ficus religiosa*, and leaves of *Aloe barbadensis* [64]. Regarding neuroprotection, some publications are the related to genus *Peucedanum* [65] or *Bacopa monnieri* [66]. This cluster is among the clusters of traditional medicine (1-1) and drug efficacy (1-5).

Finally, the seventh orange cluster (1-7) is of small relative importance within this cluster analysis and is focused on malaria. As it is known, malaria is one of the most lethal diseases in the world every year [67]. Malaria causes nearly half a million deaths and was estimated at over 200 million cases, 90 per cent of which occurred in African countries [68]. Of the *Plasmodium* species affecting humans, *Plasmodium falciparum* causes the most deaths, although *Plasmodium vivax* is the most widely spread except in sub-Saharan Africa [69]. On the other hand, this cluster cites *Plasmodium berghei*, which mainly affects mice, and is often used as a model for testing medicines or vaccines [70].

The second period under study, from 2015 to 2019, is shown in Figure 10, where five clusters have been identified, Table 7, as opposed to the previous period which was seven. Now, there is no cluster focusing on malaria. In Figure 10, the colors of the cluster have been unified with those of Figure 9, when the clusters have the same topic as in the previous period.

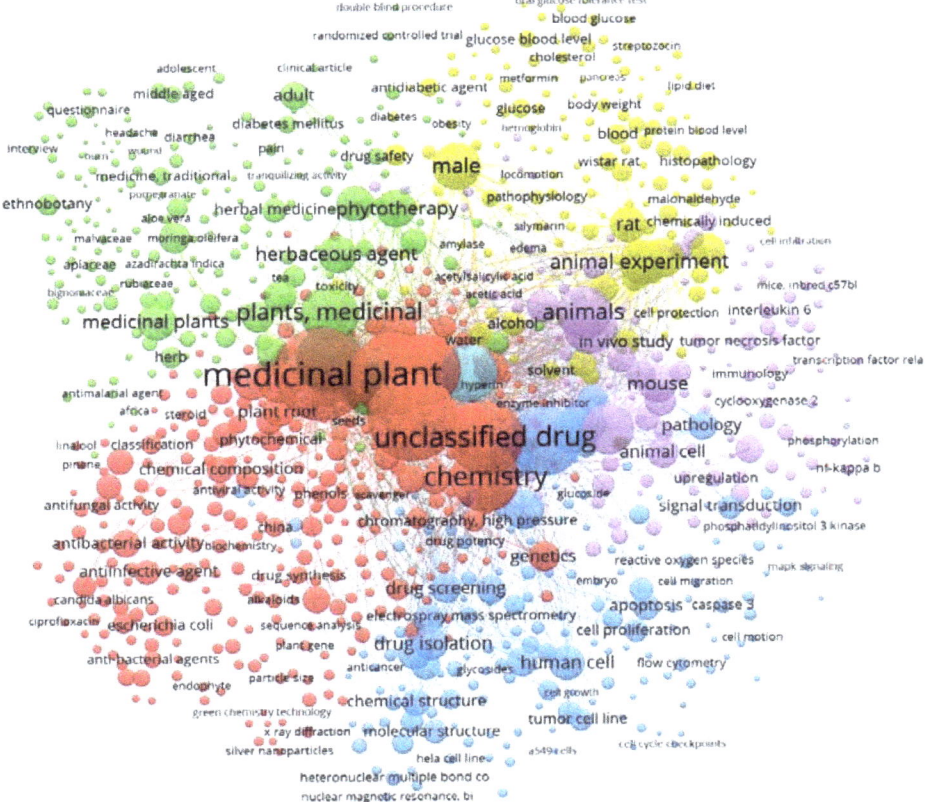

Figure 10. Network of keywords in medical plants publications: Clusters between 2015–2019.

Table 7. Main keywords used by the communities detected in the topic in the period 2015–2019.

Cluster	Color	Main Keywords	Topic
2-1	Red	Unclassified drug, chemistry, plant extract, phytochemistry, flavonoid	Unclassified drug
2-2	Green	Traditional medicine, herbaceous agent, phytotherapy, ethnopharmacology, drug efficacy	Traditional medicine
2-3	Blue	In vitro study, human cell, antineoplastic agent, cytotoxicity, apoptosis	Cancer
2-4	Cyan	In vivo study, male, oxidative stress, animal tissue, rat, antidiabetic activity, liver protection	In vivo study- antidiabetic activity
2-5	Purple	Metabolism, animal, anti-inflammatory activity, mouse, dose response	Animals- Anti-inflammatory activity

The first cluster in order of importance (2-1), the red one in Figure 10, can be seen to be that of unclassified drug, which has gone from fourth place (1-4) to first in this last period. In this period, research works include one on the therapeutic potential of spirooxindoles as antiviral agents [71], or the antimicrobial peptides from plants [72].

The second cluster of this last period (2-2), the one in green in Figure 10, is the one assigned to traditional medicine, which has now moved up to second place (1-1) in decreasing order of significance. It seems that this cluster of traditional medicine is now the merging with the drug efficacy cluster of the previous period (1-4). This cluster includes research such as oxidative stress and Parkinson's disease [73].

The cluster from the previous period that was devoted to animals-in vivo study (1-3), we assume is now divided into three new clusters. The first of these would be the third cluster (2-3), blue in Figure 10, which can be considered to be dedicated to cancer. One of the works in this cluster is "Anticancer activity of silver nanoparticles from Panax ginseng fresh leaves in human cancer cells" [74]. Then, the other two are committed to in vivo studies or with animals. The first one seems to be more engaged in vivo study at antidiabetic activity [75,76], would be the cyan-colored cluster 4 (2-4). The other cluster (2-5) involved in testing anti-inflammatory activity, with plants such as Curcumin [77], *Rosmarinus officinalis* [78], would be the purple cluster in Figure 10.

3.8. Collaboration Network of Countries

Figure 11 shows the collaborative network between countries doing research on medicinal plants. Table 8 lists the countries of each cluster identified and the main country of each cluster. The countries that are most central to this network of collaboration between countries are India, Iran, Indonesia, and the USA. The largest cluster is led by Brazil, which is also not restricted to its own geographical area as it has strong collaborative links with European countries as well as with neighboring countries such as Argentina. The second cluster led by South Africa also presents the same features as the previous one, some collaborations with nearby countries, Tanzania, Congo, or Sudan, but also with European countries such as France, Belgium, or the Netherlands.

The third cluster is led by India and has very strong collaboration with Iran, but it could also be considered as the central country in the whole international collaboration network. The cooperation with European countries comprises mainly Eastern countries like Poland, Serbia, or Croatia.

The fourth cluster, led by Germany and Pakistan, includes Middle Eastern countries such as Jordan, Saudi Arabia, and United Arab Emirates, which are quite related to the cluster led by China. The fifth cluster seems to have a geographical consideration within Asia by including countries such as Indonesia, Malaysia, Thailand, and Australia. The sixth cluster includes very technologically advanced countries such as USA, UK, Japan, Canada, or South Korea. The seventh cluster is very small in the number of countries. It is made up of very different countries like some in Africa: Cameroon and Kenya; some of Europe as Denmark, and some from Asia like Nepal. In this sense, most of the research linked to African countries in general and to Cameroon particularly is linked to the most frequent parasitic diseases [79], such as African trypanosomiasis [80], diarrhea [81] or tuberculosis [82]. Finally, the China cluster is made up of nearby areas of influence such as Taiwan, Singapore, Hong Kong, Macau, or Taiwan.

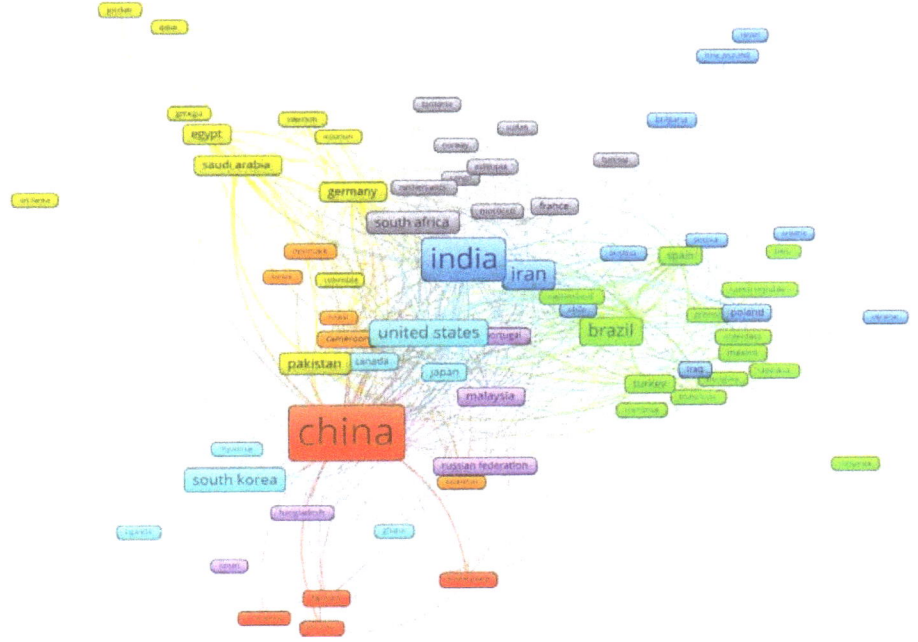

Figure 11. Countries network collaboration.

Table 8. Countries collaboration in the period 2009–2019.

Cluster	Color	Main Countries	Number of Countries	Leader
1	Green	Brazil, Italy, Turkey, Spain	16	Brazil
2	Grey	South Africa, Belgium, France, Morocco	14	South Africa
3	Blue	India, Iran, Iraq, Chile	12	India
4	Yellow	Germany, Pakistan, Saudi Arabia, Egypt	12	Pakistan
5	Purple	Indonesia, Malaysia, Thailand, Australia	10	Indonesia
6	Cian	USA, UK, Japan, Canada, South Korea	8	USA
7	Orange	Cameroon, Kenya, Denmark, Nepal	5	Cameroon
8	Red	China, Taiwan, Singapore, Hong Kong	5	China

4. Conclusions

The use of plants as a source of research in the search for active compounds for medicine has been proven to have a significant scientific output. An analysis of the scientific literature indexed in the Scopus database concerning medicinal plants clearly shows that in the last 20 years, progress has been rapid, with a peak in 2010. From this year onwards, publications have stabilized at just over 5000 per year.

The research of products derived from the plants shows great collaboration between the countries of the first world and the countries with a traditional use of these plants from Asia, Africa or Latin America, all this to produce new medicines with scientific tests of safety and effectiveness. Within the analysis of the different clusters of collaboration between countries, there are four from Asia, led by China, India, Indonesia and Pakistan; two from Africa, led by South Africa and Cameroon, and then one from Latin America, led by Brazil and another from North America, led by the USA. It has been proven that there is no cluster of European countries, but that they generally collaborate with countries with which they have a commercial relationship. The research of medicinal plants in Africa is greatly underdeveloped, in contrast with China and India. In fact, there is no African country among the countries that published the most in this field. Among the first 25 institutions there is only one that belongs to the African continent. From this top 25, 13 are from China (including the first 7), 3 from Brazil, 2 from South Korea, and 1 of Saudi Arabia, Pakistan, Iran, Mexico, Cameroon, France, and Malaysia.

The most widely used search terms by the main institutions researching in this field are Unclassified Drug, Plant Extract, and Controlled Study. From the study of the keywords in the period from 2009 to 2014, seven clusters have been found, those dedicated to: Traditional medicine, Drug determination, Animals-in vivo study, Unclassified drug, Drug efficacy, Effect of extraction solvent, and Malaria. Subsequently, from the period 2015 to 2019, the clusters are reduced to five, and those focused on: Unclassified drug, Traditional medicine, Cancer, In vivo study—antidiabetic activity, and Animals—anti-inflammatory activity.

This is proven by the fact that of the total number of publications analyzed, more than 100,000, only 11% are in the Agricultural and Biological Sciences category, while more than 50% are grouped in the Pharmacology, Toxicology and Pharmaceutics category and Medicine. This study highlights the scarce research from the agronomic perspective regarding domestication, production or genetic or biotechnological research on breeding of medicinal plants.

Author Contributions: E.S.-M., J.A.G.-C. and F.M.-A. conceived the research, designed the search, and wrote the manuscript. All authors have read and agreed to the published version of the manuscript.

Funding: This research received no external funding.

Acknowledgments: The authors would like to thank to the CIAIMBITAL (University of Almeria, CeiA3) for its support.

Conflicts of Interest: The authors declare no conflict of interest.

References

1. Fonnegra, F.G. *Plantas Medicinales Aprobadas en Colombia*; University of Antioquia: Antioquia, Colombia, 2007.
2. Joppa, L.N.; Roberts, D.L.; Myers, N.; Pimm, S.L. Biodiversity hotspots house most undiscovered plant species. *Proc. Natl. Acad. Sci. USA* **2011**, *108*, 13171–13176. [CrossRef] [PubMed]
3. Pimm, S.L.; Jenkins, C.N.; Abell, R.; Brooks, T.M.; Gittleman, J.L.; Joppa, L.N.; Sexton, J.O. The biodiversity of species and their rates of extinction, distribution, and protection. *Science* **2014**, *344*, 1246752. [CrossRef] [PubMed]
4. Grover, J.K.; Yadav, S.; Vats, V. Medicinal plants of India with anti-diabetic potential. *J. Ethnopharmacol.* **2002**, *81*, 81–100. [CrossRef]
5. Kunle, O.F.; Egharevba, H.O.; Ahmadu, P.O. Standardization of herbal medicines-A review. *Int. J. Biodivers. Conserv.* **2012**, *4*, 101–112. [CrossRef]
6. WHO. World Health Organization. General Guidelines for Methodologies on Research and Evaluation of Traditional Medicine. 2000. Available online: https://apps.who.int/iris/bitstream/handle/10665/66783/WHO_EDM_TRM_2000.1.pdf (accessed on 12 May 2020).
7. Gurib-Fakim, A. Medicinal plants: Traditions of yesterday and drugs of tomorrow. *Mol. Asp. Med.* **2006**, *27*, 1–93. [CrossRef]
8. Houghton, P.J. The role of plants in traditional medicine and current therapy. *J. Altern. Complementary Med.* **1995**, *1*, 131–143. [CrossRef]
9. Kinghorn, A.D.; Seo, E.K. Plants as Sources of Drugs. ACS Symposium Series, Vol. 647. Agricultural Materials as Renewable Resources, Chapter 12, pp. 179–193. Available online: https://pubs.acs.org/doi/abs/10.1021/bk-1996-0647.ch012 (accessed on 12 May 2020).
10. Jones, W.P.; Chin, Y.W.; Kinghorn, A.D. The role of pharmacognosy in modern medicine and pharmacy. *Curr. Drug Targets* **2006**, *7*, 247–264. [CrossRef]

11. Faridi, P.; Zarshenas, M.M.; Abolhassanzadeh, Z.; Mohagheghzadeh, A. Collection and storage of medicinal plants in The Canon of Medicine. *Pharmacogn. J.* **2010**, *2*, 216–218. [CrossRef]
12. Koh, G. The Canon of Medicine (Al-Qanun fi'l-tibb) By Ibn Sina (Avicenna) 11th century. *BMJ* **2009**, *339*, b5358. [CrossRef]
13. Reeds, K.M. Renaissance humanism and botany. *Ann. Sci.* **1976**, *33*, 519–542. [CrossRef]
14. Atanasov, A.G.; Waltenberger, B.; Pferschy-Wenzig, E.M.; Linder, T.; Wawrosch, C.; Uhrin, P.; Rollinger, J.M. Discovery and resupply of pharmacologically active plant-derived natural products: A review. *Biotechnol. Adv.* **2015**, *33*, 1582–1614. [CrossRef] [PubMed]
15. Gertsch, J. How scientific is the science in ethnopharmacology? Historical perspectives and epistemological problems. *J. Ethnopharmacol.* **2009**, *122*, 177–183. [CrossRef] [PubMed]
16. Arceusz, A.; Radecka, I.; Wesolowski, M. Identification of diversity in elements content in medicinal plants belonging to different plant families. *Food Chem.* **2010**, *120*, 52–58. [CrossRef]
17. Salmerón-Manzano, E.; Manzano-Agugliaro, F. Worldwide Research on Low Cost Technologies through Bibliometric Analysis. *Inventions* **2020**, *5*, 9. [CrossRef]
18. Chan, K. Some aspects of toxic contaminants in herbal medicines. *Chemosphere* **2003**, *52*, 1361–1371. [CrossRef]
19. Adoum, O.A. Determination of toxicity levels of some savannah plants using brine shrimp test (BST). Bayero. *J. Pure Appl. Sci.* **2009**, *2*, 135–138.
20. Li, S.Y.; Zhang, B.L.; Tan, F.P. Glycopenia coma caused by taking both dimethylbiguanide and Momordica charantia buccal tablet in one patient. *Chin. J. New Drugs Clin. Remedies* **2004**, *23*, 189–190.
21. Basch, E.; Gabardi, S.; Ulbricht, C. Bitter melon (Momordica charantia): A review of efficacy and safety. *Am. J. Health Syst. Pharm.* **2003**, *60*, 356–359. [CrossRef]
22. Street, R.A.; Stirk, W.A.; Van Staden, J. South African traditional medicinal plant trade—challenges in regulating quality, safety and efficacy. *J. Ethnopharmacol.* **2008**, *119*, 705–710. [CrossRef]
23. Masondo, N.A.; Makunga, N.P. Advancement of analytical techniques in some South African commercialized medicinal plants: Current and future perspectives. *S. Afr. J. Bot.* **2019**, *126*, 40–57. [CrossRef]
24. Viljoen, A.; Sandasi, M.; Vermaak, I. The role of the South African Journal of Botany as a vehicle to promote medicinal plant research–A bibliometric appraisal. *S. Afr. J. Bot.* **2019**, *122*, 3–10. [CrossRef]
25. Masondo, N.A.; Stafford, G.I.; Aremu, A.O.; Makunga, N.P. Acetylcholinesterase inhibitors from southern African plants: An overview of ethnobotanical, pharmacological potential and phytochemical research including and beyond Alzheimer's disease treatment. *S. Afr. J. Bot.* **2019**, *120*, 39–64. [CrossRef]
26. TchuifonTchuifon, D.; Fu, H.Z.; Ho, Y.S. Cameroon publications in the Science Citation Index Expanded: Bibliometric analysis. *Revista De Biología Trop.* **2017**, *65*, 1582–1591. [CrossRef]
27. Thomford, N.E.; Dzobo, K.; Chopera, D.; Wonkam, A.; Skelton, M.; Blackhurst, D.; Dandara, C. Pharmacogenomics implications of using herbal medicinal plants on African populations in health transition. *Pharmaceuticals* **2015**, *8*, 637–663. [CrossRef]
28. Fernández, B.E.; Armas, R.C. Cuban scientific production about medicinal plants and natural products from PlantMedCUBA database, 1967–2010. *Revista Cubana De Plantas Medicinales* **2013**, *18*, 348–360.
29. Zhang, G.; Si, J.; Zhu, Y. Bibliometrics of woody medical plants in China. *China J. Chin. Mater. Med.* **2010**, *35*, 654–657.
30. Xu, W.; Zou, Z.; Pei, J.; Huang, L. Longitudinal trend of global artemisinin research in chemistry subject areas (1983–2017). *Bioorg. Med. Chem.* **2018**, *26*, 5379–5387. [CrossRef]
31. Gupta, B.M.; Ahmed, K.M.; Dhawan, S.M.; Gupta, R. Aloe Vera (Medicinal Plant) research: A scientometric assessment of global publications output during 2007-16. *Pharmacogn. J.* **2018**. [CrossRef]
32. Xu, W.; Choi, H.K.; Huang, L. State of Panax ginseng research: A global analysis. *Molecules* **2017**, *22*, 1518. [CrossRef]
33. Al-Qallaf, C.L. A bibliometric analysis of the Punica grantum L. literature. *Malays. J. Libr. Inf. Sci.* **2017**, *14*, 83–103.
34. Ram, S. A bibliometric assessment of apocynin (Apocynum cannabinum) research. *Ann. Libr. Inf. Stud. (ALIS)* **2013**, *60*, 149–158.
35. Gupta, B.M.; Ahmed, K.M.; Bansal, J.; Bansal, M. Andrographis paniculata Global Publications Output: A Bibliometric Assessment during 2003-18. *Int. J. Pharm. Investig.* **2019**, *9*, 101–108. [CrossRef]

36. Ortega-Cuadros, M.; Tofiño-Rivera, A.P. Exploratory review of the antibacterial and antifungal activity of Lippia alba (Mill.) N. E. Br (bushy matgrass). *Revista Cubana De Plantas Medicinales.* 2019, 24. Available online: http://www.revplantasmedicinales.sld.cu/index.php/pla/article/view/771/361 (accessed on 12 May 2020).
37. Ahmed, K.M.; Gupta, B.M. India's contribution on antioxidants: A bibliometric analysis, 2001–2010. *Scientometrics* 2013, *94*, 741–754. [CrossRef]
38. Basu, T.; Mallik, A.; Mandal, N. Evolving importance of anticancer research using herbal medicine: A scientometric analysis. *Scientometrics* 2017, *110*, 1375–1396. [CrossRef]
39. Yeung, A.W.K.; El-Demerdash, A.; Berindan-Neagoe, I.; Atanasov, A.G.; Ho, Y.S. Molecular responses of cancers by natural products: Modifications of autophagy revealed by literature analysis. *Crit. Rev. ™ Oncog.* 2018, *23*, 5–6. [CrossRef]
40. Du, J.; Tang, X.L. Natural products against cancer: A comprehensive bibliometric study of the research projects, publications, patents and drugs. *J. Cancer Res. Ther.* 2014, *10*, 27.
41. Gimenez, E.; Salinas, M.; Manzano-Agugliaro, F. Worldwide research on plant defense against biotic stresses as improvement for sustainable agriculture. *Sustainability* 2018, *10*, 391. [CrossRef]
42. Montoya, F.G.; Alcayde, A.; Baños, R.; Manzano-Agugliaro, F. A fast method for identifying worldwide scientific collaborations using the Scopus database. *Telemat. Inform.* 2018, *35*, 168–185. [CrossRef]
43. Novas, N.; Alcayde, A.; El Khaled, D.; Manzano-Agugliaro, F. Coatings in Photovoltaic Solar Energy Worldwide Research. *Coatings* 2019, *9*, 797. [CrossRef]
44. la Cruz-Lovera, D.; Perea-Moreno, A.J.; la Cruz-Fernández, D.; Alvarez-Bermejo, J.A.; Manzano-Agugliaro, F. Worldwide research on energy efficiency and sustainability in public buildings. *Sustainability* 2017, *9*, 1294. [CrossRef]
45. Cai, Y.; Luo, Q.; Sun, M.; Corke, H. Antioxidant activity and phenolic compounds of 112 traditional Chinese medicinal plants associated with anticancer. *Life Sci.* 2004, *74*, 2157–2184. [CrossRef]
46. Lobo, V.; Patil, A.; Phatak, A.; Chandra, N. Free radicals, antioxidants and functional foods: Impact on human health. *Pharmacogn. Rev.* 2010, *4*, 118. [CrossRef]
47. Devasagayam, T.P.A.; Tilak, J.C.; Boloor, K.K.; Sane, K.S.; Ghaskadbi, S.S.; Lele, R.D. Free radicals and antioxidants in human health: Current status and future prospects. *J. Assoc. Physicians India* 2004, *52*, 4.
48. Zheng, W.; Wang, S.Y. Antioxidant activity and phenolic compounds in selected herbs. *J. Agric. Food Chem.* 2001, *49*, 5165–5170. [CrossRef]
49. Hammer, K.A.; Carson, C.F.; Riley, T.V. Antimicrobial activity of essential oils and other plant extracts. *J. Appl. Microbiol.* 1999, *86*, 985–990. [CrossRef]
50. Baker, E.J.; Valenzuela, C.A.; De Souza, C.O.; Yaqoob, P.; Miles, E.A.; Calder, P.C. Comparative anti-inflammatory effects of plant-and marine-derived omega-3 fatty acids explored in an endothelial cell line. *Mol. Cell Biol. Lipids* 2020, *1865*, 158662. [CrossRef]
51. Rocha, F.G.; de Mello Brandenburg, M.; Pawloski, P.L.; da Silva Soley, B.; Costa, S.C.A.; Meinerz, C.C.; Cabrini, D.A. Preclinical study of the topical anti-inflammatory activity of Cyperus rotundus L. extract (Cyperaceae) in models of skin inflammation. *J. Ethnopharmacol.* 2020, *254*, 112709. [CrossRef]
52. Ranilla, L.G.; Kwon, Y.I.; Apostolidis, E.; Shetty, K. Phenolic compounds, antioxidant activity and in vitro inhibitory potential against key enzymes relevant for hyperglycemia and hypertension of commonly used medicinal plants, herbs and spices in Latin America. *Bioresour. Technol.* 2010, *101*, 4676–4689. [CrossRef]
53. Gullett, N.P.; Amin, A.R.; Bayraktar, S.; Pezzuto, J.M.; Shin, D.M.; Khuri, F.R.; Kucuk, O. Cancer prevention with natural compounds. *Semin. Oncol.* 2010, *37*, 258–281. [CrossRef]
54. Patel, D.K.; Prasad, S.K.; Kumar, R.; Hemalatha, S. An overview on antidiabetic medicinal plants having insulin mimetic property. *Asian Pac. J. Trop. Biomed.* 2012, *2*, 320–330. [CrossRef]
55. Cragg, G.M.; Newman, D.J. Natural products: A continuing source of novel drug leads. *Biochim. Biophys. Acta (BBA)* 2013, *1830*, 3670–3695. [CrossRef] [PubMed]
56. Tiwari, B.K.; Valdramidis, V.P.; O'Donnell, C.P.; Muthukumarappan, K.; Bourke, P.; Cullen, P.J. Application of natural antimicrobials for food preservation. *J. Agric. Food Chem.* 2009, *57*, 5987–6000. [CrossRef] [PubMed]
57. Riella, K.R.; Marinho, R.R.; Santos, J.S.; Pereira-Filho, R.N.; Cardoso, J.C.; Albuquerque-Junior, R.L.C.; Thomazzi, S.M. Anti-inflammatory and cicatrizing activities of thymol, a monoterpene of the essential oil from Lippia gracilis, in rodents. *J. Ethnopharmacol.* 2012, *143*, 656–663. [CrossRef] [PubMed]

58. Babu, N.P.; Pandikumar, P.; Ignacimuthu, S. Anti-inflammatory activity of Albizia lebbeck Benth, an ethnomedicinal plant, in acute and chronic animal models of inflammation. *J. Ethnopharmacol.* **2009**, *125*, 356–360. [CrossRef]
59. López-Lázaro, M. Distribution and biological activities of the flavonoid luteolin. *Mini Rev. Med. Chem.* **2009**, *9*, 31–59. [CrossRef]
60. Kumar, S.; Pandey, A.K. Chemistry and biological activities of flavonoids: An overview. *Sci. World J.* **2013**, 162750. [CrossRef]
61. Shang, X.; He, X.; He, X.; Li, M.; Zhang, R.; Fan, P.; Jia, Z. The genus Scutellaria an ethnopharmacological and phytochemical review. *J. Ethnopharmacol.* **2010**, *128*, 279–313. [CrossRef]
62. Ma, H.; He, X.; Yang, Y.; Li, M.; Hao, D.; Jia, Z. The genus Epimedium: An ethnopharmacological and phytochemical review. *J. Ethnopharmacol.* **2011**, *134*, 519–541. [CrossRef]
63. Toyang, N.J.; Verpoorte, R. A review of the medicinal potentials of plants of the genus Vernonia (Asteraceae). *J. Ethnopharmacol.* **2013**, *146*, 681–723. [CrossRef]
64. Sultana, B.; Anwar, F.; Ashraf, M. Effect of extraction solvent/technique on the antioxidant activity of selected medicinal plant extracts. *Molecules* **2009**, *14*, 2167–2180. [CrossRef]
65. Sarkhail, P. Traditional uses, phytochemistry and pharmacological properties of the genus Peucedanum: A review. *J. Ethnopharmacol.* **2014**, *156*, 235–270. [CrossRef]
66. Saini, N.; Singh, D.; Sandhir, R. Neuroprotective effects of Bacopa monnieri in experimental model of dementia. *Neurochem. Res.* **2012**, *37*, 1928–1937. [CrossRef]
67. Garrido-Cardenas, J.A.; González-Cerón, L.; Manzano-Agugliaro, F.; Mesa-Valle, C. Plasmodium genomics: An approach for learning about and ending human malaria. *Parasitol. Res.* **2019**, *118*, 1–27. [CrossRef]
68. Garrido-Cardenas, J.A.; Manzano-Agugliaro, F.; González-Cerón, L.; Gil-Montoya, F.; Alcayde-Garcia, A.; Novas, N.; Mesa-Valle, C. The Identification of Scientific Communities and Their Approach to Worldwide Malaria Research. *Int. J. Environ. Res. Public Health* **2018**, *15*, 2703. [CrossRef]
69. Garrido-Cardenas, J.A.; Cebrián-Carmona, J.; González-Cerón, L.; Manzano-Agugliaro, F; Mesa-Valle, C. Analysis of Global Research on Malaria and Plasmodium vivax. *Int. J. Environ. Res. Public Health* **2019**, *16*, 1928. [CrossRef]
70. Garrido-Cardenas, J.A.; Mesa-Valle, C.; Manzano-Agugliaro, F. Genetic approach towards a vaccine against malaria. *Eur. J. Clin. Microbiol. Infect. Dis.* **2018**, *37*, 1829–1839. [CrossRef]
71. Ye, N.; Chen, H.; Wold, E.A.; Shi, P.Y.; Zhou, J. Therapeutic potential of spirooxindoles as antiviral agents. *ACS Infect. Dis.* **2016**, *2*, 382–392. [CrossRef]
72. Broekaert, W.F.; Cammue, B.P.; De Bolle, M.F.; Thevissen, K.; De Samblanx, G.W.; Osborn, R.W.; Nielson, K. Antimicrobial peptides from plants. *Crit. Rev. Plant Sci.* **1997**, *16*, 297–323. [CrossRef]
73. Sarrafchi, A.; Bahmani, M.; Shirzad, H.; Rafieian-Kopaei, M. Oxidative stress and Parkinson's disease: New hopes in treatment with herbal antioxidants. *Curr. Pharm. Des.* **2016**, *22*, 238–246. [CrossRef]
74. Castro-Aceituno, V.; Ahn, S.; Simu, S.Y.; Singh, P.; Mathiyalagan, R.; Lee, H.A.; Yang, D.C. Anticancer activity of silver nanoparticles from Panax ginseng fresh leaves in human cancer cells. *Biomed. Pharmacother.* **2016**, *84*, 158–165. [CrossRef]
75. Ríos, J.L.; Francini, F.; Schinella, G.R. Natural products for the treatment of type 2 diabetes mellitus. *Planta Med.* **2015**, *81*, 975–994. [CrossRef] [PubMed]
76. Xu, L.; Li, Y.; Dai, Y.; Peng, J. Natural products for the treatment of type 2 diabetes mellitus: Pharmacology and mechanisms. *Pharmacol. Res.* **2018**, *130*, 451–465. [CrossRef] [PubMed]
77. Pulido-Moran, M.; Moreno-Fernandez, J.; Ramirez-Tortosa, C.; Ramirez-Tortosa, M. Curcumin and health. *Molecules* **2016**, *21*, 264. [CrossRef]
78. Rocha, J.; Eduardo-Figueira, M.; Barateiro, A.; Fernandes, A.; Brites, D.; Bronze, R.; Fernandes, E. Anti-inflammatory effect of rosmarinic acid and an extract of Rosmarinus officinalis in rat models of local and systemic inflammation. *Basic Clin. Pharmacol. Toxicol.* **2015**, *116*, 398–413. [CrossRef]
79. Garrido-Cardenas, J.A.; Mesa-Valle, C.; Manzano-Agugliaro, F. Human parasitology worldwide research. *Parasitology* **2018**, *145*, 699–712. [CrossRef]
80. Kamte, S.L.N.; Ranjbarian, F.; Campagnaro, G.D.; Nya, P.C.B.; Mbuntcha, H.; Woguem, V.; Benelli, G. Trypanosoma brucei inhibition by essential oils from medicinal and aromatic plants traditionally used in Cameroon (Azadirachta indica, Aframomum melegueta, Aframomum daniellii, Clausena anisata, Dichrostachys cinerea and Echinops giganteus). *Int. J. Environ. Res. Public Health* **2017**, *14*, 737. [CrossRef]

81. Njume, C.; Goduka, N.I. Treatment of diarrhoea in rural African communities: An overview of measures to maximise the medicinal potentials of indigenous plants. *Int. J. Environ. Res. Public Health* **2012**, *9*, 3911–3933. [CrossRef] [PubMed]
82. Garrido-Cardenas, J.A.; de Lamo-Sevilla, C.; Cabezas-Fernández, M.T.; Manzano-Agugliaro, F.; Martínez-Lirola, M. Global tuberculosis research and its future prospects. *Tuberculosis* **2020**, *121*, 101917. [CrossRef]

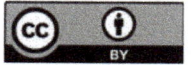

© 2020 by the authors. Licensee MDPI, Basel, Switzerland. This article is an open access article distributed under the terms and conditions of the Creative Commons Attribution (CC BY) license (http://creativecommons.org/licenses/by/4.0/).

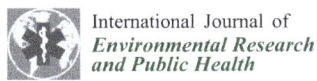 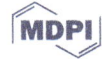

Article

Characterizing Obesity Interventions and Treatment for Children and Youths during 1991–2018

Bach Xuan Tran [1,2,*], Son Nghiem [3], Clifford Afoakwah [3], Carl A. Latkin [2], Giang Hai Ha [4], Thao Phuong Nguyen [5], Linh Phuong Doan [6], Hai Quang Pham [4], Cyrus S.H. Ho [7] and Roger C.M. Ho [8,9,10]

1. Institute for Preventive Medicine and Public Health, Hanoi Medical University, Hanoi 100000, Vietnam
2. Bloomberg School of Public Health, Johns Hopkins University, Baltimore, MD 21205, USA; carl.latkin@jhu.edu
3. Centre for Applied Health Economics (CAHE), Griffith University, Brisbane, QLD 4222, Australia; s.nghiem@griffith.edu.au (S.N.); c.afoakwah@griffith.edu.au (C.A.)
4. Institute for Global Health Innovations, Duy Tan University, Da Nang 550000, Vietnam; giang.ighi@gmail.com (G.H.H.); qhai.ighi@gmail.com (H.Q.P.)
5. Center of Excellence in Evidence-based Medicine, Nguyen Tat Thanh University, Ho Chi Minh City 700000, Vietnam; thao.coentt@gmail.com
6. Center of Excellence in Pharmacoeconomics and Management, Nguyen Tat Thanh University, Ho Chi Minh City 700000, Vietnam; linh91.coentt@gmail.com
7. Department of Psychological Medicine, National University Hospital, Singapore 119074, Singapore; cyrushosh@gmail.com
8. Center of Excellence in Behavioral Medicine, Nguyen Tat Thanh University, Ho Chi Minh City 700000, Vietnam; pcmrhcm@nus.edu.sg
9. Department of Psychological Medicine, Yong Loo Lin School of Medicine, National University of Singapore, Singapore 119228, Singapore
10. Institute for Health Innovation and Technology (iHealthtech), National University of Singapore, Singapore 119228, Singapore
* Correspondence: bach.ipmph@gmail.com; Tel.: +84-982228662

Received: 12 August 2019; Accepted: 26 October 2019; Published: 31 October 2019

Abstract: Overweight and obesity have become a serious health problem globally due to its significant role in increased morbidity and mortality. The treatments for this health issue are various such as lifestyle modifications, pharmacological therapies, and surgery. However, little is known about the productivity, workflow, topics, and landscape research of all the papers mentioning the intervention and treatment for children with obesity. A total of 20,925 publications from the Web of Science database mentioning interventions and treatment in reducing the burden of childhood overweight and obesity on physical health, mental health, and society published in the period from 1991 to 2018 were in the analysis. We used Latent Dirichlet Allocation (LDA) for identifying the topics and a dendrogram for research disciplines. We found that the number of papers related to multilevel interventions such as family-based, school-based, and community-based is increasing. The number of papers mentioning interventions aimed at children and adolescents with overweight or obesity is not high in poor-resource settings or countries compared to the growth in the prevalence of overweight and obesity among youth due to cultural concepts or nutrition transition. Therefore, there is a need for support from developed countries to control the rising rates of overweight and obesity.

Keywords: scientometrics; obesity; interventions; children; youths; pediatrics

1. Introduction

Obesity is defined as the "abnormal or excessive fat accumulation" that may seriously have an impact on health [1] and is considered one of the most significant health challenges of the 21st century. There are several definitions used in research regarding childhood obesity [2–4], yet, none of them are ideal for all studies and the use of definition is based on "practical aspects" [5].

Globally, the prevalence of overweight and obesity in children and youth continues to rise. According to World Health Organization (WHO) data, in 2016, nearly one in five children and adolescents between the ages of 5–19 were affected by overweight or obesity [6]. Furthermore, 38.3 million children under the age of five were estimated to be overweight in 2017 [2]. Several low and middle-income settings are leading at this rate, such as Egypt, Fiji, Jordan, Lebanon, and Nicaragua [6,7]. Notably, there was a 48% increase in the prevalence of children and adolescents with overweight and obesity from 2010–2016 in the South-East Asia region alone [8].

Childhood overweight and obesity is not only associated with immediate health risks but can progress into adulthood, leading to the development of a host of non-communicable diseases [9–13], or mental health illness [14,15]. Children or adolescents with overweight or obesity are also more likely to be bullied at school [16]. Moreover, overweight and obesity can have deleterious consequences in the later life of children and adolescents. Stigmatization in the workplace [17] increases the chance of being unemployed and having lower income among women with obesity and overweight [18,19].

Another matter is the economic impact of childhood overweight and obesity. In the Republic of Ireland, the annual healthcare costs amongst children and adolescents with overweight and obesity were on average €1,709,703 [20]. Research from Australia suggests that the cost to the government as a consequence of children affected by overweight and obesity between the ages of 6–13 is over AUD $43 million per annum [21]. Moreover, even more staggering is the annual direct health cost of childhood overweight and obesity in the USA, which has been estimated to be USD $14 billion [22].

Tackling childhood overweight and obesity requires a multifaceted approach. The WHO proposes that prevention should start before birth, emphasizing the importance of healthy maternal nutrition and gestational weight gain [8,23]. The adage "breast is best" is also true in the prevention of childhood obesity, while also providing the best nutrients for infants during this stage of their life [24]. However, food environments also play an integral role in childhood overweight and obesity, and the WHO has previously recommended policy actions to promote restrictions on the marketing strategies that food and beverage industries target at children. These include, for example, preventing the marketing of foods high in saturated and trans-fats, sugar and salt in any form, in places where children gather (e.g., local sports grounds); internalizing positive emotional food memories being used to develop a healthy lifestyle [25], and ensuring that schools promote physical activity and provide health education [26,27].

Treatment targeted towards individuals is also recommended. Diet therapy, for example, can include the introduction of low-fat diets, calorie-controlled diets, or meal replacements. A previously published systematic review has evidenced that there is some merit behind the effectiveness of diet therapy [28]. Physical activity is also crucial for the prevention of childhood overweight and obesity and maintaining healthy body weight. Moreover, there is strong evidence to support the impacts of regular physical activity for the reduction of a risk factor for CVD and diabetes [29,30]. The family and the food environment that a child grows up around can also contribute to promoting weight loss and sustained weight maintenance for children [31,32].

Reviews of childhood overweight and obesity literature can help summarize evidence and guide policy development for addressing this global epidemic. Previously, several systematic reviews and meta-analyses in the field of treatment and intervention of obesity for children and adolescents have been conducted [28,33]. These studies provided insights on a defined research question by synthesizing evidence from previous research. However, a limitation of this approach is that these reviews tend to emphasize a unidimensional topic, which makes it difficult to compare with other research domains over time.

Previously, researchers have applied scientometric analytic approaches to literature reviewing. This method generates a profile of publications for an area of research, and describes the number of publications, citations, downloads, type of journals where this research is published, and patterns of co-authorship, to understand the growth in research productivity and trends specific to that area of research [34,35]. However, scientometric analyses lack essential implications for clinical research, health services improvement, and community interventions, as they do not aim to understand the landscape of topics being researched. Thus, this study aims to describe the growth of research publications regarding interventions for childhood overweight and obesity and to understand the current research landscape. By combining scientometric and content analysis approaches, the authors categorize interdisciplinary topics and interests of the research community regarding interventions for overweight and obesity among children, that can be used to drive future policies.

2. Materials and Methods

2.1. Search Strategy and Eligibility

We used the online database Web of Science (WOS) to identify research papers regarding interventions to treat children and adolescents with obesity. The search was conducted in June 2019 and included articles published between January 1991 and December 2018. The WOS database was selected because it is suitable for our objectives, including (1) 254 various disciplines [36], (2) Higher impact journals [37]. Moreover, WOS allows us to download a large amount of data with important information for our analysis, such as the number of times the papers were downloaded and research areas which were assigned by WOS.

The WOS database search, using keywords, was divided into two steps. Specialists in the field of nutrition and adolescent health found keywords related to "obesity" and "children". In step 1, they were used to collect research articles and reviews from WOS. The database search process is shown in Table S1. These papers were then downloaded under the .txt format and imported into STATA (version 14.0, STATA Corp., TX, the USA). Using a STATA syntax, we searched specifically for papers that included the terms "trial*", and "intervention*" in the title or abstract (step 2).

Papers written in languages other than English were excluded. Additionally, papers other than original research articles or reviews (e.g., editorial, book chapter, letters to the editor or conference proceedings), and papers where the authors were anonymous or unlisted were also excluded from the current study (Figure S1).

2.2. Data Extraction

Two independent researchers extracted the following data from the final library of papers: (1) author names, (2) publication title, (3) publication year, (4) journal's title of publication, (5) authors' keywords, (6) author affiliations, (7) corresponding author details, (8) number of citations, (9) research areas and (10) abstract. Any inconsistencies in the extracted data by the two researchers were resolved by discussion.

2.3. Data Analysis

Data extracted by the independent researchers were transferred into STATA (version 14.0, STATA Corp., TX, the USA). Descriptive statistics were used to generate results for the following publication characteristics: (1) the number of publications produced per year, (2) the number of publications per country (from 1991–2018), (3) the average number of citations for all published papers per year, (4) the frequency of publication downloads in the last six months of 2018 and in the period of 2014–2018, and (5) the average number of publication downloads in the last six months of 2018 and during the period of 2014–2018. Latent Dirichlet Allocation (LDA) was chosen as the method of classifying papers into comparable topics [38–42]. A STATA syntax was used to assign papers to 10 major topics. The data were exported into Microsoft Excel for reading titles and abstracts.

Two researchers independently reviewed the titles and abstracts of most cited papers within each research topic to assign the labels correctly for each topic. After that, an expert would discuss with two researchers to unify the name of topics. Besides providing the total number and percentage of research studies by each topic, we ranked the research interests of these research topics based on the total number of its publications in the past five years. Table 1 identifies how the inputs and outputs of each of these analytical methods.

Table 1. Type of data, methods and the results.

Type of Data	Unit of Analysis	Analytical Methods	Presentations of Results
Keywords, Countries	Words	Frequency of co-occurrence	(1) Map of keyword clusters
Abstracts	Papers	Latent Dirichlet Allocation	(2) 10 classifications of research topics
Web of Science (WOS) classification of research areas	WOS research areas	Frequency of co-occurrence	(3) Dendrogram of research disciplines (WOS classification)

3. Results

Table 2 shows the general characteristics of research publications. Between the years 1991 to 2018, there were 20,925 papers related to interventions and treatments for children and adolescents with overweight or obesity. On average, the number of publications each year increased. There was a notable jump in the number of publications between the years 2010 and 2011; 852 and 1,432 publications respectively (roughly a 68% increase in 2011). This phenomenon may be explained by the impact of the "Let's Move!" campaign [43] and the Affordable Care Act (ACA) on childhood obesity [44]. The total number of usages and the mean use rate of the last five years of papers published in 2013 were the highest compared with that of other years, which shows the recent interest of readers, was significantly higher within the past five years (Figure 1).

Table 2. General characteristics of publications.

Year Published	Total Number of Papers	Total Citations	Mean Cite Rate Per Year	Total Usage * Last 6 Months	Total Usage * Last 5 Years	Mean Use Rate ** Last 6 Months	Mean Use Rate ** Last 5 Years
2018	2333	2032	0.87	7750	12,590	3.32	1.08
2017	2147	8532	1.99	3507	20,822	1.63	1.94
2016	2147	15,174	2.36	2704	30,954	1.26	2.88
2015	2103	28,147	3.35	2363	36,240	1.12	3.45
2014	1838	29,916	3.26	1597	33,525	0.87	3.65
2013	1560	36,230	3.87	1140	35,573	0.73	4.56
2012	1459	38,440	3.76	976	27,891	0.67	3.82
2011	1432	42,896	3.74	998	22,267	0.70	3.11
2010	852	33,522	4.37	508	11,302	0.60	2.65
2009	963	39,974	4.15	541	11,023	0.56	2.29
2008	812	39,424	4.41	425	9002	0.52	2.22
2007	668	38,459	4.80	323	8008	0.48	2.40
2006	529	35,718	5.19	284	7142	0.54	2.70
2005	415	32,184	5.54	188	4187	0.45	2.02
2004	307	22,925	4.98	126	3368	0.41	2.19
2003	254	21,127	5.20	99	2187	0.39	1.72
2002	187	16,138	5.08	97	1778	0.52	1.90
2001	151	14,033	5.16	82	2160	0.54	2.86
2000	141	10,951	4.09	96	1610	0.68	2.28
1999	130	11,093	4.27	72	1226	0.55	1.89
1998	117	10,223	4.16	51	1155	0.44	1.97
1997	87	4801	2.51	13	448	0.15	1.03
1996	65	3886	2.60	10	336	0.15	1.03
1995	60	4438	3.08	13	315	0.22	1.05
1994	36	2212	2.46	11	153	0.31	0.85
1993	51	2475	1.87	10	167	0.20	0.65
1992	43	1639	1.41	10	113	0.23	0.53
1991	38	1634	1.54	10	104	0.26	0.55

* Total usage: Total number of downloads. ** Mean use rate: Total number of downloads/Total number of papers.

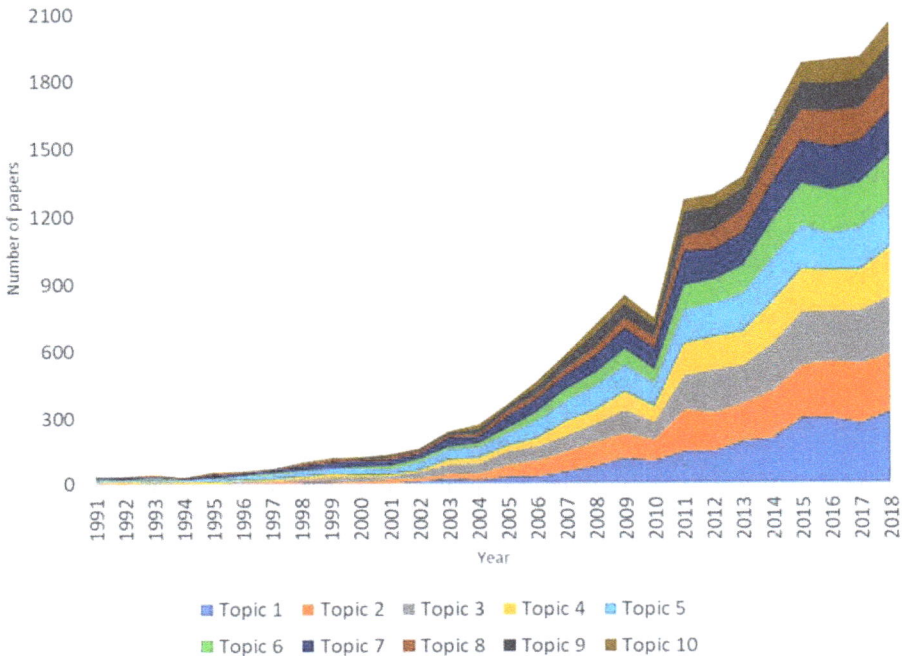

Figure 1. Changes in research topics development in obesity interventions among children and youths. Note: Topic 1: Communities interventions; Topic 2: Pharmacotherapeutic interventions; Topic 3: Epidemiological studies; Topic 4: Family-based, multidisciplinary interventions; Topic 5: Treatment of obesity-related diseases; Topic 6: Psychological and social impairments related to obesity; Topic 7: Treatment of chronic conditions with complications by obesity; Topic 8: Biomedical and preclinical research of obesity-related issues; Topic 9: Community interventions to promote physical activity; Topic 10: Dietary interventions. Topic 1, Topic 2, and Topic 3 received the highest number of papers; meanwhile, Topic 10 had the lowest number of publications.

Table 3 presents the top 60 countries where the research was conducted. Two-thirds of the studies were conducted in the USA with 1394 papers (20.61%). In the top 10 countries, there were three Asian countries, India, China, and Oman, each of which contributed 4.9%, 3.4%, and 2.9% of the publications, respectively. In Africa, a high percentage of children with apparently healthy BMI-for-age have excessive body fatness [45], such as South Africa (9.4%–school-age children and adolescents 5–19 years, 2016), and Ghana (15%–school children 9–15 years, 2012).

The top ten research topics are presented in Table 4. Topics with the highest volumes of publications included Topic 2: Pharmacotherapeutic interventions on obesity and complications (n = 2475 publications); Topic 1: Community Interventions among Children and Youths (n = 2371 publications); and Topic 3: Epidemiological studies of obesity among children and youth (n = 2350 publications).

Table 3. Number of papers by countries as study settings.

Rank	Country Settings	Frequency	%	Rank	Country Settings	Frequency	%
1	United States	1394	20.6%	31	Poland	41	0.6%
2	Australia	672	9.9%	32	Chile	40	0.6%
3	India	329	4.9%	33	Malaysia	39	0.6%
4	United Kingdom	268	4.0%	34	Israel	38	0.6%
5	China	230	3.4%	35	Saudi Arabia	37	0.5%
6	Canada	222	3.3%	36	Thailand	36	0.5%
7	Ireland	204	3.0%	37	Switzerland	34	0.5%
8	Oman	197	2.9%	38	Singapore	33	0.5%
9	Brazil	177	2.6%	39	Indonesia	30	0.4%
10	Germany	140	2.1%	40	Wallis and Futuna	30	0.4%
11	Japan	131	1.9%	41	Colombia	29	0.4%
12	Mexico	128	1.9%	42	Viet Nam	29	0.4%
13	Iran	125	1.8%	43	Portugal	28	0.4%
14	New Zealand	125	1.8%	44	Bangladesh	27	0.4%
15	Spain	117	1.7%	45	Niger	25	0.4%
16	Netherlands	116	1.7%	46	Austria	23	0.3%
17	South Africa	107	1.6%	47	Georgia	23	0.3%
18	Sweden	88	1.3%	48	Kuwait	23	0.3%
19	Italy	86	1.3%	49	Nigeria	23	0.3%
20	Taiwan	66	1.0%	50	Argentina	22	0.3%
21	Greece	63	0.9%	51	Egypt	22	0.3%
22	Belgium	62	0.9%	52	Cuba	21	0.3%
23	France	62	0.9%	53	Czech	20	0.3%
24	Denmark	53	0.8%	54	Hungary	20	0.3%
25	Norway	53	0.8%	55	Bulgaria	18	0.3%
26	Turkey	46	0.7%	56	Jersey	18	0.3%
27	Finland	44	0.6%	57	Estonia	17	0.3%
28	Pakistan	44	0.6%	58	Guatemala	17	0.3%
29	Peru	43	0.6%	59	Lebanon	17	0.3%
30	Hong Kong	42	0.6%	60	Ghana	16	0.2%

Table 4. The top ten research topics classified using the Latent Dirichlet Allocation method.

Rank by the Highest Volume	Research Topics	n	Percent
Topic 2	Pharmacotherapeutic interventions on obesity and complications	2475	13.30%
Topic 1	Community Interventions among Children and Youths	2371	12.80%
Topic 3	Epidemiological studies of obesity among children and youths	2350	12.70%
Topic 5	Treatment of obesity-related diseases	2296	12.40%
Topic 7	Treatment of chronic conditions with complications by obesity	2082	11.20%
Topic 4	Family-based, multidisciplinary interventions	1889	10.20%
Topic 6	Psychological and social impairments related to obesity	1688	9.10%
Topic 8	Biomedical and preclinical research of obesity-related issues	1276	6.90%
Topic 9	Community interventions to promote physical activity	1264	6.80%
Topic 10	Dietary interventions	851	4.60%

Figure 1 depicts the changes in publication volume related to the top ten research topics. In the last five years, Topic 1: School, Community, and System Approaches to Obesity Interventions among Children and Youths, and Topic 2: Pharmacotherapeutic interventions on obesity and related chronic conditions, have attracted the most attention amongst researchers. Notably, treatment for health issues related to obesity (Topic 5 or Topic 7) was one of the main concerns in this field of research.

Figure 2 presents the hierarchical clustering of research disciplines in the intervention and treatment of children and adolescents with obesity. The horizontal axis of the dendrogram shows the distance or dissimilarity between clusters while the vertical represents the research disciplines.

Figure 2 shows that research landscapes in the intervention and treatment of children and adolescents with obesity and overweight are rooted in pediatrics and psychology disciplines. These research areas had a close connection with other clinic fields such as Hepatology, Urology, or Dentistry. In the top, we found the integration of (a) Psychiatry, (b) Psychology clinical, and (c) Psychology. This shows a looser connection between Pediatrics and Psychology clinical; meanwhile, associations between obesity and psychiatric disorders has been proved in some studies [46,47].

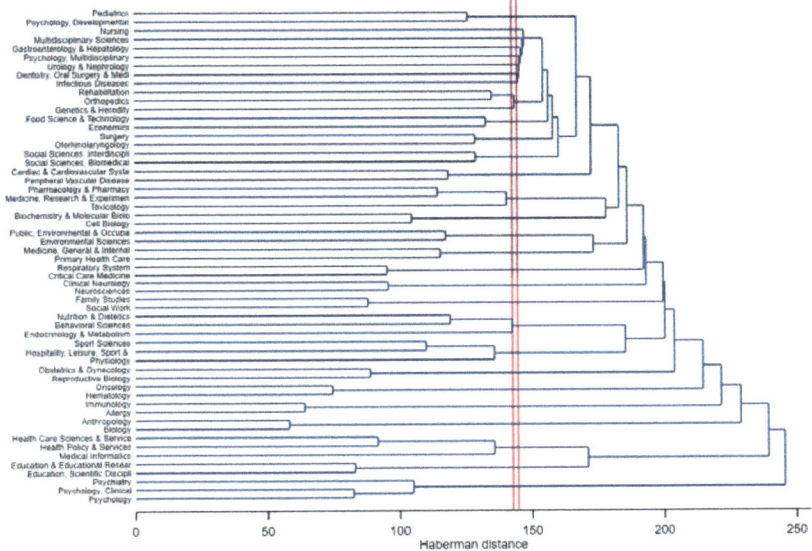

Figure 2. Dendrogram of coincidence of research areas using the WOS classifications.

4. Discussion

This study aimed to describe the growth of research publications regarding interventions for childhood overweight and obesity and to understand the current research landscape by grouping publications according to similarities in the topic areas being researched. By quantifying the scientometrics profile of publications, it is evident that over time, there has been a gradual increase in the publication of research related to interventions and treatments for children with obesity. Applying the LDA technique, we found that the number of publications related to school and community-based intervention has increased over the period. Moreover, the results highlighted the importance of research support in lower-middle-income countries (LMICs), especially, where the prevalence of childhood obesity has been increased [45].

Unsurprisingly, the majority of the research related to interventions and treatment for childhood obesity was conducted in the United States. India and China were the two lower-middle-income countries that appeared the most in the abstracts (Table 2). However, it should be noticed that the majority of children with overweight and obesity live in lower-setting countries, where the rates are rising faster than in high-income countries [48]. The possible causes of this are various, including the Western diet [49], the low activity level [50], or regarding the cultural perspective, where obesity means beauty, better health, power, and higher socioeconomic status [51]. Each LMIC needs to investigate the causes of this phenomenon due to the difference in the contextual background. Yet, due to the limitation in research funding and facilities, human resources, or communication [52], the contextualized evidence might not be found in the short term. Thus, LMICs might benefit from the active research collaboration with developed countries or countries in the same region, such as India and China.

By applying our proposed approach, the combination of scientometrics and content analysis, the present study has identified that there has been a wealth of research conducted globally focusing on the development of the pharmacotherapeutic, family-based, school-based, and community-based interventions, especially in the last five years. Meanwhile, seemingly unidimensional approaches, such as diet or nutrition-related interventions, have reduced. This suggests a definite shift in research towards multifaceted intervention and treatment approaches, particularly those that focus on children's immediate environments. Besides, our studies found that 13.3% of the total papers mentioned pharmacotherapeutic interventions and related chronic conditions. Pharmacotherapy is recommended as a combination method when lifestyle intervention and support from a specialist alone are not enough due to extreme excess weight and related chronic conditions [53]. However, this method should be carefully applied under the supervision of health staff due to some side-effects this may cause to health [54].

The findings suggest some implications for designing interventions, health research, and policy. The number of articles related to the treatment and intervention in poor-resource countries were not high compared with that of high-income countries; meanwhile, the prevalence of obesity and overweight in those settings is increasing. These countries should actively collaborate with other developed countries and countries in the same region (either through their own government or through the support of neighboring/higher-income countries) in order to combat their rising rates of overweight and obesity. Health system strengthening and capacity building, especially in developing countries, will remain as core components of international and national strategies. The developed countries might note the increasing number in the publication regarding the interventions and treatment of childhood obesity. Further research needs to be done to find the most effective strategies of intervention, and treatment of childhood obesity.

Some limitations should be acknowledged. Firstly, the Web of Sciences was the only database used in the analysis. There is a likelihood the low-impact journals, which publish articles from the developing countries, are not being included in the WOS database. Therefore, that may not reflect the development of publications on interventions among children with obesity in developing countries. Future research should consider expanding to other databases to cover the larger number of publications, which contributes more meaningful knowledge to the research field. Secondly, the language of selected papers was restricted to only English. However, there were only 121 papers in other languages, which was a quite small number compared with the total number of papers associated with overweight and obesity in children and youth. Finally, only titles and abstracts were used in the content analysis. However, by quantifying different layers of information (documents by years, citation, and countries where studies conducted) and applying an advanced analytic technique, the Latent Dirichlet Allocation for titles and abstracts analysis [55], we could discover the trend and hidden themes of the research studies [56].

5. Conclusions

Research regarding interventions and treatment for children and adolescents with overweight or obesity is still of great interest to researchers over the world. By applying LDA, we identified ten major topics research related to the intervention and treatment of overweight and obesity among children and adolescents. Notably, is the development in the number of publications that mentioned family-based, school-based, and community-based. Besides, the active collaboration from the LMICs' side, and the support as well as further research on treatments and intervention from developed countries, are needed to reduce the increasing prevalence of childhood obesity.

Supplementary Materials: Supplemental Table S1: Search query for Overweight and Obesity in Children and Adolescents, Figure S1: Selection of papers.

Author Contributions: Conceptualization, B.X.T., S.N., C.A., C.A.L., G.H.H., H.Q.P., C.S.H.H. and R.C.M.H.; Data curation, B.X.T., S.N., C.A.L., T.P.N., L.P.D. and H.Q.P.; Formal analysis, C.A., C.A.L. and R.C.M.H.; Investigation, B.X.T., S.N., C.A., T.P.N. and L.P.D.; Methodology, B.X.T., S.N., C.A., G.H.H., T.P.N., L.P.D. and C.S.H.H.; Project administration, B.X.T.; Software, C.A., G.H.H., T.P.N., L.P.D. and H.Q.P.; Supervision, B.X.T., S.N., C.A.L., C.S.H.H. and R.C.M.H.; Validation, B.X.T., S.N., C.A.L., C.S.H.H. and R.C.M.H.; Visualization, G.H.H., T.P.N., L.P.D. and H.Q.P.; Writing—original draft, B.X.T., G.H.H. and H.Q.P.; Writing—review & editing, B.X.T., S.N., C.A., C.A.L., G.H.H., C.S.H.H. and R.C.M.H.

Funding: This research received no external funding.

Acknowledgments: Not applicable.

Conflicts of Interest: The authors declare no conflict of interest.

References

1. World Health Organization (WHO). Key Facts—Obesity and Overweight. Available online: https://www.who.int/news-room/fact-sheets/detail/obesity-and-overweight (accessed on 26 June 2019).
2. United Nations Children's Fund (UNICEF); World Health Organization (WHO); International Bank for Reconstruction and Development/The World Bank. *Levels and Trends in Child Malnutrition: Key Findings of the 2018 Edition of the Joint Child Malnutrition Estimates*; WHO: Geneva, Switzerland, 2018.
3. Centres for Disease Control and Prevention (CDC). Defining Childhood Obesity. Available online: https://www.cdc.gov/obesity/childhood/defining.html (accessed on 26 June 2019).
4. Cole, T.J.; Bellizzi, M.C.; Flegal, K.M.; Dietz, W.H. Establishing a standard definition for child overweight and obesity worldwide: International survey. *BMJ* **2000**, *320*, 1240–1243. [CrossRef] [PubMed]
5. Rolland-Cachera, M.F.; Group, E.C.O. Childhood obesity: Current definitions and recommendations for their use. *Int. J. Pediatr. Obes.* **2011**, *6*, 325–331. [CrossRef] [PubMed]
6. World Health Organization (WHO). Global Health Observatory (GHO) Data. Available online: https://www.who.int/gho/ncd/risk_factors/overweight_obesity/obesity_adolescents/en/ (accessed on 26 June 2019).
7. Organisation for Economic Co-Operation and Development (OECD). DAC List of ODA Recipients. Available online: http://www.oecd.org/dac/financing-sustainable-development/development-finance-standards/daclist.htm (accessed on 26 June 2019).
8. World Health Organization (WHO). *Taking Action on Childhood Obesity*; WHO: Geneva, Switzerland, 2018.
9. Lloyd, L.J.; Langley-Evans, S.C.; McMullen, S. Childhood obesity and risk of the adult metabolic syndrome: A systematic review. *Int. J. Obes.* **2012**, *36*, 1–11. [CrossRef] [PubMed]
10. Bacha, F.; Gidding, S.S. Cardiac Abnormalities in Youth with Obesity and Type 2 Diabetes. *Curr. Diabetes Rep.* **2016**, *16*, 62. [CrossRef]
11. Mohanan, S.; Tapp, H.; McWilliams, A.; Dulin, M. Obesity and asthma: Pathophysiology and implications for diagnosis and management in primary care. *Exp. Biol. Med.* **2014**, *239*, 1531–1540. [CrossRef]
12. Narang, I.; Mathew, J.L. Childhood obesity and obstructive sleep apnea. *J. Nutr. Metab.* **2012**, *2012*, 134202. [CrossRef]
13. Africa, J.A.; Newton, K.P.; Schwimmer, J.B. Lifestyle Interventions Including Nutrition, Exercise, and Supplements for Nonalcoholic Fatty Liver Disease in Children. *Digest. Dis. Sci.* **2016**, *61*, 1375–1386. [CrossRef]
14. Morrison, K.M.; Shin, S.; Tarnopolsky, M.; Taylor, V.H. Association of depression & health related quality of life with body composition in children and youth with obesity. *J. Affect. Disord.* **2015**, *172*, 18–23. [CrossRef]
15. Halfon, N.; Larson, K.; Slusser, W. Associations between obesity and comorbid mental health, developmental, and physical health conditions in a nationally representative sample of US children aged 10 to 17. *Acad. Pediatr.* **2013**, *13*, 6–13. [CrossRef]
16. Bacchini, D.; Licenziati, M.R.; Garrasi, A.; Corciulo, N.; Driul, D.; Tanas, R.; Fiumani, P.M.; Di Pietro, E.; Pesce, S.; Crinò, A. Bullying and victimization in overweight and obese outpatient children and adolescents: An Italian multicentric study. *PLoS ONE* **2015**, *10*, e0142715. [CrossRef]
17. Flint, S.W.; Snook, J. Obesity and discrimination: The next 'big issue'? *Int. J. Discrim. Law* **2014**, *14*, 183–193. [CrossRef]
18. Lee, H.; Ahn, R.; Kim, T.; Han, E. Impact of Obesity on Employment and Wages among Young Adults: Observational Study with Panel Data. *Int. J. Environ. Res. Public Health* **2019**, *16*, 139. [CrossRef] [PubMed]

19. Härkönen, J.; Räsänen, P.; Näsi, M. Obesity, unemployment, and earnings. *Nord. J. Work. Life Stud.* **2011**, *1*, 23–38. [CrossRef]
20. Perry, I.J.; Millar, S.R.; Balanda, K.P.; Dee, A.; Bergin, D.; Carter, L.; Doherty, E.; Lorraine, F.; Hamilton, D.; Jaccard, A.; et al. *What Are the Estimated Costs of Childhood Overweight and Obesity on the Island of Ireland?* Safefood: Cork, Ireland, 2017.
21. Black, N.; Hughes, R.; Jones, A.M. The health care costs of childhood obesity in Australia: An instrumental variables approach. *Econ. Hum. Biol.* **2018**, *31*, 1–13. [CrossRef] [PubMed]
22. Marder, W.; Chang, S. *Childhood Obesity: Costs, Treatment Patterns, Disparities in Care, and Prevalent Medical Conditions*; Thomson Medstat Research Brief: Stamford, CT, USA, 2006.
23. Haire-Joshu, D.; Tabak, R. Preventing Obesity Across Generations: Evidence for Early Life Intervention. *Annu. Rev. Public Health* **2016**, *37*, 253–271. [CrossRef]
24. Moreno, M.A.; Furtner, F.; Rivara, F.P. Breastfeeding as Obesity Prevention. *Arch. Pediatr. Adol. Med.* **2011**, *165*, 772. [CrossRef] [PubMed]
25. Von Essen, E.; Martensson, F. Young adults' use of emotional food memories to build resilience. *Appetite* **2017**, *112*, 210–218. [CrossRef]
26. Lobelo, F.; Garcia de Quevedo, I.; Holub, C.K.; Nagle, B.J.; Arredondo, E.M.; Barquera, S.; Elder, J.P. School-based programs aimed at the prevention and treatment of obesity: Evidence-based interventions for youth in Latin America. *J. Sch. Health* **2013**, *83*, 668–677. [CrossRef]
27. The State of Obesity. The State of Childhood Obesity. Available online: https://www.stateofobesity.org/childhood/ (accessed on 27 June 2019).
28. Flodmark, C.E.; Marcus, C.; Britton, M. Interventions to prevent obesity in children and adolescents: A systematic literature review. *Int. J. Obes.* **2006**, *30*, 579–589. [CrossRef]
29. Agarwal, S.K. Cardiovascular benefits of exercise. *Int. J. Gen. Med.* **2012**, *5*, 541–545. [CrossRef]
30. Buttar, H.S.; Li, T.; Ravi, N. Prevention of cardiovascular diseases: Role of exercise, dietary interventions, obesity and smoking cessation. *Exp. Clin. Cardiol.* **2005**, *10*, 229–249.
31. Berge, J.M. A review of familial correlates of child and adolescent obesity: What has the 21st century taught us so far? *Int. J. Adolesc. Med. Health* **2009**, *21*, 457–484. [CrossRef] [PubMed]
32. Kitzmann, K.M.; Beech, B.M. Family-based interventions for pediatric obesity: Methodological and conceptual challenges from family psychology. *J. Fam. Psychol.* **2011**, *20*, 175–189. [CrossRef]
33. Rajjo, T.; Mohammed, K.; Alsawas, M.; Ahmed, A.T.; Farah, W.; Asi, N.; Almasri, J.; Prokop, L.J.; Murad, M.H. Treatment of Pediatric Obesity: An Umbrella Systematic Review. *J. Clin. Endocrinol. Metab.* **2017**, *102*, 763–775. [CrossRef] [PubMed]
34. Tran, B.X.; Dang, K.A.; Le, H.T.; Ha, G.H.; Nguyen, L.H.; Nguyen, T.H.; Tran, T.H.; Latkin, C.A.; Ho, C.S.H.; Ho, R.C.M. Global Evolution of Obesity Research in Children and Youths: Setting Priorities for Interventions and Policies. *Obes. Facts* **2019**, *12*, 137–149. [CrossRef]
35. Vioque, J.; Ramos, J.M.; Navarrete-Munoz, E.M.; Garcia-de-la-Hera, M. A bibliometric study of scientific literature on obesity research in PubMed (1988–2007). *Obes. Rev.* **2010**, *11*, 603–611. [CrossRef]
36. Clarivate Analytics. Web of Science Core Collection. Available online: https://clarivate.com/webofsciencegroup/solutions/web-of-science-core-collection/ (accessed on 11 October 2019).
37. Aghaei Chadegani, A.; Salehi, H.; Yunus, M.; Farhadi, H.; Fooladi, M.; Farhadi, M.; Ale Ebrahim, N. A comparison between two main academic literature collections: Web of Science and Scopus databases. *Asian Soc. Sci.* **2013**, *9*, 18–26. [CrossRef]
38. Li, Y.; Rapkin, B.; Atkinson, T.M.; Schofield, E.; Bochner, B.H. Leveraging Latent Dirichlet Allocation in processing free-text personal goals among patients undergoing bladder cancer surgery. *Qual. Life Res.* **2019**. [CrossRef]
39. Valle, D.; Albuquerque, P.; Zhao, Q.; Barberan, A.; Fletcher, R.J., Jr. Extending the Latent Dirichlet Allocation model to presence/absence data: A case study on North American breeding birds and biogeographical shifts expected from climate change. *Glob. Chang. Biol.* **2018**, *24*, 5560–5572. [CrossRef] [PubMed]
40. Chen, C.; Zare, A.; Trinh, H.N.; Omotara, G.O.; Cobb, J.T.; Lagaunne, T.A. Partial Membership Latent Dirichlet Allocation for Soft Image Segmentation. *IEEE Trans. Image Process.* **2017**, *26*, 5590–5602. [CrossRef]
41. Lu, H.M.; Wei, C.P.; Hsiao, F.Y. Modeling healthcare data using multiple-channel latent Dirichlet allocation. *J. Biomed. Inf.* **2016**, *60*, 210–223. [CrossRef] [PubMed]

42. Gross, A.; Murthy, D. Modeling virtual organizations with Latent Dirichlet Allocation: A case for natural language processing. *Neural Netw.* **2014**, *58*, 38–49. [CrossRef] [PubMed]
43. Andersen, J.A.; Wylie, L.E.; Brank, E.M. Public health framing and attribution: Analysis of the first lady's remarks and news coverage on childhood obesity. *Cogent Soc. Sci.* **2017**, *3*, 1268748. [CrossRef]
44. Diane Pilkey, L.S.; Gee, E.; Finegold, K.; Amaya, K.; Robinson, W. *The Affordable Care Act and Adolescents ASPE research brief*; Office of the Assistant Secretary for Planning and Evaluation: Washing, DC, USA, 2013.
45. Diouf, A.; Adom, T.; Aouidet, A.; Hamdouchi, A.E.; Joonas, N.I.; Loechl, C.U.; Leyna, G.H.; Mbithe, D.; Moleah, T.; Monyeki, A.; et al. Body mass index vs deuterium dilution method for establishing childhood obesity prevalence, Ghana, Kenya, Mauritius, Morocco, Namibia, Senegal, Tunisia and United Republic of Tanzania. *Bull. World Health Organ.* **2018**, *96*, 772–781. [CrossRef] [PubMed]
46. Devlin, M.J.; Yanovski, S.Z.; Wilson, G.T. Obesity: What Mental Health Professionals Need to Know. *Am. J. Psychiatry* **2000**, *157*, 854–866. [CrossRef]
47. Değirmenci, T.; Kalkan-Oğuzhanoğlu, N.; Sözeri-Varma, G.; Özdel, O.; Fenkçi, S. Psychological Symptoms in Obesity and Related Factors. *Noro. Psikiyatr. Ars.* **2015**, *52*, 42–46. [CrossRef]
48. World Health Organization (WHO). Facts and Figures on Childhood Obesity. Available online: https://www.who.int/end-childhood-obesity/facts/en/ (accessed on 13 October 2019).
49. Cordain, L.; Eaton, S.B.; Sebastian, A.; Mann, N.; Lindeberg, S.; Watkins, B.A.; O'Keefe, J.H.; Brand-Miller, J. Origins and evolution of the Western diet: Health implications for the 21st century. *Am. J. Clin. Nutr.* **2005**, *81*, 341–354. [CrossRef]
50. Bhurosy, T.; Jeewon, R. Overweight and obesity epidemic in developing countries: A problem with diet, physical activity, or socioeconomic status? *ScientificWorldJournal* **2014**, *2014*, 964236. [CrossRef]
51. Nour, N.N. Obesity in resource-poor nations. *Rev. Obstet. Gynecol.* **2010**, *3*, 180–184.
52. Vose, P.; Cervellini, A. Problems of scientific research in developing countries. *IAEA Bull.* **1983**, *25*, 37–40.
53. Joo, J.K.; Lee, K.S. Pharmacotherapy for obesity. *J. Menopausal. Med.* **2014**, *20*, 90–96. [CrossRef] [PubMed]
54. Gadde, K.M.; Apolzan, J.W.; Berthoud, H.-R. Pharmacotherapy for Patients with Obesity. *Clin. Chem.* **2018**, *64*, 118–129. [CrossRef] [PubMed]
55. Baghaei Lakeh, A.; Ghaffarzadegan, N. Global Trends and Regional Variations in Studies of HIV/AIDS. *Sci. Rep.* **2017**, *7*, 4170. [CrossRef] [PubMed]
56. Wang, H.; Wu, F.; Lu, W.; Yang, Y.; Li, X.; Li, X.; Zhuang, Y. Identifying Objective and Subjective Words via Topic Modeling. *IEEE Trans. Neural Netw. Learn. Syst.* **2018**, *29*, 718–730. [CrossRef]

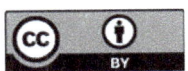

© 2019 by the authors. Licensee MDPI, Basel, Switzerland. This article is an open access article distributed under the terms and conditions of the Creative Commons Attribution (CC BY) license (http://creativecommons.org/licenses/by/4.0/).

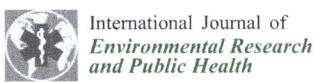 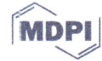

Review

Musculoskeletal Risks: RULA Bibliometric Review

Marta Gómez-Galán [1], Ángel-Jesús Callejón-Ferre [1,2,*], José Pérez-Alonso [1], Manuel Díaz-Pérez [1] and Jesús-Antonio Carrillo-Castrillo [3]

[1] Department of Engineering, University of Almería, Research Center CIMEDES (CeiA3), 04120 Almería, Spain; mgg492@ual.es (M.G.-G.); jpalonso@ual.es (J.P.-A.); madiaz@ual.es (M.D.-P.)
[2] Laboratory-Observatory Andalusian Working Conditions in the Agricultural Sector (LASA), 41092 Seville, Spain
[3] School of Industrial Engineering, University of Seville, 41092 Seville, Spain; jcarrillo3@us.es
* Correspondence: acallejo@ual.es; Tel.: +34-950-214-236; Fax: +34-950-015-491

Received: 30 May 2020; Accepted: 15 June 2020; Published: 17 June 2020

Abstract: The objective of this study was to reveal RULA method applications in terms of the knowledge, country, year and journal categories. The search was performed using the "Web of Science Core Collection". The period from 1993 to April 2019 was selected. Eight hundred nine results were obtained, of which 226 were used. The largest number of publications was determined to be in the fields of industry and health and social assistance, which coincides with the OWAS and Standardized Nordic Questionnaire methods. By country, the USA stands out for its greater number of research studies and categories that are encompassed. By date, 2016 was the year when more studies were carried out, again coinciding with the Standardized Nordic Questionnaire. By journal, "Work—A Journal of Prevention Assessment and Rehabilitation" is highlighted, as it is for the REBA method as well. It was concluded that RULA can be applied to workers in different fields, usually in combination with other methods, while technological advancement provides benefits for its application.

Keywords: biomechanics; musculoskeletal disorders; RULA; ergonomics; applications

1. Introduction

1.1. Musculoskeletal Disorders (MSD)

One of the most common work diseases in Europe are musculoskeletal disorders. These appear in various areas of the body, the most common developing in the back and upper extremities [1].

Among the causes that stand out for their appearance are the physical (manual, forced or frequently repeated movements, harmful postures and vibrations, etc.) and those relating to work organisation (high work rate, schedule, routine work, etc.) [2].

This type of disorder has numerous consequences for the affected worker, but also for businesses and countries (at the economic level) [3].

To prevent this occupational disease, it is necessary to identify all the risk factors that occur during work. Once determined, preventive measures should be taken to avert them, or actions taken to reduce them [2]. Some authors propose measures such as rotating workers between different jobs [4], providing ergonomic training to workers [5], designing ergonomic tools for MSD analysis in the workplace [6], redesigning work equipment from the ergonomic perspective [7], etc.

1.2. Assessment Methods

There are numerous methods for assessing musculoskeletal disorders. These can be classified into three main groups: direct, semi-direct and indirect (Table 1 [8]).

Table 1. Types of MSD assessment methods [8].

Direct	Semi-Direct	Indirect
Placing sensors on workers' bodies as they perform tasks.	Observing the task being carried out and using software to analyse it.	Employing questionnaires.

Of the three groups above, the most economical methods are the indirect ones since they are based solely on completing questionnaires. The opposite is true in the other two cases as software licenses are required and sensors have to be purchased. Direct methods are the most accurate because they provide virtually automatic information. In terms of complexity, direct and indirect methods stand out—in the former because the use of sensors can be a nuisance for the worker and, in the latter, because of the subsequent statistical analysis [8].

When selecting a method for a particular study, it is advisable to consider several criteria (cost, accuracy, complexity, application time, etc.) and to analyse the advantages and disadvantages of each.

1.3. Examples of Direct, Semi-Direct and Indirect Methods

The following are some examples of direct, semi-direct, and indirect assessment methods (Figure 1; Figure 2; [9–13]; [14–30]).

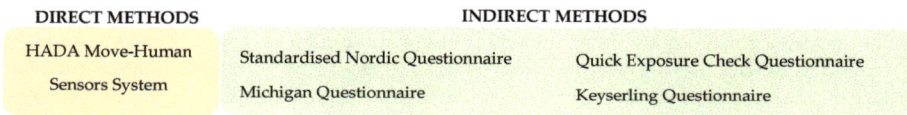

Figure 1. Examples of direct and indirect methods.

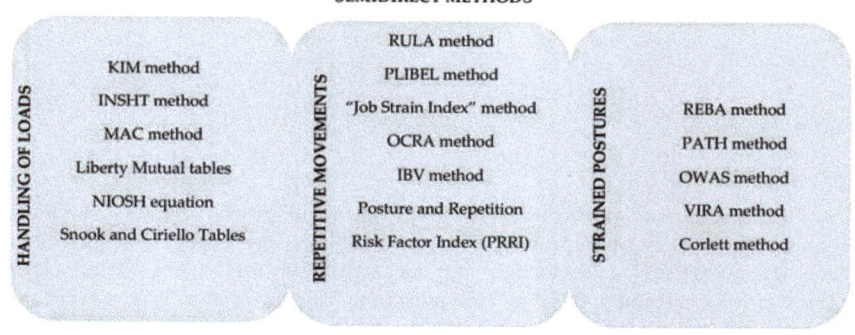

Figure 2. Examples of semi-direct methods (see Appendix A).

1.4. Rapid Upper Limb Assessment (RULA) Method

The RULA method was designed in 1993 by McAtamney and Corlett. Its objective is to know if workers are exposed to MSD risk factors in the upper extremities during the performance of their work [20].

The method assesses three factors: the posture of the different areas of the body, the load or force exerted and the muscle activity (static posture or repetitive movements). The body regions which RULA focuses on are divided into two groups [31]:

- Group A: arm, forearm, wrist and wrist turn.
- Group B: neck, torso and legs.

- Three main stages [20,31] are performed to carry out the assessment using this method:
- Observation of postures. This is done while the worker performs the task and can be realised in three ways: direct observation or by taking images or videos. The postures to be assessed (those most repeated, those performed for more than 10% or 15% of the task and those that are most harmful) are selected. Only one side of the body is analysed, namely the one which suffers most harm; however, if they are very different, then both sides are assessed.
- Scores. For the postures to be assessed, the angle must be measured between each of the body areas and the vertical. The lower extremities are not measured, although it is taken into account whether the posture is balanced and supported. Using these data, which are modified by different criteria and considering the load factors and muscle activity, the RULA scores are calculated (Figure 3).
- Action levels. From the final scores, one obtains the action level. RULA differentiates four levels:

  ➢ Level 1 (Score: 1–2). No action is needed.
  ➢ Level 2 (Score: 3–4). Measures should be taken, but not in the short term.
  ➢ Level 3 (Score 5–6). Measures should be taken in the short term.
  ➢ Level 4 (Score 7). Urgent action must be taken.

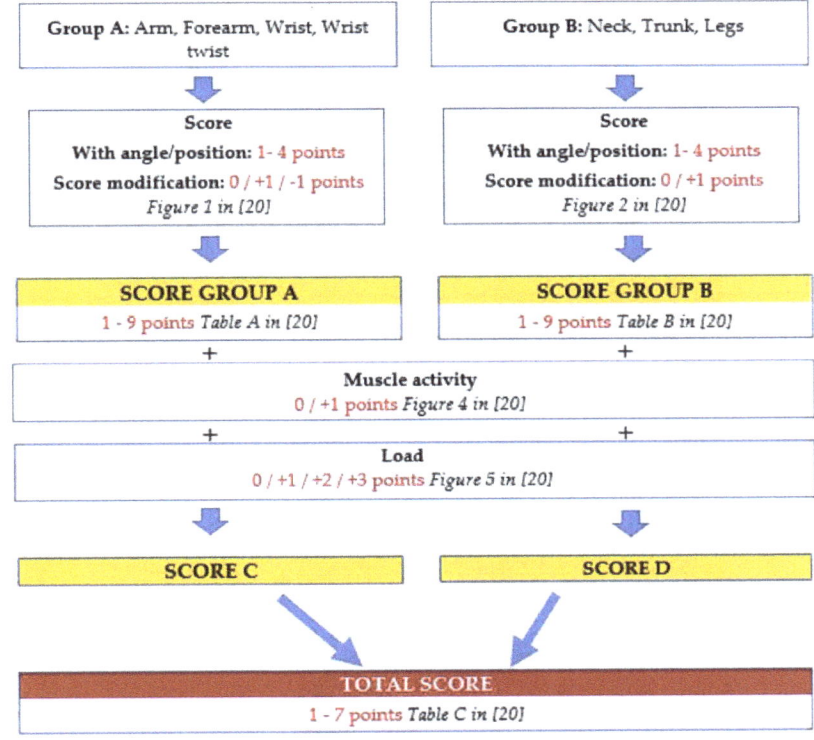

Figure 3. RULA Scores [20,31].

1.4.1. Advantages

Some advantages of the RULA method include:

- It is a reliable method to use for repetitive tasks, mainly in the upper limbs [31].
- It has been applied to workers across very different areas [31].
- The assessor needs no experience in order to apply it during the observation phase [20].
- It is not very complex to apply. The method is simple to use [32].
- It can be applied with the help of software [31,32].

1.4.2. Limitations

Among the disadvantages of the RULA method are the following:

- It results in a high-level risk for non-permanent jobs [31].
- The left and right side of the body are assessed independently [32].
- It does not take into account the time the worker takes to carry out the task [32].

1.5. Objective

The aim of this work is to review all the studies in which the RULA method has been applied from 1993 to April 2019 and to analyse them according to the following categories: knowledge, country, year and journal.

2. Materials and Methods

To search for information about the different RULA method applications, the University of Almería's library website was accessed. There, we used the "Web of Science" (WoS) database, the license of which is managed by the Spanish Foundation for Science and Technology (FECYT).

The search was done by selecting the "Web of Science Core Collection" and the advanced search option, in which "so = Applied Ergonomics" was introduced. The "Create Citation Reports" option was selected. In this way, the total number of available citations was consulted for the original article proposing the RULA method by McAtamney and Corlett [20].

The number of studies obtained was 809, in the period from 1993 to 29 April 2019. Of these, using the title and abstract of each study, we finally selected a total of 226 results, discarding those that did not include the method's application. The final studies were from 1998 to 2019.

It should be noted that the main limitation of the information search is that we only used the Web of Science Core Collection; no other databases were accessed. Therefore, some studies may have been overlooked with the search method used.

3. Results and Discussion

The studies obtained from the search have been analysed and classified according to the categories of knowledge, location (countries), publication date (years) and journals.

3.1. Classification by Knowledge Categories

A particular classification [33] has been used to order the RULA studies according to the knowledge categories. Table 2 shows the different areas presented, the designated nomenclature and the number of published studies.

Table 2. Knowledge categories [33].

Knowledge Category	Number of Studies
Agriculture, forestry and fishing	18
Mining and quarrying	2
Manufacturing	74
Water supply; sewerage, waste management and remediation activities	1
Construction	4
Wholesale and retail trade; repair of motor vehicles and motorcycles	3
Transportation and storage	12
Accommodation and food service activities	3
Information and communication	9
Financial and insurance activities	1
Professional, scientific and technical activities	2
Administrative and support service activities	12
Public administration and defence; compulsory social security	2
Education	12
Human health and social work activities	38
Arts, entertainment and recreation	3
Other service activities	3
Activities of households as employers; undifferentiated goods and services producing activities of households for own use	2
Other scopes not previously included *	25

* The category "Other areas not previously included" is not part of the classification used; it is a section that encompasses studies that have not been considered in the other fields.

In total, 19 categories are differentiated. One can observe that "Manufacturing" stands out as having more studies than the rest, a total of 74. This is followed by 38 and 25 publications corresponding to "Human health and social work activities" and "Other areas not previously included ", respectively (Table 2).

In contrast, two fields are differentiated in which only one research study is recorded—"Water supply, sewerage, waste management and remediation activities" and "Financial and insurance activities" (Table 2).

Figure 4 shows the different areas of knowledge based on the frequency of the published studies.

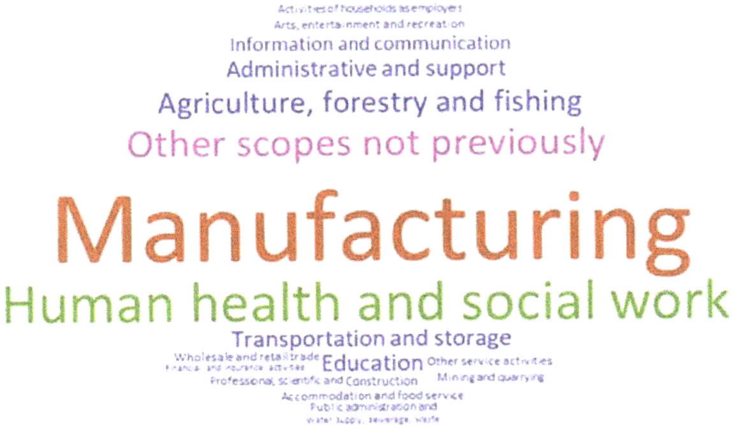

Figure 4. Knowledge categories and frequency.

Below is a description of each of these categories [33].

3.1.1. Agriculture, Forestry and Fishing

Table 3 summarises the studies related to this category.

Table 3. Agriculture, forestry and fishing.

Reference	Year	Country	Study Objective
[34]	2019	Italy	RULA and REBA assessment of a forestry worker using a wood-chipper machine.
[35]	2018	Thailand	Design of a knife to improve the ergonomics for workers who collect rubber. BCTQ and RULA were used for the assessment.
[36]	2018	USA	Use of RULA and other ergonomic tools on blueberry harvesters.
[37]	2018	India	Application of OWAS, RULA, REBA, QEC and others on rice growing workers.
[38]	2018	Thailand	Use of the Musculoskeletal Nordic Questionnaire, RULA and a tasks checklist in hazardous places for fruit farmers.
[39]	2018	India	Implementation of the modified Standardized Nordic Questionnaire and the RULA method on farm workers performing manual tasks.
[40]	2018	Spain	Use of RULA, REBA and OWAS on olive farm workers during the task of pruning with a chainsaw.
[41]	2018	India	Use of the Musculoskeletal Nordic Questionnaire and the RULA method on farm workers engaged in manual harvesting.
[42]	2018	South Korea	Comparison of the ALLA method with RULA, REBA and OWAS using the assessment of postures developed in agriculture.
[43]	2017	Turkey	Application of REBA, RULA, QEC and OWAS on nursery workers.
[44]	2016	Indonesia	RULA assessment on workers who use threshing machines for rice cultivation.
[45]	2016	Spain	Application of RULA on farm workers performing crop stringing
[46]	2016	Malaysia	Assessment using RULA and other ergonomic tools on workers responsible for cutting oil palm.
[47]	2014	Malaysia	Application of RULA on workers charged with oil palm collection.
[48]	2013	Malaysia	Use of RULA on oil palm harvesters.
[49]	2013	Thailand	Use of the Industrial Ergonomics Screening Tool, based on HAL (Hand Activity Level) and RULA methods on workers during rice cultivation ploughing with a cultivator.
[50]	2012	Italy	Conducting a study with the aim of redesigning the space for the driver of an agricultural tractor. Catia V5 software and other tools, including RULA, were used.
[51]	2012	Thailand	Use of a survey, a form and RULA on rubber harvesters.

Crop and Animal Production, Hunting and Related Service Activities

The RULA method has been used for the ergonomic assessment of farm workers working on various crops or specific tasks.

In fruit crops, Thetkathuek et al. [38] applied it together with the Nordic Musculoskeletal Questionnaire and a tasks checklist. In total, 861 farm workers took part in Thailand. They showed that men with more than 10 years of experience had their necks most affected and women their lower backs. In blueberry harvesting, Kim et al. [36] used it in conjunction with the Borg CR10 scale, electromyography, the Cumulative Trauma Disorders (CTD) index and NIOSH (National Occupational Institute for Safety and Health). They concluded that the risk was reduced by carrying out the work with the help of machinery.

Three studies were carried out on oil palm harvesting. In two of them, other ergonomic tools were also used. In the first study, 109 workers were assessed, while three and seven were assessed in the other two. The results for all three showed that most workers were exposed to a very high level of risk when carrying out the tasks. Changes were required as a matter of urgency [46–48].

Three other studies were conducted into rice cultivation. Pal and Dhara [37] studied 166 workers in India. They also used other methods such as REBA (The Rapid Entire Body Assessment), OWAS (The Ovako Working Analysis System), etc. The results showed the frequent appearance of MSD, with the most affected areas being the lumbar, hip, wrist, shoulder and knee regions. In the other two studies, farm workers were assessed when using machinery during the tasks: in one case using threshing machines and in the other using a cultivator. For both, it was concluded that there was a high risk of MSD [44,49].

In olive cultivation, Pardo-Ferreira et al. [40] assessed farm workers performing pruning with a chainsaw. Other methods were also used, in particular REBA and OWAS. They determined that change was needed, as workers were exposed to ergonomic risks.

Another series of studies was conducted using the RULA method to assess different tasks. Jain et al. [39,41] carried out two studies focusing on manual tasks, also using a questionnaire The first concluded the frequent development of musculoskeletal disorders in workers; this coincided with the second, which indicated a score (RULA) of 5 or above for 92% of the workers.

Vazquez-Cabrera [45] investigated farm workers during crop stringing. They simulated different ways to do it in a laboratory according to the height, crop weight and guides used. Among other findings, heights of 1.4 m were shown to be acceptable, with 1.2 and 1.6 m heights also being possible. Weights over 2 kg were found not to be suitable.

Finally, some authors set out specific objectives. Kong et al. [42] used RULA to assess Korean farm workers as they adopted 96 postures. The aim was to apply RULA along with the REBA, OWAS and ALLA (Agricultural Lower Limb Assessment) methods in order to compare the last one with the previous three, proving it to be the most correct. Di Gironimo et al. [50] set out to redesign and improve the ergonomics of an agricultural tractor's driver space. In addition to RULA, this was done using Catia V5 software (as well as other ergonomic tools) to design a 3D model. Some devices in the cab needed to be corrected to provide better ergonomics.

Forestry and Logging

Studies in this category using the RULA method have only been carried out in forestry.

Several authors focused on rubber harvesting workers (tappers). Meksawi et al. [51] also used a survey and a form. According to the RULA results, an action Level 3 was obtained, so changes needed to be made to the work. Pramchoo et al. [35] assessed the ergonomics of a new knife designed for tapping. Two groups participated, one of them using the new knife. In each group, half of the workers suffered discomfort related to the carpal tunnel syndrome. The Boston Carpal Tunnel Syndrome Questionnaire (BCTQ) was also applied. The new knife, among other advantages, reduced the discomfort from carpal tunnel syndrome in sufferers and improved the wrist posture.

Regarding forestry activity, two studies were performed to assess workers. Cremasco et al. [34] focused on tasks performed with a wood-chipper; they also used REBA in their assessment. Unver-Okan et al. [43] focused on forestry nurseries; they also employed REBA, OWAS and QEC (Quick Exposure Check). In both cases, it was determined that the RULA method was the most suitable for such assessments.

3.1.2. Mining and Quarrying

Table 4 presents the only two studies related to this category.

Table 4. Mining and quarrying.

Reference	Year	Country	Study Objective
[52]	2010	India	Use of REBA, RULA, OCRA and other ergonomic tools on stone carving workers.
[53]	2016	Malaysia	Application of RULA on mine workers.

In this field of knowledge, there are only two studies available in which the RULA method was applied—one for the ergonomic assessment of mine workers and the other, together with the REBA and OCRA (Occupational Repetitive Action) methods, in stone-carving workers. Both studies concluded that very high risks existed that required immediate changes [52,53].

3.1.3. Manufacturing

Table 5 sets out the different publications available in the field of manufacturing.

Table 5. Manufacturing.

Reference	Year	Country	Study Objective
[54]	2019	Turkey	The design of a cell in an industry using virtual reality and an ergonomic study with RULA.
[55]	2019	Malaysia	Application of RULA and interviews on workers in a car factory.
[56]	2018	India	Application of a questionnaire, RULA and REBA on brick kiln workers.
[57]	2018	Tunisia	Application of RULA and REBA on milling, turning and drilling workers.
[58]	2018	Canada	Use of the RULA method and certain devices on baristas responsible for tamping the espresso coffee.
[59]	2018	Iran	Application of a questionnaire and RULA on assembly workers in an electronic components factory.
[60]	2018	Malaysia	Use of the modified Nordic questionnaire, REBA and RULA on assembly workers in an electronics factory.
[61]	2018	Iran	Use of RULA, LUBA (Loading on the Upper Body Assessment) and NERPA (New Ergonomic Posture Assessment) on automotive, pharmaceutical and assembly workers.
[62]	2018	United Kingdom	Design and analysis of a system allowing workers to control an industrial robot. RULA was also used for its design.
[63]	2017	Malaysia	A car seat was designed with CATIA and then RULA was used for the ergonomic assessment.
[64]	2017	Iran	Use of RULA and another computer tool on sugar factory workers who manually moved the bags.
[65]	2017	Malaysia	Use of RULA and REBA on food industry workers.
[66]	2017	USA	Use of RULA and the Strain Index on aircraft factory workers.
[67]	2017	Italy	Immersive virtual reality for assembling an aircraft's wing. RULA and REBA were used for the ergonomic assessment.
[68]	2017	United Kingdom	The development of a tool for the analysis of aircraft maintenance work. RULA, OWAS and LBA were employed for the ergonomic assessment.
[69]	2017	India	Use of RULA to assess pump-assembly workers who are submerged in wells.
[70]	2017	Ecuador	Application of OWAS and RULA on workers in a shoe factory.
[71]	2017	Iran	Use of the Nordic Questionnaire and RULA on workers in a pharmaceutical company.
[72]	2017	Australia	Use of Kinect and RULA on assembly workers.
[73]	2016	Brazil	Use of the Nordic Musculoskeletal Questionnaire and RULA on chemical industry workers.
[74]	2016	India	Design of a new crane cab in the steel industry. Ergonomic assessment with RULA.
[75]	2016	Portugal	RULA and the Strain Index were applied on 3 assembly posts manned by electronic production workers in the automotive industry.
[76]	2016	India	Use of an interview, questionnaire and RULA on workers who peel pineapples.
[77]	2016	Thailand	Use of RULA and other tools, such as the Nordic Questionnaire, on workers in a frozen food company.
[78]	2016	Iran	Use of interviews, the Nordic Musculoskeletal questionnaire and RULA on shoe sole production workers.
[79]	2016	Iran	Use of RULA and the Nordic Questionnaire in packaging workers in the pharmaceutical industry.
[80]	2016	Iran	Use of the Nordic Musculoskeletal Questionnaire and RULA on sewing workers.
[81]	2016	India	Application of RULA and questionnaires in textile industry workers.
[82]	2016	Indonesia	Use of RULA on workers in a batik cap factory.
[83]	2016	Cambodia	Conducting interviews and applying RULA to textile factory workers.
[84]	2016	Portugal	Use of OSHA, RULA and the NIOSH equation in industrial workers.
[85]	2016	China	Ergonomic assessment using DELMIA of assembly in the robotics industry. Using RULA.
[86]	2015	Portugal	Application of RULA on workers in charge of maintaining an oven.
[87]	2015	Iran	Use of a questionnaire and RULA on sewing machine workers.
[88]	2015	Indonesia	Study with RULA and the Nordic Body Map Questionnaire on industry workers tasked with producing batik caps.
[89]	2015	Mexico	Use of RULA on industrial and construction workers.
[90]	2014	Malaysia	Design of a new CNC milling machine. Ergonomic assessment of this machine, and the previous machine, using RULA.
[91]	2014	Iran	Use of a questionnaire and RULA on workers who sew shoes manually.
[92]	2014	Portugal	Application of RULA and the Nordic Musculoskeletal Questionnaire on footwear factory workers.
[93]	2014	Brazil	Use of a questionnaire and RULA on workers in a transformer factory.
[94]	2014	Portugal	Use of the OSHA Checklist, RULA and the NIOSH equation on factory workers.
[95]	2013	Spain	Use of RULA, REBA and virtual simulation in metal industry workers.
[96]	2013	Malaysia	Use of the RULA method and the Cornell Musculoskeletal Discomfort Questionnaire on manual handling workers in a metal stamping factory.
[97]	2013	Turkey	Use of a questionnaire and RULA on textile workers.
[98]	2013	Malaysia	Use of questionnaires based on the Standardized Nordic Questionnaire as well as the RULA and REBA methods on batik cap factory workers.
[99]	2013	Thailand	The ergonomic assessment of clothing assembly line workers using RULA.
[100]	2013	Malaysia	Application of RULA in packaging industry workers.
[101]	2013	Germany	Development of a system to ergonomically analyse workers in the industrial sector. The assessment was carried out using RULA.
[102]	2013	Portugal	Three different studies on factory workers, each using a method, which included RULA.
[103]	2013	Australia	The use of Kinect together with RULA on assembly workers.
[104]	2012	Brazil	Shoulder study on workers in a meat packing business. Using RULA, a human body diagram and anthropometric measurements.

Table 5. *Cont.*

Reference	Year	Country	Study Objective
[105]	2012	Taiwan	Study using 3D simulation to introduce humans into a robot workplace, working with fruits and vegetables. Ergonomic analysis using LBA and RULA.
[106]	2012	USA	Application of the RULA method and two other tools on mobile phone assembly workers.
[107]	2012	Netherlands	Ergonomic assessment with RULA on laptop manufacturing workers.
[108]	2012	Iran	Use of RULA and the Nordic Musculoskeletal Questionnaire on textile workers.
[109]	2012	Thailand	Application of REBA, RULA and OWAS on rubber sheet manufacturing workers.
[110]	2012	China	Development of a method to configure the manipulation of articulated robots. Using RULA.
[111]	2012	Canada	Use of 8 methods, including RULA, on industrial workers.
[112]	2012	Germany	Use of RULA to assess a humanoid robot arm with human-like postures.
[113]	2011	Turkey	Use of the adapted Nordic Musculoskeletal Questionnaire and RULA on textile workers.
[114]	2011	Indonesia	Use of a virtual space with a human model to ergonomically assess workers in a textile business. One of the methods used was RULA.
[115]	2010	Spain	Applying RULA through a Digital Human Model to assess roof slate manufacturing workers.
[116]	2010	Portugal	Use of RULA on cutlery polishing workers.
[117]	2010	Netherlands	Use of RULA and other tools on mobile phone assembly workers.
[118]	2010	USA	Use of 5 assessment methods, including RULA, on sawmill workers.
[119]	2010	India	Ergonomic assessment with RULA of assembly line workers.
[120]	2008	Canada	Use of various methods, including RULA, on sawmill workers.
[121]	2007	Canada	Use of 5 assessment methods, including RULA, on sawmill workers.
[122]	2007	South Korea	Use of REBA, RULA and OWAS on workers from various industries such as the electronics, steel, chemical and automotive industries.
[123]	2006	Portugal	Using RULA, Surface EMG, a questionnaire, and a clinical examination on paint workers in the automotive industry.
[124]	2004	Germany	Study of the benefits of employing a human digital model in the automotive industry and ergonomic assessment with RULA.
[125]	2004	Iran	Ergonomic analysis with RULA of workers in rug-fixing workshops.
[126]	2003	Spain	Application of RULA on workers in the metallurgical industry
[127]	2003	United Kingdom	Research to establish QEC action categories through the ergonomic assessment of industry workers, simultaneously applying QEC and RULA.

Manufacture of Motor Vehicles, Trailers and Semi-Trailers

The RULA method was used in four research studies to ergonomically assess automotive workers. Each focused on various tasks such as painting, assembly and others. One of the studies used a human digital model, obtaining some benefits from its use [124]. In the others, in addition to the RULA method, other assessment tools were applied. It was concluded that the risk of musculoskeletal disorders existed. Two of them yielded high-level risks [55,75,123]. On the other hand, Mat et al. [63] used RULA to ergonomically assess a car seat. The seat was analysed after being designed with CATIA software and optimisation was performed. This showed a decrease in the level of risk.

Manufacture of Other Non-Metallic Mineral Products

Sain and Meena [56] used RULA, REBA and a questionnaire to perform an ergonomic analysis on brick furnace personnel. They concluded that some tasks needed to be modified as there was a risk of musculoskeletal disorders. Coinciding with this need to take action, Monteil et al. [115] employed RULA via a digital human model on roof slate manufacturing workers.

Manufacture of Fabricated Metal Products, Except Machinery and Equipment

The RULA method was used by Boulila et al. [57] along with REBA and a survey on milling, turning and drilling workers. Twelve postures were determined to negatively influence job performance. In relation to this, other authors redesigned a CNC milling machine to take worker ergonomics into account. They used RULA to analyse the postures assumed in the initial machine and those in the new design, with the latter being less harmful [90].

In addition, two studies found high risk levels according to the RULA method. The first was carried out on workers performing manual handling work in a metal stamping business. The Cornell

Musculoskeletal Discomfort Questionnaire (CMDQ) [96] was also used. The second study focused on cutlery polishing workers [116].

Finally, some authors [126] studied the relationship between ergonomics at work and product quality in the metallurgical industry. RULA was used and, as a result, the work carried out was modified. Quality improvements were identified in the newly-produced products.

Food Product Manufacture

The RULA method was used in conjunction with REBA in the food industry. It was concluded that workers adopted postures that could lead to musculoskeletal disorders [65]. Similar results were obtained by applying RULA together with other assessment tools on pineapple peeling workers, obtaining a risk Level 3 assessment [76]. It was also applied in a sugar factory assessing the bag movement task. A high-risk level was determined [64].

In two other cases, negative results were shown for certain body regions. One of them applied the method to a frozen food business, along with other tools such as the Nordic Questionnaire. This was applied to both production and office workers. The greatest discomfort appeared at the elbow [77]. The other focused on workers in a meat packing factory. RULA, a human body diagram and anthropometric measurements were used. The shoulder was shown to be at risk. It was concluded that corrective measures were required [104].

Other authors used 3D simulation and the I-DEAS programme to replace the work of a robot (used for processing fruits and vegetables) with a worker. RULA and LBA (Lower Back Analysis) were employed for the ergonomic analysis. The results found a particular posture that the seated worker could adopt to avoid a high risk to the lower back and upper limbs [105].

Finally, a study was carried out on baristas tasked with tamping espresso coffee. RULA was used in conjunction with sensors placed on the column and a force plate. Lower scores were shown when using a flat tamper rather than a traditional one [58].

Manufacture of Computer, Electronic and Optical Products

According to RULA, assembly tasks in the electronics industry indicate high levels of risk for the workers who perform them. Two studies demonstrated this, the first applied the RULA method along with a questionnaire while carrying out an intervention to achieve more comfortable postures. The other supplemented it with REBA and the modified Nordic Questionnaire. Both agreed that the body areas most affected by MSD were the lumbar region and the wrists. However, one of them also included the hands and neck while the other included the shoulders [59,60].

Other authors set out to reduce neck discomfort in mobile phone assembly workers. To do this, they performed an ergonomic intervention. An assessment, using the RULA method and other tools, was carried out before and after the intervention. Improved worker ergonomics were achieved following the intervention [106,117].

Something similar was done during the manufacture of laptops. Materials were reused and two carts were created, one for refuse collection and the other for sorting and distributing labels. An assessment was carried out with RULA before and after using the new carts. Better ergonomic and work results were obtained [107].

Manufacture of Other Transport Equipment

The RULA method was used in three studies developed in the same year which looked into aircraft manufacturing. The purpose was to assess worker ergonomics. One of the studies also used the Strain Index demonstrating a relationship among work design, performance and ergonomics [66]. In another, RULA was used in conjunction with REBA to assess aircraft wing component assembly using immersive virtual reality to perform the task [67]. Finally, a maintenance work analysis tool was developed using CATIA software. RULA, OWAS and LBA [68] were employed together.

Manufacture of Machinery and Equipment N.E.C.

In this area, the RULA method was used in a single study. It was concluded that high-risk postures were present in pump assembly workers diving into wells [69].

Manufacture of Leather and Related Products

There has been repeated use of the RULA method for the postural assessment of shoe factory workers. In some studies, it has been combined with the OWAS method and in others with the Nordic Musculoskeletal Questionnaire. In all the cases studied, negative results were obtained for some of the postures adopted [70,78,92].

These conclusions coincided with those obtained in a study on manual shoe-sewing workers. The RULA method was used together with a questionnaire. The need for postural correction was demonstrated; in some cases, it was required immediately [91].

Manufacture of Basic Pharmaceutical Products and Pharmaceutical Preparations

Two studies were developed in the pharmaceutical industry using the RULA method and the Nordic Questionnaire. One concluded that RULA was not a very successful method for assessing this type of industry. The other aimed to assess lumbar and neck discomfort [71,79].

Textile Manufacture

In the textile industry, two research studies were carried out using the RULA method and questionnaires. Approximately 380 workers participated. The results concluded that MSD was common. One of the studies found that the body areas suffering the greatest discomfort were the neck, knees and lumbar region [81,97]. Using the same ergonomic tools, Dianat et al. [87] also established that the neck and back were the body regions most affected in sewing machine workers. They also pointed to other areas such as the shoulders, wrists and hands.

Other authors also employed RULA in the textile industry along with the Nordic Musculoskeletal Questionnaire, or an adaptation of it. They assessed 566 workers in one study and 283 in the other. Both studies concluded that high levels of risk were present in their results and therefore there was a need to take corrective actions, in some cases immediately. They agreed that the affected body areas included the torso, neck and arms, amongst others [108,113].

Other assessments were carried out in industries located in Indonesia and Cambodia. In the first of these, a virtual space with a human model was used and four tasks were analysed: cutting, sewing, putting on buttons and finishing. The Posture Evaluation Index (PEI) was used, which includes the LBA, OWAS and RULA scores. The second was performed using interviews and RULA. In both cases, workers could develop musculoskeletal disorders [83,114].

Analysis was also carried out on people working in rug-fixing workshops. They usually performed their tasks squatting. Using a survey, it was possible to deduce the most affected body regions, and then to design a new work posture from this information. This posture was subsequently assessed with RULA, demonstrating it to be less harmful [125].

Other authors found a way to organise clothing assembly tasks at particular workstations. To do this, they assessed both productivity and ergonomics; RULA was used for the latter [99].

Using the same ergonomic tools, Dianat et al. [80] concluded from the studies described above that there is a high onset rate of musculoskeletal disorders among sewing workers.

Finally, several ergonomic studies have also been carried out in the batik cap industry. One demonstrated the emergence of MSD among the workers, and the other two determined new work postures for specific tasks that were less harmful [82,88,98].

Manufacture of Basic Metals

Garcia-Garcia et al. [95] used RULA and REBA along with virtual simulation to assess workers in a metal factory. Kushwaha and Kane [74] utilised the method to ergonomically assess two crane cabs (the usual one and a new design) in the steel industry. The new cab was designed with CATIA software and was shown to improve worker ergonomics.

Manufacture of Chemicals and Chemical Products

The Nordic Musculoskeletal Symptoms Questionnaire (NMSQ) and the RULA method were used to study ergonomics in chemical industry workers when performing various tasks. RULA showed that they were suffering from MSD. Automation and work modification [73] were proposed as a solution.

Repair and Installation of Machinery and Equipment

The risks that occur during the maintenance of a REHM V8 furnace were analysed using a modification of the NTP 330 method. The ergonomic risks were also contemplated using the RULA method and interviews. It was concluded that the ergonomic risks, amongst others, were detrimental to workers [86].

Manufacture of Electrical Equipment

At a transformer factory in Brazil, worker ergonomics were studied using RULA and a questionnaire. Risk factors were shown to be related to the posture adopted and the work rate. Immediate changes to the tasks [93] were required.

Manufacture of Paper and Paper Products

CATIA P33 V5R14 software was used to recreate the posture adopted by workers in a packaging business. RULA was used for the ergonomic assessment. Certain harmful postures were determined, mainly in tasks where heavy loads were lifted, or tasks which included bending [100].

Manufacture of Rubber and Plastic Products

In total, 25 rubber sheet manufacturing workers were ergonomically assessed using RULA, REBA and OWAS, specifically looking at nine9 different tasks. Most of the postures adopted were repeated continuously and the job was not particularly comfortable for the workers. High scores for these working postures [109] were determined according to the methods applied.

Manufacture of Wood, and Wood and Cork Products, Except Furniture; Manufacture of Articles Made from Wicker and Plaiting Materials

Several research studies were conducted on sawmill workers, using RULA in conjunction with other assessment methods and ergonomic tools. The objective was to compare the results using the different methods to find if there was any agreement among them [118,120,121].

Other

This section includes studies that are also within the scope of industry, but which cannot be included in any of the classification groups used.

Most of these studies were carried out in the past 17 years. The first one performed aimed to establish the QEC method action categories. To do this, several industry jobs were analysed using QEC and RULA, and then the results were compared [127]. RULA was also compared to other methods (OWAS and REBA) by analysing 301 worker postures in industries such as the electronics, steel, chemical and automotive industries, as well as in a hospital. OWAS and REBA ranked 21% of the postures in Categories 3 and 4, while RULA ranked 56% of them [122]. This method was also compared to seven others by performing an ergonomic assessment of 567 industrial tasks. The results were shown to be different for the same work post depending on the method used. RULA determined a high risk for nearly 80% of the jobs [111].

Eswaramoorthi et al. [119] used RULA with CATIA V5 software to assess assembly line workers. This assessment led to changes in job design to reduce or eliminate waste, as these could cause an increase in the heavy physical burden on the worker. The method was also used in another assessment of this type, but in this case on a humanoid robot arm with similar postures to those adopted by a human. The goal was to assess the robot arm's configurations [112]. Related to the above, a method was developed allowing one to configure the manipulation of articulated robots which moved similarly to humans. RULA was used to analyse the coincidence between the robot and the human [110]. Continuing in the field of robotics, one study focused on the design and analysis of a system based on gesture control. The goal was to allow workers to control an industrial-type robot. The RULA [62] method was also used for its design.

Moreover, RULA was combined with other advanced tools to carry out new research. To improve industrial production, an ergonomic study was combined with virtual reality. The design of a cell was carried out to reduce worker fatigue [54]. Conversely, RULA was combined with Kinect to collect information on the movements made by workers during mounting and assembly tasks [72,103]. Likewise, an ergonomic assessment was performed using the DELMIA (Digital Enterprise Manufacturing Interactive Application) simulation tool for assembly tasks in the robotics industry. RULA determined the harmful postures and the necessary redesign of the work to improve them [85]. Finally, a system was developed using sensors placed on the workers' bodies. RULA was used by a computer in real time, displaying the results on a screen. When these were very harmful, acoustic and visual signals were initiated. It was concluded that this system, which showed the information to the worker, reduced the occurrence of MSD [101].

Rivero et al. [89] carried out an assessment of industrial and construction workers using RULA. They explained that increased productivity is closely linked to good worker ergonomics. Other authors also used it in conjunction with OSHA and the NIOSH equation. They concluded that rapid changes were required in 65% of the industrial tasks [84,94].

Baptista et al. [102] conducted three studies with three methods, including RULA. In total, 109 factory workers participated. The results showed that there were workers suffering from MSD, although no indications were presented. Finally, Yazdanirad et al. [61] also used three assessment methods to assess 210 people in three industries (the automotive, pharmaceutical and assembly industries). The results concluded that RULA was the most suitable method.

3.1.4. Water Supply; Sewerage, Waste Management and Remediation Activities

Table 6 presents a single study belonging to this category.

Table 6. Water supply; sewerage, waste management and remediation activities.

Reference	Year	Country	Study Objective
[128]	2015	Turkey	RULA and REBA assessment of workers in waste collection.

Cakit [128] conducted a study to analyse waste collection workers. A programme was used to assess the postures adopted during loading and unloading. In addition, the RULA and REBA methods were used. They concluded the need for urgent changes in the postures adopted.

3.1.5. Construction

Table 7 presents studies conducted in the construction field using RULA.

Table 7. Construction.

Reference	Year	Country	Study Objective
[129]	2019	Canada	Development of a 3D system to simulate the working environment in the construction field. Use of RULA in the ergonomic assessment.
[130]	2018	Canada	Development of a 3D visualisation tool for the construction field. Use of RULA in ergonomic assessment.
[131]	2016	Canada	Development of a new way to measure the angles that form the postures to apply RULA.
[132]	2013	Canada	Assessment with RULA, REBA and the Strain Index on construction workers.

Shanahan et al. [132] analysed the usefulness of three assessment methods (RULA, REBA and the Strain Index) when used in non-fixed tasks and comparing them with four psychophysical scales from Borg 10. Fourteen construction workers without MSD were followed up. They concluded that the best method for this type of task was the Strain Index.

Another study proposed a more accurate way of measuring the angles in the postures adopted by construction workers in order to use the RULA method [131].

Finally, Li et al. [129,130] also focused on the field of construction. They developed a 3D system that allows one to simulate the working environment and perform an ergonomic assessment. They also applied REBA and RULA for the analysis.

3.1.6. Wholesale and Retail Trade; Repair of Motor Vehicles and Motorcycles

In this category, only three studies are presented (Table 8).

Table 8. Wholesale and retail trade; repair of motor vehicles and motorcycles.

Reference	Year	Country	Study Objective
[133]	2014	Malaysia	Assessment using RULA, the modified Nordic Questionnaire and other tools on car repair mechanics.
[134]	2017	Italy	Assessment using RULA, REBA, the Strain Index and OCRA on clothing store vendors.
[135]	2016	Italy	Development of a portable and wireless tool based on the RULA method and the Strain Index for postural assessment.

Wholesale and Retail Trade and Repair of Motor Vehicle and Motorcycles

Risk factors and the onset of MSD were studied in car repair mechanics. In total, 191 workers participated. The modified Nordic Questionnaire was used with RULA, in addition to other tools. Most workers were shown to have this type of disorder [133].

Retail Trade, Except Motor Vehicles and Motorcycles

Capodaglio [134] conducted an ergonomic study on 70 clothing store vendors. RULA, REBA, the Strain Index and OCRA were used. The results showed a high risk in the upper extremities for the postures adopted. Another study was carried out at supermarket check-outs. A tool was developed to carry out a postural assessment of the workers. It was a portable and wireless system based on RULA and the Strain Index. It allowed the assessment to be performed as the task was being undertaken [135].

3.1.7. Transportation and Storage

Table 9 contains the studies available in the Transportation and Storage category.

Table 9. Transportation and storage.

Reference	Year	Country	Study Objective
[136]	2018	Brazil	Assessment with RULA and a survey on dangerous goods drivers.
[137]	2017	France	Application of RULA and measurement of angles with sensors in material handling workers.
[138]	2017	China	Development of a new method based on the RULA method.
[139]	2016	Iran	Development of a new nozzle for fuel hoses and assessment with RULA of the people who used it.
[140]	2016	India	Assessment with RULA, REBA and other tools on industrial vehicle drivers.
[141]	2016	Cambodia	Assessment of the use of a new tool using RULA for storage in supermarkets.
[142]	2015	Saudi Arabia	Application of RULA and other tools on supermarket warehouse workers.
[143]	2012	Venezuela	Assessment with RULA and OCRA of workers of a transport company.
[144]	2012	USA	Assessment with RULA, REBA, PLIBEL and iLMM of bus drivers responsible for handling wheelchairs.
[145]	2008	Slovenia	Application of goniometry and OWAS, RULA and CORLETT on car drivers.
[146]	2005	United Kingdom	RULA and OWAS were applied in addition to other tools on forklift drivers.
[147]	2003	Italy	RULA assessment of garbage truck and road cleaning drivers.

Land Transport and Transport via Pipelines

The RULA method was used in various studies to analyse drivers of different vehicles, such as garbage trucks and road-cleaning trucks. In total, 77 workers participated. The study concluded that the neck was the most affected area. The scores obtained varied depending on whether an adjustable seat was used [147]. Drivers of dangerous goods vehicles also suffered discomfort in the neck region, as well as in the feet, ankles, hands, etc. According to RULA, immediate changes to the tasks were required [136]. Similarly, car drivers were assessed, but this time RULA was used along with other methods such as OWAS and CORLETT. Goniometry was applied on some workers. The results showed different levels of discomfort in various parts of the body [145]. The method was used together with OCRA to assess workers in five transport company posts. In addition, a group interview was carried out. RULA demonstrated action Levels 1 and 2 [143].

Hoy et al. [146] studied the vibrations and postures to which forklift drivers were exposed. RULA, OWAS and a questionnaire were applied, and the vibrations were measured. The posture test results showed frequent lumbar discomfort. The highest risk level postures were those comprising a bent or twisted torso.

Another such study focused on wheelchair-support bus drivers. The assessment involved four workers and one passenger. Three different wheelchairs were used. The RULA, REBA, PLIBEL and iLMM methods were employed. High-level risks were determined during this task [144].

Balaji and Alphin [140] focused on drivers of industrial vehicles. Their objective was to optimise the worker's area in the vehicle in order to reduce discomfort from the postures adopted. The software analysis was performed using RULA and REBA. Nearly half of the workers performed the task at a high-risk level. The areas most affected were the arm, wrist and torso.

Lastly, a new type of nozzle was developed for fuel refilling hoses. One hundred people were assessed using RULA while putting fuel in their vehicles. The postures were shown to be less harmful with the new design [139].

Warehousing and Support Activities for Transportation

In total, 92 workers from a supermarket warehouse were ergonomically assessed, specifically in two tasks—lifting boxes and pulling them. RULA was used in conjunction with other tools. Lifting the boxes affected the workers' lower back, while the other task affected the lower arm and wrist [142]. Using the same method in the same workplace, they assessed the effect caused by a new storage tool. They concluded that it allowed for better work completion and resulted in less back and shoulder risks [141].

Finally, material handling workers were assessed. Sensors capable of measuring angles during a work task were used and, from these data, RULA was applied. The results showed high levels of risk in the postures adopted [137].

Air Transport

Some authors performed a study in which a new RULA method was developed. This allowed astronauts to be posturally assessed [138].

3.1.8. Accommodation and Food Service Activities

Three studies are differentiated in this field of knowledge (Table 10).

Table 10. Accommodation and food service activities.

Reference	Year	Country	Study Objective
[148]	2018	Brazil	Use of a survey and REBA, RULA and OWAS methods in industrial kitchen workers.
[149]	2014	China	Application of OWAS, RULA and the NIOSH equation in cooks at a Chinese restaurant.
[150]	2005	Canada	Use of 4 ergonomic tools, including RULA in pub workers.

Workers in an industrial kitchen, chefs at a Chinese restaurant and pub workers were assessed. RULA was used in all of these along with other ergonomic methods or tools. In the first case, RULA obtained more harmful results than for the other methods applied. The second showed that repetitive actions were performed on the upper extremities. The third concluded that very harmful tasks existed that required corrective actions [148–150].

3.1.9. Information and Communication

Table 11 is composed of the different studies that have been carried out in the area of Information and Communication.

Table 11. Information and communication.

Reference	Year	Country	Study Objective
[151]	2019	Turkey	Testing using RULA and other tools of the effectiveness of ergonomic training to people who make regular use of the computer.
[152]	2014	Israel	Application of the RULA method and a modification of it (mRULA) in computer workers, to check if mRULA was valid.
[153]	2012	Iran	Testing using RULA of whether there was an improvement or not in the ergonomic results in VDT workers after training.
[154]	2009	USA	Application of RULA to know the results of an ergonomic intervention in a worker who used the computer.
[155]	2005	Israel	Application of a questionnaire and RULA on workers of a technology company.
[156]	2003	United Kingdom	Use of RULA in workers who used the computer and were visually impaired.
[157]	2002	Turkey	The benefits of ergonomic training and physiotherapy sessions in VDT operators were studied. Use of RULA and other tools.
[158]	1999	USA	Use of RULA in workers who entered data with VDT screens and others that classified and sorted documents.
[159]	1998	Australia	Application of RULA and surface electromyography on computer workers.

Several studies have been carried out on people who work regularly on a computer. One of these studies investigated whether the position where the mouse was placed with respect to the keyboard influenced the arm and shoulder postures adopted. RULA and surface electromyography were used. Some results showed that the position taken by right-handed people was less damaging if the number keyboard was not used [159]. Another similar analysis was performed on 10 workers who were also visually impaired. Harmful postures were identified for all the participants, and several recommendations [156] were made. Ekinci et al. [151] carried out an assessment very similar to the previous cases, using other tools in addition to RULA. The objective was to check the effectiveness of pre-use ergonomic computer training. Ergonomic risk was shown to decrease as a result. One of the workers carrying out this same task was followed up. They indicated discomfort in the neck and upper right extremity. They received physiotherapy sessions and ergonomic intervention, after which RULA indicated an improvement in the results [154].

Other authors used RULA [158] to assess workers carrying out two specific tasks, one based on entering data using VDT (Visual Display Terminal) screens and another on document classification and sorting. The results showed that the first task required further assessment. The second had to be modified after identifying harmful postures. Another group of VDT workers had the ergonomic training they received assessed using the method. The results improved after this, reducing the action levels [153]. To this end, RULA was used in conjunction with the Visual Analog Scale (VAS) to test the benefits of ergonomic training and physiotherapy sessions. VDT operators from the Software Corporation participated. It was observed that the methods were beneficial as they decreased the risk factors and the development of musculoskeletal disorders [157].

Other authors ergonomically assessed workers at a technology company, focusing on programming, management, administration and marketing tasks. RULA deduced high action levels with no risk-free postures [155]. Lastly in this area, the RULA method was applied, along with a modified version of it (mRULA), on 29 people working in computer science. The goal was to know if mRULA was valid for ergonomic assessment. They concluded that it could be used, and that it was only necessary to make an observation [152].

3.1.10. Financial and Insurance Activities

Table 12 encompasses a single research study.

Table 12. Financial and insurance activities.

Reference	Year	Country	Study Objective
[160]	2012	Brazil	Application of the RULA method on workers in the financial department of a hospital.

An ergonomic study was carried out in the financial department of a hospital using the RULA method. The results showed the need for ergonomic actions. This could reduce the grounds for absenteeism due to work-related accidents and increase well-being at work [160].

3.1.11. Professional, Scientific and Technical Activities

Publications relating to this category are presented below (Table 13).

Table 13. Professional, scientific and technical activities.

Reference	Year	Country	Study Objective
[161]	2016	Spain	Application of OWAS and other tools to evaluate veterinarians.
[162]	2008	China	Ergonomic analysis using software based on the RULA method of people who perform their work on desktops.

Other Professional, Scientific and Technical Activities

A study was carried out to establish a procedure for product design managers to perform an ergonomic assessment at the start of the design. This was developed for work carried out on desktops. To this end, information on the movement of workers was collected and a digital human model was created. Software incorporating the RULA method was used to perform the ergonomic analysis [162].

Veterinary Activities

The work of 12 veterinarians was assessed while performing four different tasks. Several tools were used, including a modification of RULA, to assess the wrist. It was concluded that, of the four tasks, only the posture adopted for suturing was not detrimental to the wrist [161].

3.1.12. Administrative and Support Service Activities

In this field of knowledge, 12 studies have been analysed (Table 14).

Table 14. Administrative and support service activities.

Reference	Year	Country	Study Objective
[163]	2019	Iran	Assessment of the benefits of an ergonomic programme performed on office workers in a petrochemical company using a questionnaire and RULA.
[164]	2017	Netherlands	To verify an upper extremity assessment questionnaire, with the help of RULA.
[165]	2017	Brazil	Application of ROSA, RULA and the Maastricht questionnaire to assess office workers.
[166]	2016	Philippines	Use of the Standardized Nordic Questionnaire, and the RULA and REBA methods on cleaning workers.
[167]	2015	USA	Application of RULA and a lighting study on office workers.
[168]	2015	USA	RULA was applied, among other tools, to office workers who used a computer.
[169]	2015	Brazil	RULA, along with other methods and questionnaires, was applied to office workers.
[170]	2014	Portugal	RULA was applied to administrative workers.
[171]	2014	Turkey	The effectiveness of web ergonomic training for office workers was assessed. The RULA method and surveys were used.
[172]	2012	Australia	Use of ManTRA, QEC and RULA on cleaning workers.
[173]	2012	Israel	Application of RULA on office workers who use computers in order to assess the usefulness of a training method.
[174]	2011	Portugal	The RULA method was applied to office workers.

Building Services and Landscape Activities

Two studies were carried out on cleaning workers using the RULA method. The first was used in conjunction with the REBA method and the Standardized Nordic Questionnaire. The results indicated risks ranging from medium to very high [166]. The second also made use of the Manual Task Risk Assessment (ManTRA) and QEC and the cleaning task was assessed. The results showed that the staff developed musculoskeletal disorders [172].

Office Administration, Office Support and Other Business Support Activities

Several research studies were conducted on the risks of MSD for office workers. One of these focused on computer staff. The workers were divided into two groups, one of which contained workers already suffering from discomfort. The ROSA (Rapid Office Strain Assessment), RULA and Maastricht questionnaire methods were used. RULA indicated worse scores for workers suffering discomfort [165]. Two similar studies were performed (one of which was determined with RULA) showing that more than half the workers suffered from musculoskeletal disorders and that the most injured areas of the body were the back and upper limbs. The other study proposed corrective actions for the work carried out [169,174]. Administrative workers were ergonomically studied in the same way. In addition to using RULA, measurements were taken of the workers and the office furniture. The study concluded that the subjects were developing MSD. Corrective actions were necessary over the short term [170].

Two further studies were carried out with RULA using an intervention group and a control group. In one of them, two groups were created containing 100 workers, and lighting data and information were collected. It was determined that the use of adjustable lights improved both the ergonomics and vision while the tasks were carried out [167]. In the other study, the intervention group used a particular keyboard, mouse and touchscreen. RULA showed a decrease in harmful upper limb postures although this worsened for the hands [168].

Several works were also carried out, the objective of which was to assess ergonomic programmes. One of them was performed in Iran on office workers in a petrochemical business. A questionnaire and the RULA method were used for the assessment. Improvements were made to the postures affecting the neck, shoulders, upper back and lumbar area thanks to the ergonomic programme [163]. With the same purpose in mind, Taieb-Maimon et al. [173] assessed three groups of workers who used computers in offices, one the control group and two that had received different types of training. Workers were assessed with RULA before, during and after the training. It was observed that the two groups with training improved their postures in a short period of time. Dalkilinc and Kayihan [171] also demonstrated that ergonomic training improved the postures adopted by office workers; they used RULA and surveys. In this case, it was web training.

Finally, in this field of knowledge, Cavalini et al. [164] verified an upper extremity assessment questionnaire called the Upper Extremity Work Demand (UEWD-R). The assessment was carried out using RULA with the help of office workers who used computers. The results indicated that the questionnaire was valid for assessing postural load on upper extremities.

3.1.13. Public Administration and Defence; Compulsory Social Security

Table 15 presents the research developed in this field.

Table 15. Public administration and defence; compulsory social security.

Reference	Year	Country	Study Objective
[175]	2017	South Korea	Application of OWAS, RULA and REBA on soldiers.
[176]	2010	USA	Application of REBA, RULA and the NIOSH equation on firefighters and emergency physicians.

Nam et al. [175] assessed the postural load on soldiers when cleaning cannons in two different ways: manually and with an automated tool. OWAS, RULA and REBA were applied. They concluded that there was a lower risk (Level 2) when using the tool than with manual cleaning (Level 4). Another assessment of this type was developed for firefighters and emergency physicians. RULA, REBA and the NIOSH equation were used. The results showed high risks, indicating the need for corrective action [176].

3.1.14. Education

Table 16 consists of 12 studies developed in education.

Table 16. Education.

Reference	Year	Country	Study Objective
[177]	2018	South Africa	Use of RULA and a questionnaire on students using the computer.
[178]	2018	Philippines	Application of RULA and REBA on students in a chemistry laboratory.
[179]	2015	South Africa	Use of RULA and VAS to assess ergonomic training carried out with school students who used a computer.
[180]	2014	Australia	Ergonomic assessment with RULA of children using ICT (Information and Communications Technology) to ascertain if the assessor's experience is relevant in this method.
[181]	2014	Iran	Use of the Nordic Musculoskeletal Questionnaire, the RULA method and other methods as well as interviews on people who used computers at two universities.
[182]	2014	Malaysia	The use of RULA and other tools on elementary school students.
[183]	2012	Iran	Assessing a training programme using RULA and other tools on university workers using computers.
[184]	2012	Malaysia	Application of a questionnaire, REBA and RULA on students between 13 and 15 years old.
[185]	2011	Indonesia	Use of a virtual environment for ergonomic analysis of a bicycle. PEI was used, containing methods such as RULA.
[186]	2009	USA	Application of the modified RULA method and the University of California Computer Use Checklist on university students using computers.
[187]	2009	Ireland	The RULA method and other tools were used on high school students using computers.
[188]	2007	Ireland	Application of RULA, the body discomfort chart and VAS on school children using computers.

Breen et al. [188] and Kelly et al. [187] used RULA and other tools to study the postures adopted by students on the computer. Some authors focused on primary schools and others on high schools. They concluded that about 60% of the postures belonged to action Level 2. Sellschop et al. [177,179] provided ergonomic training to students with the same characteristics. They assessed effectiveness using two groups (the intervention and control groups) with the same method and other tools. In the intervention group, the risk decreased according to RULA, with action Level 4 disappearing. Other authors found that the assessor's experience of using RULA and task observation was not relevant. They demonstrated this by assessing children while they took part in ICT. The study was performed by two groups of assessors, one of them experienced in applying the method [180].

Some authors [181,186] ergonomically analysed students at the university level, also while using computers. Two studies are differentiated, one using the RULA method and the other a modification of it (mRULA) in addition to other tools. It was shown that, at an engineering university, 30.8% of participants were exposed to a Level 3 risk. In medicine, 42.9% were exposed to a Level 2 risk. On the other hand, when employed at the Qazyin University of Medical Sciences on workers using the computer, it was intended to assess a training programme. This was done in stages, through a control group and an intervention group. RULA, VAS and the Nordic Questionnaire were used. The intervention group improved. The programme proved beneficial to the workers [183].

Furthermore, in the field of education, other ergonomic analyses were carried out using RULA and other tools. They focused on students at different levels. In some cases, harmful postures were adopted due to, among other causes, the furniture used. New furniture designs were required [178,182]. Students aged between 13 and 15 were also assessed in a total of 104 positions. It was concluded that the 13-year-olds were more at risk [184].

Finally, other authors used a virtual environment to perform an ergonomic analysis on a folding bike. This was designed at the University of Indonesia. RULA was used along with other methods. The goal was to obtain the best design, which was completed when the handlebars were 32 cm high and the saddle at 83 cm [185].

3.1.15. Human Health and Social Work Activities

Table 17 presents the studies according to the "Human health and social work activities" category.

Table 17. Human health and social work activities.

Reference	Year	Country	Study Objective
[189]	2019	Canada	To check the usefulness of a training course for ophthalmologists on the placement of a slit lamp, using RULA.
[190]	2019	Netherlands	Use of RULA, among other tools, on operating room nurses using the da Vinci robot.
[191]	2019	Iran	Assessment using RULA of workers performing a task in a traditional way and with a newly designed instrument.
[192]	2018	USA	Application of RULA on otolaryngologists.
[193]	2018	Ireland	Use of RULA and other tools on ICU nurses.
[194]	2018	United Kingdom	Use of RULA and statistical analysis on dental students.
[195]	2018	Netherlands	To check if it was effective to give ergonomic training to surgical personnel in using robots, performed with RULA and other tools.
[196]	2017	United Kingdom	Ergonomic assessment with RULA on plastic surgeons who used magnifying glasses.
[197]	2017	India	Postural assessment of surgeons during a laparoscopic operation.
[198]	2017	Italy	Use of RULA and another method on dentists while carrying out an operation.
[199]	2017	USA	The RULA method was used to assess postures adopted by otolaryngologists.
[200]	2016	USA	Ergonomic assessment (including the RULA method) on gynaecology surgeons using 4 different chairs and several tools.
[201]	2016	France	Use of RULA together with a tool to assess the use of a new instrument designed for use by surgeons.
[202]	2016	United Kingdom	Study on the methods used, such as RULA, to analyse ergonomics in health-related jobs.
[203]	2016	Iran	Ergonomic assessment of dental students using RULA and a questionnaire.
[204]	2016	Portugal	Ergonomic study of workers in a hospital laboratory, using RULA.
[205]	2016	Brazil	Ergonomic assessment using 3 methods, including RULA, of emergency pharmacy workers.
[206]	2015	South Korea	Application of RULA and QEC on dentists.
[207]	2015	Turkey	Use of a form and RULA on intensive care nurses.
[208]	2015	Iran	Use of the RULA method and other tools on dentists.
[209]	2015	Poland	Integration of different ergonomic methods or tools, such as RULA, in nursing and surgery workers.
[210]	2015	Iran	Use of a questionnaire, RULA and the Nordic Musculoskeletal Questionnaire on dentists.
[211]	2014	Brazil	Use of RULA to assess upper limb postures in dental students.
[212]	2014	India	Use of RULA and other ergonomic tools on laboratory technicians.
[213]	2014	USA	Ergonomic study using RULA on workers performing ultrasounds.
[214]	2013	Brazil	Use of OWAS and RULA on students in the last year of dental studies.

Table 17. Cont.

Reference	Year	Country	Study Objective
[215]	2013	USA	Ergonomic study using RULA and other ergonomic tools on surgeons manipulating a robot.
[216]	2013	South Korea	Use of REBA, RULA and the Strain Index on dental hygienists.
[217]	2012	USA	Ergonomic analysis using RULA, amongst other tools, on office-based surgery workers.
[218]	2011	USA	Using a virtual reality simulator on surgeons performing a laparoscopic cholecystectomy. Ergonomic assessment with RULA.
[219]	2011	Taiwan	RULA assessment of one of the tasks performed during blood tests.
[220]	2010	USA	Application of RULA and three-dimensional imaging on surgeons who perform laryngeal microsurgery.
[221]	2010	Spain	Data collection using CyberGlove (R) and assessment using an adapted RULA method.
[222]	2008	United Kingdom	Application of the RULA method on mammogram radiologists.
[223]	2007	United Kingdom	Ergonomic assessment using RULA on dental students using two different armchairs.
[224]	2005	USA	Use of the Job Strain Index and RULA to assess surgeons performing an endoscopy manually and with the help of a robot.
[225]	2001	Canada	Use of an optoelectronic system to collect posture data on surgeons, and then assessing them with a modified RULA.
[226]	2000	Ireland	Ergonomic intervention in biomedical workers. RULA was used in the ergonomic assessment, among others.

This field is divided into different specialties to show the available studies in a more ordered fashion.

- Ophthalmology

Ratzlaff et al. [189] tested the usefulness of an ergonomic training course given to 10 ophthalmologists. They focused on a task that consisted of positioning a slit lamp. It was assessed before and after training, using RULA applied with software. Risk levels were shown to be lower after training.

- Radiology

In the United Kingdom, mammogram radiologists were ergonomically assessed. Three work posts were analysed, one for digital mammograms, one for film mammograms and the third for both. The RULA method was used. It was determined that no more MSDs developed as a result of performing the mammograms digitally [222].

- Nursing

Sezgin and Esin [207] evaluated 1,515 intensive care nurses. They mainly used the RULA method. They showed that the hardest-hit areas of the body were the back and legs. They also concluded that the scores for this method were lowered by giving the Ergonomic Risk Management Programme (ERMP) to workers [193].

Sung et al. [219] decided to use an armrest and mirror to observe the tubes after each blood test. These proposals reduced the RULA score from 7 to 2. Therefore, the postures of the workers improved, mainly in the neck and shoulders.

As a last study, Garosi et al. [191] designed and developed a new instrument for a nursing task that used to be done manually. According to RULA, the level of risk decreased from 3 to 2 in the upper extremities when using this new tool.

- Otolaryngology

Goyil et al. [192,199] analysed the postures adopted by the otolaryngologists when the patient was placed in position (sitting or lying on their back). The RULA method was used. Higher risk levels were determined for sitting patients.

- Ultrasounds

Workers performing ultrasounds were assessed because they often suffer from musculoskeletal discomfort. RULA was used on five participants and on 24 ultrasounds; other parameters were also taken into account. The results showed awkward postures for the upper limbs [213].

- Laboratory

Some authors found that lab workers in hospitals developed MSD from performing their tasks. In these studies, they applied RULA, sometimes with other methods or tools [204,212].

- Surgery

The use of robots in surgery does not always lead to correct postures in the workers. Several authors assessed surgical personnel during their work using RULA and other tools. They found detrimental results and the need to modify the tasks [190,215]. One solution could be to provide ergonomic training to workers who perform surgery with robots. According to RULA, this improved the levels of risk [195]. The use of robot in other cases led to ergonomic improvements. One of these was when performing endoscopies. Surgeons obtained lower RULA scores when using robots than when performing the operation manually [224].

Other authors focused their studies (using the RULA method) on surgeons performing laparoscopies. They showed that there was a risk regarding the postures the surgeons developed [197]. In some cases, they combined these studies with the use of new technologies. For example, Youssed et al. [218] used a virtual reality simulator in this type of study, whereas Sanchez-Margallo et al. [221] used a glove called a CyberGlove (R). This glove allowed one to measure the movements made by the wrist, which can then be applied to an adapted RULA method. Bensignor et al. [201] designed a robotic needle holder for this type of surgery. Using RULA, they demonstrated that surgeon's postures were less harmful than when performing the technique in the traditional way.

Other ergonomic analyses were performed on surgeons carrying out various tasks. Li et al. [196] used RULA to assess plastic surgeons who used magnifying glasses, and who suffered discomfort in the upper extremities. They indicated that modifying the height of the table or the distance of the magnifying glass from the workplace could lessen these problems. Person et al. [225] used an optoelectronic system to take posture data and obtain results using a modified RULA. They found harmful results mainly at the wrist. Hermandon and Choi [217] agreed that the wrist was one of the hardest-hit areas. They used RULA and other tools on office-based surgery (OBS) workers. They concluded that these workers were at high risk of musculoskeletal disorders. In addition, they highlighted other areas of the body that were harmed such as the arms, shoulder, neck and back.

Other authors assessed surgeons' postures using RULA when they performed the same procedure in different ways. For example, Statham et al. [220] focused on laryngeal microsurgery surgeons. They assessed them while performing the task adopting three different postures, one with the arms unsupported and the other two with different supports. They deduced the levels of risk to which the surgeons were exposed. Singh et al. [200] assessed gynaecology surgeons using four different chairs. They determined a medium-to-high risk in the neck and shoulders. They showed that the chairs did not influence the scores.

Finally, some authors presented the idea of integrating different ergonomic methods and tools to assess nursing and surgery workers. OWAS, REBA, RULA and NIOSH were used, amongst other methods [209].

- Dentistry

Several authors focused on ergonomically assessing dental students while they were doing their internships. This was done using RULA, sometimes together with other methods or questionnaires. They concluded that there was a high level of risk regarding musculoskeletal disorders [203,211,214]. Ergonomic improvements in this area showed that using a Bambach Saddle armchair resulted in lower risk than when using a conventional chair [223], and that using magnifying glasses was beneficial for adopting lower-risk postures [194].

This type of study was also conducted on dentists to assess their postures. RULA was used in conjunction with other methods in most cases. Marcon et al. [198] compared the difference between using a magnifying glass, a microscope or not using anything at all during operations. They showed that using a microscope led to more harmful postures. In addition, these dentists are usually harmed by the postures they adopt during their tasks. Therefore, it is necessary to establish changes, some of which are required immediately. The most affected parts of the body are the lumbar region and neck [206]. This coincides with that determined by Tirgar et al. [208], although they added that another area affected was the shoulders, as inferred by Rafie et al. [210].

To conclude this group, the ergonomics of dental hygienists were also studied. They used RULA, REBA and the Strain Index. It was concluded that the postures the hygienists adopted contributed to the onset of musculoskeletal disorders [216].

- Other

An ergonomic assessment of workers in an emergency pharmacy was carried out using three methods, including RULA. This led to some improvements in their work [205]. Another series of improvements was made for women workers in the biomedical field. An intervention was carried out based on changes to the workplace and recommendations. According to RULA, this was beneficial as it led to lower scores for more than half of the postures [226]. Finally, methods for analysing ergonomics in health-related jobs were studied. It was concluded that RULA could be used to attain more accurate results [202].

3.1.16. Arts, Entertainment and Recreation

Table 18 includes only three studies.

Table 18. Arts, entertainment and recreation.

Reference	Year	Country	Study Objective
[227]	2013	India	The modified Nordic Questionnaire, REBA and RULA were applied to potters and sculptors.
[228]	2011	Israel	RULA and questionnaires were used on orchestral musicians.
[229]	2010	India	RULA, REBA, OVAKO, OCRA and the Strain Index were applied to craft workers.

In the field of music, some authors demonstrated, with RULA and other tools, that musicians often suffer MSD mainly in the upper extremities. The risk is higher in those who play string instruments [228]. The development of such disorders was also confirmed in potters, sculptors and craft workers in India. They made use of RULA and other assessment methods. For all cases, harmful postures were deduced as well as the need to make changes to avoid them, immediately for the crafts workers [227,229].

3.1.17. Other Service Activities

Only three studies are presented in this category as well (Table 19).

Table 19. Other service activities.

Reference	Year	Country	Study Objective
[230]	2017	USA	Use of a survey and the RULA method on tattocists.
[231]	2015	India	REBA, RULA and OCRA were used on bicycle repair workers.
[232]	2011	Portugal	An ergonomic study using RULA and QEC was conducted on workers from four spas.

Repair of Computers, and Personal and Household Goods

An ergonomic assessment was carried out on bicycle repair workers. The RULA, REBA and OCRA methods were used, along with other parameter measurement. The tasks assessed were shown to be at a high-risk level, and that immediate improvement actions were required [231].

Other Personal Service Activities

Some authors focused on spa workers, with the aim of preventing them from developing MSD during three of their tasks. An assessment was carried out with RULA and QEC. The results showed that ergonomic information and training would improve the postures adopted [232]. A similar study, using only RULA and a survey, was conducted on tattooists. It was concluded that 71% of the postures adopted had a high level of risk and therefore urgent corrective measures were needed [230].

3.1.18. Activities of Households as Employers; Undifferentiated Goods- and Services-Producing Activities of Households for Own Use

Table 20 summarises the publications in this category.

Table 20. Activities of households as employers; undifferentiated goods-and services-producing activities of households for own use.

Reference	Year	Country	Study Objective
[233]	2016	Ecuador	Assessment of people in wheelchairs who performed some domestic or work activity, using the RULA method and MAPFRE.
[234]	2012	Italy	5 ergonomic methods or tools were used, including RULA, on people performing household chores.

Domestic workers are also exposed to the onset of musculoskeletal disorders, although, according to Apostoli et al. [234], at a medium or low level. This was deduced by research in which RULA and other assessment methods or tools were applied. Another similar study was carried out using the RULA and MAPFRE methods, but in this case the workers were in wheelchairs. It was inferred that there were risks caused by the postures that had to be adopted in the chair in order to carry out the tasks [233].

3.1.19. Other Areas Not Previously Included

Finally, a category (Table 21) is presented that is not covered by the classification used but has applications that cannot be included in the above fields of knowledge.

Table 21. Other scopes not previously included.

Reference	Year	Country	Study Objective
[235]	2019	Ecuador	New way to perform ergonomic analysis using the Kinect V2 sensor together with the RULA method.
[236]	2018	Brazil	RULA and the deformation rate (SI) were studied, and the analysis of various jobs was carried out.
[237]	2018	Malaysia	Conducting a study to assess the utility of the RULA-Kinect (TM) system.
[238]	2018	Malaysia	Research to compare the RULA method with the RULA-Kinect system.
[239]	2018	Thailand	Ergonomic study using a questionnaire and the RULA method on people who use mobile phones.
[240]	2017	France	A study using Kinect with the RULA method.
[241]	2017	Turkey	Development of the ARULA (Advanced RULA) method, which improves the advantages of RULA.
[242]	2017	Italy	Development of a software called K2RULA.
[243]	2017	South Korea	Use of RULA in conjunction with Quick Rating (QRating) to assess people making gestures while communicating.
[244]	2016	Australia	Using sensors, including Kinect for the RULA application.
[245]	2015	Sweden	Ergonomic assessment with RULA on children while they are using ICT devices.
[246]	2015	France	Development of a method for performing ergonomic assessments using a virtual mannequin and RULA scores.
[247]	2015	Iran	RULA employed on box office sales workers.
[248]	2014	Japan	Study of the relationship between upper limb discomfort and each degree of freedom. Using RULA.
[249]	2014	Taiwan	Use of RULA on workers at a gas bottle company.
[250]	2013	South Korea	Attempt to adopt gestures for virtual environment commands. RULA was used in the analysis.
[251]	2012	Ireland	Employing RULA on children who are computer users.
[252]	2011	Germany	Adapts the RULA method with Virtual Human to control human movements.
[253]	2011	Portugal	Development of a semi-automatic system with two video cameras and RULA.
[254]	2011	Portugal	Application of RULA and OCRA on workers using machines and other equipment.
[255]	2010	Portugal	Development of a semi-automatic system for ergonomic assessment using RULA and two synchronised cameras.
[256]	2009	Italy	Assessment performed with several methods, including RULA.
[257]	2008	United Kingdom	Study of two biometric-type devices. RULA was used.
[258]	2007	USA	Influence of orientation and placement of tool handles on gripping force. RULA was used.
[259]	2007	USA	Two methods were developed and a modified RULA method was also used.

The different studies available are divided into groups according to the topic covered:

- Sensors

The Kinect sensor has been used in several studies together with the RULA method for ergonomic analysis. Some of them have compared the results by performing the assessment without the sensor and were similar. With Kinect, you can reduce the assessment time or subjectivity with professional analysis [235,244].

- Use of mobile phones and computers

Some authors assessed people who sent SMS using their mobile phones. They used a questionnaire and the RULA method. The latter exposed a risk Level 3 for the right and left area of the body, so modifications [239] were required. Employing the same method, other authors assessed the postures of children using computers or other ICT devices. They deduced risk categories of Level 2 or higher for the latter. In the case of computers, it was inferred that the RULA method was not recommended for applying to girls under eight years of age [245,251].

- Methods

Can and Figlali [241] developed a new assessment method from RULA, called ARULA (Advanced RULA). This was characterised as improving the advantages of the initial method, such as its high pre-observation time, assessment, etc.

One assessment was carried out using various methods such as the State of Washington method, OCRA, RULA, the Strain Index, etc. A high or very high level of risk for the upper limbs [256] was obtained with all. Two of the above methods, the Strain Index and RULA, were also studied from the perspective of validity, reliability, etc. The analysis of various jobs that included static positions or repetitive tasks was carried out, concluding that training was necessary to apply the [236] methods. Finally, a study was conducted on perceived discomfort in the different postures of the upper extremities. The RULA method [248] was used.

- Technological Evolution

Technology was used to apply the RULA method in several studies. Manghisi et al. [242] developed software called K2RULA capable of assessing workers during the task or with subsequent analysis. Goncalves and Fernandes [253,255] developed a semi-automatic system for performing ergonomic assessments using the RULA method. It was based on two synchronised video recording cameras for observing the worker's tasks. From these recordings, RULA automatically calculated the scores, obtaining the action level for each of the observations. Plantard et al. [246] developed a method for performing ergonomic assessments using a virtual mannequin and RULA scores. They noted that the results of this new method coincided with those that had actually been obtained. Finally, Schlette and Rossmann [252] adapted the RULA method with Virtual Human in order to control human movements. The goal was to control the movements of a humanoid robot that are similar to those performed by a human.

- Gestures

One study used RULA in conjunction with another method called Quick Rating (QRating) to ergonomically assess people who made typical gestures when communicating. Physical discomfort during these gestures should be controlled [243].

In another study, gestures were required for 18 commands used in the movement of objects in a virtual environment. To do this, they were determined using Korean sign language and others created by the user. All these gestures were analysed and the RULA method [250] was used for this purpose.

- Other works

Razavi and Behbudi [247] ergonomically analysed box office workers with the RULA method, following the adoption of a series of improvements. It was concluded that there was a reduced level of risk. The same type of study was carried out on workers at a gas bottle company. It determined the existence of postures with an action Level 3 risk, and the need for changes in a short period of time [249]. It was also carried out on workers who used machines and other equipment during their work. Anthropometric information and the OCRA method were also used [254].

On the other hand, Ward et al. [257] used RULA to assess the ergonomics of postures adopted in the use of biometric devices (fingerprints and veins on the palm of the hand). They concluded that the positions in which they were placed (angles and heights) influenced the postures adopted. McGorry and Lin [258] studied the influence on grip strength of the orientation and placement (height and distance) of tool handles. They used RULA to carry out an ergonomic assessment.

Finally, several authors developed two assessment methods, one that considered frequent and harmful postures and the other the time. An assessment was made, using these methods and a modified RULA method, of the postures adopted by a group of people. They deduced that there was no coincidence between the methods [259].

3.2. Country-by-Country Ranking

The revised applications are also classified according to their location, taking into account the fields of knowledge (Figure 5).

There are 34 countries where the RULA method has been used. The USA stands out with 23 studies, followed by Iran with 21, Malaysia with 17, India with 16, Portugal with 15, Brazil with 12 and Canada and the United Kingdom with 11. All other countries have 10 or fewer research studies. Eight locations have a single publication: Saudi Arabia, Japan, Mexico, Poland, Slovenia, Sweden, Tunisia and Venezuela (Figure 5).

In addition to the USA having the largest number of studies, it is also the country where the most knowledge categories have been covered. This comprises a total of 10 areas. "Human health and social work activities" stand out with nine studies, followed by "Manufacturing" with three (Figure 5). Both categories match the ones that have the most published studies at the general level (Figure 4 and Table 2).

The places following the USA are Turkey, Italy, Iran, India and Brazil, with seven different locations. In all of them, except Italy, the largest number of publications also corresponds to "Manufacturing". Iran stands out with 11 studies in this category.

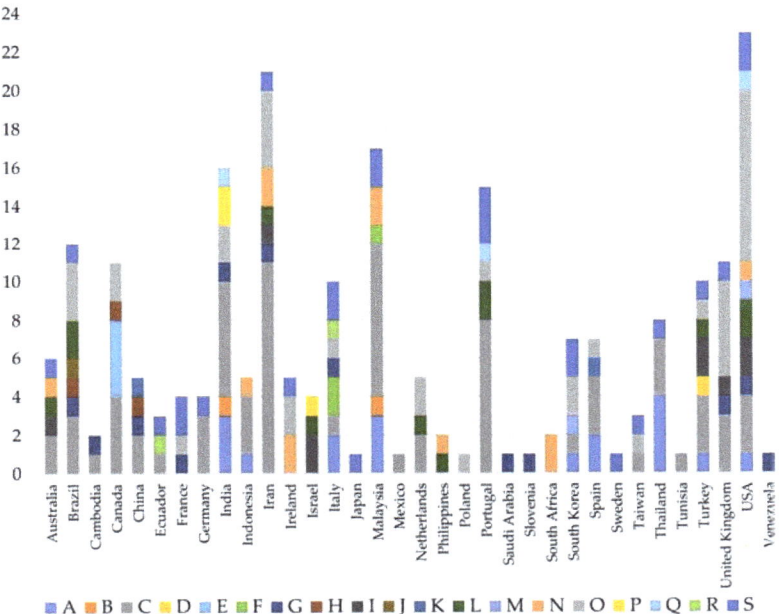

Figure 5. Number of studies classified by knowledge categories and countries: Agriculture, forestry and fishing (**A**); Mining and quarrying (**B**); Manufacturing (**C**); Water supply; sewerage, waste management and remediation activities (**D**); Construction (**E**); Wholesale and retail trade; repair of motor vehicles and motorcycles (**F**); Transportation and storage (**G**); Accommodation and food service activities (**H**); Information and communication (**I**); Financial and insurances activities (**J**); Professional, scientific and technical activities (**K**); Administrative and support service activities (**L**); Public administration and defiance; compulsory social security (**M**); Education (**N**); Human health and social work activities (**O**); Arts, entertainment and recreation (**P**); Other service activities (**Q**); Activities of households as employers; undifferentiated goods and services producing activities of households for own use (**R**); and Other scopes not previously included (**S**).

Countries such as Venezuela, Tunisia, Sweden South Africa, Slovenia, Poland, Mexico, Japan and Saudi Arabia only cover one area (Figure 5).

The United Kingdom is the location where the RULA method originated. However, it is not a place where it has been most applied, as only 11 studies have been performed there. The method originated with assessments carried out on workers in the industry [20]. Despite this, RULA has not been widely used in industry in the United Kingdom; it presents only three studies. "Human health and social work activities" stands out with five publications (Figure 5).

Figure 6 shows the different countries according to the frequency of the published studies.

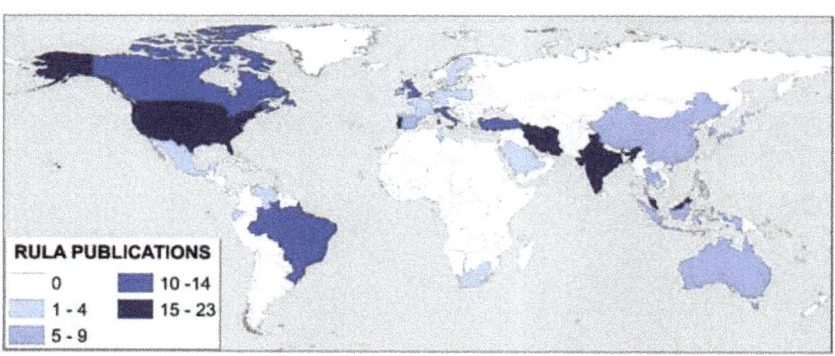

Figure 6. Map with frequencies.

3.3. Classification by Years

Figure 7 shows the period of time in which RULA has been used and in which areas of knowledge.

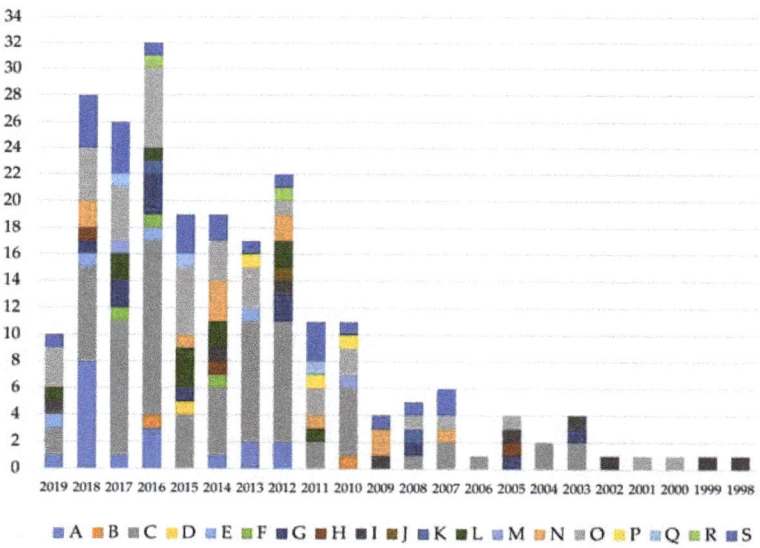

Figure 7. Number of studies classified by knowledge and year categories: Agriculture, forestry and fishing (**A**); Mining and quarrying (**B**); Manufacturing (**C**); Water supply; sewerage, waste management and remediation activities (**D**); Construction (**E**); Wholesale and retail trade; repair of motor vehicles and motorcycles (**F**); Transportation and storage (**G**); Accommodation and food service activities (**H**); Information and communication (**I**); Financial and insurances activities (**J**); Professional, scientific and technical activities (**K**); Administrative and support service activities (**L**); Public administration and defiance; compulsory social security (**M**); Education (**N**); Human health and social work activities (**O**); Arts, entertainment and recreation (**P**); Other service activities (**Q**); Activities of households as employers; undifferentiated goods and services producing activities of households for own use (**R**); and Other scopes not previously included (**S**).

The RULA method was created in 1993; however, according to the review carried out, it was not until 1998 that it was first applied.

From 1998 to 2019, the method has been applied every year. It should be noted that the year 2019 includes only the studies developed up until April.

The year 2016 stands out for the largest number of research studies (32). This is followed by the year 2018 with 28, 2017 with 26, 2012 with 22, 2014 and 2015 with 19 each, 2013 with 17 and 2010 and 2011 with 11 each. All other years have 10 or fewer studies.

Over the past 10 years, there has been an increase in such research. This may be due to the importance and awareness that occupational hazard prevention has received in recent times. In addition, it might be linked to the development of new technologies. These allow the method to be applied more quickly and efficiently (Figure 7).

It is noted (Figure 7) that over the past 10 years, the number of categories investigated has also increased compared to the previous 12 years. The year 2016 is characterised not only as having the largest number of publications, but also by the largest number of areas studied (11). "Manufacturing" stands out for representing 13 of the 32 research studies, followed by "Human health and social work activities" with 6. There are seven years with a single category (1998–2002, 2004 and 2006).

3.4. Classification by Journal

Table 22 presents all the journals available in this review, the number of articles published in each, knowledge categories (Web of Science), impact factor, rank and quartile. In total, 163 studies are differentiated. The rest of those that have been reviewed do not correspond to journal articles.

Table 22. Number of publications (N) by scientific journal, knowledge categories (Web of Science), impact factor, rank and quartile (2018).

Journal	N	Impact Factor	Categories	Rank	Quartile
Advanced Science Letters	1	1.253	Multidisciplinary Sciences—SCIE	15/59	Q2
Agronomy	1	2.259	Agronomy—SCIE Plant Sciences—SCIE	19/89 78/228	Q1 Q2
American Journal of Obstetrics and Gynecology	1	6.120	Obstetrics & Gynecology SCIE	2/83	Q1
American Journal of Veterinary Research	1	1.070	Veterinary Sciences—SCIE	65/141	Q2
Applied Ergonomics	16	2.610	Ergonomics—SSCI Psychology, applied—SSCI Engineering, industrial—SCIE	3/16 25/82 20/46	Q1 Q2 Q2
Archives of Environmental & Occupational Health	1	1.483	Environmental Sciences—SCIE Public, environmental & occupational health—SCIE	181/251 124/186	Q3 Q3
Automation in Construction	1	4.313	Construction & Building Technology—SCIE Engineering, Civil—SCIE	8/63 7/132	Q1 Q1
Balkan Medical Journal	1	1.203	Medicine, General & Internal—SCIE	94/160	Q3
Behaviour & Information Technology	1	1.429	Computer Science, Cybernetics—SCIE Ergonomics—SSCI	13/23 8/16	Q3 Q2
Brazilian Journal of Physical Therapy	1	1.879	Orthopedics—SCIE Rehabilitation—SCIE	38/76 27/65	Q2 Q2
British Dental Journal	2	1.438	Dentistry, Oral Surgery & Medicine—SCIE	59/91	Q3
British Journal of Biomedical Science	1	2.365	Medical Laboratory Technology—SCIE	12/29	Q2
Canadian Journal of Civil Engineering	1	0.742	Engineering, Civil—SCIE	111/132	Q4
Canadian Journal of Ophtalmology—Journal Canadien D Ophtalmologie	1	1.305	Ophthalmology—SCIE	49/60	Q4
Ciencia UNEMI	1	No impact factor.			
Clinical Biomechanics	1	1.977	Engineering, Biomedical—SCIE Orthopedics—SCIE Sport Sciences—SCIE	53/80 35/76 39/83	Q3 Q2 Q2
Cogent Engineering	1	No impact factor.			
Collegium Antropologicum	1	0.609	Anthropology—SSCI	48/82	Q3
Design Journal	1	No impact factor.			
DYNA-Colombia	1	No impact factor.			

Table 22. Cont.

Journal	N	Impact Factor	Categories	Rank	Quartile
Ergonomics	7	2.181	Engineering, industrial—SCIE Ergonomics—SSCI Psychology—SCIE Psychology, applied—SSCI	21/46 5/16 38/77 35/82	Q2 Q2 Q2 Q2
European Journal of Dental Education	1	1.531	Dentistry, Oral Surgery & Medicine—SCIE Education, Scientific Disciplines—SCIE	48/91 23/41	Q3 Q3
Fresenius Environmental Bulletin	1	0.691	Environmental Sciences—SCIE	240/251	Q4
Global Nest Journal	1	0.869	Environmental sciences—SCIE	232/251	Q4
Health Promotion Perspectives	1	No impact factor.			
Health Scope	2	No impact factor.			
Human Factors and Ergonomics in Manufacture & Service Industries	2	1.000	Ergonomics—SSCI Engineering, manufacturing—SCIE	13/16 45/49	Q4 Q4
Independent Journal of Management & Production	1	No impact factor.			
Indian Journal of Community Health	1	No impact factor.			
Indian Journal of Occupational and Environmental Medicine	3	No impact factor.			
Industrial Health	1	1.319	Environmental Sciences—SCIE Public, environmental & occupational health—SCIE Toxicology	201/251 143/186 86/93	Q4 Q4 Q4
Intelligent Decision Technologies-Netherlands	1	No impact factor.			
Intensive and Critical Care Nursing	1	1.652	Nursing—SSCI Nursing—SCIE	30/118 33/120	Q2 Q2
International Archives of Occupational and Environmental Health	1	2.025	Public, environmental & occupational health—SCIE	90/186	Q2
International Journal of Environmental Research and Public Health	1	2.468	Environmental Sciences—SCIE Public, environmental & occupational health—SSCI Public, environmental & occupational health—SCIE	112/251 38/164 67/186	Q2 Q1 Q2
International Journal of Industrial Engineering—Theory Applications and Practice	1	0.532	Engineering, industrial—SCIE Engineering, Manufacturing—SCIE	45/46 47/49	Q4 Q4
International Journal of Industrial Ergonomics	12	1.571	Ergonomics—SSCI Engineering, industrial—SCIE	7/16 28/46	Q2 Q3
International Journal of Injury Control and Safety Promotion	1	0.870	Public, environmental & occupational health—SSCI	146/164	Q4
International Journal of Integrated Engineering	1	No impact factor.			
International Journal of Interactive Design and Manufacturing—IJIDEM	1	No impact factor.			
International Journal of Occupational Safety and Ergonomics	8	1.377	Ergonomics—SSCI Public, environmental & occupational health—SSCI	9/16 110/164	Q3 Q3
International Journal of Productivity and Performance Management	1	No impact factor.			
International Journal of Technology	1	No impact factor.			
International Journal of Working Conditions	1	No impact factor.			
International Journal of Workplace Health Management	1	No impact factor.			
International Nursing Review	1	1.562	Nursing—SSCI Nursing—SCIE	36/118 38/120	Q2 Q2
Iranian Journal of Public Health	2	1.225	Public, environmental & occupational health—SSCI Public, environmental & occupational health—SCIE	122/164 149/186	Q3 Q4
Journal of Advanced Simulation in Science and Engineering	1	No impact factor.			
Journal of Agricultural Safety and Health	1	No impact factor.			
Journal of Back and Musculoskeletal Rehabilitation	4	0.814	Orthopedics—SCIE Rehabilitation—SCIE	65/76 60/65	Q4 Q4
Journal of Bionic Engineering	1	2.463	Engineering, Multidisciplinary—SCIE Materials Science, Biomaterials—SCIE Robotics—SCIE	28/88 21/32 13/26	Q2 Q3 Q2
Journal of Construction Engineering and Management	1	2.734	Construction & Building Technology—SCIE Engineering, civil—SCIE Engineering, industrial—SCIE	15/63 32/132 17/46	Q1 Q1 Q2
Journal of Engineering Science and Technology	1	No impact factor.			
Journal of Environmental and Public Health	1	No impact factor.			
Journal of Health and Safety at Work	1	No impact factor.			

Table 22. *Cont.*

Journal	N	Impact Factor	Categories	Rank	Quartile
Journal of Minimal Access Surgery	1	0.966	Surgery—SCIE	168/203	Q4
Journal of Minimally Invasive Gynecology	1	2.547	Obstetrics & Gynecology- SCIE	25/83	Q2
Journal of Musculoskeletal Pain	1	No impact factor.			
Journal of Occupational Health	2	1.800	Public, environmental & occupational health—SCIE	105/186	Q3
Journal of Physical Therapy Science	2	0.392	Rehabilitation—SCIE	61/64	Q4
Journal of Robotics	1	No impact factor.			
Journal of Robotic Surgery	1	No impact factor.			
Journal of Sound and Vibration	1	3.123	Acoustics—SCIE Engineering, Mechanical—SCIE Mechanics—SCIE	5/31 27/129 21/134	Q1 Q1 Q1
Journal of the Faculty of Engineering and Architecture of Gazi University	1	0.652	Engineering, multidisciplinary—SCIE	76/88	Q4
Laryngoscope	1	2.343	Medicine, research & experimental- SCIE Otorhinolaryngology—SCIE	78/136 12/42	Q3 Q2
Makara Journal of Technology	1	No impact factor.			
Medicina del Lavoro	2	0.583	Public, environmental & occupational health—SCIE	179/186	Q4
Occupational and Environmental Medicine	2	3.556	Public, environmental & occupational health—SCIE	1/186	Q1
Occupational Medicine-Oxford	1	1.222	Public, environmental & occupational health—SCIE	150/186	Q4
Otolaryngology-Head and Neck Surgery	1	2.310	Otorhinolaryngology—SCIE Surgery—SCIE	13/42 72/203	Q2 Q2
Otology & Neurotology	1	2.063	Clinical Neurology—SCIE Otorhinolaryngology—SCIE	134/199 15/42	Q3 Q2
Pain Clinic	1	No impact factor.			
Physical Therapy	1	3.043	Orthopedics—SCIE Rehabilitation—SCIE	16/76 7/65	Q1 Q1
PLOS ONE	2	2.776	Multidisciplinary Sciences—SCIE	24/69	Q2
Safety and Health at Work	1	1.431	Public, environmental & occupational health—SSCI Public, environmental & occupational health—SCIE	102/164 131/186	Q3 Q3
Safety Science	1	3.619	Engineering, industrial—SCIE Operations research & management science—SCIE	10/46 16/84	Q1 Q1
Sensors	1	3.031	Chemistry, Analytical—SCIE Electrochemistry—SCIE Instruments & Instrumentation—SCIE	23/84 12/26 15/61	Q2 Q2 Q1
South African Journal of Physiotherapy	1	No impact factor.			
Surgical Endoscopy and Other Interventional Techniques	4	3.209	Surgery—SCIE	39/203	Q1
Surgical Endoscopy—Ultrasound and Interventional Techniques	1	No impact factor.			
Turkish Journal of Physical Medicine and Rehabilitation	1	0.223	Rehabilitation—SCIE	65/65	Q4
Work—A Journal of Prevention Assessment & Rehabilitation	26 *	1.009	Public, environmental & occupational health—SSCI	138/164	Q4
Workplace Health & Safety	1	0.922	Nursing—SSCI Nursing—SCIE	91/118 93/120	Q4 Q4

* Mode.

Of all the journals, there are four with a greater number of articles published: "Work—A Journal of Prevention Assessment & Rehabilitation" with 26 studies, followed by "Applied Ergonomics" with 16, "International Journal of Industrial Ergonomics" with 12 and "International Journal of Occupational Safety and Ergonomics" with 8 (Table 22).

3.5. Comparing Results with Other Methods

Some bibliographic reviews similar to this one have already been carried out. They have focused on other indirect and semi-direct assessment methods. Some matches are presented in the results obtained.

The RULA method matches the OWAS method and the Standardized Nordic Questionnaire in the most common knowledge categories. The field of industry and health and social assistance are the most researched, with one or the other being highlighted depending on the method [8,260]. The REBA method has also been highlighted in industry, although the health-related field ranks fourth [261].

For countries with the highest number of publications, none of the methods coincided with RULA, since REBA excelled in India, OWAS in Finland and the Nordic Questionnaire in Iran. However, for REBA, the second country with the most studies was the USA [8,260,261].

By date, the Nordic Questionnaire matches RULA. The year 2016 was when more studies were published for both [260].

Finally, with regards to journals, information is only available for the REBA method. The journal with the largest number of publications on this method is "Work—A Journal of Prevention Assessment & Rehabilitation"; this is also the case for RULA [261].

It should be noted that this comparison is general since the date range selected in each of the studies is not the same.

3.6. Sustainability and the RULA Method

By integrating ISO 45001 with ISO 9001 and ISO 14001, organisations seek to implement quality management, occupational safety and health and the environment in a single system (Figure 8). The three systems, operating together, allow the organisation to optimise:

- The quality of the product or service
- Customer satisfaction
- The disposal of waste that has an impact on the environment
- The efficiency of the processes
- The health and safety of workers

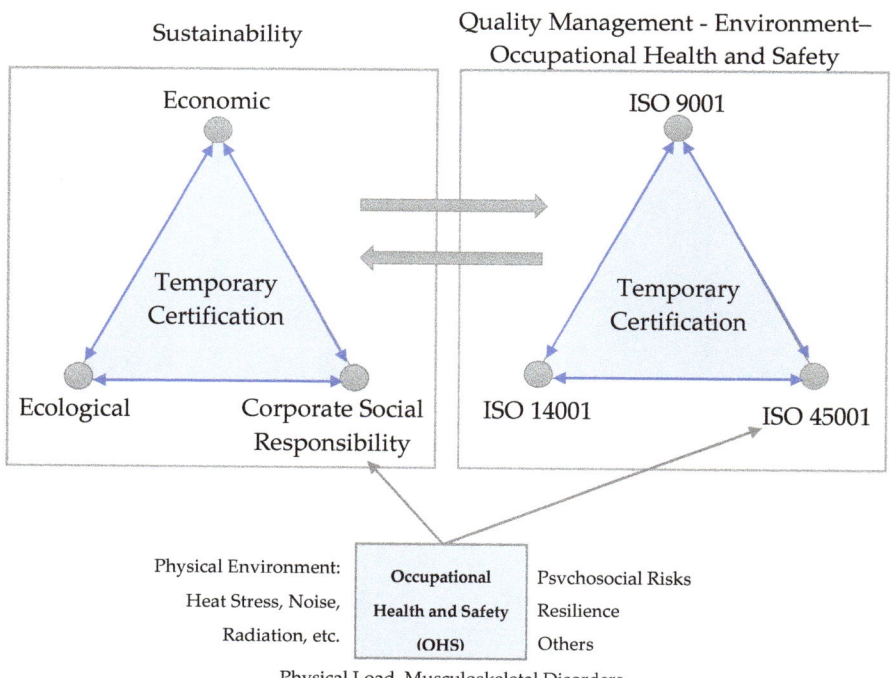

Figure 8. Parts of sustainability.

Sustainability is a set of three fundamental parts: economic, social and environmental [262].

Sustainability, therefore, is not only focused on natural resources, but also plays a very important role in companies and contracted staff [263]. It fosters a relationship between healthy living and caring for nature [262]. For this reason, it is very important to also focus on the care of workers, carrying out assessments in order to obtain improvements in their health and safety [264].

The RULA method pursues this objective, as it focuses on the study of musculoskeletal disorders. Therefore, the use of this method contributes to the production of sustainable products.

3.7. Limitations

The country classification in this document has been based on the origin of the authors, as not all studies are clear about their location. The locations selected in each study have been those to which the greatest number of authors belong. In cases where it was not possible to follow this criterion, the location of the first author was selected.

4. Conclusions

The RULA method has been used in two main areas, "Manufacturing" and "Human health and social work activities". However, it has been found not to be a sector-specific method. It can be applied to workers in any field.

Its use has been increasing over the last 10 years, perhaps indicating it is an effective method which is being tested more and more. This is also coupled with a growing awareness of workers' health and safety. The year that stands out for the number of studies published is 2016 with a total of 32, followed by 2018 with a total of 28.

Countries such as the USA and Iran excel at applying the method and encompassing numerous fields of knowledge. The journal with the most publications is "Work—A Journal of Prevention Assessment & Rehabilitation", with a total of 26. This journal is followed by "Applied Ergonomics" with 16 published studies.

RULA is usually used in combination with other ergonomic methods or tools to provide better and more reliable results. In this way, it is possible to contemplate different risk factors and evaluate numerous body areas. In addition, technological advancement is also appreciated in all sectors, since in many studies the method is combined with the use of sensors, software, virtual reality, etc.

Author Contributions: Conceptualisation, M.G.-G., Á.-J.C.-F., J.P.-A., M.D.-P. and J.-A.C.-C.; methodology, M.G.-G., Á.-J.C.-F., J.P.-A., M.D.-P. and J.-A.C.-C.; software, M.G.-G., Á.-J.C.-F., J.P.-A., M.D.-P. and J.-A.C.-C.; validation, M.G.-G., Á.-J.C.-F., J.P.-A., M.D.-P. and J.-A.C.-C.; formal analysis, M.G.-G., Á.-J.C.-F., J.P.-A., M.D.-P. and J.-A.C.-C.; investigation, M.G.-G., Á.-J.C.-F., J.P.-A., M.D.-P. and J.-A.C.-C.; resources, M.G.-G., Á.-J.C.-F., J.P.-A., M.D.-P. and J.-A.C.-C.; data curation, M.G.-G., Á.-J.C.-F., J.P.-A., M.D.-P. and J.-A.C.-C.; writing—original draft preparation, M.G.-G., Á.-J.C.-F., J.P.-A., M.D.-P. and J.-A.C.-C.; writing—review and editing, M.G.-G., Á.-J.C.-F., J.P.-A., M.D.-P. and J.-A.C.-C.; visualisation, M.G.-G., Á.-J.C.-F., J.P.-A., M.D.-P. and J.-A.C.-C.; supervision, M.G.-G., Á.-J.C.-F., J.P.-A., M.D.-P. and J.-A.C.-C.; and project administration, M.G.-G., Á.-J.C.-F., J.P.-A.. M.D.-P. and J.-A.C.-C. All authors have read and agreed to the published version of the manuscript.

Funding: This research received no external funding.

Acknowledgments: We acknowledge Laboratory-Observatory Andalusian Working Conditions in the Agricultural Sector (LASA; C.G. 401487) and the Research Own Plan of the University of Almería.

Conflicts of Interest: The authors declare no conflict of interest.

Appendix A

The following table shows a summary of the meanings of the abbreviations.

Table A1. Abbreviations.

Abbreviations	Meaning
ALLA	Agricultural Lower Limb Assessment
BCTQ	Boston Carpal Tunnel Syndrome Questionnaire
CMDQ	Cornell Musculoskeletal Discomfort Questionnaire
CTD	Cumulative Trauma Disorders
DELMIA	Digital Enterprise Manufacturing Interactive Application
EMG	Electromyograpgy
FECYT	Spanish Foundation for Science and Technology
HAL	Hand Activity Level
IBV	Instituto de Biomecánica de Valencia (In Spanish)
ICT	Information and Communications Technology
iLMM	Industrial Lumbar Motion Monitor
INSHT	Instituto Nacional de Seguridad e Higiene en el Trabajo (In Spanish)
KIM	Key Indicator Method
LBA	Lower Back Analysis
LUBA	Loading on the Upper Body Assessment
MAC	Manual Handling Assessment Charts
ManTRA	Manual Task Risk Assessment
MSD	Musculoskeletal Disorders
NERPA	New Ergonomic Posture Assessment
NIOSH	National Institute of Occupational Safety and Health
NMSQ	Nordic Musculoskeletal Symptoms Questionnaire
OBS	Office-based Surgery
OCRA	Occupational Repetitive Action
OSHA	Occupational Safety & Health Administration
OWAS	Ovako Working Analysis System
PATH	Posture, Activity, Tools and Handling
PEI	Posture Evaluation Index
PLIBEL	Method for the identification of musculoskeletal stress factors which may have injurious effects
PRRI	Posture and Repetition Risk Factor Index
QEC	Quick Exposure Check
QRating	Quick Rating
REBA	Rapid Entire Body Assessment
ROSA	Rapid Office Strain Assessment
RULA	Rapid Upper Limb Assessment
SI	Strain Index
UEWD-R	Upper Extremity Work Demand
VAS	Visual Analog Scale
VDT	Visual Display Terminal
VIRA	Video film technique for Registration and Analysis of working postures and movements
WoS	Web of Science

References

1. European Agency for Safety and Health at Work (EU-OSHA). Trastornos Musculoesqueléticos. Available online: https://osha.europa.eu/es/themes/musculoskeletal-disorders (accessed on 21 January 2020).
2. European Agency for Safety and Health at Work (EU-OSHA). Preventing Work-Related Musculoskeletal Disorders. FACTS 4. Available online: https://osha.europa.eu/es/publications/factsheet-4-preventing-work-related-musculoskeletal-disorders/view (accessed on 21 January 2020).
3. European Agency for Safety and Health at Work (EU-OSHA). Introduction to Work-Related Musculoskeletal Disorders. FACTS 71. Available online: https://osha.europa.eu/es/publications/factsheet-71-introduction-work-related-musculoskeletal-disorders/view (accessed on 21 January 2020).

4. Asensio-Cuesta, S.; Diego-Mas, J.A.; Canos-Daros, L.; Andres-Romano, C. A genetic algorithm for the design of job rotation schedules considering ergonomic and competence criteria. *Int. J. Adv. Manuf. Tech.* **2012**, *60*, 1161–1174. [CrossRef]
5. Ilonca, I.; Stanciu, A.; Rosulescu, E.; Zavaleanu, M.; Cosma, G. Ergonomics and exercises program as practical solutions for the prevention of musculoskeletal disorders in clinical dentistry. In Proceedings of the 3rd International Multidisciplinary Scientific Conference on Social Sciences and Arts, SGEM 2016, Albena, Bulgaria, 24–30 August 2016; pp. 445–452.
6. Nunes, I.L. FAST ERGO_X-A tool for ergonomic auditing and work-related musculoskeletal disorders prevention. *Work* **2009**, *34*, 133–148. [CrossRef] [PubMed]
7. Batubara, H.; Dharmastiti, R. Redesign of liquid aluminum pouring tool based on participatory ergonomics to improve productivity, workload, and musculoskeletal disorders. *Int. J. Technol.* **2017**, *8*, 352–361. [CrossRef]
8. Gomez-Galan, M.; Perez-Alonso, J.; Callejon-Ferre, A.J.; Lopez-Martinez, J. Musculoskeletal disorders: OWAS review. *Ind. Health* **2017**, *55*, 314–337. [CrossRef]
9. Alvarez-Zarate, J.M.; Marin-Zurdo, J.J.; Sistema HADA Move-Human Sensors. Sistema Portátil para Captura y Análisis Tridimensional del Movimiento Humano en Puestos de Trabajo Basado en Sensores Inerciales de Movimiento y Simulación 3D con Modelos Biomecánicos. Available online: http://www.seguridad-laboral.es/prevencion/ergonomia/sistema-hada-move-human-sensors (accessed on 22 January 2020).
10. Kuorinka, I.; Jonsson, B.; Kilbom, A.; Vinterberg, H.; Biering-Sorensen, F.; Andersson, G.; Jorgensesn, K. Standardised Nordic questionnaires for the analysis of musculoskeletal symptoms. *Appl. Ergon.* **1987**, *18*, 233–237. [CrossRef]
11. Lifshitz, Y.; Amstrong, T. A design checklist for control and prediction of cumulative trauma disorders in hand intensive manual jobs. In Proceedings of the 30th Annual Meeting of Human Factors Society, Dayton, OH, USA, 29 September–3 October 1986; pp. 837–841. [CrossRef]
12. David, G.; Woods, V.; Li, G.; Buckle, P. The development of the Quick Exposure Check (QEC) for assessing exposure to risk factors for work-related musculoskeletal disorders. *Appl. Ergon.* **2008**, *39*, 57–69. [CrossRef] [PubMed]
13. Keyserling, W.M.; Stetson, D.S.; Silverstein, B.A.; Brouwer, M.L. A checklist for evaluating ergonomic risk factors associated with upper extremity cumulative trauma disorders. *Ergonomics* **1993**, *36*, 807–831. [CrossRef] [PubMed]
14. Jürgens, W.W.; Mohr, D.; Pangert, R.; Pernack, E.; Schultz, K.; Steinberg, U. *Handlungsanleitung zur Beurteilung der Arbeitsbedingungen beim Heben und Tragen von Lasten*; LASI Veröffentlichung: Wiesbaden, Germany, 2001; Volume 9.
15. Instituto Nacional de Seguridad y Salud en el Trabajo (INSST). *Guía Técnica para la Evaluación y Prevención de los Riesgos Relativos a la Manipulación Manual de Cargas. Guías Técnicas*; INSST: Madrid, Spain, 1998.
16. Monnington, S.; Quarrie, C.; Pinder, A.; Morris, L. Development of Manual Handling Assessment Charts (MAC) for health and safety inspectors. In *Contemporary Ergonomics*; Taylor & Francis: London, UK, 2003.
17. Liberty-Mutual. Manual Materials Handling Tables. Available online: https://libertymmhtables.libertymutual.com/CM_LMTablesWeb/taskSelection.do?action=initTaskSelection (accessed on 22 January 2019).
18. National Institute for Occupational Safety and Health (NIOSH). *Work Practices Guide for Manual Lifting*; NIOSH Technical Report; NIOSH: Cincinnaty, OH, USA, 1981; pp. 81–122.
19. Snook, S.H.; Ciriello, V.M. The design of manual handling tasks: Revised tables of maximum acceptable weights and forces. *Ergonomics* **1991**, *34*, 1197–1213. [CrossRef]
20. McAtamney, L.; Corlett, E.N. RULA–A survey method for the investigation of work-related upper limb disorders. *App. Ergon.* **1993**, *24*, 91–99. [CrossRef]
21. Kemmlert, K. A method assigned for the identification of ergonomic hazards–PLIBEL. *Appl. Ergon.* **1995**, *26*, 199–211. [CrossRef]
22. Moore, J.S.; Garg, A. The Strain Index: A proposed method to analyze jobs for risk of distal upper extremity disorders. *Am. Ind. Hyg. Assoc. J.* **1995**, *56*, 443–458. [CrossRef] [PubMed]
23. Colombini, D. An observational method for classifying exposure to repetitive movements of the upper limbs. *Ergonomics* **1998**, *41*, 1261–1289. [CrossRef] [PubMed]
24. García, C.; Chirivela, C.; Page del Pozo, A.; Moraga, R.; Jorquera, J. *Método Ergo IBV. Evaluación de Riesgos Laborales Asociados a la Carga Física*; Instituto de Biomecánica de Valencia (IBV): Valencia, Spain, 1997.

25. James, C.P.A.; Harburn, K.L.; Kramer, J.F. Cumulative trauma disorders in the upper extremities: Reliability of the Postural and Repetitive Risk-Factors Index. *Arch. Phys. Med. Rehab.* **1997**, *78*, 860–866. [CrossRef]
26. Hignett, S.; McAtamney, L. Rapid Entire Body Assessment (REBA). *Appl. Ergon.* **2000**, *31*, 201–205. [CrossRef]
27. Buchholz, B.; Paquet, V.; Punnett, L.; Lee, D.; Moir, S. PATH: A work sampling-based approach to ergonomic job analysis for construction and other non-repetitive work. *Appl. Ergon.* **1996**, *27*, 177–187. [CrossRef]
28. Karhu, O.; Kansi, P.; Kuorinka, I. Correcting working postures in industry: A practical method for analysis. *Appl. Ergon.* **1977**, *8*, 199–201. [CrossRef]
29. Kilbom, A.; Persson, J.; Jonsson, B. Risk factors for work-related disorders of the neck and shoulder–With special emphasis on working postures and movements. In *The Ergonomics of Working Postures*; Corlett, E.N., Wilson, J., Manenica, I., Eds.; Taylor & Francis: London, UK, 1986; pp. 44–53.
30. Corlett, E.; Madeley, S.; Manenica, I. Posture targeting: A technique for recording working postures. *Ergonomics* **1979**, *22*, 357–633. [CrossRef]
31. Instituto de Ergonomía (INERMAP). Ergomet 3.0. Available online: http://www.inermap.com/software/ergomet.html (accessed on 22 January 2020).
32. Takala, E.P.; Pehkonen, I.; Forsman, M.; Hansson, G.A.; Mthiassen, S.E.; Neumann, W.P.; Sjogaard, G.; Veiersted, K.B.; Westgaard, R.H.; Winkel, J. Systematic evaluation of observational methods assessing biomechanical exposures at work. *Scand. J. Work. Environ. Health.* **2010**, *36*, 3–24. [CrossRef]
33. Eurostat. NACE Rev. 2. Structure and Explanatory Notes. Available online: https://ec.europa.eu/eurostat/documents/1965800/1978839/NACE_rev2_explanatory_notes_EN.pdf/b09f2cb4-5dac-4118-9164-bcc39b791ef5 (accessed on 4 October 2019).
34. Cremasco, M.M.; Giustetto, A.; Caffaro, F.; Colantoni, A.; Cavallo, E.; Grigolato, S. Risk assessment for musculoskeletal disorders in forestry: A comparison between RULA and REBA in the manual feeding of a wood-chipper. *Int. J. Environ. Res. Public Health* **2019**, *16*, 793. [CrossRef]
35. Pramchoo, W.; Geater, A.F.; Harris-Adamson, C.; Tangtrakulwanich, B. Ergonomic rubber tapping knife relieves symptoms of carpal tunnel syndrome among rubber tappers. *Int. J. Ind. Ergonom.* **2018**, *68*, 65–72. [CrossRef]
36. Kim, E.; Freivalds, A.; Takeda, F.; Li, C. Ergonomic evaluation of current advancements in blueberry harvesting. *Agronomy* **2018**, *8*, 266. [CrossRef]
37. Pal, A.; Dhara, P.C. Work related musculoskeletal disorders and postural stress of the women cultivators engaged in uprooting job of rice cultivation. *Ind. J. Occup. Environ. Med.* **2018**, *22*, 163–169. [CrossRef]
38. Thetkathuek, A.; Meepradit, P.; Sangiamsak, T. A cross-sectional study of musculoskeletal symptoms and risk factors in Cambodian fruit farm workers in Eastern Region, Thailand. *Saf. Health Work* **2018**, *9*, 192–202. [CrossRef]
39. Jain, R.; Meena, M.L.; Dangayach, G.S.; Bhardwaj, A.K. Association of risk factors with musculoskeletal disorders in manual-working farmers. *Arch. Environ. Occup. Health* **2018**, *73*, 19–28. [CrossRef] [PubMed]
40. Pardo-Ferreira, M.C.; Zambrana-Ruiz, A.; Carrillo-Castrillo, J.A.; Rubio-Romero, J.C. Ergonomic risk management of pruning with chainsaw in the olive sector. In Proceedings of the 6th International Symposium on Occupational Safety and Hygiene (SHO), Guimaraes, Portugal, 26–27 March 2018; Arezes, P.M., Baptista, J.S., Barroso, M.P., Carneiro, P., Cordeiro, P., Costa, N., Melo, R.B., Miguel, A.S., Perestrelo, G., Eds.; pp. 517–522.
41. Jain, R.; Meena, M.L.; Dangayach, G.S.; Bhardwaj, A.K. Risk factors for musculoskeletal disorders in manual harvesting farmers of Rajasthan. *Ind. Health* **2018**, *56*, 241–248. [CrossRef] [PubMed]
42. Kong, Y.K.; Lee, S.Y.; Lee, K.S.; Kim, D.M. Comparisons of ergonomic evaluation tools (ALLA, RULA, REBA and OWAS) for farm work. *Int. J. Occup. Saf. Ergo.* **2018**, *24*, 218–223. [CrossRef]
43. Unver-Okan, S.; Acar, H.H.; Kaya, A. Determination of work postures with different ergonomic risk assessment methods in forest nurseries. *Fresen. Environ. Bull.* **2017**, *26*, 7362–7371.
44. Putri, N.T.; Susanti, L.; Tito, A.; Sutanto, A. Redesign of thresher machine for farmers using Rapid Upper Limb Assessment (RULA) method. In Proceedings of the IEEE International Conference on Industrial Engineering and Engineering Management (IEEM), Bali, Indonesia, 4–7 December 2016; pp. 1304–1309.
45. Vazquez-Cabrera, F.J. Ergonomic evaluation, with the RULA method, of greenhouse task of trellising crops. *Work* **2016**, *54*, 517–531. [CrossRef]

46. Mohd Nasir, N.S.; Mohd Tamrin, S.B.; Subramanian, K.; Shukoor, N.S.; Zolkifli, N.; Ng, G.S.; Muhamad Akir, N.F.; Ananta, G.P. Association of workplace stressors with salivary alpha-amylase activity levels among fresh fruit bunch cutters in Selangor. *Iran. J. Public Health* **2016**, *45*, 68–76.
47. Deros, B.M.; Khamis, N.K.; Mohamad, D.; Kabilmiharbi, N.; Daruis, D.D.I. Investigation of oil palm harvesters' postures using RULA analysis. In Proceedings of the IEEE International Conference on Biomedical Engineering and Sciences, Miri, Malaysia, 8–10 December 2014; pp. 287–290.
48. Mokhtar, M.M.; Deros, B.M.; Sukadarin, E.H. Evaluation of musculoskeletal disorders prevalence during oil palm fresh fruit bunches harvesting using RULA. In Proceedings of the 2nd International Conference on Ergonomics (ICE 2013), Kuala Lumpur, Malaysia, 2–4 September 2013; Yusuff, R.M., Ahmad, S.A., Daruis, D.D.I., Deros, B.M., Dawal, S.Z.M., Eds.; pp. 110–150.
49. Swangnetr, M.; Namkorn, P.; Phimphasak, C.; Saenlee, K.; Kaber, D.; Buranruk, O.; Puntumetakul, R. Ergonomic analysis of rice field plowing. In *Advanced in Physical Ergonomics and Safety*; Ahram, T.Z., Karwowski, W., Eds.; CRC Press: Boca Raton, FL, USA, 2013; pp. 565–574.
50. Di Gironimo, G.; Lanzotti, A.; Melemez, K.; Renno, F. A top-down approach for virtual redesign and ergonomic optimization of an agricultural tractor's driver cab. In Proceedings of the 11th ASME Biennial Conference on Engineering Systems Design and Analysis, (ESDA 2012), Nantes, France, 2–4 July 2012; pp. 801–811.
51. Meksawi, S.; Tangtrakulwanich, B.; Chongsuvivatwong, V. Musculoskeletal problems and ergonomic risk assessment in rubber tappers: A community-based study in southern Thailand. *Int. J. Ind. Ergonom.* **2012**, *42*, 129–135. [CrossRef]
52. Mukhopadhyay, P.; Srivastava, S. Evaluating ergonomic risk factors in non-regulated stone carving units of Jaipur. *Work* **2010**, *35*, 87–99. [CrossRef] [PubMed]
53. Norhidayah, M.S.; Mohamed, N.M.Z.N.; Mansor, M.A.; Ismail, A.R. RULA: Postural loading assessment tools for Malaysia mining industry. *J. Eng. Sci. Technol.* **2016**, *11*, 1–8.
54. Azizi, A.; Yazdi, P.G.; Hashemipour, M. Interactive design of storage unit utilizing virtual reality and ergonomic framework for production optimization in manufacturing industry. *Int. J. Interact. Des. Manuf. IJIDEM* **2019**, *13*, 373–381. [CrossRef]
55. Fazi, H.B.M.; Mohamed, N.M.Z.B.N.; Bin Basri, A.Q. Risks assessment at automotive manufacturing company and ergonomic working condition. In Proceedings of the 1st International Postgraduate Conference on Mechanical Engineering (IPCME), Pahang, Malaysia, 31 October 2018.
56. Sain, M.K.; Meena, M.L. Exploring the musculoskeletal problems and associated risk-factors among brick kiln workers. *Int. J. Workpl. Health Manag.* **2018**, *11*, 395–410. [CrossRef]
57. Boulila, A.; Ayadi, M.; Mrabet, K. Ergonomics study and analysis of workstations in Tunisian mechanical manufacturing. *Hum. Factor. Ergon. Man.* **2018**, *28*, 166–185. [CrossRef]
58. Gregory, D.E.; Romero, S.E. Can the use of an alternatively designed tamper alter spine posture and risk of upper limb injury while tamping espresso? *Int. J. Ind. Ergonom.* **2018**, *65*, 103–109. [CrossRef]
59. Daneshmandi, H.; Kee, D.; Kamalinia, M.; Oliaei, M.; Mohammadi, H. An ergonomic intervention to relieve musculoskeletal symptoms of assembly line workers at an electronic parts manufacturer in Iran. *Work* **2018**, *61*, 515–521. [CrossRef]
60. Yahya, N.M.; Zahid, M.N.O. Work-related musculoskeletal disorders (WMDs) risk assessment at core assembly production of electronic components manufacturing company. In Proceedings of the 4th Asia Pacific Conference on Manufacturing Systems/3rd International Manufacturing Engineering Conference (APCOMS-iMEC), Yogyakarta, Indonesia, 7–8 December 2017.
61. Yazdanirad, S.; Khoshakhlagh, A.H.; Habibi, E.; Zare, A.; Zeinodini, M.; Dehghani, F. Comparing the effectiveness of three ergonomic risk assessment methods–RULA, LUBA and NERMA–To predict the upper extremity musculoskeletal disorders. *Ind. J. Occup. Environ. Med.* **2018**, *22*, 17–21. [CrossRef]
62. Tang, G.; Webb, P. The design and evaluation of an ergonomic contactless gesture control system for industrial robots. *J. Robotic* **2018**, 9791286. [CrossRef]
63. Mat, S.; Abdullah, M.A.; Dullah, A.R.; Shamsudin, S.A.; Hussin, M.F. Car seat design using RULA analysis. In Proceedings of the 4th Mechanical Engineering Research Day (MERD), Melaka, Malaysia, 30 March 2017; BonAbdoollah, M.F., Tuan, T.B., Salim, M.A., Akop, M.Z., Ismail, R., Musa, H., Eds.; pp. 130–131.

64. Ziaei, M.; Ziaei, H.; Hosseini, S.Y.; Gharagozlou, F.; Keikshamoghaddam, A.A.; Laybidi, M.I.; Moradinazar, M. Assessment and virtual redesign of a manual handling Workstation by computer-aided three-domensional interactive application. *Int. J. Occup. Saf. Ergo.* **2017**, *23*, 169–174. [CrossRef]
65. Fazi, H.M.; Mohamed, N.M.Z.N.; Ab Rashid, M.F.F.; Rose, A.N.M. Ergonomics study for workers at food production industry. In Proceedings of the 2nd International Conference on Automotive Innovation and Green Vehicle (AiGEV), Cyberjaya, Malaysia, 2–3 August 2016; Ghani, S.A.C., Hamzah, W.A.W., Alias, A., Eds.;
66. Alabdulkarim, S.; Nussbaum, M.A.; Rashedi, E.; Kim, S.; Agnew, M.; Gardner, R. Impact of task design on task performance and injury risk: Case study of a simulated drilling task. *Ergonomics* **2017**, *60*, 851–866. [CrossRef] [PubMed]
67. Vosniakos, G.C.; Deville, J.; Matsas, E. On inmersive virtual environments for assessing human-driven assembly of large mechanical parts. In Proceedings of the 27th International Conference on Flexible Automation and Intelligent Manufacturing (FAIM), Modena, Italy, 27–30 June 2017; Pellicciari, M., Peruzzini, M., Eds.; pp. 1263–1270.
68. Lockett, H.L.; Arvanitopoulos-Darginis, K. An Automated Maintainability Prediction Tool Integrated with Computer Aided Design. In Proceedings of the 27th CIRP Design Conference, Cranfield, UK, 10–12 May 2017; Shehab, E., Tomiyama, T., Lockett, H., Salonitis, K., Roy, R., Tiwari, A., Eds.; pp. 440–445.
69. Binoosh, S.A.; Mohan, G.M.; Ashok, P.; Sekaran, K.D. Virtual postural assessment of an assembly work in a small scale submersible pump manufacturing industry. *Work* **2017**, *58*, 567–578. [CrossRef] [PubMed]
70. Carlos, S.R.; Cesar, R.M.; Rosa, G.P.; Edwin, P. Evaluation factors musculoskeletal risk area shoe fitting. *Ciencia UNEMI* **2017**, *10*, 69–80.
71. Labbafinejad, Y.; Danesh, H.; Imanizade, Z. Assessment of upper limb musculoskeletal pain and posture in workers of packaging units of pharmaceutical industries. *Work* **2017**, *56*, 337–344. [CrossRef]
72. Nahavandi, D.; Hossny, M. Skeleton-free RULA ergonomic assessment using Kinect sensors. *Intel. Decis. Technol.* **2017**, *11*, 275–284. [CrossRef]
73. Monteiro, L.; Santos, J.; Santos, V.; Franca, V.; Alsina, O. Analysis of overload in the musculoskeletal system of women developing repetitive tasks in fluid filling process in chemical industry. In Proceedings of the 12th International Symposium on Occupational Safety and Hygiene of Portuguese-Society-of-Occupational-Safety-and-Hygiene (SHO), Guimaraes, Portugal, 23–24 March 2016; Arezes, P.M., Baptista, J.S., Barroso, M.P., Carneiro, P., Cordeiro, P., Costa, N., Melo, R.B., Miguel, A.S., Perestrelo, G., Eds.; pp. 29–33.
74. Kushwaha, D.K.; Kane, P.V. Ergonomic assessment and workstation design of shipping crane cabin in steel industry. *Int. J. Ind. Ergonom.* **2016**, *52*, 29–39. [CrossRef]
75. Silva, L.; Carneiro, P.; Braga, A.C. Work-related musculoskeletal disorders of the upper limbs in an auto components company. In Proceedings of the 12th International Symposium on Occupational Safety and Hygiene of Portuguese-Society-of-Occupational-Safety-and-Hygiene (SHO), Guimaraes, Portual, 23–24 March 2016; Arezes, P.M., Baptista, J.S., Barroso, M.P., Carneiro, P., Cordeiro, P., Costa, N., Melo, R.B., Miguel, A.S., Perestrelo, G., Eds.; pp. 463–468.
76. Kumar, P.; Chakrabarti, D.; Patel, T.; Chowdhuri, A. Work-related pains among the workers associated with pineapple peeling in small fruit processing units of North East India. *Int. J. Ind. Ergonom.* **2016**, *53*, 124–129. [CrossRef]
77. Thetkathuek, A.; Meepradit, P.; Jaidee, W. Factors affecting the musculoskeletal disorders of workers in the frozen food manufacturing factories in Thailand. *Int. J. Occup. Saf. Ergo.* **2016**, *22*, 49–56. [CrossRef]
78. Veisi, H.; Choobineh, A.R.; Ghaem, H. Musculoskeletal problems in Iranian hand-woven shoe-sole making operation and developing guidelines for workstation design. *Int. J. Occup. Environ. Med.* **2016**, *7*, 87–97. [CrossRef]
79. Labbafinejad, Y.; Imanizade, Z.; Danesh, H. Ergonomic risk factors and their association with lower back and neck pain among pharmaceutical employees in Iran. *Workpl. Health Saf.* **2016**, *64*, 586–595. [CrossRef]
80. Dianat, I.; Karimi, M.A. Musculoskeletal symptoms among handicraft workers engaged in hand sewing tasks. *J. Occup. Health* **2016**, *58*, 644–652. [CrossRef] [PubMed]
81. Ravichandran, S.P.; Shah, P.B.; Lakshminarayanan, K.; Ravichandran, A.P. Musculoskeletal problems among workers in a garment industry, at Tirupur, Tamil Nadu. *Ind. J. Community Health* **2016**, *28*, 269–274.

82. Sutari, W.; Andias, R.; Doyoyekti, Y.N.; Dwiastuti, M.; Mufidah, I. Musculoskeletal disorder: An Indonesian "Batik Cap" industry case study. *Adv. Sci. Lett.* **2016**, *22*, 1824–1826. [CrossRef]
83. Van, L.; Chaiear, N.; Sumananont, C.; Kannarath, C. Prevalence of musculoskeletal symptoms among garment workers in Jandal province, Cambodia. *J. Occup. Health* **2016**, *58*, 107–117. [CrossRef]
84. Coelho, C.; Oliveira, P.; Maia, E.; Maia, J.; Dias-Teixeira, M. The importance of ergonomics analysis in prevention of MSDs: A pilot study. In Proceedings of the International Conference on Safety Management and Human Factors, Orlando, FL, USA, 27–31 July 2016; Arezes, P., Ed.; pp. 139–151.
85. Zhao, L.Z.; Zhang, Y.H.; Wu, X.H.; Yan, J.H. Virtual assembly simulation and ergonomics analysis for the industrial manipulator based on DELMIA. In Proceedings of the 6th International Asia Conference on Industrial Engineering and Management Innovation (IEMI), Tianjin, China, 25–26 July 2015; Qi, E., Ed.; pp. 527–538.
86. Almeida, M.D.; Laranieira, P.; Rebelo, M. Risk assessment in maintenance of a rehm reflow oven V8. In Proceedings of the International Symposium on Occupational Safety and Hygiene (SHO), Guimaraes, Portugal, 12–13 February 2015; Arezes, P., Baptista, J.S., Barroso, M.P., Carneiro, P., Cordeiro, P., Costa, N., Melo, R., Miguel, A.S., Perestrelo, G., Eds.; pp. 6–8.
87. Dianat, I.; Kord, M.; Yahyazade, P.; Karimi, M.A.; Stedmon, A.W. Association of individual and work-related risk factors with musculoskeletal symptoms among Iranian sewing machine operators. *Appl. Ergon.* **2015**, *51*, 180–188. [CrossRef]
88. Sutari, W.; Yekti, Y.N.D.; Astuti, M.D.; Sari, Y.M. Analysis of working posture on muscular skeleton disorders of operator in stamp scraping in 'batik cap' industry. In Proceedings of the International Conference on Industrial Engineering and Service Science (IESS), Yogyakarta, Indonesia, 1–2 September 2015; Puiawan, N., Ciptomulyono, U., Baihaqi, I., Santosa, B., Eds.; pp. 133–138.
89. Rivero, L.C.; Rodriguez, R.G.; Perez, M.D.; Mar, C.; Juarez, Z. Fuzzy logic and RULA method for assessing the risk of working. In Proceedings of the 6th International Conference on Applied Human Factors and Ergonomics (AHFE), Las Vegas, NV, USA, 26–30 July 2015; Ahram, T., Karwowski, W., Schmorrow, D., Eds.; pp. 4816–4822.
90. Halim, I.; Mahmood, A.R.; Hasan, H.; Sihombing, H.; Saptari, A.; Abu Bakar, B.; Ahmad, S. Ergonomic design of CNC milling machine for safe working posture. In Proceedings of the 4th International Conference on Mechanical and Manufacturing Engineering (ICME 2013), Bangi Putrajaya, Malaysia, 17–18 December 2013; Ismail, A.E., Nor, N.H.M., Ali, M.F.M., Ahmad, R., Masood, I., Tobi, A.L.M., Ghafir, M.F.A., Muhammad, M., Wahab, M.S., Zain, B.A.M., Eds.; pp. 60–64.
91. Dianat, I.; Salimi, A. Working conditions of Iranian hand-sewn shoe workers and associations with musculoskeletal symptoms. *Ergonomics* **2014**, *57*, 602–611. [CrossRef]
92. Mendes, A.C.; Moreira, J.; Maia, R.; Goncalves, M.A. Ergonomic work analysis of swing arm cutting machine by RULA method. In Proceedings of the 10th Annual Congress of the Portuguese-Society-of-Occupational-Safety-and-Hygiene on Occupational Safety and Hygiene (SPOSHO), Guimaraes, Portugal, 13–14 February 2014; Arezes, P.M., Baptista, J.S., Barroso, M.P., Carneiro, P., Cordeiro, P., Costa, N., Melo, R.B., Miguel, A.S., Perestrelo, G., Eds.; pp. 743–748.
93. Bolzan, G.N.; Freitas, G.S.; Franz, L.A.S. A study regarding the ergonomic conditions in an area of winding transformers. In Proceedings of the 10th Annual Congress of the Portuguese-Society-of-Occupational-Safety-and-Hygiene on Occupational Safety and Hygiene (SPOSHO), Guimaraes, Portugal, 13–14 February 2014; Arezes, P.M., Baptista, J.S., Barroso, M.P., Carneiro, P., Cordeiro, P., Costa, N., Melo, R.B., Miguel, A.S., Perestrelo, G., Eds.; pp. 247–252.
94. Coelho, C.; Oliveira, P.; Maia, E.; Rangel, R.; Dias-Teixeira, M. The importance of ergonomics analysis in prevention of MSDs: Exploratory study in Swedwood-Portugal. In Proceedings of the 10th Annual Congress of the Portuguese-Society-of-Occupational-Safety-and-Hygiene on Occupational Safety and Hygiene (SPOSHO), Guimaraes, Portugal, 13–14 February 2014; Arezes, P.M., Baptista, J.S., Barroso, M.P., Carneiro, P., Cordeiro, P., Costa, N., Melo, R.B., Miguel, A.S., Perestrelo, G., Eds.; pp. 725–729
95. Garcia-Garcia, M.; Sanchez-Lite, A.; Camacho, A.M.; Domingo, R. Analysis of postural assessment methods and virtual simulation tools into manufacturing engineering. *DYNA* **2013**, *80*, 5–15.
96. Vathna, M.; Abdullah, N.S.; Dawal, S.Z.M.; Aoyama, H.; Sothea, K. Investigation on musculoskeletal symptoms and ergonomic risk factors at metal stamping industry. In Proceedings of the 2nd International Conference on Ergonomics (ICE 2013), Kuala Lumpur, Malaysia, 2–4 September 2013; Yusuff, R.M., Ahmad, S.A., Daruis, D.D.I., Deros, B.M., Dawal, S.Z.M., Eds.; p. 293.

97. Berberoglu, U.; Tokuc, B. Work-related musculoskeletal disorders at two textile factories in Edirne, Turkey. *Balk. Med. J.* **2013**, *30*, 23–27. [CrossRef]
98. Yusof, N.; Yusof, R.; Basri, F.M.F.A.; Soin, N. Ergonomic evaluation of postural assessment among "canting" batik workers. In Proceedings of the 2nd International Conference on Ergonomics (ICE 2013), Kuala Lumpur, Malaysia, 2–4 September 2013; Yusuff, R.M., Ahmad, S.A., Daruis, D.D.I., Deros, B.M., Dawal, S.Z.M., Eds.; p. 226.
99. Jaturanonda, C.; Nanthavanij, S.; Das, S.K. Heuristic procedure for the assembly line balancing problem with postural load smoothness. *Int. J. Occup. Saf. Ergo.* **2013**, *19*, 531–541. [CrossRef]
100. Mohamad, D.; Deros, B.M.; Ismail, A.R.; Daruis, D.D.I.; Sukadarin, E.H. RULA analysis of work-related disorder among packaging industry worker using digital human modelong (DHM). In Proceedings of the 2nd International Conference on Ergonomics (ICE 2013), Kuala Lumpur, Malaysia, 2–4 September 2013; Yusuff, R.M., Ahmad, S.A., Daruis, D.D.I., Deros, B.M., Dawal, S.Z.M., Eds.; pp. 9–15.
101. Vignais, N.; Miezal, M.; Bleser, G.; Mura, K.; Gorecky, D.; Marin, F. Innovative system for real-time ergonomic feedback in industrial manufacturing. *Appl. Ergon.* **2013**, *44*, 566–574. [CrossRef]
102. Baptista, J.S.; Costa, J.T.; Conceicao, F.; Vaz, M.; Pinto, S.; Guedes, J.; Silva, J.P. Diagnosis of musculoskeletal disorders in manufacturing workers. In Proceedings of the 9th International Symposium on Occupational Safety and Hygiene (SHO), Guimaraes, Portugal, 14–15 February 2013; Arezes, P., Baptista, J.S., Barroso, M.P., Carneiro, P., Costa, N., Melo, R., Miguel, A.S., Perestrelo, G., Cordeiro, P., Eds.; pp. 49–51.
103. Haggag, H.; Hossnv, M.; Nahavandi, S.; Creighton, D. Real time ergonomic assessment for assembly operations using Kinect. In Proceedings of the UKSim-AMSS 15th International Conference on Computer Modelling and Simulation (UKSim), Cambridge, UK, 10–12 April 2013; AlDabass, D., Orsoni, A., Yunus, J., Cant, R., Ibrahim, Z., Eds.; pp. 495–500.
104. Reis, P.F.; Peres, L.S.; Tirloni, A.S.; dos Reis, D.C.; Estrazulas, J.A.; Rossato, M.; Moro, A.R.P. Influence of anthropometry on meat-packing plant workers: An approach to the shoulder joint. *Work* **2012**, *41*, 4612–4617. [CrossRef] [PubMed]
105. Chiu, Y.C.; Chen, S.; Wu, G.J.; Lin, Y.H. Three-dimensional computer-aided human factors engineering analysis of a grafting robot. *J. Agric. Saf. Health* **2012**, *18*, 181–194. [CrossRef] [PubMed]
106. Miguez, S.A.; Halbeck, M.S.; Vink, P. Participatory ergonomics and new work: Reducing neck complaints in assembling. *Work* **2012**, *41*, 5108–5113. [CrossRef] [PubMed]
107. Miguez, S.A.; Pires, C.R.; Domingues, J.L.R. New ways of working in a notebook manufacturing. In *Advances in Social and Organizational Factors*; Vink, P., Ed.; 2012; pp. 692–700.
108. Naiarkola, S.A.M.; Mirzaei, R. Evaluation of upper limb musculoskeletal loads due to posture, repetition, and force by Rapid Upper Limb Assessment in a textile factory. *Health Scope* **2012**, *1*, 18–24. [CrossRef]
109. Wintachai, P.; Charoenchai, N. The comparison of ergonomics postures assessment methods in rubber sheet production. In Proceedings of the IEEE International Conference on Industrial Engineering and Engineering Management (IEEM), Hong Kong, China, 10–13 December 2012; pp. 1257–1261.
110. Gan, Y.H.; Dai, X.Z. Human-like manipulation planning for articulated manipulator. *J. Bionic. Eng.* **2012**, *9*, 434–445. [CrossRef]
111. Chiasson, M.E.; Imbeau, D.; Aubry, K.; Delisle, A. Comparing the results of eight methods used to evaluate risk factors associated with musculoskeletal disorders. *Int. J. Ind. Ergonom.* **2012**, *42*, 478–488. [CrossRef]
112. Zacharias, F. Knowledge representations for planning manipulation tasks. In *Knowledge Representations for Planning Manipulation Tasks*; 2012; Volume 16, pp. 1–143.
113. Ozturk, N.; Esin, M.N. Investigation of musculoskeletal symptoms and ergonomic risk factors among female sewing machine operators in Turkey. *Int. J. Ind. Ergonom.* **2011**, *41*, 585–591. [CrossRef]
114. Muslim, E.; Nurtjahyo, B.; Ardi, R. Ergonomic analysis of garment industry using Posture Evaluation Index (PEI) in virtual environment. *Makara J. Technol.* **2011**, *15*, 75–81.
115. Monteil, N.R.; Vilas, D.D.; Pereira, D.C.; Prado, R.R. A simulation-based ergonomic evaluation for the operational improvement of the slate splitters work. In Proceedings of the 22nd European Modeling and Simulation Symposium (EMSS), Fes, Morocco, 13–15 October 2010; Bruzzone, A., Frydman, C., Longo, F., Mekouar, K., Piera, M.A., Eds.; pp. 191–200.
116. Lopes, O.; Rosario, R. Ergonomic study of a workplace. In Proceedings of the 6th International Symposium on Occupational Safety and Hygiene (SHO 2010), Guimaraes, Portugal, 11–12 February 2010; Arezes, P., Baptista, J.S., Barroso, M.P., Carneiro, P., Cordeiro, P., Costa, N., Melo, R., Miguel, A.S., Perestrelo, G.P., Eds.; pp. 397–400.

117. Miguez, S.A.; Vink, P.; Hallbeck, M.S. Participatory ergonomics in a mobile factory: Ergonomic device to decrease neck pain. In *Advanced in Occupational, Social, and Organizational Ergonomics*; Vink, P., Kantola, J., Eds.; 2010; pp. 1–9.
118. Jones, T.; Kumar, S. Comparison of ergonomic risk assessment output in four sawmill jobs. *Int. J. Occup. Saf. Ergo.* **2010**, *16*, 105–111. [CrossRef]
119. Eswaramoorthi, M.; John, M.; Rajagopal, C.A.; Prasad, P.S.S.; Mohanram, P.V. Redesigning assembly stations using ergonomic methods as a lean tool. *Work* **2010**, *35*, 231–240. [CrossRef]
120. Jones, T.; Kumar, S. Comparison of ergonomic risk assessment output in a repetitive sawmill occupation: Trim-saw operator. *Work* **2008**, *31*, 367–376. [PubMed]
121. Jones, T.; Kumar, S. Comparison of ergonomic risk assessments in a repetitive high-risk sawmill occupation: Saw-filer. *Int. J. Ind. Ergonom.* **2007**, *37*, 744–753. [CrossRef]
122. Kee, D.; Karwowski, W. A comparison of three observational techniques for assessing postural loads in industry. *Int. J. Occup. Saf. Ergo.* **2007**, *13*. [CrossRef] [PubMed]
123. Carnide, F.; Veloso, A.; Gamboa, H.; Caldeira, S.; Fragoso, I. Interaction of biomechanical and morphological factors on shoulder workload in industrial paint work. *Clin. Biomech.* **2006**, *21*, S33–S38. [CrossRef] [PubMed]
124. Berger, U.; Lepratti, R.; Otte, H. Application of digital human modelling concepts for automotive production. In Proceedings of the 5th International Symposium on Tools and Methods of Competitive Engineering, Lausanne, Switzerland, 13–17 April 2004; Horyath, I., Xirouchakis, P., Eds.; pp. 365–373.
125. Choobineh, A.; Tosian, R.; Alhamdi, Z.; Davarzanie, M. Ergonomic intervention in carpet mending operation. *Appl. Ergon.* **2004**, *35*, 493–496. [CrossRef] [PubMed]
126. Gonzalez, B.A.; Adenso-Diaz, B.; Torre, P.G. Ergonomic performance and quality relationship: An empirical evidence case. *Int. J. Ind. Ergonom.* **2003**, *31*, 33–40. [CrossRef]
127. Brown, R.; Li, G.Y. The development of action levels for the 'quick exposure check' (QEC) system. *Contemp. Ergon.* **2003**, *1*, 41–46.
128. Cakit, E. Assessment of the physical demands of waste collection tasks. *Glob. Nest J.* **2015**, *17*, 426–438.
129. Li, X.M.; Han, S.; Gul, M.; Al-Hussien, M. Automated post-3D visualization ergonomic analysis system for rapid workplace design in modular construction. *Automat. Constr.* **2019**, *98*, 160–174. [CrossRef]
130. Li, X.M.; Han, S.; Gul, M.; Al-Hussein, M.; El- Rich, M. Assessment and Work Modification Framework and its Validation for a Lifting Task. *J. Constr. Eng. Manag.* **2018**, *144*. [CrossRef]
131. Golabchi, A.; Han, S.; Fayek, A.R. A fuzzy logic approach to posture-based ergonomic analysis for field observation and assessment of construction manual operations. *Can. J. Civil Eng.* **2016**, *43*, 294–303. [CrossRef]
132. Shanahan, C.J.; Vi, P.; Salas, E.A.; Reider, V.L.; Hochman, L.M.L.; Moore, A.E. A comparison of RULA, REBA and Strain Index to four psychophysical scales in the assessment of non-fixed work. *Work* **2013**, *45*, 367–378. [CrossRef] [PubMed]
133. Ahmad Nasaruddin, A.F.; Mohd Tamrin, S.B.; Karuppiah, K. The prevalence of musculoskeletal disorder and the association with risk factors among auto repair mechanics in Klang Valley, Malaysia. *Iran. J. Public Health* **2014**, *43*, 34–41.
134. Capodaglio, E.M. Occupational risk and prolonged standing work in apparel sales assistants. *Int. J. Ind. Ergonom.* **2017**, *60*, 53–59. [CrossRef]
135. Peppoloni, L.; Filippeschi, A.; Ruffaldi, E.; Avizzano, C.A. (WMSDs issue) A novel wearable system for the online assessment of risk for biomechanical load in repetitive efforts. *Int. J. Ind. Ergonom.* **2016**, *52*, 1–11. [CrossRef]
136. Rabello, M.V.T.; Costa, D.M.B.; Morgado, C.V. Work-related musculoskeletal disorders in the transportation of dangerous goods. In Proceedings of the 6th International Symposium on Occupational Safety and Hygiene (SHO), Guimaraes, Portugal, 26–27 March 2018; Arezes, P.M., Baptista, J.S., Barroso, M.P., Carneiro, P., Cordeiro, P., Costa, N., Melo, R.B., Miguel, A.S., Perestrelo, G., Eds.; pp. 331–334.
137. Vignais, N.; Bernard, F.; Touvenot, G.; Sagot, J.C. Physical risk factors identification based on body sensor network combined to videotaping. *Appl. Ergon.* **2017**, *65*, 410–417. [CrossRef]
138. Wang, W.; Zhang, W.; Feng, W.J. The astronaut ergonomics assessment methodology in microgravity environment. In Proceedings of the 2nd International Conference on Reliability System Engineering (ICRSE), Beijing, China, 10–12 July 2017.

139. Sayyahi, Z.; Mirzaei, R.; Mirzaei, R. Improving body posture while fueling with a newly designed pump nozzle. *Int. J. Occup. Saf. Ergo.* **2016**, *22*, 327–332. [CrossRef]
140. Balaji, K.K.; Alphin, M.S. Computer-aided human factors analysis of the industrial vehicle driver cabin to improve occupational health. *Int. J. Injury. Control Saf.* **2016**, *23*, 240–248. [CrossRef]
141. Blackwell, C.J.; Wasas, J.S.; Flanagan, S.P.; Norman, B.A.; Haight, J.M. Grocery shelf stocking tool: Analysis of productivity and human factors. *Int. J. Prod. Perform. Manag.* **2016**, *65*, 554–570. [CrossRef]
142. Basahel, A.M. Investigation of work-related musculoskeletal disorders (MSDs) in warehouse workers in Saudi Arabia. In Proceedings of the 6th International Conference on Applied Human Factors and Ergonomics (AHFE), Las Vegas, NV, USA, 26–30 July 2015; Ahram, T., Karwowski, W., Schmorrow, D., Eds.; pp. 4643–4649.
143. Escalona, E.; Hernandez, M.; Yanes, L.; Yanes, L.; Yanes, L. Ergonomic evaluation in a values transportation company in Venezuela. *Work* **2012**, *41*, 710–713. [CrossRef]
144. Ahmed, M.; Campbell-Kyureghyan, N.; Frost, K.; Bertocci, G. Ergonomic evaluation of a wheelchair transportation securement system. *Work* **2012**, *41*, 4924–4930. [CrossRef]
145. Ravnik, D.; Otahal, S.; Fikfak, M.D. Using different methods to assess the discomfort during car driving. *Collegium Antropol.* **2008**, *32*, 267–276.
146. Hoy, J.; Mubarak, N.; Nelson, S.; de Landas, M.S.; Magnusson, M.; Okunribido, O.; Pope, M. Whole body vibration and posture as risk factors for low back pain among forklift truck drivers. *J. Sound. Vib.* **2005**, *284*, 933–946. [CrossRef]
147. Massaccesi, M.; Pagnotta, A.; Soccetti, A.; Masali, M.; Masiero, C.; Greco, F. Investigation of work-related disorders in truck drivers using RULA method. *Appl. Ergon.* **2003**, *34*, 303–307. [CrossRef]
148. Costa, D.M.B.; Ferreira, R.V.; Galante, E.B.F.; Nobrega, J.S.W.; Alves, L.A.; Morgado, C.V. Comparative assessment of work-related musculoskeletal disorders in an industrial kitchen. In Proceedings of the 6th International Symposium on Occupational Safety and Hygiene (SHAO), Guimaraes, Portugal, 26–17 Mars 2018; Arezes, P.M., Baptista, J.S., Barroso, M.P., Carneiro, P., Cordeiro, P., Costa, N., Melo, R.B., Miguel, A.S., Perestrelo, G., Eds.; pp. 325–329.
149. Xu, Y.W.; Cheng, A.S.K. An onsite ergonomics assessment for risk of work-related musculoskeletal disorders among cooks in a Chinese restaurant. *Work* **2014**, *48*, 539–545. [CrossRef] [PubMed]
150. Jones, T.; Strickfaden, M.; Kumar, S. Physical demands analysis of occupational tasks in neighborhood pubs. *Appl. Ergon.* **2005**, *36*, 535–545. [CrossRef]
151. Ekinci, Y.; Uysal, S.A.; Kabak, V.Y.; Duger, T. Does ergonomics training have an effect on body posture during computer usage? *J. Back Musculoskelet.* **2019**, *32*, 191–195. [CrossRef] [PubMed]
152. Levanon, Y.; Lerman, Y.; Gefen, A.; Ratzon, N.Z. Validity of the modified RULA for computer workers and reliability of one observation compared to six. *Ergonomics* **2014**, *57*, 1856–1863. [CrossRef]
153. Rasoulzadeh, Y.; Gholamnia, R. Effectiveness of an ergonomics training program on decreasing work-related musculoskeletal disorders risk among video display terminals users. *Health Promot. Persp.* **2012**, *2*, 89–95. [CrossRef]
154. Fabrizio, P. Ergonomic intervention in the treatment of a patient with upper extremity and neck pain. *Phys. Ther.* **2009**, *89*, 351–360. [CrossRef]
155. Shuval, K.; Donchin, M. Prevalence of upper extremity musculoskeletal symptoms and ergonomic risk factors at a Hi-Tech company in Israel. *Int. J. Ind. Ergonom.* **2005**, *35*, 569–581. [CrossRef]
156. Douglas, G.; Long, R. An observation of adults with visual impairments carrying out copy-typing tasks. *Behav. Inform. Technol.* **2003**, *22*, 141–153. [CrossRef]
157. Dalkilinc, M.; Bumin, G.; Kayihan, H. The effects of ergonomic training and preventive physiotherapy in musculo-skeletal pain. *Pain Clin.* **2002**, *14*, 75–79. [CrossRef]
158. Mohammed, O.; Shell, R.; Swanson, N. Investigating the postural stress associated with sedentary work. In Proceedings of the XIVth Annual International Occupational Ergonomics and Safety Conference 1999, Orlando, FL, USA, 6–9 June 1999; Lee, G.C.H., Ed.; pp. 401–406.
159. Cook, C.J.; Kothival, K. Influence of mouse position on muscular activity in the neck, shoulder and arm in computer users. *Appl. Ergon.* **1998**, *29*, 439–443. [CrossRef]
160. Monteiro, L.F.; Martins, F.A.; Felipe, A.; Mattosinho, C.M.D.; Cavalcanti, S.L.; Santos, M.B.G.; Franca, V.V. Ergonomic problem analysis: Applying the Rapid Upper Limb Assessment method in a hospital of the Paulo Afonso /BA/ Brazil. In Proceedings of the 8th International Symposium on Occupational Safety and Hygiene (SHAO), Guimaraes, Portugal, 9–10 February 2012; Arezes, P., Baptista, J.S., Barroso, M.P., Carneiro, P., Cordeiro, P., Costa, N., Melo, R., Miguel, A.S., Perestrelo, G.P., Eds.; pp. 397–402.

161. Tapia-Araya, A.E.; Uson-Gargallo, J.; Sanchez-Margallo, J.A.; Perez-Duarte, F.J.; Martin-Portugues, I.D.G.; Sanchez-Margallo, F.M. Muscle activity and hand motion in veterinarians performing laparoscopic training tasks with a box trainer. *Am. J. Vet. Res.* **2016**, *77*, 186–193. [CrossRef]
162. Lau, N.; Wong, B. Engineering assessment in biomechanics and ergonomic adoptable for designer at early product design phase. In Proceedings of the 12th World Multi-Conference on Systemics, Cybernetics and Indformatics/14th International Conference on Information Systems Analysis and Synthesis, Orlando, FL, USA, 29 June–2 July 2008; Callaos, N., Lesso, W., Zinn, C.D., Baralt, J., Yoshida, E., Eds.; pp. 124–129.
163. Bazazan, A.; Dianat, I.; Feizollahi, N.; Mombeini, Z.; Shirazi, A.M.; Castellucci, H.I. Effect of a posture correction based intervention on musculoskeletal symptoms and fatigue among control room operators. *Appl. Ergon.* **2019**, *76*, 12–19. [CrossRef] [PubMed]
164. Cavalini, M.A.; Berduszek, R.J.; Van der Sluis, C.K. Construct validity and test-retest reliability of the revised Upper Extremity Work Demands (UEWD-R) Scale. *Occup. Environ. Med.* **2017**, *74*, 763–768. [CrossRef]
165. Rodrigues, M.S.; Leite, R.D.V.; Lelis, C.M.; Chaves, T.C. Differences in ergonomic and workstation factors between computer office workers with and without reported musculoskeletal pain. *Work* **2017**, *57*, 563–572. [CrossRef]
166. Tantuco, J.T.; Mirasol, I.V.O.; Oleta, T.A.C.; Custodio, B.P. Postural analysis and assessment of perceived musculoskeletal pain of cleaners in Metro Manila, Philippines. In Proceedings of the International Conference on Physical Ergonomics and Human Factors, Orlando, FL, USA, 27–31 July 2016; Goonetilleke, R., Karwowski, W., Eds.; pp. 255–263.
167. Joines, S.; James, T.; Liu, S.W.; Wang, W.J.; Dunn, R.; Cohen, S. Adjustable task lighting: Field study assesses the benefits in an office environment. *Work* **2015**, *51*, 471–481. [CrossRef]
168. Dropkin, J.; Kim, H.; Punnet, L.; Wegman, D.H.; Warren, N.; Buchholz, B. Effect of an office ergonomic randomized controlled trial among workers with neck and upper extremity pain. *Occup. Environ. Med.* **2015**, *72*, 6–14. [CrossRef]
169. Quemelo, P.R.V.; Gasparato, F.D.; Vieira, E.R. Prevalence, risks and severity of musculoskeletal disorder symptoms among administrative employees of a Brazilian company. *Work* **2015**, *52*, 533–540. [CrossRef]
170. Macedo, A.C.; Azhena, C.F.; Brito, A.P. A case study of ergonomics encompassing white-collar workers: Anthropometry, furniture dimensions, working posture and musculoskeletal disorders. *Int. J. Work. Condit.* **2014**, *8*, 31–43.
171. Dalkilinc, M.; Kayihan, H. Efficacy of web-based [e-learning] office ergonomics training: A test study. *J. Musculoskelet. Pain* **2014**, *22*, 275–285. [CrossRef]
172. Bell, A.F.; Steele, J.R. Risk of musculoskeletal injury among cleaners during vacuuming. *Ergonomics* **2012**, *55*, 237–247. [CrossRef] [PubMed]
173. Taieb-Maimon, M.; Cwilek, J.; Shapira, B.; Orenstein, I. The effectiveness of a training method using self-modeling webcam photos for reducing musculoskeletal risk among office workers using computers. *Appl. Ergon.* **2012**, *43*, 376–385. [CrossRef] [PubMed]
174. Lima, T.M.; Coelho, D.A. Prevention of musculoskeletal disorders (MSDs) in office work: A case study. *Work* **2011**, *39*, 397–408. [CrossRef] [PubMed]
175. Nam, K.H.; Lee, S.; Kyung, G.; An, J.; An, S. Development of ergonomic gun barrel cleaning method: Automation and its advantages. *Hum. Factor. Ergon. Man.* **2017**, *27*, 243–248. [CrossRef]
176. Gentzler, M.; Stader, S. Posture stress on firefighters and emergency medical technicians (EMTs) associated with repetitive reaching, bending, lifting, and pulling tasks. *Work* **2010**, *37*, 227–239. [CrossRef]
177. Sellschop, I.V.; Myezwa, H.; Mudzi, W.; Musenge, E. Ergonomic behavior of learners in a digitally driven school environment: Modification using an ergonomic intervention programme. *S. Afr. J. Physiother.* **2018**, *74*, a348. [CrossRef]
178. Santiago, J.T.S.; Dizon, P.H.P.; Espina, M.A.C.; Tamayao, M.M. An ergonomic design of senior high school science laboratories in the Philippines. In Proceedings of the AHFE International Conference on Ergonomics in Design, Los Angeles, CA, USA, 17–21 July 2017; Rebelo, F., Soares, M., Eds.; pp. 869–881.
179. Sellschop, I.; Myezwa, H.; Mudzi, W.; Mbambo-Kekana, N. The effect of a computer-related ergonomic intervention program on leaners in a school environment. *Work* **2015**, *51*, 869–877. [CrossRef]
180. Chen, J.D.; Falkmer, T.; Parsons, R.; Buzzard, J.; Ciccarelli, M. Impact of experience when using the Rapid Upper Limb Assessment to assess postural risk in children using information and communication technologies. *Appl. Ergon.* **2014**, *45*, 398–405. [CrossRef]

181. Mirzaei, R.; Naiarkola, S.A.M.; Khanoki, B.A.; Ansari, H. Comparative assessment of upper limbs musculoskeletal disorders by Rapid Upper Limb Assessment among computer users of Zahedan universities. *Health Scope* **2014**, *3*. [CrossRef]
182. Yahya, M.S.; Palaniandy, T.; Zainun, N.Y.; Mohammad, M. Development of Malaysian primary school children anthropometrics data for designing school furniture parameters. In Proceedings of the 4th International Conference on Mechanical and Manufacturing Engineering (ICME 2013), Bangi Putrajaya, Malaysia, 17–18 December 2013; Ismail, A.E., Nor, N.H.M., Ali, M.F.M., Ahmad, R., Masood, I., Tobi, A.L.M., Ghafir, M.F.A., Muhammad, M., Wahab, M.S., Zain, B.A.M., Eds.; p. 1191.
183. Tavafian, S.S.; Zeidi, I.I.M.; Heidarnia, A.R. Theory-based education and postural ergonomic behaviours of computer operators: A randomized controlled trial from Iran. *Turk. Fiz. Tip. Rehab. Dergisi* **2012**, *58*, 312. [CrossRef]
184. Hashim, A.M.; Dawal, S.Z.M.; Yusogg, N. Ergonomic evaluation of postural stress in school workshop. *Work* **2012**, *41*, 827–831. [CrossRef] [PubMed]
185. Muslim, E.; Nurtjahyo, B.; Ardi, R. Ergonomic evaluation of a folding bike design using virtual environment modelling. *Int. J. Technol.* **2011**, *2*, 122–129.
186. Menendez, C.C.; Amick, B.C.; Chang, C.H.; Harrist, R.B.; Jenkins, M.; Robertson, M.; Janowitz, I.; Rempel, D.M.; Katzh, J.N.; Dennerlein, J.T. Evaluation of two posture survey instruments for assessing computing postures among college students. *Work* **2009**, *34*, 421–430. [CrossRef] [PubMed]
187. Kelly, G.; Dockrell, S.; Galvin, R. Computer use in school: Its effect on posture and discomfort in schoolchildren. *Work* **2009**, *32*, 321–328. [CrossRef] [PubMed]
188. Breen, R.; Pyper, S.; Rusk, Y.; Dockrell, S. An investigation of children's posture and discomfort during computer use. *Ergonomics* **2007**, *50*, 1582–1592. [CrossRef]
189. Ratzlaff, T.D.; Diesbourg, T.L.; McAllister, M.J.; von Hacht, M.; Brissette, A.R.; Bona, M.D. Evaluating the efficacy of an educational ergonomics module for improving slit lamp positioning in ophthalmology residents. *Can. J. Ophthalmol.* **2019**, *54*, 159–163. [CrossRef]
190. Van't Hullenaar, C.D.P.; Bos, P.; Broeders, I.A.M.J. Ergonomic assessment of the first assistant during robot-assisted surgery. *J. Robot. Surg.* **2019**, *13*, 283–288. [CrossRef]
191. Garosi, E.; Mazloumi, A.; Kalantri, R.; Vahedi, Z.; Shirzhiyan, Z. Design and ergonomic assessment of an infusion set connector tool used in nursing work. *Appl. Ergon.* **2019**, *75*, 91–98. [CrossRef]
192. Goyil, N.; DeMayo, W.M.; Hirsch, B.E.; McCall, A.A. Patient positioning during in-office otologic procedures impacts physician ergonomics. *Otol. Neurotol.* **2018**, *39*, E883–E888. [CrossRef]
193. Sezgin, D.; Esin, M.N. Effects of a PRECEDE-PROCEED model based ergonomic risk management programme to reduce musculoskeletal symptoms of ICU nurses. *Intens. Crit. Care. Nur.* **2018**, *47*, 89–97. [CrossRef] [PubMed]
194. McLaren, W.; Parrott, L. Do dental students have acceptable working posture? *Brit. Dent. J.* **2018**, *225*, 59–67. [CrossRef] [PubMed]
195. Van't Hullenaar, C.D.P.; Mertens, A.C.; Ruurda, J.P.; Broeders, I.A.M.J. Validation of ergonomic instructions in robot-assisted surgery simulator training. *Surg. Endosc.* **2018**, *32*, 2533–2540. [CrossRef]
196. Li, Z.L.; Baber, C.; Li, F.X.; Macdonald, C.; Godwin, Y. Predicting upper limb discomfort for plastic surgeons wearing loupes based on multi-objective optimization. *Cogent Eng.* **2017**, *4*. [CrossRef]
197. Dabholkar, T.Y.; Yardi, S.S.; Oak, S.N.; Ramchandani, S. Objective ergonomic risk assessment of wrist and spine with motion analysis technique during simulated laparoscopic cholecystectomy in experienced and novice surgeons. *J. Minim. Access. Surg.* **2017**, *13*, 124–130. [CrossRef]
198. Marcon, M.; Pispero, A.; Pignatelli, N.; Lodi, G.; Tubaro, S. Postural assessment in dentistry based on multiple markers tracking. In Proceedings of the 16th IEEE International Conference on Computer Vision (ICCV), Venice, Italy, 22–29 October 2017; pp. 1408–1415.
199. Govil, N.; DeMayo, W.M.; Hirsch, B.E.; McCall, A.A. Optimizing positioning for in-office otology procedures. *Otolaryng. Head Neck* **2017**, *156*, 156–160. [CrossRef]
200. Singh, R.; Carranza, D.; Morrow, M.M.; Vos-draper, T.L.; Mcgree, M.; Weaver, A.; Woolley, S.M.; Hallbeck, S.; Gebhart, J. Effect of different chairs on work-related musculoskeletal discomfort during vaginal surgery. *Am. J. Obstet. Gynecol.* **2016**, *214*, S456–S457. [CrossRef]
201. Bensignor, T.; Morel, G.; Reversat, D.; Fuks, D.; Gayet, B. Evaluation of the effect of a laparoscopic robotized needle hoder on ergonomics and skills. *Surg. Endosc.* **2016**, *30*, 446–454. [CrossRef]

202. Shafti, A.; Lazpita, B.U.; Elhage, O.; Wurdemann, H.A.; Althoefer, K. Analysis of comfort and ergonomics for clinical work environments. In Proceedings of the 38th Annual International Conference of the IEEE-Engineering-in-Medicine-and-Biology-Society (EMBC), Orlando, FL, USA, 16–20 August 2016; Patton, J., Barbieri, R., Ji, J., Jabbari, E., Dokos, S., Mukkamala, R., Guiraud, D., Jovanov, E., Dhaher, Y., Panescu, D., et al., Eds.; pp. 1894–1897.
203. Movahhed, T.; Dehghani, M.; Arghami, S.; Arghami, A. Do dental students have a neutral working posture? *J. Back Musculoskelet.* **2016**, *29*, 859–864. [CrossRef]
204. Carvalho, F.; Melo, R.B.; Costa, V. Ergonomic work analysis of a pathological anatomy service in a portuguese hospital. In Proceedings of the International Conference on Safety Management and Human Factors, Orlando, FL, USA, 27–31 July 2016; Arezes, P., Ed.; pp. 449–462.
205. Rosso, C.B.; Vieira, L.C.; da Silva, S.L.C.; Amaral, F.G. Work analysis of drug-dispensing process in a hospital emergency pharmacy. *Indepen. J. Manag. Prod.* **2016**, *7*, 134–150. [CrossRef]
206. Park, H.S.; Kim, J.; Roh, H.L.; Namkoong, S. Analysis of the risk factors of musculoskeletal disease among dentists induced by work posture. *J. Phys. Ther. Sci.* **2015**, *27*, 3651–3654. [CrossRef] [PubMed]
207. Sezgin, D.; Esin, M.N. Predisposing factors for musculoskeletal symptoms in intensive care unit nurses. *Int. Nurs. Rev.* **2015**, *62*, 92–101. [CrossRef] [PubMed]
208. Tirgar, A.; Javanshir, K.; Talebian, A.; Amini, F.; Parhiz, A. Musculoskeletal disorders among a group of Iranian general dental practitioners. *J. Back Musculoskelet.* **2015**, *28*, 755–759. [CrossRef]
209. Bartnicka, J. Knowledge-based ergonomic assessment of working conditions in surgical ward-A case study. *Saf. Sci.* **2015**, *71*, 178–188. [CrossRef]
210. Rafie, F.; Jam, A.Z.; Shahravan, A.; Raoof, M.; Eskandarizadeh, A. Prevalence of upper extremity musculoskeletal disorders in dentists: Symptoms and risk factors. *J. Environ. Public Health* **2015**. [CrossRef]
211. Corrocher, P.A.; Presoto, C.D.; Campos, J.A.D.B.; Garcia, P.P.N.S. The association between restorative pre-clinical activities and musculoskeletal disorders. *Eur. J. Dent. Educ.* **2014**, *18*, 142–146. [CrossRef]
212. Maulik, S.; Iqbal, R.; De, A.; Chandra, A.M. Evaluation of the working posture and prevalence of musculoskeletal symptoms among medical laboratory technicians. *J. Back Musculoskelet.* **2014**, *27*, 453–461. [CrossRef]
213. Roll, S.C.; Selhorst, L.; Evans, K.D. Contribution of positioning to work-related musculoskeletal discomfort in diagnostic medical sonographers. *Work* **2014**, *47*, 253–260. [CrossRef]
214. Garcia, P.P.N.S.; Polli, G.S.; Campos, J.A.D.B. Working postures of dental students: Ergonomic analysis using the Ovako Working Analysis System and Rapid Upper Limb Assessment. *Med. Lav.* **2013**, *104*, 440–447.
215. Craven, R.; Franasiak, J.; Mosaly, P.; Gehrig, P.A. Ergonomic deficits in robotic gynecologic oncology surgery: A need for intervention. *J. Minim. Invas. Gyn.* **2013**, *20*, 648–655. [CrossRef] [PubMed]
216. Noh, H.; Roh, H. Approach of industrial physical therapy to assessment of the musculoskeletal system and ergonomic risk factors of the dental hygienist. *J. Phys. Ther. Sci.* **2013**, *25*, 821–826. [CrossRef] [PubMed]
217. Hermandon, J.E.; Choi, S.D. Study of musculoskeletal risks of the office-based surgeries. *Work* **2012**, *41*, 1940–1943. [CrossRef] [PubMed]
218. Youssed, Y.; Lee, G.; Godinez, C.; Sutton, E.; Klein, R.V.; George, I.M.; Seagull, F.J.; Park, A. Laparoscopic cholecystectomy poses physical injury risk to surgeons: Analysis of hand technique and standing position. *Surg. Endosc.* **2011**, *25*, 2168–2174. [CrossRef]
219. Sung, P.C.; Lee, H.Y.; Ong, C.C.; Chen, C.Y. An ergonomic intervention of the blood testing task for the prevention of WMSDs. In Proceedings of the 9th Pan-Pacific Conference on Ergonomics (PPCOE, Kaohsiung, Taiwan, 7–10 November 2010; Lin, D.Y.M., Chen, H.C., Eds.; pp. 261–265.
220. Statham, M.M.; Sukits, A.L.; Redfern, M.S.; Smith, L.J.; Sok, J.C.; Rosen, C.A. Ergonomic analysis of microlaryngoscopy. *Laryngoscope* **2010**, *120*, 297–305. [CrossRef]
221. Sanchez-Margallo, F.M.; Sanchez-Margallo, J.A.; Pagador, J.B.; Moyano, J.L.; Moreno, J.; Uson, J. Ergonomic assessment of hand movements in laparoscopic surgery using the Cyberglove (R). In Proceedings of the Computational Biomechanics Medicine IV, London, UK, 24 September 2009; Miller, K., Nielsen, P.M.F., Eds.; p. 121.
222. Taylor-Phillips, S.; Wallis, M.G.; Gale, A.G. Mammography workstation design: Effect on mammographer behavior and the risk of musculoskeletal disorders-art. No. 69171G. In Proceedings of the Medical Imaging 2008 Conference, San Diego, CA, USA, 17–19 February 2008; Sahiner, B., Manning, D.J., Eds.: p. 9171.

223. Gandavadi, A.; Ramsay, J.R.E.; Burke, F.J.T. Assessment of dental student posture in two seating conditions using RULA methodology-a pilot study. *Brit. Dent. J.* **2007**, *203*, 601–605. [CrossRef]
224. Lee, E.C.; Rafiq, A.; Merrell, R.; Ackerman, R.; Dennerlein, J.T. Ergonomics and human factors in endoscopic surgery: A comparison of manual vs telerobotic simulation systems. *Surg. Endosc.* **2005**, *19*, 1064–1070. [CrossRef]
225. Person, J.G.; Hodgson, A.J.; Nagy, A.G. Automated high-frequency posture sampling for ergonomic assessment of laparoscopic surgery. *Surg Endosc-Ultras.* **2001**, *15*, 997–1003. [CrossRef]
226. Kilrov, N.; Dockrell, S. Ergonomic intervention: Its effect on working posture and musculoskeletal symptoms in female biomedical scientists. *Brit. J. Biomed. Sci.* **2000**, *57*, 199–206.
227. Sahu, S.; Moitra, S.; Maity, S.; Pandit, A.K.; Roy, B. A comparative ergonomics postural assessment of potters and sculptors in the unorganized sector in West Bengal, India. *Int. J. Occup. Saf. Ergo.* **2013**, *19*, 455–462. [CrossRef]
228. Kaufman-Cohen, Y.; Ratzon, N.Z. Correlation between risk factors and musculoskeletal disorders among classical musicians. *Occup. Med.* **2011**, *61*, 90–95. [CrossRef] [PubMed]
229. Mukhopadhyay, P.; Sriyastaya, S. Ergonomic design issues in some craft sectors of Jaipur. *Des. J.* **2010**, *13*, 99–124. [CrossRef]
230. Keester, D.L.; Sommerich, C.M. Investigation of musculoskeletal discomfort, work postures, and muscle activation among practicing tattoo artist. *Appl. Ergon.* **2017**, *58*, 137–143. [CrossRef] [PubMed]
231. Mukhopadhyay, P.; Jhodkar, D.; Kumar, P. Ergonomic risk factors in bicycle repairing units at Jabalpur. *Work* **2015**, *51*, 245–254. [CrossRef] [PubMed]
232. Oliveira, A.C.; Silva, R.; Domingues, J.P. Work-related musculoskeletal disorders in balneotherapy practitioners. In Proceedings of the 7th International Symposium on Occupational Safety and Hygiene (SHO), Guimaraes, Portugal, 10–11 February 2011; Arezes, P., Baptista, J.S., Barroso, M.P., Carneiro, P., Cordeiro, P., Costa, N., Melo, R., Miguel, A.S., Perestrelo, G.P., Eds.; pp. 447–451.
233. San Antonio, T.; Urrutia, F.; Larrea, A. Ergonomic analysis for people with physical disbilities when the wheelchair is considered as their workstation. In Proceedings of the IEEE Ecuador Technical Chapters Meeting (ETCM), Guayaquil, Ecuador, 12–14 October 2016.
234. Apostoli, P.; Sala, E.; Curti, S.; Cooke, R.M.T.; Violante, F.S.; Mattioli, S. Loads of housework? Biomechanical assessments of the upper limbs in women performing common household tasks. *Int. Arch. Occup. Environ. Health* **2012**, *85*, 421–425. [CrossRef] [PubMed]
235. Marino, C.; Santana, R.; Vargas, J.; Morales, L.; Cisneros, L. Reliability and validity of postural evaluations with Kinect v2 sensor ergonomic evaluation system. In Proceedings of the 6th Conference on Information and Communication Technologies of Ecuador (TIC-EC), Riobamba, Ecuador, 21–23 November 2018; BottoTobar, M., BarbaMaggi, L., GonzalezHuerta, J., VillacresCevallos, P., Gomez, O.S., UyidiaFassler, M.I., Eds.; pp. 86–99.
236. Valentim, D.P.; Sato, T.D.; Comper, M.L.C.; da Silva, A.M.; Boas, C.V.; Padula, R.S. Reliability, construct validity and interpretability of the Brazilian version of the Rapid Upper Limb Assessment (RULA) and Strain Index (SI). *Braz. J. Phys. Ther.* **2018**, *22*, 198–204. [CrossRef] [PubMed]
237. Halim, I.; Umar, R.Z.R.; Ahmad, N.; Jamli, M.R.; Mohamed, M.S.S.; Albawab, T.M.M.; Abdullah, M.H.L.; Padmanathan, V. Usability study of integrated RULA.-Kinect (TM) system for work posture assessment. *Int. J. Integr. Eng.* **2018**, *10*, 175–184. [CrossRef]
238. Umar, R.Z.R.; Ling, C.F.; Ahmad, N.; Halim, I.; Lee, F.A.M.A.; Abdullasim, N. Initial validation of RULA-Kinect system-comparing assessment results between system and human assessors. In Proceedings of the 5th Mechanical Engineering Research Day (MERD), Melaka, Malaysia, 3 May 2018; BinAbdollah, M.F., Ed.; pp. 67–68.
239. Namwongsa, S.; Puntumetakul, R.; Neubert, M.S.; Chaiklieng, S.; Boucaut, R. Ergonomic risk aassessment of smartphone users using the Rapid Upper Limb Assessment (RULA) tool. *PLoS ONE* **2018**, *13*, e0203394. [CrossRef]
240. Plantard, P.; Shum, H.P.H.; Le Pierres, A.S.; Multon, F. Validation of an ergonomic assessment method using Kinect data in real workplace conditions. *Appl. Ergon.* **2017**, *65*, 562–569. [CrossRef]
241. Can, G.F.; Figlali, N. Image processing based rapid upper limb assessment method. *J. Fac. Eng. Archit. Gazi Univ.* **2017**, *32*, 719–731. [CrossRef]

242. Manghisi, V.M.; Uva, A.E.; Fiorentino, M.; Bevilacqua, V.; Trotta, G.F.; Monno, G. Real time RULA assessment using Kinect v2 sensor. *Appl. Ergon.* **2017**, *65*, 481–491. [CrossRef] [PubMed]
243. Son, M.; Jung, J.; Park, W. Evaluating the utility of two gestural discomfort evaluation methods. *PLoS ONE* **2017**, *12*. [CrossRef] [PubMed]
244. Nahavandi, D.; Hossny, M. Skeleton-free task-specific Rapid Upper Limb ergonomic assessment using depth imaging sensors. In Proceedings of the 15th IEEE Sensors Conference, Orlando, FL, USA, 30 October–3 November 2016.
245. Ciccarelli, M.; Chen, J.D.; Vaz, S.; Cordier, R.; Falkmer, T. Managing children's postural risk when using mobile technology at home: Challenges and strategies. *Appl. Ergon.* **2015**, *51*, 189–198. [CrossRef] [PubMed]
246. Plantard, P.; Auvinet, E.; Le Pierres, A.S.; Multon, F. Pose estimation with a Kinect for ergonomic studies: Evaluation of the accuracy using a virtual mannequin. *Sensors* **2015**, *15*, 1785–1803. [CrossRef] [PubMed]
247. Razavi, H.; Behbudi, A. Ergonomic assessment and design of electronic ticket booths in Mashhad city. *J. Health Saf. Work* **2015**, *5*, 5.
248. Chihara, T.; Seo, A.; Izumi, T. Total perceived discomfort function for upper limbs based on joint moment. *J. Adv. Simulat. Sci. Eng.* **2014**, *1*, 36–50. [CrossRef]
249. Chen, Y.L.; Chiang, H.T. A tilt rolling movement of a gas cylinder: A case study. *Work* **2014**, *49*, 473–481. [CrossRef]
250. Son, M.; Park, W.; Jung, J.; Hwang, D.; Park, J. Utilizing sign language gestures for gesture-based interaction: A usability evaluation study. *Int. J. Ind. Eng. Theory* **2013**, *20*, 548–561.
251. Dockrell, S.; O'Grady, E.; Bennett, K.; Mullarkey, C.; McConnell, R.; Ruddy, R.; Twomey, S.; Flannery, C. An investigation of the reliability of Rapid Upper Limb Assessment (RULA) as a method of assessment of children's computing posture. *Appl. Ergon.* **2012**, *43*, 632–636. [CrossRef]
252. Schlette, C.; Rossmann, J. Motion control strategies for humanoids based on ergonomics. In Proceedings of the 4th International Conference on Intelligent Robotics and Applications (ICIRA 2011), Aachen, Germany, 6–8 December 2011; Jeschke, S., Liu, H.H., Schilberg, D., Eds.; pp. 229–240.
253. Goncalves, P.J.S.; Fernandes, N.O.G. A semi-automatic system for posture risk assessment. In Proceedings of the 16th Annual Scientific Conference on Web Technology, New Media Communications and Telematic Theory Methods, Tools and Applications, London, UK, 18–20 April 2011; AlSaedy, H., Ed.; pp. 64–69.
254. Pires, C.; Lima, F. The contribution of ergonomics in the safety of machinery and equipment. In Proceedings of the 7th International Symposium on Occupational Safety and Hygiene (SHO), Guimaraes, Portugal, 10–11 February 2011; Arezes, P., Baptista, J.S., Barroso, M.P., Carneiro, P., Cordeiro, P., Costa N., Melo, R., Miguel, A.S., Perestrelo, G.P., Eds.; pp. 527–531.
255. Goncalves, P.J.S.; Fernandes, N.O. RULAmatic—A semi-automatic posture recognition system for RULA risk evaluation method. In Proceedings of the 2nd International Conference on Innovations, Recent Trends and Challenges in Mechatronics, Mechanical Engineering and New High-Tech Products Development (MECAHITECH), Bucharest, Romania, 23–24 September 2010; pp. 266–271.
256. Apostoli, P.; Sala, E. Evidence of work-related musculoskeletal disorders of the upper extremities and current methods of risk assessment: Can Charlie Chaplin give us any suggestions in "Modern Times". *La Medicina del lavoro* **2009**, *100*, 384–395.
257. Ward, J.; Riley, C.; Johnson, G. Posture, position & biometrics: Guidelines for self-service technology. In Proceedings of the Annual Meeting of the Ergonomics-Society, Nottingham, UK; Bust, P.D., Ed.; 2008; pp. 121–126.
258. McGorry, R.W.; Lin, J.H. Power grip strength as a function of tool handle orientation and location. *Ergonomics* **2007**, *50*, 1392–1403. [CrossRef] [PubMed]
259. Bao, S.; Howard, N.; Spielholz, P.; Silverstein, B. Two posture analysis approaches and their application in a modified Rapid Upper Limb Assessment evaluation. *Ergonomics* **2007**, *50*, 2118–2136. [CrossRef] [PubMed]
260. Lopez-Aragon, L.; Lopez-Liria, R.; Callejon-Ferre, A.J.; Gomez-Galan, M. Applications of the Standardized Nordic Questionnaire: A review. *Sustainability* **2017**, *9*, 1514. [CrossRef]
261. Hita-Gutierrez, M.; Gomez-Galan, M.; Diaz-Perez, M.; Callejon-Ferre, A.J. An overview of REBA method applications in the world. *Int. J. Environ. Res. Public Health* **2020**, *17*, 2635. [CrossRef]
262. Zink, K.J. Designing sustainable work systems: The need for a systems approach. *Appl. Ergon.* **2014**, *45*, 126–132. [CrossRef]

263. Haslam, R.; Waterson, P. Ergonomics and Sustainability. *Ergonomics* **2013**, *56*, 343–347. [CrossRef]
264. Gomez-Galan, M.; Callejon-Ferre, A.J.; Perez-Alonso, J.; Diaz-Perez, M.; Golasi, I. Repetitive movements in melon cultivation workers under greenhouses. *Agriculture* **2019**, *9*, 236. [CrossRef]

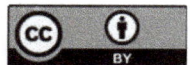

© 2020 by the authors. Licensee MDPI, Basel, Switzerland. This article is an open access article distributed under the terms and conditions of the Creative Commons Attribution (CC BY) license (http://creativecommons.org/licenses/by/4.0/).

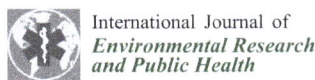 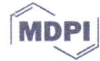

Article

Current State and Future Trends: A Citation Network Analysis of the Academic Performance Field

Clara Martinez-Perez *, Cristina Alvarez-Peregrina, Cesar Villa-Collar and Miguel Ángel Sánchez-Tena

School of Biomedical and Health Science, Universidad Europea de Madrid, 28670 Madrid, Spain; cristina.alvarez@universidadeuropea.es (C.A.-P.); villacollarc@gmail.com (C.V.-C.); miguelangel.sanchez@universidadeuropea.es (M.Á.S.-T.)
* Correspondence: claramarperez@hotmail.com

Received: 6 June 2020; Accepted: 22 July 2020; Published: 24 July 2020

Abstract: *Background*: In recent years, due to its complexity and relevance, academic performance has become a controversial research topic within the health and educational field. The main purposes of this study were to analyze the links between publications and authors via citation networks, to identify the different research areas and to determine the most cited publications. *Methods*: The publication search was performed through the Web of Science database, using the term "Academic Performance" for a time interval from 1952 to 2019. The software used to analyze the publications was the Citation Network Explorer. *Results*: We found a total of 16,157 publications with 35,213 citations generated in the network, and 2018 had the highest number of publications of any year. The most cited publication was published in 2012 by Richardson et al. with a citation index score of 352. By using the clustering function, we found nine groups related to different areas of research in this field: health, psychology, psychosociology, demography, physical activity, sleep patterns, vision, economy, and delinquency. *Conclusions*: The citation network showed the main publications dealing with the different factors that affect academic performance, and it was determined that psychological and psychosocial factors were the most relevant.

Keywords: academic performance; citation network; motivation

---

1. Introduction

Academic performance is frequently associated with a country's social and economic development [1]. Numerous studies have concurred that academic achievements are the result of cognitive and non-cognitive abilities, as well as the socio-cultural environment in which the learning takes place [2,3]. In this sense, academic performance is associated with intellectual factors, for example, long-term memory or the ability to think abstractly, and non-intellectual factors, such as motivation or self-discipline [4].

Motivation is an internal condition that influences behavior, i.e., mental power that helps people to meet their goals and achieve academic success [5–7]. To be able to motivate students, it is important to instill in them a greater desire to learn and make them enjoy studying. It has been proved that unmotivated students are not interested in learning or participating in class, and this attitude will affect their academic performance [6].

Scientific literature supports that cognitive abilities and self-efficacy can predict academic performance outcomes [8,9]. In 1983, Gardner explained [10] that self-sufficient people can organize themselves and carry out actions to meet their goals.

Furthermore, psychosocial wellbeing is strongly related to thoughts, motivation, and decision-making relating to academic effort [11,12]. According to Vilar et al., a poor psychosocial status may be the result of a poor socio-economic situation, unfavorable family circumstances, or a bad relationship with classmates [13]. Students in these situations tend to have a negative attitude towards school and the learning process. This results in a low level of self-discipline and bad performance. In contrast, students with a positive psychosocial dynamic tend to have a high socioeconomic level and a good family relationship. They are also optimistic and have a good attitude at school.

Other factors related to good performance at school include a healthy diet (rich in fiber and nutrients); practicing physical activity (as this increases metabolism, oxygenation and blood flow, delivering the hormones that promote neurological health); sleeping well (which improves cognitive functions, such as memory and learning) and good vision (visual impairment harms the development of motor skills, cognition, and language in child development) [14–17].

Citation network analysis is used to search for a specific topic within the scientific literature. By analyzing one publication, it is possible to find other relevant additional publications, to demonstrate, qualitatively, and quantitatively, the connections between articles and authors by creating groups [18]. Furthermore, it is also possible to quantify the most cited publications in each group, to study the development of a research field, or to focus the literature search on a specific topic [19,20].

Given the numerous factors that affect academic performance, this study aimed to identify the different areas of research and to discover the most cited publications. The connection between publications and research groups was also analysed using CitNetExplorer, software which enables the study of how the scientific literature in a particular field of has evolved.

2. Materials and Methods

2.1. Data Source

The search was performed using the Web of Science (WOS) database, by entering the main descriptor: "Academic performance", as this is the most commonly used expression in both fields, education and health. The search was limited to a topical search (TS) on article, keywords, and abstract, linked with the OR Table. Time was limited to the interval 1952–2019.

Likewise, the Web of Science database allows the adding of references to its library when performing bibliographical searches directly in external databases or library catalogues.

With regards to the citation indices, the Social Sciences Citation Index, Science Citation Index Expanded and Emerging Sources Citation Index were used.

On the other hand, and due to the differences in citation styles among authors and institutions, CiteSpace software was used with a view to standardizing the data. The search and download date of the publications was the 25 April 2020.

2.2. Data Analyisis

All the publications were analyzed using the Citation Network Explorer software. This software is used for analyzing and visualizing the citation networks of scientific publications. It allows the researcher to download citation networks directly from Web of Science. Likewise, it makes it possible to manage citation networks which include millions of publications and related citations. In this way, a citation network comprising millions of publications can be initiated so a deeper analysis can then be performed in order to obtain a smaller subnetwork of 100 publications on the same topic.

By using the citation score as an attribute, a quantitative analysis of the most cited publications within a specific time interval was performed. Through this, internal connections within the WOS database were quantified. By considering other databases, included in the WOS, the external connections were also quantified [20].

CitNetExplorer offers a number of techniques to analyze the citation networks of publications. The clustering function is achieved using the formula developed by Van Eck in 2012 [20].

$$V(c_1,\ldots,c_n) = \sum_{i<j} \delta\left(c_i,c_j\right)\left(s_{ij}-\gamma\right) \quad (1)$$

The clustering function was used to establish a group for each publication. This function grouped those publications with a greater level of association according to the citation networks [20].

Finally, the central publications were analyzed using the Identifying Core Publications function. The role of this function was to identify the publications that were considered as the core of the citation network and eliminate those which were considered insignificant. The number of connections was established by the researchers, meaning therefore that the greater this parameter was, the lower the number of central publications would be [20]. Thus, those publications that presented four or more citations within the citations network were considered.

On the other hand, the drilling down function was used, as it allows deep analysis to be carried out at different levels for each of the groups.

3. Results

The first articles on academic performance were published in 1952, so therefore it was decided that the selected time interval would be from 1952 to 2019. 16,157 publications and 35,213 citations inside the WOS were found. Out of all the publications, 77.62% were articles, 13.5% proceedings papers, 3.75% reviews, 2.16% meeting abstracts, 1.61% book chapters and the remaining 1.01% was comprised of editorial materials, letters, notes, book reviews, corrections, books, data papers, news items, reprints, amendments, additions and retracted publications.

The number of publications on this topic has increased significantly since 2015 (1952–2014: 46.77% of publications; 2015–2019: 53.23% of publications). 2018 was the year with the highest number of publications, with 1889 publications and 120 citations on the network (Figure 1).

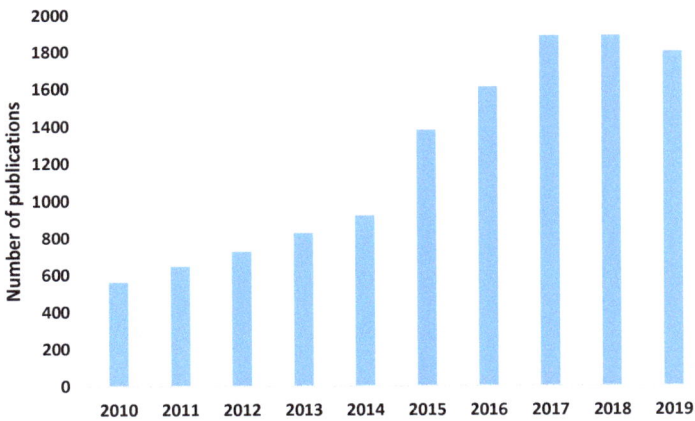

Figure 1. Number of publications per year.

Figure 2 shows the citation network and Table 1 all the details of the 20 most-cited publications. The first was an article by Richardson et al. [21], which was published in 2012 and boasted a citation index of 352. This work was a systematic review and meta-analysis of the years between 1997 and 2010 that analyzed 7167 articles on different demographic and psychosocial factors that influence academic performance in university students.

Table 1. Details of the 20 most cited publications on academic performance.

Author	Title	Year	Total Citation	Citation Rate
Richardson et al. [21]	Psychological correlates of university students' academic performance: A systematic review and meta-analysis.	2012	352	50.28
Pintrich et al. [22]	Motivational and self-regulated learning components of classroom academic performance.	1990	344	11.86
Poropat [23]	A meta-analysis of the five-factor model of personality and academic performance	2009	270	24.54
Robbins et al. [24]	Do Psychosocial and Study Skill Factors Predict College Outcomes? A Meta-Analysis	2004	239	14.94
Chamorro-Premuzic et al. [25]	Personality predicts academic performance: Evidence from two longitudinal university samples	2003	179	11.19
Duckworth et al. [26]	Self-Discipline Outdoes IQ in Predicting Academic Performance of Adolescents	2005	165	11.78
O'Connor et al. [27]	Big Five personality predictors of post-secondary academic performance	2007	159	13.25
Kirschner et al. [28]	Facebook® and academic performance	2010	127	14.11
Curcio et al. [29]	Sleep loss, learning capacity and academic performance	2006	126	9.69
Ferguson et al. [30]	Factors associated with success in medical school: systematic review of the literature	2002	125	7.35
Chemers et al. [31]	Academic self-efficacy and first year college student performance and adjustment.	2001	122	6.78
Kuncel et al. [32]	Academic Performance, Career Potential, Creativity, and Job Performance: Can One Construct Predict Them All?	2004	112	7.47
Hillman et al. [33]	Be smart, exercise your heart: exercise effects on brain and cognition	2008	104	9.45
Castelli et al. [34]	Physical Fitness and Academic Achievement in Third- and Fifth-Grade Students	2007	103	8.58
Trockel et al. [35]	Health-Related Variables and Academic Performance Among First-Year College Students: Implications for Sleep and Other Behaviors	2000	98	5.16
Chapell et al. [36]	Test Anxiety and Academic Performance in Undergraduate and Graduate Students	2005	95	6.78
Cassady et al. [37]	Cognitive Test Anxiety and Academic Performance	2002	94	5.53
Wolfson et al. [38]	Understanding adolescents' sleep patterns and school performance: a critical appraisal	2003	94	5.87
Rampersaud et al. [39]	Breakfast Habits, Nutritional Status, Body Weight, and Academic Performance in Children and Adolescents	2005	94	6.71
Dyrbye et al. [40]	Systematic Review of Depression, Anxiety, and Other Indicators of Psychological Distress Among U.S. and Canadian Medical Students	2006	94	7.23

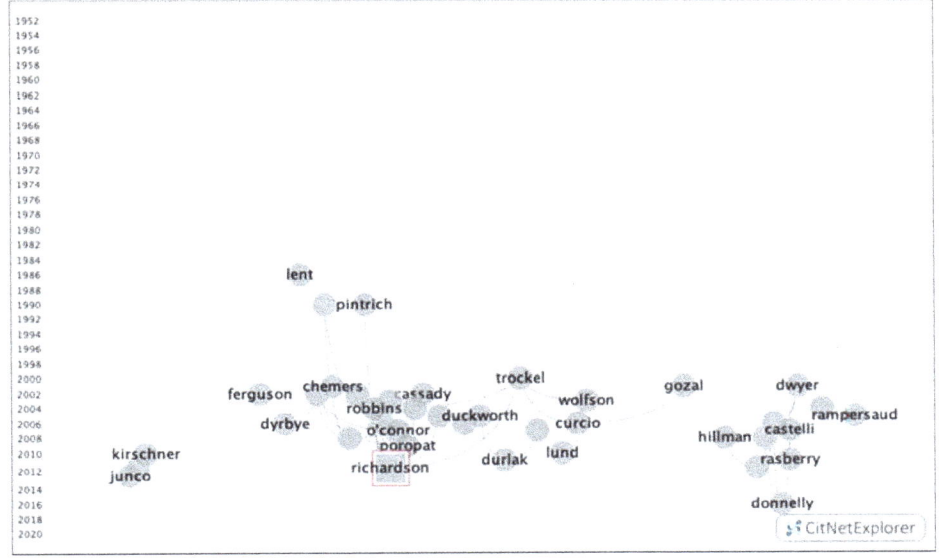

Figure 2. Citation Network of the 20 most cited publications on academic performance.

Out of the 20 most-cited articles, 11 dealt with the psychological factors that affect academic performance [21–27,31,32,36,37]. Two of the articles discussed how demographic and cognitive factors and personality can predict future academic performance [30,40]. Three articles addressed the benefits that healthy lifestyles have on academic performance [33,34,39]. The impact of sleep on academic performance was considered in three of the articles [29,35,38] and the final article focused on how the use of digital devices and social media affects academic performance [28].

3.1. Description of the Publications.

Academic performance is a multidisciplinary research field and the areas of education (36%) and psychology (28.24%) (Figure 3) are particularly worth mentioning. Figure 4 shows the 10 journals with the highest number of publications.

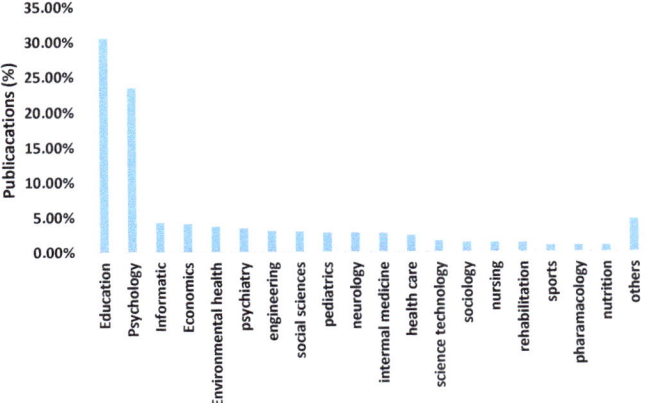

Figure 3. Percentage of publications by research field.

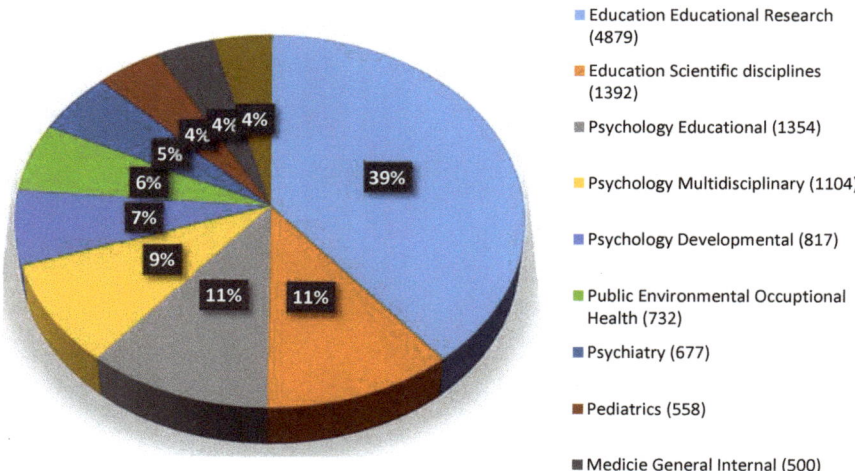

Figure 4. Top ten journals with the most publications.

The countries with the highest number of publications are the United States (39.10%), Spain (8.51%) and England (5.54%) (Figure 5).

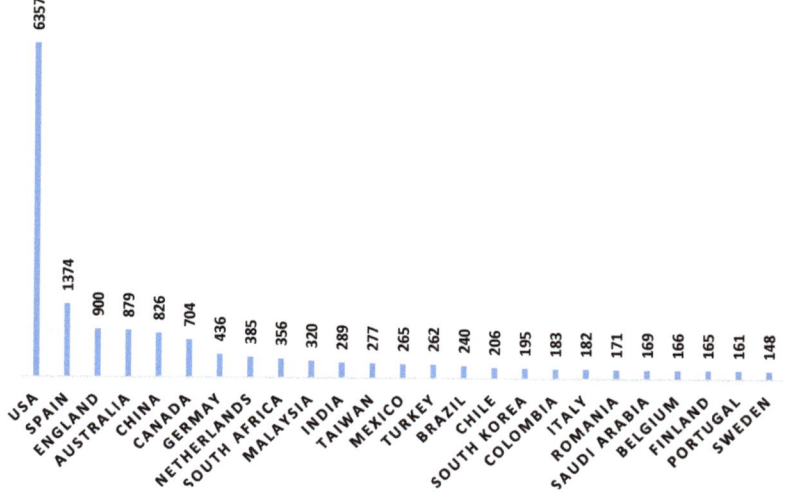

Figure 5. Number of publications by country.

3.2. Clustering Function

23 groups were found using the clustering function, with 9 of these groups containing a significant number of publications; however, the remaining 14 groups only reached 1.5% (Figure 6).

With regards to clustering parameters, a resolution value of 1.0 (default value in CitNetExplorer software) was considered, and the minimal publication size for each group was 500.

Table 2 shows the information from the citation networks on the nine main groups, ordered from largest to smallest according to their size.

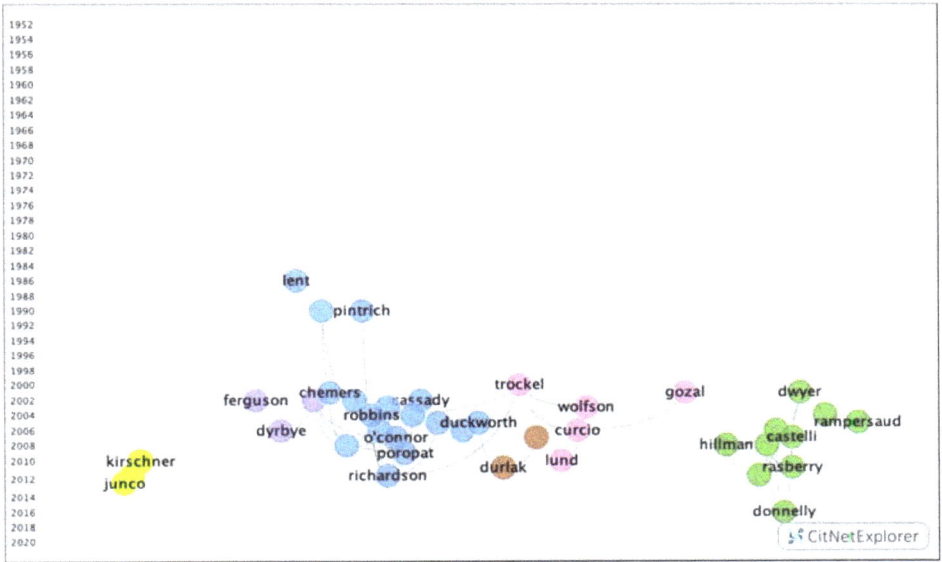

Figure 6. Clustering function in the network of citations on academic performance.

Table 2. Citation network information on the nine main groups.

Main Cluster	Number of Publications	Number of Citation Links	Number of Citations Median (Range)	Number of Publications with ≥4 Citations	Number of Publications in 100 Most Cited Publication
Group 1	3223	11,097	1 (0–352)	1734	47
Group 2	1094	4407	1 (0–104)	481	22
Group 3	971	2638	1 (0–125)	494	5
Group 4	777	1356	1 (0–35)	461	1
Group 5	734	1567	1 (0–55)	456	2
Group 6	665	1107	1 (0–21)	489	2
Group 7	640	2407	1 (0–126)	256	12
Group 8	619	1587	1 (0–35)	409	0
Group 9	591	1772	1 (0–127)	329	9

In group 1, 3223 articles and 11,097 citations were found across the network. The most cited publication was the article by Richardson et al. [21], which was published in 2012 in the Psychological Bulletin, and it also ranked first among the 20 most cited publications. In this group, the different articles analyzed the impact of personality, cognitive ability, self-discipline, motivation, and demographic and psychosocial factors on academic performance (Figure 7).

In group 2, 1095 publications and 4407 citations were found across the network. The most cited publication in this group was the article by Hillman et al. [33], which was published in 2008 in Nature Reviews Neuroscience. In this article, the authors concluded that physical exercise leads to greater physical and mental health throughout life. The articles in group 2 dealt with the influence of visual impairments, such as uncorrected refractive errors, on academic performance. The articles in this group also analyzed the association between the number of hours spent watching television and obesity, as well as the positive impact that a healthy lifestyle, such as a healthy diet or practicing physical exercise, has on cognitive skills and academic performance (Figure 8).

In group 3, 971 publications and 2638 citations were found across the network. The most cited publication was the article by Ferguson et al. [30], which was published in 2002 in the British Medical

Journal. This paper analyzed the requirements for predicting future academic performance, such as previous academic ability, personality, learning, or personal references. The common topic in this group was how personality, demographic data, and mental (depression, anxiety, and stress) and emotional (motivation) states influence academic performance. These papers also considered the academic selection process, focusing specifically on careers in the field of health (Figure 9).

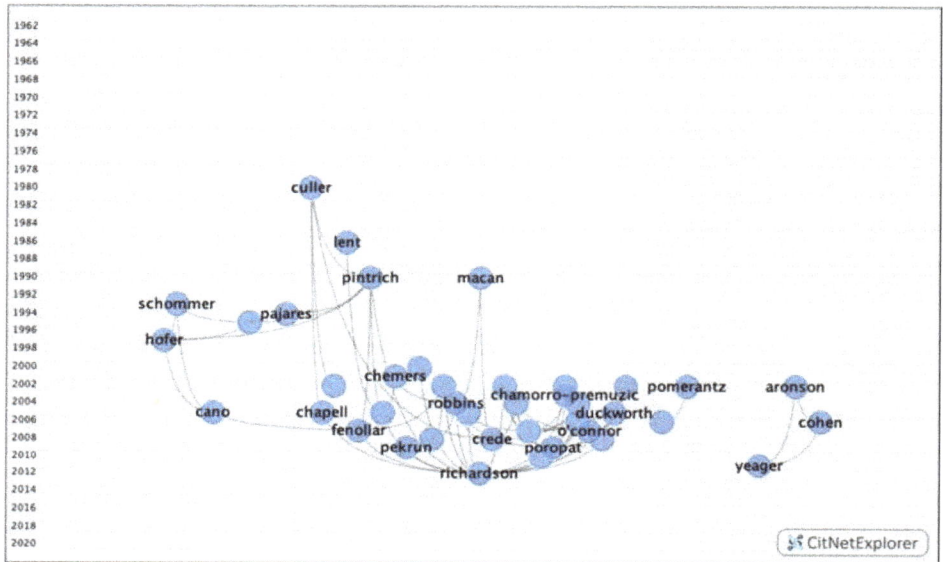

Figure 7. Group 1 citation network.

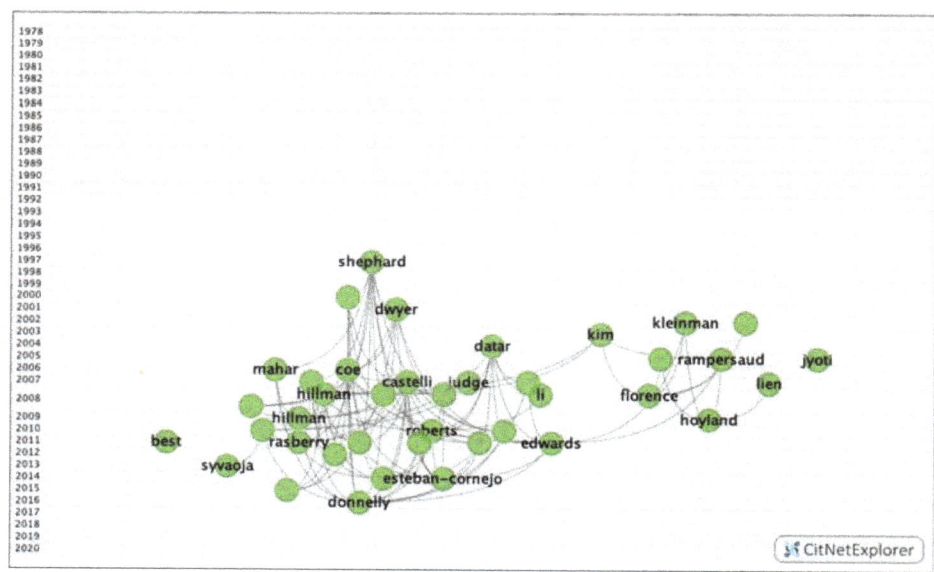

Figure 8. Group 2 citation network.

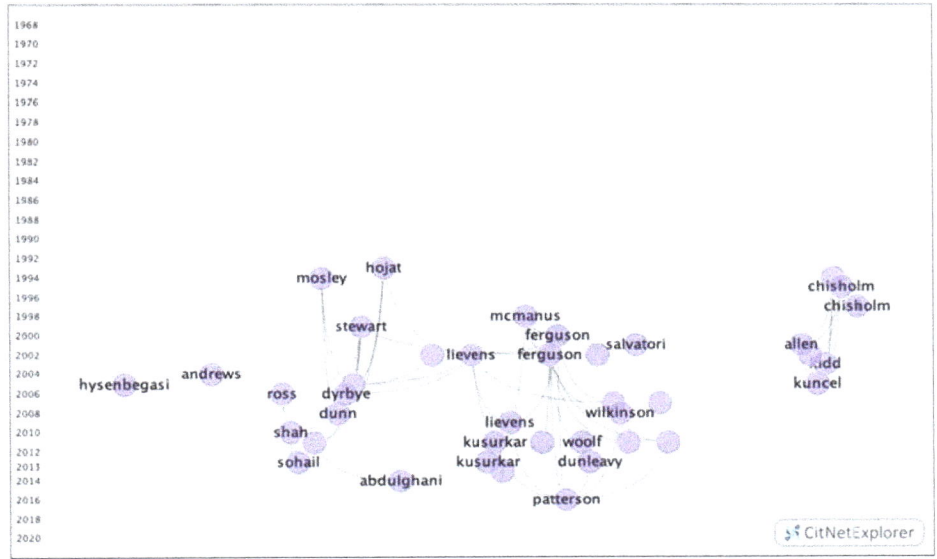

Figure 9. Group 3 citation network.

In group 4, 776 publications and 1354 citations were found throughout the network. The most cited publication was the article by Fuligni et al. [41], which was published in 1997 in Child Development. This article analyzed how family background, parental attitudes, and peer support influence the academic performance of immigrant students. The common theme in this group was the influence of psychosocial and economic factors, such as family, teachers, peers, gender, or corrected refractive errors on academic performance (Figure 10).

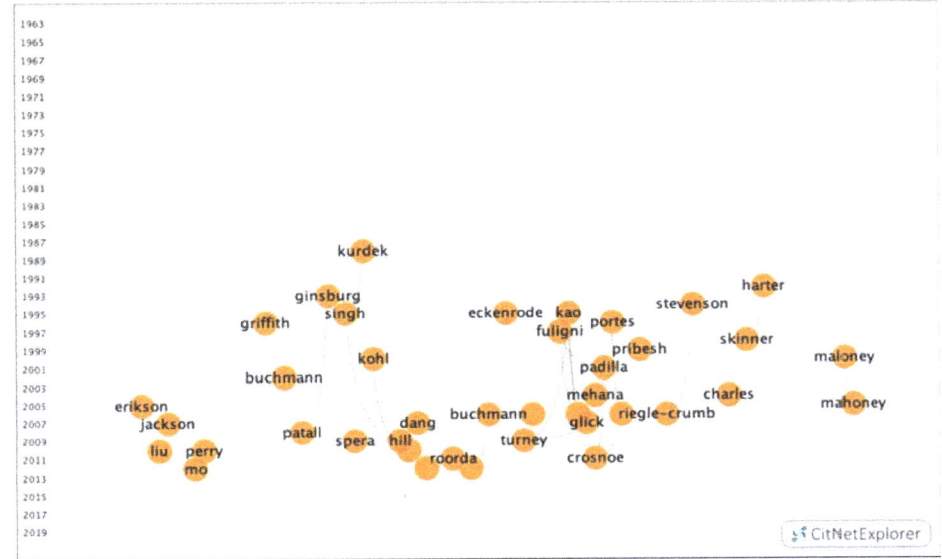

Figure 10. Group 4 citation network.

In group 5, 734 publications and 1567 citations were found throughout the network. The most cited publication was the article by Crede et al. [42], which was published in 2010 in Review of Educational Research. In this publication, the authors concluded that class attendance has a positive impact on grades. The common subject in group 5 was the relationship between students who attend class and those who work, and the impact of this on academic performance (Figure 11).

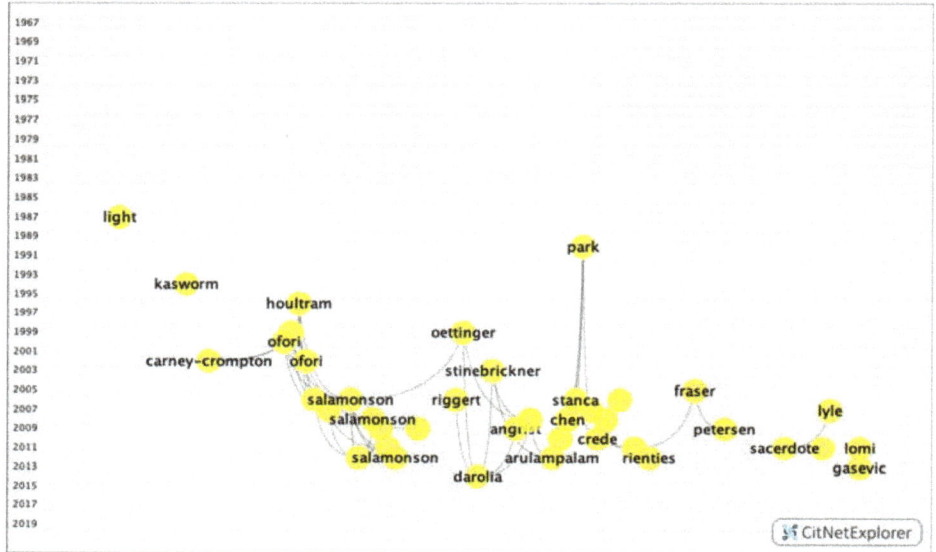

Figure 11. Group 5 citation network.

In group 6, 665 publications and 1107 citations were found throughout the network. The most cited publication was an article by Duncan et al. [43], which was published in 2007 in Developmental Psychology. In this article, the authors analyzed cognitive, attention, and socio-emotional skills in terms of academic performance. The common topic in this group was the relationship between the said skills, drug use, bullying, and delinquency, and academic performance (Figure 12).

In group 7, 640 publications and 2407 citations were found throughout the network. The most cited publication was an article by Curcio et al. [29], which was published in 2006 in the journal Sleep Medicine Reviews. In this publication, the authors analyzed the impact of sleep on academic performance. The common topic addressed by this group was the impact of sleep and stress on academic performance (Figure 13).

In group 8, 619 publications and 1587 citations were found throughout the network. The most cited publication was an article by Dupaul et al. [44], which was published in 1991 in School Psychology Review. This study analyzed the academic performance of children with behavioral disorders. The common topic in this group was how hyperactivity disorders influence academic performance (Figure 14).

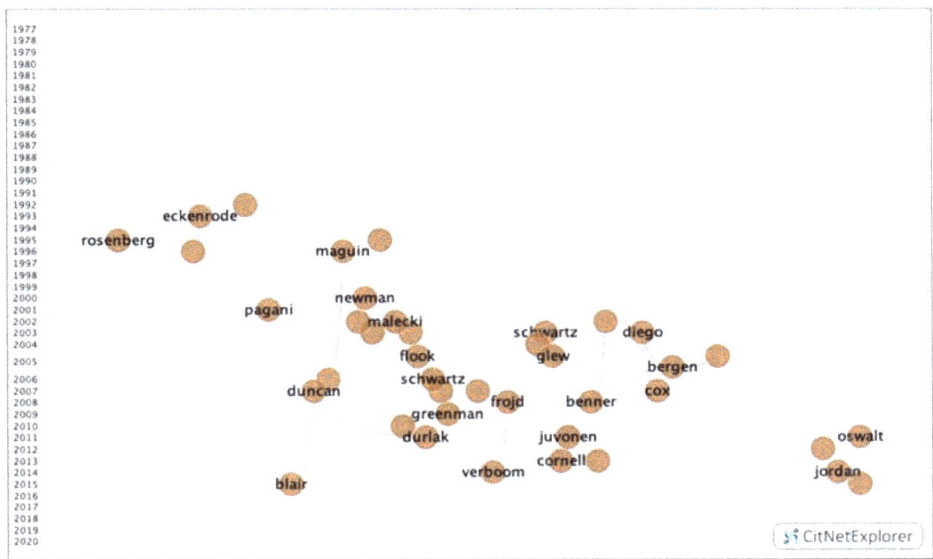

Figure 12. Group 6 citation network.

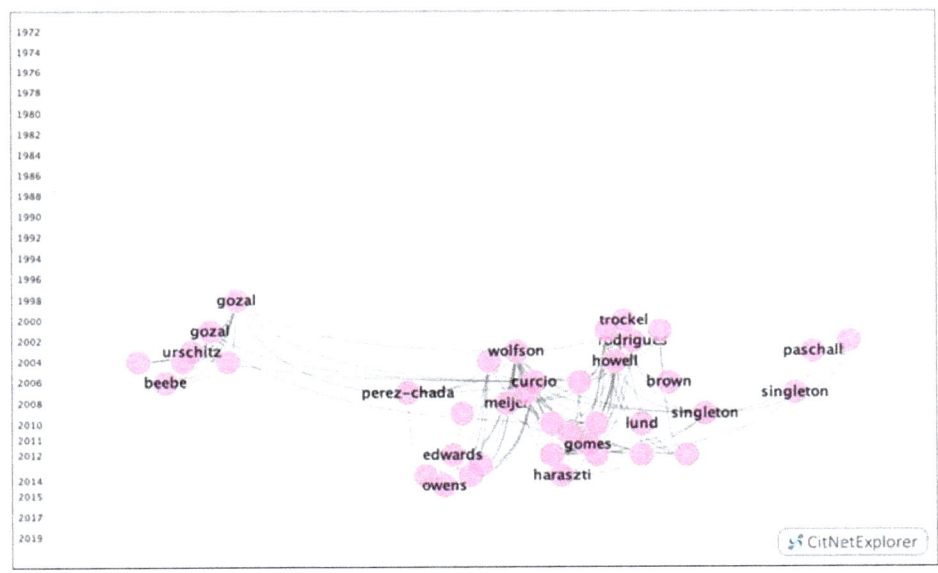

Figure 13. Group 7 citation network.

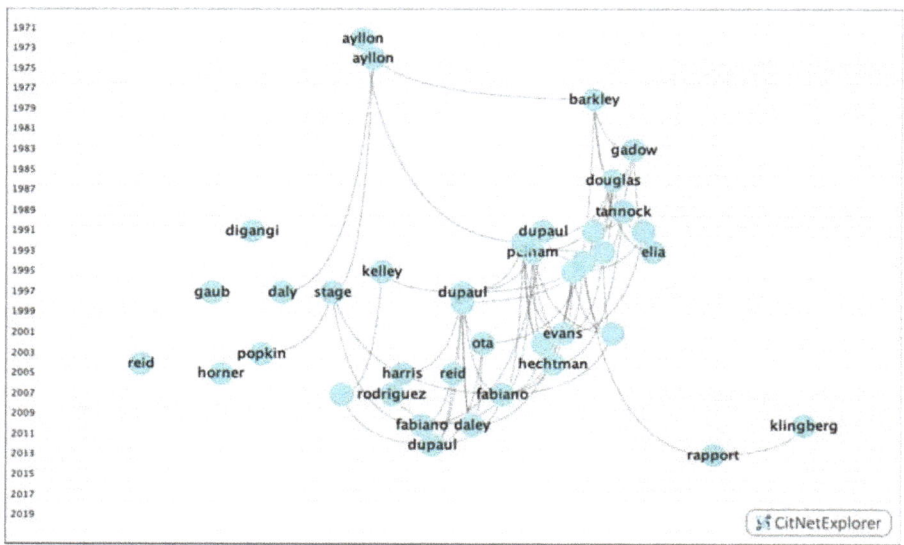

Figure 14. Group 8 citation network.

In group 9, 591 publications and 1772 citations were found throughout the network. The most cited publication was an article by Kirschner et al. [28], which was published in 2010 in Computers in Human Behavior. This study analyzed the negative impact of social networks, such as Facebook, on academic performance. The common subject in this group was the influence of digital devices and social networks on academic performance (Figure 15).

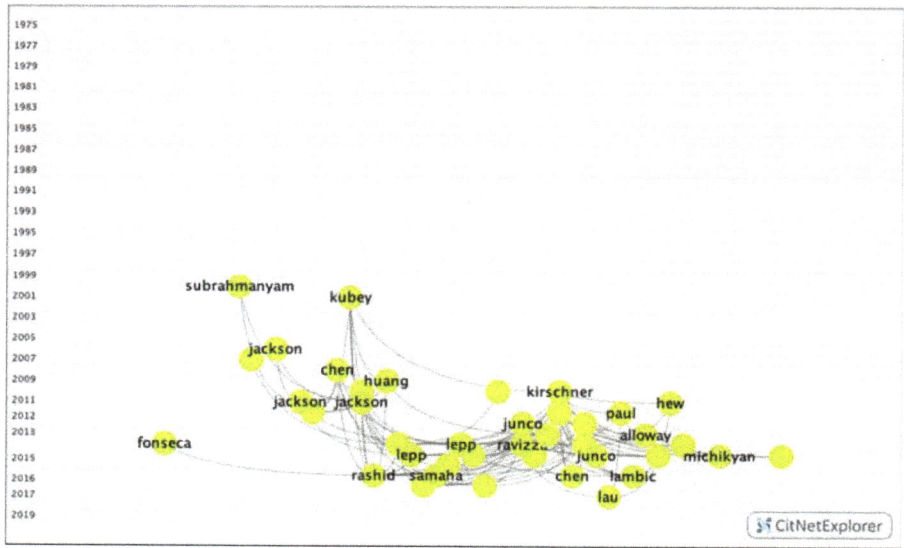

Figure 15. Group 9 citation network.

Table 3 shows a more detailed description of the oldest and most recent publications from the nine main groups.

Table 3. The oldest and most recent journal information from the nine main groups.

	Cluster	Autor	Title	Year	Total Citation
Group 1	Pioneers	Jones et al. [45]	The Individual High School as a Predictor of College Academic Performance	1962	2
	Most Recent	Carmona-Halty et al. [46]	How Psychological Capital Mediates Between Study–Related Positive Emotions and Academic Performance	2019	3
Group 2	Pioneers	Rourke et al. [47]	Neuropsychological significance of variations in patterns of academic performance: Verbal and visual-spatial abilities	1978	7
	Most Recent	Singh et al. [48]	Effects of physical activity interventions on cognitive and academic performance in children and adolescents: a novel combination of a systematic review and recommendations from an expert panel	2019	12
Group 3	Pioneers	Flook et al. [49]	Academic performance with, and without, knowledge of scores on tests of intelligence, aptitude, and personality	1968	1
	Most Recent	Hu et al. [50]	Maladaptive Perfectionism, Impostorism, and Cognitive Distortions: Threats to the Mental Health of Pre-clinical Medical Students	2019	1
Group 4	Pioneers	Finger et al. [51]	Academic performance of public and private school students	1963	1
	Most Recent	Chyn et al. [52]	Housing Voucher Take-Up and Labor Market Impacts	2018	1
Group 5	Pioneers	Henry et al. [53]	Part-time employment and academic performance of freshmen	1967	3
	Most Recent	Nordamann et al. [54]	Turn up, tune in, don't drop out: the relationship between lecture attendance, use of lecture recordings, and achievement at different levels of study	2019	1
Group 6	Pioneers	Bewley et al. [55]	Academic-performance and social-factors related to cigarette-smoking by schoolchildren	1977	3
	Most Recent	Pörhölä et al. [56]	Bullying and social anxiety experiences in university learning situations	2019	1
Group 7	Pioneers	Lucas et al. [57]	Interaction in University Selection, Mental Health and Academic Performance	1972	3
	Most Recent	Adelantado-Renau et al. [58]	The effect of sleep quality on academic performance is mediated by Internet use time: DADOS study	2019	2
Group 8	Pioneers	Chadwick et al. [59]	Systematic reinforcement: academic performance of underachieving students	1971	2
	Most Recent	Kortekaas-rijaarsdam et al. [60]	Does methylphenidate improve academic performance? A systematic review and meta-analysis	2019	1
Group 9	Pioneers	Cooper et al. [61]	The importance of race and social class information in the formation of expectancies about academic performance	1975	1
	Most Recent	Al-Rahmi et al. [62]	Massive Open Online Courses (MOOCs): Data on higher education	2019	1

Figure 16 shows that, after analyzing the relationship among the different groups by means of the drilling down function, no connection has been found between the main publications in different groups.

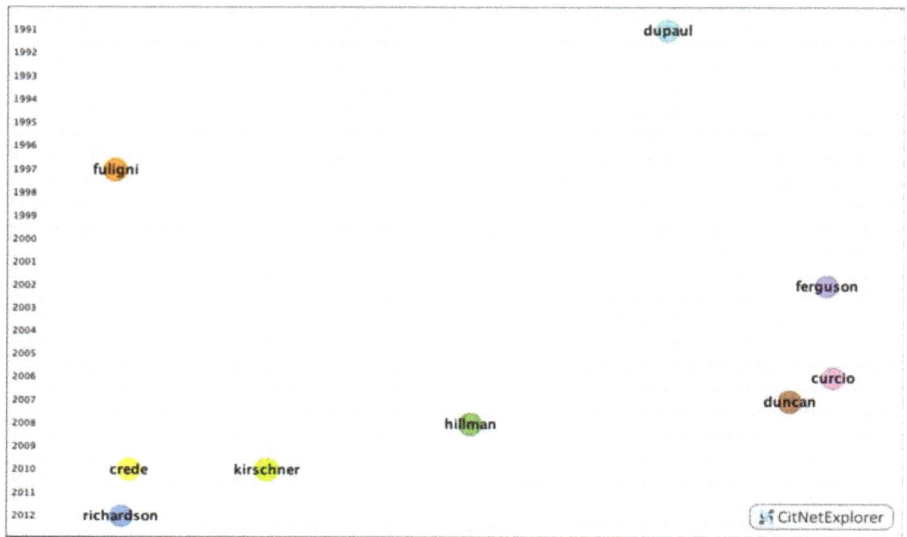

Figure 16. Relationship between the nine major groups.

3.2.1. Group 1—Subclusters

10 subclusters have been found (Figure 17), five of which boast a significant number of publications (Table 4). The remaining groups are relatively small with less than 200 publications and 1778 citation networks.

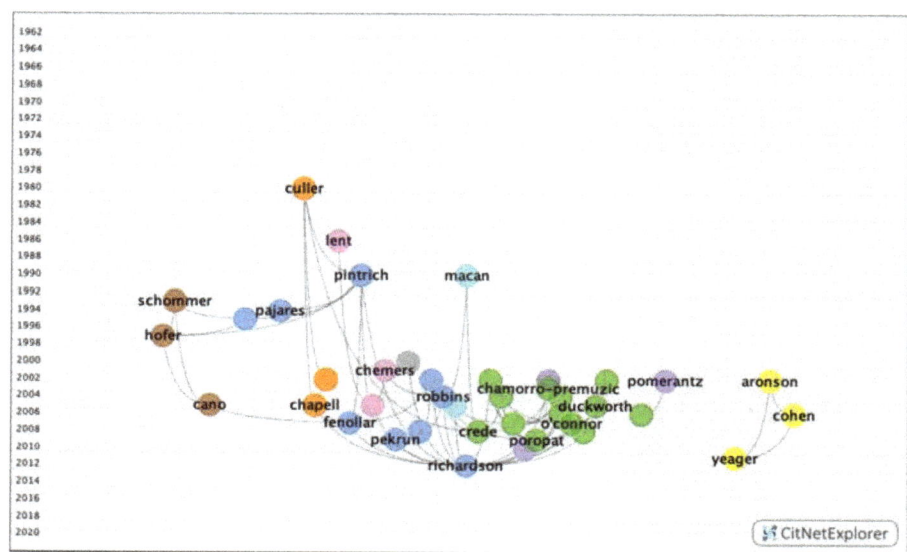

Figure 17. Group 1-subclusters citation network.

Table 4. The most important subclusters from group 1.

Sub-Cluster	1	2	3	4	5
No. of publications	727	665	284	280	251
No. of citation links	1985	2447	495	704	708
Pioneers	Schultz et al., 1993 [63]	Savage et al., 1962 [64]	Greiner et al., 1997 [65]	Carrier et al., 1966 [66]	Kennelly et al., 1975 [67]
Most cited	Richardson et al., 2012 [21]	Poropat et al., 2009 [23]	Schaufeli et al., 2002 [68]	Chapell et al., 2005 [36]	Aronson et al., 2002 [69]
Most Recent	Trigeros Ramos et al., 2019 [70]	Proyer et al., 2019 [71]	Carmona et al., 2019 [46]	Alammari et al., 2018 [72]	Wang et al., 2019 [73]
Topic of discussion	Influence of motivation on academic performance	Influence of personality on academic performance	Influence of self-discipline and emotions on academic performance	Influence of anxiety on academic performance	Influence of demographic psychology on academic performance
Conclusion	Motivation has a positive influence on academic performance	Research into this group is still being carried out, therefore consensus has not yet been reached	Self-control strategies have a positive influence on academic performance	Anxiety has a negative influence on final grades; therefore self-control strategies are necessary.	Intelligence is malleable; therefore the negative stereotypes of immigrant children and academic performance must be eliminated

3.2.2. Group 2—Subclusters

10 subclusters have been found (Figure 18), three of which boast a significant number of publications (Table 5). The remaining groups are relatively small with less than 90 publications and 464 citation networks.

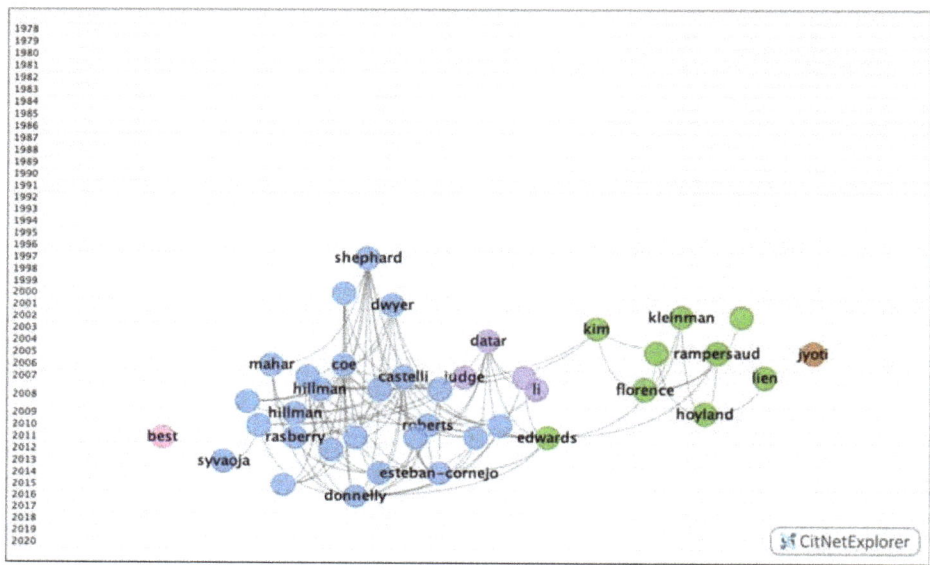

Figure 18. Group 2-subclusters citation network.

Table 5. The most important subclusters from group 2.

Sub-Cluster	1	2	3
No. of publications	431	186	141
No. of citation links	2324	571	359
Pioneers	Nelson et al., 1993 [74]	Nidich et al., 1993 [75]	Kovacs et al., 1992 [76]
Most cited	Hillman et al., 2008 [33]	Rampersaud et al., 2005 [39]	Datar et al., 2004 [77]
Most Recent	Singh et al., 2019 [48]	Adelantado-Renau et al., 2019 [78]	Allison et al., 2019 [79]
Topic of discussion	The benefits of physical exercise on academic performance	The benefits of a healthy diet on academic performance	The link between state of health and academic performance
Conclusion	Physical exercise improves mental and physical health throughout life.	A diet that is rich in fiber, nutrients, fruits and dairy products is recommended.	Poor mental and physical health has a negative impact on academic performance

3.3. Core Function

4660 publications with four or more citations (28.8% of all publications) and a citation network of 23,747 were found (Figure 19).

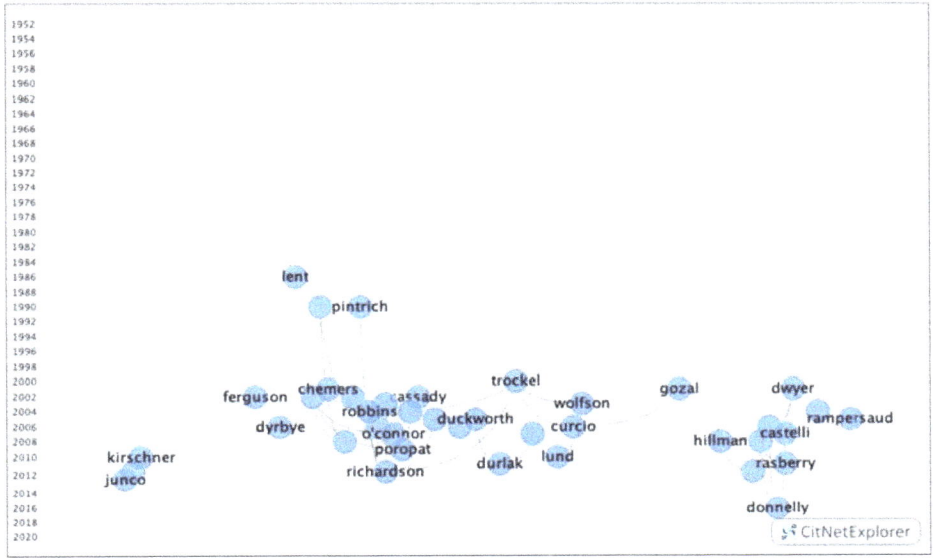

Figure 19. Core Function in the academic performance citation network.

4. Discussion

The main databases, such as WOS and Scopus, allow for the exploration of citation networks. However, these databases do not offer a general overview of the connection between citations from a group of publications. Thus, their usefulness is limited to carrying out a systematic review of all existing literature. This is the reason why we used CitNetExplorer software to visualize, analyze, and explore citation networks of scientific publications. CitNetExplorer offers a more detailed analysis of the citation networks in comparison with other databases such as WOS or Scopus [20].

As our main objective was to analyze all the existing literature on the different factors that influence academic performance, we used the WOS database to perform our bibliographic search, given that it is the only database for which the search range begins in 1900. However, it is important to point out that WOS only accepts journals with an international presence, and these are only admitted following a rigorous selection process.

In this way, the CitNetExplorer software allowed us to gather and analyze all of the literature available on academic performance up to the present date. Furthermore, the connection between the fields of study and the different research groups was also found by using citation network analysis.

In order to obtain the results, the following functionalities were used: the clustering functionality, as it allows the publications to be grouped by citation relationship; the drilling down functionality, which provides a deeper analysis of the existing bibliography for each of the groups; and the core publications functionality, which shows the most relevant publications, i.e., those which have a minimum citation number. Therefore, these functionalities enable the researcher to conduct a complete analysis of the studies published on a particular subject.

In recent years, the number of publications on academic performance has significantly increased. In the past, research carried out on this topic focused predominantly on the influence of psychological factors on academic performance [80,81]. From the year 2000, the advent of digital devices brought about scientific research into their influence on academic performance. These devices were responsible for the growth of a more sedentary lifestyle which resulted in numerous studies on the impact of such behaviour.

Since 2015, the number of publications on psychological and psychosocial factors has increased by 52.83% and they have taken a multidisciplinary turn. As such, multiple factors that affect academic performance, such as demographic, psychosocial, psychological, lifestyle, and mental and physical health factors, have been analysed. [82–85].

With regards to the authors, Kirk is worth mentioning in the early years, for having published over 70 papers on academic performance between 1952 and 1982. Currently, Rozelle and Salamonson are considered as two of the most prominent authors in this field of study, as they have published 40 and 33 papers respectively in the period between the years 2005 and 2010 and up to date.

2018 has been identified as a "key year", given the large number of publications and the content of the documents, in which the main topic of study was the importance of mental and physical health on academic performance [86,87]. In the study conducted by Stajkovic et al. [86], published in 2018, the authors confirmed that awareness and emotional stability predict self-efficacy and this is positively related to academic performance. In the study by de Greeff et al. [87], published in 2018, it was determined that physical activity has a positive effect on attention, while long-term physical activity programs have a positive impact on executive functions, attention, and academic performance. Therefore, this study has confirmed that all of the factors that influence academic performance are interrelated, with psychological and psychosocial factors considered to be the most prevalent.

The countries with a greater number of publications are the United States, Spain and Britain. The educational systems of these countries are intense, which places students at a higher risk of anxiety and stress. Furthermore, and with regards to psychosocial factors, the students are more competitive. Consequently, many studies have focused on analyzing risk factors for academic performance in these countries. Nevertheless, it must be taken into consideration that, in the case of China, students are showing symptoms of anxiety and depression more often, and therefore the number of publications is expected to increase over the coming years.

In the United States, the number of publications is significantly higher than in other countries. This is due to increased interest in the topics related to student learning. Likewise, the trend for the number of publications to increase in the field of education in countries like the United States or Britain has been associated with a combination of factors, such as being English-speaking countries and the possible connections among the various research groups in the scientific community [88,89].

With regards to the journals with the larger numbers of publications, it is worth mentioning that they are mainly Psychology and Educational Science journals, as psychological and psychosocial factors are those with the greatest influence. Moreover, the majority of the journals are from the United States and Britain.

Nowadays, students are more competitive and are therefore at a greater risk of suffering from stress. Several authors have defined stress as "an adverse reaction that people have to excessive pressures and demands placed on them. In other words, stress arises when people find themselves in an overwhelming situation and believe they are unable to cope with it" [90,91]. The study by Aafreen et al. [92], which was published in 2018, corroborated that students who are unable to manage stress are affected mentally, physically and emotionally and as such they tend to present anxiety and depression, which leads to a decline in academic performance. At the same time, the articles by Chapell et al. [36] and Cassady et al. [37], published in 2005 and 2002, respectively, focused on the relationship between stress and final grades. Both of the studies concluded that higher levels of anxiety were associated with lower grades and vice versa. That is to say, stress has a negative impact on academic performance and, likewise, the results demonstrated that female students present higher levels of anxiety than male students. Nowadays, the preparation of students is not only based on their studying for an undergraduate degree, but also on the idea that they at least have to have a master's degree, which can lead to a higher prevalence of stress, anxiety and depression.

Health professionals recommend physical exercise and a balanced diet to prevent stress. Several studies have shown that people who exercise are less likely to suffer from anxiety and depression, and that stress symptoms can be improved by doing exercise [93,94]. Another study carried out in Spain among university students demonstrated that having a poor diet and being overweight are strongly associated with higher levels of stress, especially in women, and these factors have a negative impact on academic performance [95]. Consequently, scientific evidence reveals a significant relationship between academic performance and health status, therefore vision problems, nutrition, stress, obesity, anxiety, behavioral disorders and aggression are associated with a poor academic performance [96]. It should be noted that the personality of students with psychosocial well-being is characterized by determination and pragmatism in their academic efforts, therefore enabling them to establish high-level objectives that they pursue successfully [13].

In the future, health and welfare programs must be established in schools to reduce the incidence of behaviors that could have a detrimental effect on the physical and mental health of young people, as this could result in improved academic performance. In the study by Van Loon et al. [97], published in 2019, two school programs were created to improve the control of anxiety and social abilities. These programs were aimed at preventing mental health problems that have a negative impact on academic performance. It is also important to consider that as students get older they become more competitive, therefore meaning that they are more likely to suffer from physical and mental damage. As a result, the content of programs aimed at controlling stress in order to improve academic performance will be different in both primary and secondary education and at university.

This study provides a brand new approach which can guide researchers in the revision of the wealth of literature that exists on academic performance. Over the coming years, research in this field will continue to focus mainly on the impact of psychological factors on academic performance as a consequence of the constant increase in competitiveness among students. In this way, research questions based on this data posed by future studies will focus mainly on how psychological and psychosocial factors could be improved in order to increase academic performance.

Likewise, the number of studies on the impact of the use of devices on academic performance is also likely to increase, given that constant changes in lifestyle are becoming more and more frequent. With regards to citation network studies, they are also likely to become more numerous as it is the only method of analysis which provides a global overview of the different research fields within a particular subject. Moreover, the CitNetExplorer software facilitates the analysis of all existing studies on a given topic, thus allowing for detailed research to be conducted, which might change the way in which research is carried out in different fields of study.

5. Conclusions

In this study, 16,157 publications on academic performance were analysed, which were obtained from the Web of Science (WOS) database between 1952 and 2019. All of the publications were analysed using the Citation Network Explorer software, which makes it possible to visualize, analyze and explore the citation networks of scientific publications.

Academic performance may be influenced by various factors, including psychological, psychosocial, economic, environmental or personal factors. Self-sufficient students present learning and self-control skills which facilitate studying, and as a consequence increase their motivation. This means that they have the skills and willingness to learn. Likewise, the personality of the students with psychosocial wellbeing is often characterized by determination and pragmatism in academic effort, which enables them to set high-level goals for themselves, which they successfully pursue. On the other hand, scientific evidence suggests a significant relationship between academic performance and health, meaning that vision problems, nutrition, stress, obesity, anxiety, behavioral disorders or aggression are associated with poor academic performance. This is why it is necessary to establish health and wellbeing programs in schools, which are aimed at preventing behaviors that put the mental and physical health of young people at risk, and at improving their academic performance.

The citation network showed the main publications on the different factors that affect academic performance, and it was determined that psychological and psychosocial factors were the most relevant.

This study offers a global overview of the number of publications for each of the years and field of study, as well as a general description of the 20 most-cited publications.

Author Contributions: Conceptualization, C.A.-P., M.A.S.-T., C.M.-P. and C.V.-C.; methodology, C.A.-P., M.Á.S.-T., C.M.-P. and C.V.-C.; software, C.A.-P., M.Á.S.-T., C.M.-P. and C.V.-C.; validation, C.A.-P., M.Á.S.-T., C.M.-P. and C.V.-C.; formal analysis, C.A.-P., M.Á.S.-T., C.M.-P. and C.V.-C.; investigation, C.A.-P., M.Á.S.-T., C.M.-P. and C.V.-C.; resources, C.A.-P., M.Á.S.-T., C.M.-P. and C.V.-C.; data curation, C.A.-P., M.Á.S.-T., C.M.-P. and C.V.-C.; writing—original draft preparation, C.A.-P., M.Á.S.-T., C.M.-P. and C.V.-C.; writing—review and editing, C.A.-P., M.Á.S.-T., C.M.-P. and C.V.-C.; visualization, C.A.-P., M.Á.S.-T., C.M.-P. and C.V.-C.; supervision, C.A.-P., M.Á.S.-T., C.M.-P. and C.V.-C.; project administration, C.A.-P., M.Á.S.-T., C.M.-P. and C.V.-C.; funding acquisition, C.A.-P., M.Á.S.-T., C.M.-P. and C.V.-C. All authors have read and agreed to the published version of the manuscript.

Funding: This research received no external funding.

Conflicts of Interest: The authors declare no conflict of interest.

References

1. Ali, N.; Jusoff, K.; Ali, S.; Mokhtar, N.; Salamat, A.S.A. The Factors Influencing Students' Performance at Universiti Teknologi MARA Kedah, Malaysia. *Manag. Sci. Eng.* **2009**, *3*, 81–90.
2. Lee, J.; Stankov, L. *Non-Cognitive Psychological Processes and Academic Achievement*, 1st ed.; Routledge: New York, NY, USA, 2016.
3. Liem, G.A.D.; Tan, S.H. *Asian Education Miracles: In Search of Sociocultural and Psychological Explanations*, 1st ed.; Routledge: New York, NY, USA, 2019.
4. Jung, K.R.; Zhou, A.Q.; Lee, R.M. Self-efficacy, self-discipline and academic performance: Testing a context-specific mediation model. *Learn. Individ. Differ.* **2017**, *60*, 33–39. [CrossRef]
5. Sternberg, R.J.; Williams, W.M. *Educational Psychology*, 2nd ed.; Pearson: Somerset, NJ, USA, 2009.
6. Slavin, R.E. *Educational Psychology Theory and Practise*, 8th ed.; Pearson: Boston, MA, USA, 2006.
7. Alderman, M.K. *Motivation for Achievement: Possibilities for Teaching and Learning*, 2nd ed.; Lawrence Erlbaum Associates Publishers: Hillsdale, NJ, USA, 2004.
8. Schunk, D. *Learning Theories: An Educational Perspective*, 4th ed.; Merrill/Prentice-Hall: Columbu, OH, USA, 2004.
9. Murphy, P.; Alexander, P. A motivated Exploration of Motivation Terminalogy. *Contemp. Educ. Psychol.* **2000**, *25*, 3–53. [CrossRef] [PubMed]
10. Gardner, H. *Frames of Mind: The Theory of Multiple Intelligences*, 1st ed.; Basic Books: New York, USA, 1983.
11. Becker, B.E.; Luther, S.S. Social-emotional factors affecting achievement outcomes among disadvantaged students: Closing the achievement gap. *Educational Psychologist.* **2002**, *37*, 197–214. [CrossRef]
12. Park, N.; Peterson, C.; Seligman, M.E.P. Strength of character and well-being. *J. Soc. Clin. Psychol.* **2004**, *23*, 603–619. [CrossRef]
13. Vilar, G.N.; Santos, L.A.; Sobral, F.J. Quality of life, self-esteem and psychosocial factors in adolescents with acne vulgaris. *Bras. Dermatol.* **2015**, *90*, 622–629. [CrossRef]
14. Eagle, T.F.; Sheetz, A.; Gurm, R.; Woodward, A.C.; Kline-Rogers, E.; Leibowitz, R.; Durussel-Weston, J.; Palma-Davis, L.; Aaronson, S.; Fitzgerald, C.M.; et al. Understanding childhood obesity in America: Linkages between household income, community resources, and children's behaviors. *Am. Heart J.* **2012**, *163*, 836–843. [CrossRef]
15. Whiteman, A.S.; Young, D.E.; He, X.; Chen, T.C.; Wagenaar, R.C.; Stern, C.E.; Schon, K. Research report: Interaction between serum BDNF and aerobic fitness predicts recognition memory in healthy young adults. *Behav. Brain Res.* **2014**, *259*, 302–312. [CrossRef]
16. Lim, J.; Dinges, D.F. A meta-analysis of the impact of short-term sleep deprivation on cognitive variables. *Psychol. Bull.* **2010**, *136*, 375–389. [CrossRef]
17. Remígio, M.C.; Leal, D.; Barros, E.; Travassos, S.; Ventura, L.O. Achados oftalmológicos em pacientes com múltiplas deficiências. *Arq. Bras. Oftalmol.* **2006**, *69*, 929–932. [CrossRef]
18. Leydesdorff, L. Can Scientific Journals be Classified in terms of Aggregated Journal-Journal Citation Relations using the *Journal Citation Reports*? *J. Am. Soc. Inf. Sci. Tec.* **2006**, *57*, 601–613. [CrossRef]

19. González, C.M. Análisis de citación y de redes sociales para el estudio del uso de revistas en centros de investigación: An approach to the development of collections. *Ciência da Informação* **2009**, *38*, 46–55. [CrossRef]
20. Van Eck, N.J.; Waltman, L. CitNetExplorer: A new software tool for analyzing and visualizing citation networks. *J. Informetr.* **2014**, *8*, 802–823. [CrossRef]
21. Richardson, M.; Abraham, C.; Bond, R. Psychological correlates of university students' academic performance: A systematic review and meta-analysis. *Psychol. Bull.* **2012**, *138*, 353–387. [CrossRef]
22. Pintrich, P.R.; De Groot, E.V. Motivational and self-regulated learning components of classroom academic performance. *J. Educ. Psychol.* **1990**, *82*, 33–40. [CrossRef]
23. Poropat, A.E. A meta-analysis of the five-factor model of personality and academic performance. *Psychol. Bull.* **2009**, *135*, 322–338. [CrossRef]
24. Robbins, S.B.; Lauver, K.; Le, H.; Davis, D.; Langley, R.; Carlstrom, A. Do Psychosocial and Study Skill Factors Predict College Outcomes? A Meta-Analysis. *Psychol. Bull.* **2004**, *130*, 261–288. [CrossRef]
25. Chamorro-Premuzcil, T.; Furnham, A. Personality predicts academic performance: Evidence from two longitudinal university samples. *J. Res. Pers.* **2003**, *37*, 319–338. [CrossRef]
26. Duckworth, A.L.; Seligman, M.E. Self-Discipline Outdoes IQ in Predicting Academic Performance of Adolescents. *Psychol. Sci.* **2005**, *16*, 939–944. [CrossRef]
27. O'Connor, M.C.; Paunonen, S.V. Big Five personality predictors of post-secondary academic performance. *Pers. Individ. Dif.* **2007**, *43*, 971–990. [CrossRef]
28. Kirschner, P.A.; Karpinski, A.C. Facebook® and academic performance. *Comput. Hum. Behav.* **2010**, *26*, 1237–1245. [CrossRef]
29. Curcio, G.; Ferrara, M.; De Gennaro, L. Sleep loss, learning capacity and academic performance. *Sleep Med. Rev.* **2006**, *10*, 323–337. [CrossRef]
30. Ferguson, E.; James, D.; Madeley, L. Factors associated with success in medical school: Systematic review of the literature. *BMJ.* **2002**, *324*, 952–957. [CrossRef]
31. Chemers, M.M.; Hu, L.; Garcia, B.F. Academic self-efficacy and first year college student performance and adjustment. *J. Educ. Psychol.* **2001**, *93*, 55–64. [CrossRef]
32. Kuncel, N.R.; Hezlett, S.A.; Ones, D.S. Academic Performance, Career Potential, Creativity, and Job Performance: Can One Construct Predict Them All? *J. Pers. Soc. Psychol.* **2004**, *86*, 148–161. [CrossRef]
33. Hillman, C.H.; Erickson, K.I.; Kramer, A.F. Be smart, exercise your heart: Exercise effects on brain and cognition. *Nat. Rev. Neurosci.* **2008**, *9*, 58–65. [CrossRef]
34. Castelli, D.M.; Hillman, C.H.; Buck, S.M.; Erwin, H.E. Physical Fitness and Academic Achievement in Third- and Fifth-Grade Students. *J. Sport. Exerc. Psychol.* **2007**, *29*, 239–252. [CrossRef]
35. Trockel, M.T.; Barmes, M.D.; Egget, D.L. Health-Related Variables and Academic Performance Among First-Year College Students: Implications for Sleep and Other Behaviors. *J. Am. Coll Health.* **2000**, *49*, 125–131. [CrossRef]
36. Chapell, M.S.; Blanding, Z.B.; Silverstein, M.E.; Takahashi, M.; Newman, B.; Gubi, A.; McCann, N. Test Anxiety and Academic Performance in Undergraduate and Graduate Students. *J. Educ Psychol.* **2005**, *97*, 268–274. [CrossRef]
37. Cassady, J.C.; Johnson, R.E. Cognitive Test Anxiety and Academic Performance. *Contemp. Educ. Psychol.* **2002**, *27*, 270–295. [CrossRef]
38. Wolfson, A.R.; Carskadon, M.A. Understanding adolescent's sleep patterns and school performance: A critical appraisal. *Sleep Med. Rev.* **2003**, *7*, 491–506. [CrossRef]
39. Rampersaud, G.C.; Pereira, M.A.; Girald, B.L.; Adams, J.; Metzi, J.D. Breakfast Habits, Nutritional Status, Body Weight, and Academic Performance in Children and Adolescents. *J. Am. Diet. Assoc.* **2005**, *105*, 743–760. [CrossRef]
40. Dyrbye, L.N.; Thomas, M.R.; Shanafelt, T.D. Systematic Review of Depression, Anxiety, and Other Indicators of Psychological Distress Among U.S. and Canadian Medical Students. *Acad. Med.* **2006**, *81*, 354–357. [CrossRef]
41. Fuligni, A.J. The Academic Achievement of Adolescents from Immigrant Families: The Role of Family Background, Attitudes, and Behavior. *Child. Dev.* **1997**, *68*, 351–363. [CrossRef]

42. Crede, M.; Roch, S.G.; Kleszczynka, U.M. Class Attendance in College: A Meta-Analytic Review of the Relationship of Class Attendance with Grades and Student Characteristics. *Rev. Educ Res.* **2010**, *80*, 272–295. [CrossRef]
43. Duncan, G.J.; Dowsett, C.J.; Claessens, A.; Magnuson, K.; Huston, A.C.; Klebanov, P.; Pagani, L.S.; Feinstein, L.; Engel, M.; Brooks-Gunn, J.; et al. School readiness and later achievement. *Dev. Psychol.* **2007**, *43*, 1428–1446. [CrossRef]
44. DuPaul, G.J.; Rapport, M.D.; Perriello, L.M. Teacher ratings of academic skills: The development of the Academic Performance Rating Scale. *Sch. Psychol. Rev.* **1991**, *20*, 284–300.
45. Jones, R.L.; Siegel, L. The Individual High School as a Predictor of College Academic Performance. *Educ. Psychol. Meas.* **1962**. [CrossRef]
46. Carmona-Halty, M.; Salanova, M.; Llorens, S.; Schaufeli, W.B. How Psychological Capital Mediates Between Study–Related Positive Emotions and Academic Performance. *J. Happiness Stud.* **2019**, *20*, 605–617. [CrossRef]
47. Rourke, B.P.; Finlayson, M.A. Neuropsychological Significance of Variations in Patterns of Academic Performance: Verbal and Visual-Spatial Abilities. *J. Abnorm Child. Psychol.* **1978**, *6*, 121–133. [CrossRef]
48. Singh, A.S.; Saliasi, E.; Van den Berg, V.; Uijtdewilligen, L.; de Groot, R.H.M.; Jolles, J.; Andersen, L.B.; Bailey, B.R.; Chang, Y.-K.; Diamond, A.; et al. Effects of Physical Activity Interventions on Cognitive and Academic Performance in Children and Adolescents: A Novel Combination of a Systematic Review and Recommendations From an Expert Panel. *Br. J. Sports Med.* **2019**, *53*, 640–647. [CrossRef] [PubMed]
49. Flook, A.J.; Saggar, U. Academic performance with, and without, knowledge of scores on tests of intelligence, aptitude, and personality. *J. Educ Psychol.* **1968**, *59*, 395–401. [CrossRef]
50. Hu, L.S.; Chibnall, J.T.; Slavin, S.J. Maladaptive Perfectionism, Impostorism, and Cognitive Distortions: Threats to the Mental Health of Pre-clinical Medical Students. *Acad. Psychiatry* **2019**, *43*, 381–385. [CrossRef] [PubMed]
51. Finger, J.A.; Schlesser, G.E. Academic performance of public and private school students. *J. Educ. Psychol.* **1963**, *54*, 118–122. [CrossRef]
52. Chyn, E.; Hyman, J.; Kapustin, M. Housing Voucher Take-Up and Labor Market Impacts. *J. Policy Anal. Manag.* **2018**, *38*. [CrossRef]
53. Henry, J.B. Part-time employment and academic performance of freshmen. *J. Coll. Stud. Pers.* **1967**, *8*, 257–260.
54. Nordmann, E.; Calder, C.; Bishop, P.; Irwin, A.; Comber, D. urn up, tune in, don't drop out: The relationship between lecture attendance, use of lecture recordings, and achievement at different levels of study. *High. Educ.* **2019**, *77*, 1065–1084. [CrossRef]
55. Bewley, B.R.; Bland, J.M. Academic performance and social factors related to cigarette smoking by schoolchildren. *Br. J. Prev. Soc. Med.* **1977**, *31*, 18–24. [CrossRef]
56. Pörhölä, M.; Almonkari, M.; Kunttu, K. Bullying and social anxiety experiences in university learning situations. *Soc. Psychol. Educ.* **2019**, *22*, 723–742. [CrossRef]
57. Lucas, C.J.; Stringer, P. Interaction in university selection, mental-health and academic performance. *Brit. J. Psychiat.* **1972**, *120*, 189. [CrossRef]
58. Adelantado-Renau, M.; Diez-Fernandez, A.; Beltran-Valls, M.R.; Soriano-Maldonado, A.; Moliner-Urdiales, D. The Effect of Sleep Quality on Academic Performance Is Mediated by Internet Use Time: DADOS Study. *J. Pediatr. (Rio J.)* **2019**, *95*, 410–418. [CrossRef] [PubMed]
59. Chadwick, B.A.; Day, R.C. Systematic reinforcement: Academic performance of underachieving students. *J. Appl. Behav. Anal.* **1971**, *4*, 311–319. [CrossRef] [PubMed]
60. Kortekaas.Rijlaarsdam, A.F.; Luman, M.; Sonuga-Barke, E.; Oosterlaan, J. Does Methylphenidate Improve Academic Performance? A Systematic Review and Meta-Analysis. *Eur. Child. Adolesc. Psychiatry* **2019**, *28*, 155–164. [CrossRef]
61. Cooper, H.M.; Baron, R.M.; Lowe, C.A. The importance of race and social class information in the formation of expectancies about academic performance. *J. Educ. Psychol.* **1975**, *67*, 312–319. [CrossRef]
62. Al-Rahmi, W.; Aldraiweesh, A.; Yahaya, N.; Bin Kamin, Y.; Zeki, A.M. Massive Open Online Courses (MOOCs): Data on higher education. *Data Brief.* **2019**, *22*, 118–125. [CrossRef]
63. Schultz, G.F.; Switzky, H.N. The academic achievement of elementary and junior high school students with behavior disorders and their nonhandicapped peers as a function of motivational orientation. *Learn. Individ. Differ.* **1993**, *5*, 31–42. [CrossRef]

64. Savage, R.D. II.—Personality factors and academic performance. *Br. J. Educ. Psychol.* **1962**, *32*. [CrossRef]
65. Greiner, J.M.; Karoly, P. Effects of self-control training on study activity and academic-performance-analysis of self-monitoring, self-reward, and systematic-planning components. *J. Couns. Psychol.* **1997**, *6*, 495–502. [CrossRef]
66. Carrier, N.A.; Jewell, D.O. Efficiency in measuring the effect of anxiety upon academic performance. *J. Educ. Psychol.* **1966**, *57*, 23–26. [CrossRef]
67. Kennelly, K.; Kinley, S. Perceived contingency of teacher administered reinforcements and academic performance of boys. *J. Anal. Psychol.* **1975**, *12*.
68. Schaufeli, W.B.; Martínez, I.B.; Marques Pinto, A.; Salanova, M.; Bakker, A.B. Burnout and Engagement in University Students: A Cross-National Study. *J. Cross Cult.* **2002**, *33*, 464–481. [CrossRef]
69. Aronson, J.; Fried, C.B.; Good, C. Reducing the Effects of Stereotype Threat on African American College Students by Shaping Theories of Intelligence. *J. Exp. Soc. Psychol.* **2002**, *38*, 113–125. [CrossRef]
70. Trigeros Ramos, R.; Navarro Gómez, N. The influence of the teacher on the motivation, learning strategies, critical thinking and academic performance of high school students in physical education. *Psychol. Soc. Educ.* **2019**, *11*, 73–79. [CrossRef]
71. Proyer, R.T.; Tandler, N. An update on the study of playfulness in adolescents: Its relationship with academic performance, well-being, anxiety, and roles in bullying-type-situations. *Soc. Psychol. Educ.* **2019**, *23*, 73–99. [CrossRef]
72. Alammari, M.R.; Fried, C.B.; Bukhary, D.M. Factors contributing to prosthodontic exam anxiety in undergraduate dental students. *Adv. Med. Educ. Pract.* **2018**, *10*, 31–38. [CrossRef]
73. Wang, Y.; Pei, F.; Zhai, F.; Gao, Q. Academic performance and peer relations among rural-to-urban migrant children in Beijing: Do social identity and self-efficacy matter? *Asian Soc. Work Policy Rev.* **2019**, *13*. [CrossRef]
74. Nelson, M. Vitamin and mineral supplementation and academic performance in schoolchildren. *Proc. Nutr. Soc.* **1992**, *51*, 303–313. [CrossRef]
75. Nidich, S.I.; Morehead, P.; Nidich, R.J.; Sands, D.; Sharma, H. The effect of the Maharishi Student Rasayana food supplement on non-verbal intelligence. *Pers. Individ. Differ.* **1993**, *15*, 599–602. [CrossRef]
76. Kovacs, M.; Goldston, D.; Iyengar, S. Intellectual development and academic performance of children with insulin-dependent diabetes mellitus a longitudinal study. *Dev. Psychol.* **1992**, *28*, 676–684.
77. Datar, A.; Sturm, R.; Magnabosco, J.L. Childhood Overweight and Academic Performance: National Study of Kindergartners and First-Graders. *Obes Res.* **2004**, *12*, 58–68. [CrossRef]
78. Adelantado-Renau, M.; Beltran-Valls, M.R.; Esteban-Cornejo, I.; Martínez-Vizcaíno, V.; Santaliestra-Pasías, A.M.; Moliner-Urdiales, D. The influence of adherence to the Mediterranean diet on academic performance is mediated by sleep quality in adolescents. *Acta Paediatr.* **2019**, *108*, 339–346. [CrossRef]
79. Allison, M.A.; Attisha, E.; Council on School Health. The Link between School Attendance and Good Health. *Pediatrics* **2019**, *143*, e20183648. [CrossRef]
80. Hills, J.R. Transfer shock: The academic performance of the junior college transfer. *J. Exp. Educ.* **1965**, *33*, 201–215. [CrossRef]
81. Macan, T.H.; Shahani, C.; Dipboye, R.L.; Philips, A.P. College students' time management: Correlations with academic performance and stress. *J. Educ. Psychol.* **1990**, *82*, 760–768. [CrossRef]
82. Donelly, J.E.; Hillman, C.H.; Castelli, D.; Etiner, J.L.; Lee, S.; Philip, T.; Lambourne, K.; Szabo-Reed, A.N. Physical Activity, Fitness, Cognitive Function, and Academic Achievement in Children: A Systematic Review. *Med. Sci. Sports Exerc.* **2016**, *48*, 1197–1222. [CrossRef]
83. Samaha, M.; Hawi, N.S. Relationships among smartphone addiction, stress, academic performance, and satisfaction with life. *Comput. Hum. Behav.* **2016**, *57*, 321–325. [CrossRef]
84. Bailey, T.H.; Philips, L.J. The influence of motivation and adaptation on students' subjective well-being, meaning in life and academic performance. *High. Educ. Res. Dev.* **2015**, *35*, 1–16. [CrossRef]
85. Hanafi, Z.; Noor, F. Relationship between Demographic Factors and Emerging adult's Academic Achievement. *Int. J. Acad.* **2016**, *6*. [CrossRef]
86. Stajkovic, A.D.; Bandura, A.; Locke, E.A.; Lee, D.; Sergent, K. Test of three conceptual models of influence of the big five personality traits and self-efficacy on academic performance: A meta-analytic path-analysis. *Pers. Individ. Differ.* **2018**, *120*, 238–245. [CrossRef]

87. de Greef, J.W.; Bosker, R.J.; Oosterlaan, J.; Visscher, C.; Hartman, E. Effects of Physical Activity on Executive Functions, Attention and Academic Performance in Preadolescent Children: A Meta-Analysis. *J. Sci Med. Sport.* **2018**, *21*, 501–507. [CrossRef]
88. Lee, M.; Wu, Y.; Tsai, C. Research Trends in Science Education from 2003 to 2007: A content analysis of publications in selected journals. *Int. J. Sci. Educ.* **2009**, *31*, 1999–2020. [CrossRef]
89. Aparicio-Martinez, P.; Perea-Moreno, A.J.; Martinez-Jimenez, M.P.; Redel-Macías, M.D.; Vaquero-Abellan, M.; Pagliari, C. A Bibliometric Analysis of the Health Field Regarding Social Networks and Young People. *Int. J. Environ. Res. Public Health.* **2019**, *16*, 4024. [CrossRef]
90. Campbell, F. *Occupational Stress in the Construction Industry*; Chartered Institute of Building: Berkshire, UK, 2006.
91. Bataineh, M.Z. Academic stress among undergraduate students: The case of education faculty at king saud university. *Iny. Interdiscip. J. Educ.* **2013**, *2*, 82–88. [CrossRef]
92. Aafreen, M.M.; Priya, V.V.; Gayathri, R. Effect of stress on academic performance of students in different streams. *Drug Invent Today* **2018**, *10*, 1176–1780.
93. De Mello, M.T.; de Aquino Lemos, V.; Antunes, H.K.M.; Bittencourt, L.; Santos-Silva, R.; Tufik, S. Relationship between physical activity and depression and anxiety symptoms: A population study. *J. Affect. Disord.* **2013**, *149*, 241–246. [CrossRef]
94. Paluska, S.A.; Schwenk, T.L. Physical activity and mental health: Current Concepts. *Sports Med.* **2000**, *29*, 167–180. [CrossRef]
95. Chacón-Cuberos, R.; Zurita-Ortega, F.; Olmedo-Moreno, E.M.; Castro-Sánchez, M. Relationship between Academic Stress, Physical Activity and Diet in University Students of Education. *Behav. Sci. (Basel)* **2019**, *9*, 59. [CrossRef]
96. Knopf, J.A.; Finnie, R.K.; Peng, Y.; Hahn, R.A.; Truman, B.I.; Vernon-Smiley, M.; Johnson, V.C.; Johnson, R.L.; Fielding, J.E.; Muntaner, C.; et al. School-based health centres to advance health equity: A community guide systematic review. *Am. J. Prev. Med.* **2016**, *51*, 114–126. [CrossRef]
97. Van Loon, A.W.G.; Creemers, H.E.; Vogelaar, S.; Saab, N.; Miers, A.C.; Westenberg, P.M.; Asscher, J.J. The effectiveness of school-based skillstraining programs promoting mental health in adolescents: A study protocol for a randomized controlled study. *BMC Public Health.* **2019**, *19*, 712. [CrossRef]

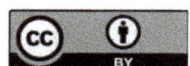

© 2020 by the authors. Licensee MDPI, Basel, Switzerland. This article is an open access article distributed under the terms and conditions of the Creative Commons Attribution (CC BY) license (http://creativecommons.org/licenses/by/4.0/).

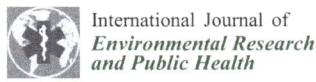 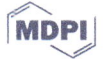

International Journal of
Environmental Research and Public Health

Article

The Contribution of Spanish Science to Patents: Medicine as Case of Study

Mila Cascajares [1], Alfredo Alcayde [1,*], José Antonio Garrido-Cardenas [2] and Francisco Manzano-Agugliaro [1]

1. Department of Engineering, University of Almeria, ceiA3, 04120 Almeria, Spain; milacas@ual.es (M.C.); fmanzano@ual.es (F.M.-A.)
2. Department of Biology and Geology, University of Almeria, 04120 Almeria, Spain; jcardena@ual.es
* Correspondence: aalcayde@ual.es; Tel.: +34-950-015-491; Fax: +34-950-015-491

Received: 19 April 2020; Accepted: 19 May 2020; Published: 21 May 2020

Abstract: Investments in research and development (R&D) and innovation are expensive, and one wishes to be assured that there is positive feedback and to receive guidance on how to direct investments in the future. The social or economic benefits of investments in R&D are of particular interest to policymakers. In this regard, public expense in research, especially through universities, is sometimes being questioned. This paper establishes a measure of how research in Spain, and specifically in its universities, is involved. In this study, we have analyzed all the literature cited in the period 1998–2018 produced by Spanish institutions and which has been cited in at least one international patent, obtaining more than 40,000 publications from more than 160,000 different authors. The data have been surprisingly positive, showing that practically all public universities contribute to this subject and that there is a great deal of international collaboration, both in terms of the number of countries with which they collaborate and the prestige of the institutions involved. Regarding the specific scientific fields in which this collaboration is most relevant, biochemistry, genetics and molecular biology, and medicine together account for almost 40% of the total works. The topics most used by these publications were those of diseases or medical problems such as: Neoplams, Carcinoma, Alzheimer Disease, or human immunodeficiency virus (HIV-1). Oncology was according to the All Science Journal Classification (ASJC) the leading and central issue. Therefore, although the result of basic research is difficult to quantify, when it is observed that there is a return in fields such as medicine or global health, it can be said that it is well employed. In terms of journals from a purely bibliometric point of view, it has been observed that some journals do not have a great impact or relative position within their categories, but they do have a great relevance in this area of patent support. Therefore, it would be worthwhile to set up a rank for scientific journals based on the citations of patents, so the percentage of articles cited in patents with Field-Weighted Citation Impact (FWCI) >1, and as an indicator of scientific transfer from universities or research centres, the transference index in patents (TIP) is also proposed.

Keywords: Scival; patents; Spain; bibliometrics; Research and Development (R&D); social returns

1. Introduction

Basic needs are all those vital necessities that contribute directly or indirectly to a person's survival, and among the most basic or subsistence necessities could be considered those of health and food. Science must respond to the needs of society and to global challenges [1]. Scientific progress enables us to have a better quality of life [2,3], for example the field of health [4] provides us with new medication to treat diseases and, if not possible [5], at least to mitigate pain [6].

Patents protect inventions that consist of products and processes that can be reproduced and replicated for industrial purposes [7]. Companies, laboratories, and individuals can apply for a patent to protect a new technology, sometimes even simply to establish technological boundaries [8]. Whatever the strategic reasons, a patent can be applied for, only if it is for industrial use [9,10]. They are extremely relevant to companies, as they are resources that serve the long-term business. The idea is to keep them in the company for a long period of time. In this way it is possible to develop or invest in a certain line of business, maintaining a certain advantage or protection against the competence. As a major source of new technology generation in developing and transition countries, universities and R&D institutions have played an increasingly active role in the technological innovation, technology transfer and commercialization of intellectual property resulting from research efforts, that finally contribute to the economic, social and cultural development of countries.

Although it is clear that patents are the engine of the industry, in the case of the biotechnology industry that has an impact on the manufacture of drugs such as vaccines [11] or some other medicines, they have a short-term impact on our health or well-being. The transfer of knowledge from research carried out in universities or research centres to the industrial sector is very complex and generally not immediate, but an important indicator is its impact on the number of patents.

Reviewing the research on the properties of the academic literature cited in the patents, it is fair to mention that one of the first works in this regard is the paper of Francisc Narin and Elliot Noma in 1985 [12]. They focused their analysis on 275 biomedical journals and the biotechnology patents in the US Patent Office classification system. As interesting data, they use as reference time for the citations the first eight years after the documents are published. The main conclusion was that science and technology were converging in key high-tech areas. Another very interesting line of research is the study of the patents that are cited by the patents [13,14], highlighting that scientometric assessments, especially of industrial activity, should include patent statistics.

Peter Collins and Suzanne Wyatt [15] studied genetics patents in the U.S. patent system granted during 1980–1985. Although the data are old, they showed that the average citations per patent to papers in basic research journals depending of the applicant country varies between 1 to 10. Another interesting data was that the age distribution of journal citations in patents granted can reach 25 years. Despite the fact that the literature in this field is extensive, focusing on the field of medicine, it is worth mentioning that it has been analyzed in specific fields since 1998 in Gastroenterology research in the United Kingdom [16] till more lately in 2019 in Cardiovascular disease research in Brazil [17].

Scientific innovation is determined by science and technology which together determine the way forward, thus, research documents and patent literature can be used to characterize scientific and technological research in a quantitative, automatic and visual way [18]. Recent studies suggest the need to improve collaboration among private and public sectors and health care organizations in research and patent activities [19]. This sort of analysis, from scientific literature and patent search data, has shown as an example that bioinformatics technology is a valuable strategy to modify, synthesize, or recombine existing antimicrobial peptides to obtain drugs against tumors with high activity and low toxicity [20].

There are some works that highlight this issue by analyzing the patents in the field of biotechnology in Spain but in a very short period of time, from 2000 to 2007 [21], or in Brazil in a longer period of time, from 1975 to 2010 [22]. In both studies, they are analyzed from the point of view of patents and not from the point of view of the science that supports them in the form of scientific publications. In any case, this work focuses on the patents obtained by these countries. In the case of the study of Brazil, only 163 patents were international, that is, from the online at World Intellectual Property Organization (WIPO) for the period from 1997 to 2010 [22]. The study of Spain shows a scarce production of patents in biotechnology, compared with European countries with similar scientific and economic capacity, which indicates a deficit in the capacity to absorb the production of new technologies generated in the public scientific sector [21]. In Spain, some recent studies in the field of medicine propose the inclusion of patent databases such as Lens.org for the assessment of the quality criteria of scientific publications [23].

The University must contribute to social and scientific progress and therefore must respond to the demands and needs of the society in which it is embedded [24,25]. Spain accounts for 87 universities of which 50 are public [26]. With respect to public universities, there is a long tradition, as the first public Spanish university that still exists was founded in 1218, the University of Salamanca (although, the first university was that of Palencia in 1209), and the last one was founded in 1998, the Polytechnic University of Cartagena. As for private universities, the first was founded in 1886, the University of Deusto, and the last three were founded in 2019. In this context, the statistics for Spain are satisfactory, with a population of almost 47 million inhabitants, there's a public university for every million inhabitants. Thus, if the age group is between 18 and 24 years, that's four million people of university age, and the rate increases to more than 12.5 public universities per million inhabitants. If private universities are also considered, the data amounts to almost 21.75 universities per million people of university age. Regarding the research funding in Spain, this was 15,000 million euros (€15 billion) in 2018.

On the other hand, the analysis of innovation systems often occurs at a national, aggregated scale, frequently based on surveys or bibliometric data derived from scientific publications such as academic papers and patents [27]. University patenting has grown most rapidly, especially in fast-growing technologies, in which university-business co-patenting is most prevalent. This suggests that rising public investment in university research is paying off, and that university research is industry-relevant [28]. In this sense, if the patents applied for by Spanish universities since they have been registered are analyzed, it can be seen that in the period from 2007 to 2018 there have been 6322, of which 327 were in 2018, the lowest amount in the whole historical period [29].

The objective of this research is twofold. On the one hand, to offer a global perspective of the knowledge transfer carried out by Spanish universities, understood as the influence that their scientific publications have on patents, that is, on those publications that are cited by the patents, and within these, the impact that this transfer has on the field of medicine, since it is one of the most important research activities in Spain. Secondly, a proposal was made to provide an index to classify universities according to their transfer, and in particular the publications cited in patents.

2. Materials and Methods

The data have been acquired using scientific databases through the different tools that these databases make available to us. Currently, access to these databases is restricted to the organizations that have subscribed to them, which limits the use of these sources. There are free access sources to access scientific publications, but the quality of the data is not the same as in the sources that are mentioned below. Logically, access to science is limited for some researchers, but the reality is that the dominance of these resources has made them indispensable for the world of research, becoming official data sources at the institutional and governmental level.

Scopus is the database developed by Elsevier that indexes the content of more than 24,600 active journal titles and more than 194,000 books from more than 5000 publishers. Its historical content dates back to 1788, and currently contains over 75 million articles, 1.4 billion references cited since 1970, over 9.5 million conference proceedings, 437 million patents from the five largest patent offices worldwide, 16 million author profiles, and around 70,000 membership profiles. Therefore, this database has been used in considerable bibliometric work in every field of knowledge [30], including medicine [31,32].

Based on the data from Scopus, Elsevier has developed its own research performance analysis tool: SciVal, offering access to the scientific output of more than 230 countries and 14,000 institutions from 1996 to the present. It should be noted that this database has also been used for studies related to the field of medicine [33]. Therefore, the main source of data for this study has been Scopus, obtained through SciVal.

In order to complete data on the ranking of scientific journals has been used:

- SCImago Journal Rank (SJR) indicator. Developed by SCImago from the widely known algorithm Google PageRank™, this indicator shows the visibility of the journals contained in the Scopus®database from 1996 [34].
- CiteScore (Scopus). This recent metric, launched in 2016 by Elsevier, is a way of measuring the citation impact of serial titles. It is an alternative to the JCR impact factor (IF) [35].
- JCR (journal citation reports), is a quality indicator of journals that measures the impact of the journals according to the citations received in the Web of Science in the SCIE (Science Citation Index Expanded) and SSCI (Social Science Citation Index) collections. JCR (Journal Citation Reports) provides a quality indicator of journals that measures the impact of the journals according to the citations received in the Web of Science in the SCIE (Science Citation Index Expanded) and SSCI (Social Science Citation Index) collections [36].

To obtain data under analysis, the following search in SciVal has been used as a starting point: "scientific publications in Spain between 1998 and 2018 filtered by ASJC categories". Journal classification approaches perform an essential function in bibliometric analysis [37]. ASJC (All Science Journal Classification) categories is the classification of subjects used by SciVal to categorise Scopus sources and the publications of each of those sources (e.g., journals). Each Scopus source can be assigned to one or more categories in the selected subject classification. Initially there are the four major subject areas: physical sciences, health sciences, social sciences, and life sciences. The ASJC classification has 27 categories (see Table 1) which are further subdivided into various subcategories. Note that multidisciplinary belongs to the four subject areas.

Table 1. ASJC (All Science Journal Classification) categories.

Subject Area	Subject Area Classifications
Physical Sciences	Chemical Engineering
	Chemistry
	Computer Science
	Earth and Planetary Sciences
	Energy
	Engineering
	Environmental Science
	Material Science
	Mathematics
	Physics and Astronomy
	Multidisciplinary
Health Sciences	Medicine
	Nursing
	Veterinary
	Dentistry
	Health Professions
	Multidisciplinary
Social Sciences	Arts and Humanities
	Business, Management and Accounting
	Decision Sciences
	Economics, Econometrics and Finance
	Psychology
	Social Sciences
	Multidisciplinary
Life Sciences	Agricultural and Biological Sciences
	Biochemistry, Genetics and Molecular Biology
	Immunology and Microbiology
	Neuroscience
	Pharmacology, Toxicology and Pharmaceutics
	Multidisciplinary

Figure 1 summarizes the methodology. Once the search was performed, it was filtered by the bibliometric marker "Patent-Cited Scholarly Output" for all publication types and for all patent offices. The result provides all publications that have been cited in at least one patent. The coverage of these patents reaches the five largest patent offices: EPO (European patent office), USPTO (U.S. patent office), UK IPO (UK intellectual property office), JPO (Japan patent office), and WIPO (World Intellectual Property Organization).

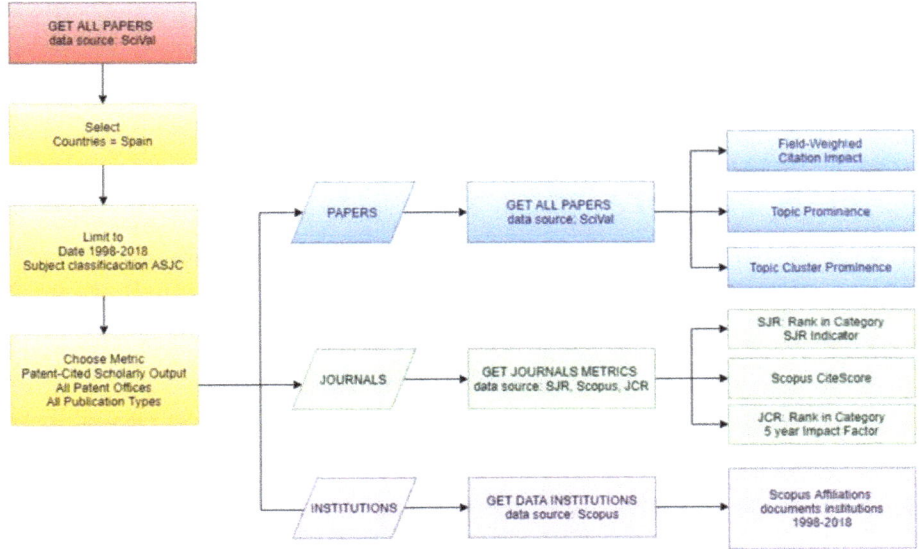

Figure 1. Methodology flowchart. Note: SJR (SCImago Journal Rank); JCR (Journal Citation Reports)

On the basis of these data, the evolution over time from 1998 to 2018 of the publications that have been cited in patents, the contribution of the authors of these publications to the development of patents, as well as the international collaboration between these authors have been analysed.

In the analysis of affiliations, the source data of the analysis has been completed with data from global publications of each affiliation between 1998 and 2018 based on Scopus. The search has been carried out by affiliation, considering the publications that as an institution have been published in each of the universities or R&D centers under study in this date range.

When analyzing the impact of the journal, it has been chosen to analyze the impact of the journal on JCR, based on data from 2018, obtaining the following metric values:

- SJR category and position within the category (rank SJR). SJR thematic categories corresponds to the classification assigned to each journal indexed in the Scopus database [34].
- Indicator SJR. It expresses the average number of weighted citations received in the selected year by the documents published in the selected journal in the three previous years
- CiteScore. Calculating CiteScore is based on the average citations received per document. CiteScore is the number of citations received by a journal in one year to documents published in the three previous years, divided by the number of documents indexed in Scopus published in those same three years [35].
- JCR category and position within the category. The JCR Category is the thematic category assigned to the journal in the Web of Science and within each category the ranking of the journal is shown, calculated according to the position of the journal in relation to the total of each category.

Each journal in JCR is assigned to at least one category and may be classified in more than one category.
- Five-year journal impact factor. This indicator shows the average number of times articles from the journal have been cited in the JCR year over the past five years. It is calculated by dividing the number of citations in the JCR year by the total number of articles published in the previous five years.

When analyzing research topics, SciVal uses so-called Topics. A Topic is a set of documents with a common interest. Topics are based on the grouping of the citation network of 95% of the Scopus content (all documents published since 1996) and are grouped within SciVal based on direct citation analysis using document reference lists, so that a document can belong to only one Topic but as newly published documents are indexed, they are added to the Topics using their reference lists. This makes the Topics dynamic and most of them increase in size over time.

They are obtained from more than one billion citation links between more than 48 million documents indexed by Scopus from 1996 onwards and more than 20 million other non-indexed documents that are cited at least twice. There are approximately 96,000 Topics. Once a year SciVal re-runs the SciVal Topics algorithm to identify newly emerging topics. A combination of the potential for emergence (recent numbers of publications vs. previous years), size of the topic, citations, and funding is considered to rank a new topic. As an example, in 2019, 37 new topics were identified and added to SciVal.

The Topics name is part of the topics cluster name. A topic cluster name is created by adding topics with similar research interests to form a broader, higher-level research area. These topic clusters can be used to gain a broader understanding of the research being carried out by a country, institution (or group) or researcher (or group). Each of the 96,000 topics has been paired with one of the 1500 cluster topics. As with topics, a researcher or institution can contribute to multiple topics, but a topic can only belong to one topic and a publication can only belong to one topic (and therefore to one cluster topic). Clusters topics are formed using the same direct citation algorithm that creates the topics. When the strength of the citation links between the topics reaches a threshold, a cluster topic is formed.

Among all the other possible metrics to evaluate the quality of the journals, it has been chosen the field-weighted citation impact, this is the average number of citations received in relation to the expected ones. Recent studies prove that the FWCI is consistent in different areas of research [38]. Expected citations are calculated for the same year of publication, same type of publication, and same discipline. The benchmark is 1, above which, the expected, and below, it has not reached what was expected.

3. Results

The results achieved from this search, of Spanish scientific papers cited by international patents from 1998 to 2018, have yielded a value of 41,068 cited publications. As expected, almost all these publications are journal articles, more than 96%, being anecdotic the case of the books (Book and Book series) with just over 1% and the conference proceedings with just over 2%. These works have been written by 313,458 co-authors, of which there are 161,046 different authors, identified by their Scopus ID. Most frequently, authors contribute to only one publication, which is the case for 35.5%, those with two are 7.5%, those with three are 3%, those with four are 1.5%, and those with five are less than 1%. By way of exception, there are 50 authors with more than 50 contributions cited by patents. This case study would be particularly interesting to study.

3.1. Global Temporal Trend

Figure 2 shows the evolution of the articles cited by patents in the period studied. The trend from 1998 to 2008 is very similar, i.e., it seems clear that the greater the research funding, the greater the number of works cited by patents. From this date the trends are different, but it must be clarified that the research does not have an immediate impact on the industry, this trend can be evaluated in the long term, so we can consider that the data up to 10 years ago, should they be representative.

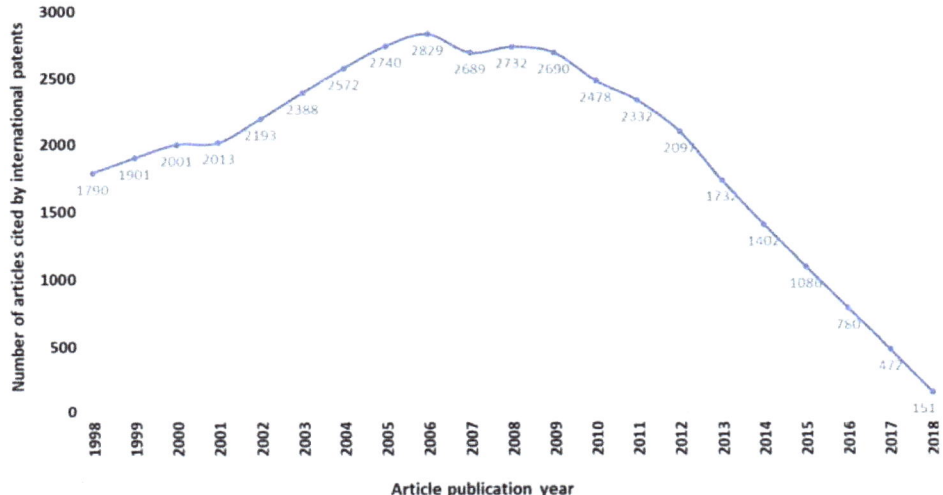

Figure 2. Publications cited by international patents and R&D funding in Spain.

3.2. Countries, Affiliations and Collaborations

The authors of these publications cited in patents belong to just over 5000 institutions around the world, proving a great collaboration with the rest of the world by the Spanish institutions. A total of 165 different countries have been involved, with the USA being the most important with almost 7500 contributions, followed by the UK with around 4200 and Germany with just over 3700. Figure 3 shows a map of Spain's international collaboration. There is scarce, or almost no, collaboration with African countries, despite the fact that, as will be seen later, the pharmaceutical industry and the area of medicine are very prominent in the domain of patents, and there are very widespread diseases in these areas, such as malaria [39], AIDS, or tuberculosis [40].

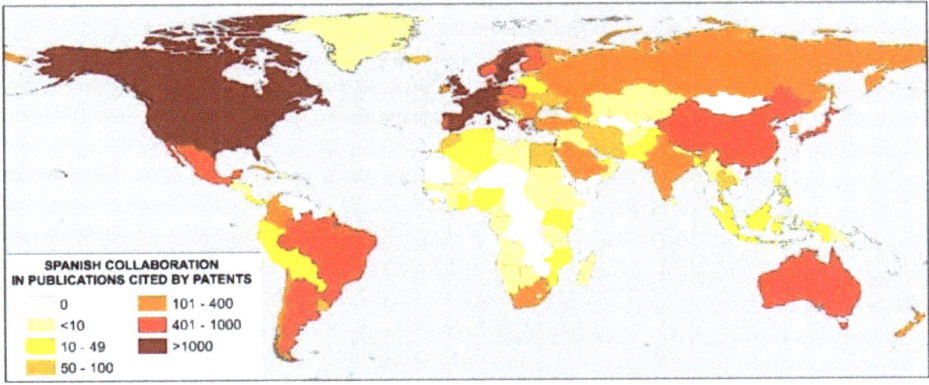

Figure 3. Worldwide collaboration with Spanish publications cited in patents.

The top 20 Spanish institutions that have contributed mostly with their publications to international patents are shown in Figure 4. It can be observed as expected that the CSIC, Consejo Superior de Investigaciones Científicas, as the Spanish state agency dedicated to scientific research and technological development, leads this ranking. An example of these studies, which is also widely cited, is a collaboration between University of Valencia, Consejo Superior de Investigaciones Científicas, Beth Israel Deaconess Medical Center, and Harvard Medical School related to the Transcranial magnetic stimulation [41].

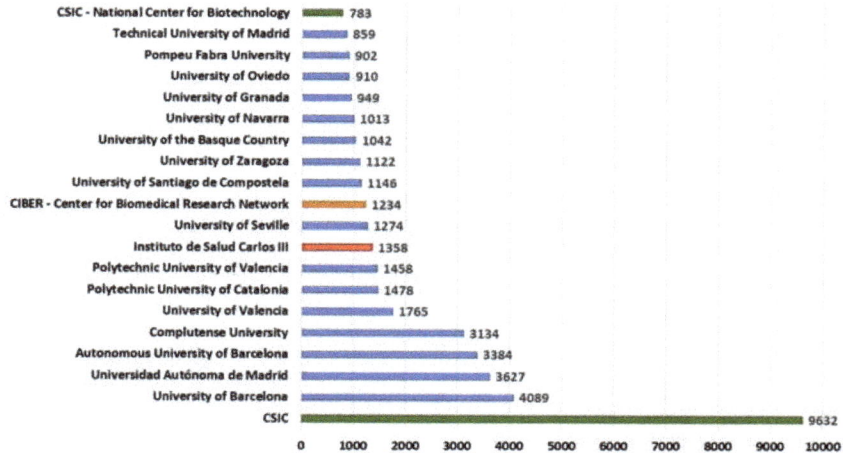

Figure 4. Top 20 Spanish institutions by publications cited in patents. Note: CSIC (Consejo Superior de Investigaciones Científicas).

Figure 4 highlights the non-university institutions, which include, apart from a specific section of the CSIC, the National Center for Biotechnology, two other autonomous health institutions, the CIBER—Center for Biomedical Research Network and the Instituto de Salud Carlos III. With respect to the universities, two of the first four stand out: The University of Barcelona and the Autonomous University of Barcelona; and two in Madrid, the Autonomous University of Madrid, and the Complutense University. In fifth place is the University of Valencia, but already distant in the number of publications. In this ranking it is remarkable that there are no other research agencies such as CIEMAT (Energy, Environmental and Technological Research Center) that in this period only appear with 251 publications cited, almost as small universities, as the University of Almeria with 210 publications cited in patents. Interestingly, these two institutions cooperate extensively in research, perhaps due to the proximity of one of the CIEMAT centres, Plataforma Solar de Almeria, to the aforementioned university, e.g., they have investigate solar reflector materials degradation due to the sand deposited on backside protective paints [42].

With the aim of having a metric of the impact of the scientific production of the universities in its transference with respect to the patents. The transference index in patents (TIP) is proposed, and this is calculated as a percentage of publications cited in patents over the total number of publications indexed. Table 2 shows this index calculated for the Top 20 Spanish universities. Those that are above 5% are considered outstanding, excellent between 4% and 5%, very good between 3% and 4%, good between 2% and 3%, average < 2%.

This TIP index shows that among this top 20, 4 universities are in the range of outstanding, apart from the three most productive, now included in this category is the University of Navarra (5.24), which is a private university. In the range of excellent there are two universities: Complutense University (4.74) and Pompeu Fabra University (4.66). Further, in the rank of very good, we find eight universities.

Table 2. Proposed Transference Index in Patents (TIP).

University	N Cited in Patents (NCP)	NCP without Collaboration	N (1998–2018)	TIP (TIP = NCP × 100/N)
University of Barcelona	4089	781	68,392	5.98
Autonomous University of Madrid	3627	314	63,288	5.73
Autonomous University of Barcelona	3384	551	65,910	5.13
Complutense University of Madrid	3134	587	66,136	4.74
University of Valencia	1765	376	52,037	3.39
Technical University of Catalonia	1478	415	51,882	2.85
Polytechnic University of Valencia	1458	339	38,660	3.77
University of Seville	1274	268	37,233	3.42
University of Santiago De Compostela	1146	412	32,766	3.77
University of Zaragoza	1122	273	32,863	3.49
University of The Basque Country	1042	311	40,071	2.80
University of Navarra	1013	315	19,324	5.39
University of Granada	949	316	43,755	2.32
University of Oviedo	910	365	25,656	3.70
Pompeu Fabra University	902	50	19,366	4.70
Technical University of Madrid	859	197	37,155	2.43
Universidad Rovira i Virgili	751	190	19,691	3.81
Universidad de Salamanca	650	114	19,411	3.35
University of Murcia	595	270	20,699	2.87
University of Málaga	539	178	19,589	2.75

What is surprising at first glance is that the most technological universities are not necessarily the best at this transfer rate: Polytechnic University of Valencia (3.77), Polytechnic University of Catalonia (2.85), and Technical University of Madrid (2.31).

In Figure 5, the top 20 non-Spanish institutions that participate in these works have been represented the ones with which most collaboration takes place. The collaboration of Spanish institutions is especially remarkable with the CNRS (Centre national de la recherche scientifique) in France with more than 1000 works. In addition, there are three other institutions in this country in the top 20: Institut national de la santé et de la recherche médicale (773), Université Paris-Saclay (498) and Sorbonne Université (416). This fact is striking since France was in fourth place in Spanish collaboration.

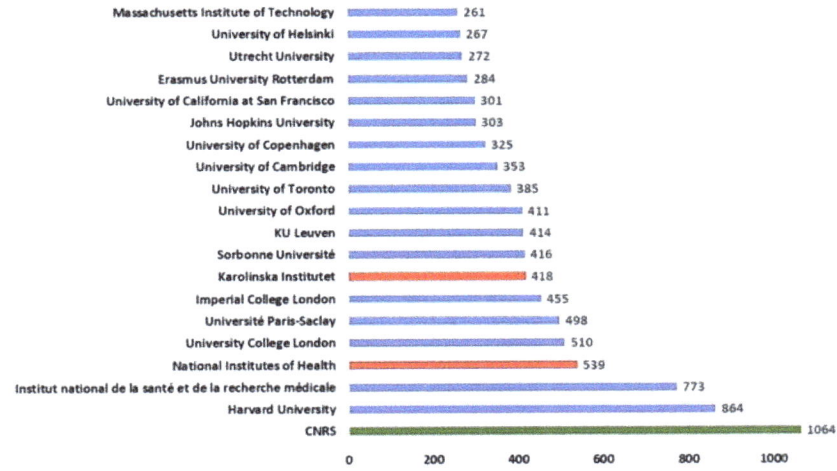

Figure 5. Top 20 Foreign institutions that collaborates with Spanish institutions.

Spanish institutions collaboration with foreign countries is significant, as 21,136 of the total number of contributions analysed are of Spanish authorship only, representing 51% of the works. Therefore, in broad terms, this means that half of the contributions cited in patents are in collaboration with foreign institutions. However, when it concerns universities, the percentage is significantly lower Table 2 shows the contributions of each university without collaboration. If the data are analyzed in relative terms, in terms of percentages, the University of Murcia has the highest percentage without collaboration with 41% and the lowest, with 5%, is the Pompeu Fabra University. But the important data is the average, which is 25%. So, only one of each four contributions cited in patents is authored by a Spanish university without collaboration.

Concerning the collaboration with the USA, the first place is taken by Harvard University (864), followed by the National Institutes of Health (539). With the UK, the institutions are universities, University College London (510), Imperial College London (455), and the University of Oxford (411). It is striking that in this top 20 of international collaboration no German institution exists, even though Germany is the third country in terms of international collaboration for Spain. Finally, it should be noted that, apart from the CNRS, the only two non-university institutions carrying out research in the field of health are the aforementioned Institut national de la santé et de la recherche médicale (France) and the Karolinska Institutet (Sweden).

3.3. Top Journals Used for the Spanish Publications Cited in Patents

The Spanish scientific studies that have been cited in patents have been published in 4579 different journals. In Table 3, the top 20 of these journals are reported, together with some of their bibliometric indicators. It can be seen that these journals are mainly in the chemical or medical field, with the clear exception of the highly recognized multidisciplinary journals such as Proceedings of the National Academy of Sciences of the United States of America (PNAS), PLoS ONE, or Nature. As an anecdote, there is only one article from the journal Science in this list of journals.

Table 3. Top 20 Journals and their metrics (Data 2018).

Journal	N	SJR Category	Rank SJR	SJR Indicator	CiteScore Scopus	JCR Category	Rank JCR	Impact Factor (5 years) JCR
Journal of Biological Chemistry	507	Biochemistry	37/446-Q1	2.403	3.92	Biology & Biochemistry	1/434-Q1	4.279
		Cell Biology	45/288-Q1					
		Molecular Biology	69/409-Q1					
Journal of Agricultural and Food Chemistry	350	Agricultural and Biological Sciences (miscellaneous)	32/272-Q1	1.111	3.8	Agriculture, Multidisciplinary	3/57-Q1	3.911
						Chemistry, Applied	14/71-Q1	
		Chemistry (miscellaneous)	56/437-Q1			Food Science &Technology	28/135-Q1	
Proceedings of the National Academy of Sciences of the United States of America (PNAS)	321	Multidisciplinary	4/120-Q1	5.601	8.58	Multidisciplinary Sciences	7/69-Q1	10.600
PLoS ONE	292	Agricultural and Biological Sciences (miscellaneous)	32/272-Q1	1.100	2.97	Multidisciplinary Sciences	24/69-Q2	3.337
		Biochemistry, Genetics and Molecular Biology (miscellaneous)	53/242-Q1					
		Medicine (miscellaneous)	474/2836-Q1					
Journal of the American Chemical Society	253	Biochemistry	5/446-Q1	7.468	14.75	Chemistry Multidisciplinary	12/172-Q1	14.491
		Catalysis	1/58-Q1					
		Colloid and Surface Chemistry	1/16-Q1					
		Chemistry (miscellaneous)	7/437-Q1					
Lecture Notes in Computer Science (including subseries Lecture Notes in Artificial Intelligence and Lecture Notes in Bioinformatics)	253	Computer Science (miscellaneous)	131/449-Q2	0.283	1.06	Computer Science, Theory & Methods (2005 is last year available)	62/71-Q4	n/a
		Theoretical Computer Science	96/160-Q3					
Nature	236	Multidisciplinary	1/120-Q1	16.345	15.21	Multidisciplinary Sciences	1/69-Q1	45.819
Journal of Organic Chemistry	233	Organic Chemistry	15/177-Q1	1.607	4.57	Chemistry, Organic	7/57-Q1	4.224

Table 3. Cont.

Journal	N	SJR Category	Rank SJR	SJR Indicator	CiteScore Scopus	JCR Category	Rank JCR	Impact Factor (5 years) JCR
Journal of Medicinal Chemistry	232	Molecular Medicine	18/173-Q1	2.287	1.05	Chemistry, Medicinal	3/61-Q1	6.060
		Drug Discovery	7/167-Q1					
Blood	221	Biochemistry	9/446-Q1	6.065	7.27	Hematology	1/73-Q1	13.206
		Cell Biology	19/288-Q1					
		Immunology	10/216-Q1					
		Hematology	2/133-Q1					
Applied and Environmental Microbiology	196	Food Science	11/301-Q1	1.663	4.18	Biotechnology & Applied Microbiology	33/162-Q1	4.701
		Biotechnology	30/328-Q1					
		Ecology	27/357-Q1			Microbiology	38/133-C2	
		Applied Microbiology and Biotechnology	11/111-Q1					
Tetrahedron	196	Biochemistry	228/446-Q3	0.709	2.39	Chemistry, Organic	26/57-Q2	2.193
		Organic Chemistry	60/177-Q2					
		Drug Discovery	56/167-Q2					
Journal of Virology	190	Insect Science	2/146-Q1	2.590	4.02	Virology	8/36-Q1	4.259
		Immunology	25/216-Q1					
		Microbiology	15/149-Q1					
		Virology	8/70-Q1					
Cancer Research	181	Cancer Research	11/216-Q1	4.047	6.94	Oncology	21/230-Q1	9.062
		Oncology	14/368-Q1					
Journal of Chromatography A	180	Biochemistry	122/446-Q2	1.188	3.78	Biochemical Research Methods	13/79-Q1	3.741
		Analytical Chemistry	14/117-Q1					
		Organic Chemistry	27/177-Q1			Chemistry, Analytical	15/84-Q1	
		Medicine (miscellaneous)	417/2836-Q1					
New England Journal of Medicine	177	Medicine (miscellaneous)	3/2836-Q1	19.524	16.1	Medicine, General & Internal	1/160-Q1	70.331
Applied Physics Letters	167	Physics and Astronomy (miscellaneous)	29/267-Q1	1.331	3.58	Physics, Applied	31/148-Q1	3.352
Clinical Cancer Research	165	Cancer Research	7/216-Q1	4.965	8.32	Oncology	16/230-Q1	9.174
		Oncology	10/368-Q1					
Chemistry—A European Journal	164	Catalysis	8/58-Q1	1.842	4.77	Chemistry, Multidisciplinary	37/172-Q1	4.843
		Chemistry (miscellaneous)	31/437-Q1					
		Organic Chemistry	8/177-Q1					
Angewandte Chemie—International Edition	159	Catalysis	2/58-Q1	5.478	11.68	Chemistry, Multidisciplinary	17/172-Q1	12.359
		Chemistry (miscellaneous)	12/437-Q1					
FEBS Letters	159	Biochemistry	63/446-Q1	1.849	3.01	Biochemistry & Molecular Biology	160/299-Q3	3.386
		Biophysics	10/133-Q1			Biophysics	30/73-Q2	
		Cell Biology	76/288-Q2					
		Genetics	60/338-Q1			Cell Biology	129/193-Q3	
		Molecular Biology	101/409-Q1					
		Structural Biology	14/53-Q2					

About the metrics of the Top 20 journals obtained, most of them belong to the first quartile (Q1), 17 of the 20 analyzed, but only four are the first of their category. Of the many metrics that can be used to analyze the journals, the field-weighted citation impact has been used, as mentioned, if the publications are above the value of 1, it is more than expected. In our case, the average of all the publications analysed is almost 4 (3.97), and 27,888 of the 41,068 papers analysed are above 1, i.e., 68%.

Three indices have been chosen to assess the articles published in the top 20 journals: field-weighted citation impact, top 10% topic, and top 10% topic cluster. The Field-Weighted Citation Impact, a Scopus-specific metric value, allows users to measure whether publications have exceeded the percentage of citations expected from them, considering the year of publication, the type of publication and the discipline. The benchmark is 1, so that higher values meet the publication's expectations and lower values below 1 do not.

Figure 6 shows the percentage of publications in each of the journals that were above 1. The data show the different percentages achieved, with the New England Journal of Medicine standing out as all the articles published exceeded the value of 1. Between 90% and 100% there are two other journals Nature and Blood, followed by the rest of the journals that are above 50%, only two titles (Lecture Notes in Computer Science, including subseries Lecture Notes in Artificial Intelligence and Lecture Notes in Bioinformatics and Tetrahedron) do not exceed 50%. Based on these data, the majority of publications not only contribute to the development and advancement of science, but also have a direct application in knowledge transfer by being cited in patents. They have surpassed the perspectives expected from them and have had a practical application in research transfer.

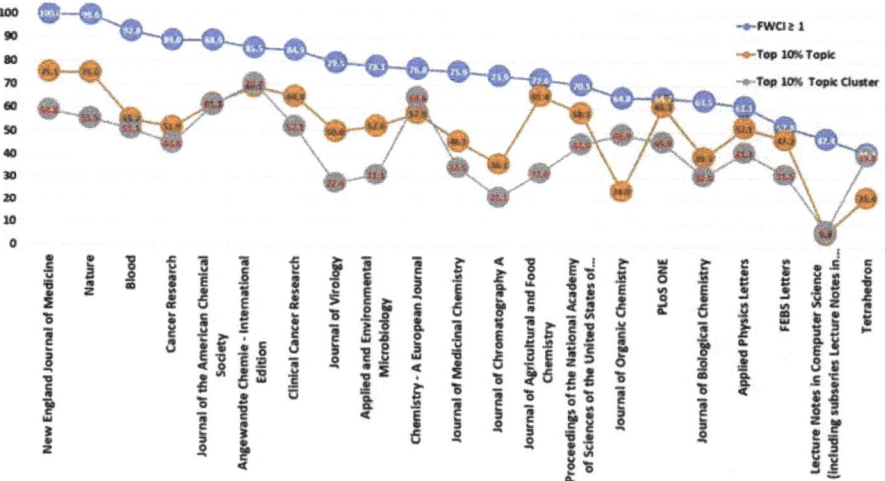

Figure 6. Percentage of articles Field-Weighted Citation Impact (FWCI) ≥ 1, Top 10% Topic y Topic Cluster.

The second index considered was the percentage of publications within each journal that contributed to the top 10% of topic and topic cluster. Being in the Top 10% of these values is indicative of the momentum of the Topics that have been assigned to these publications, thus promoting the visibility of these fields of research. Journals such as the New England Journal of Medicine or Nature place more than 75% of their publications in the top 10% of topics, as well as Angewandte Chemie—International Edition, Chemistry—A European Journal or Journal of the American Chemical Society and Angewandte Chemie—International Edition, which place more than 60% of their publications in the top 10% of topic clusters.

3.4. Subject Area Classifications of the Publications Cited in Patents

Although the journals are an early indicator of the topics covered, if one uses the classification of the database itself, namely the all science journal classification (ASJC) field name, these contributions appear in four subject areas, which in turn are divided into the 30 categories indicated in Table 1, and this classification allows a third level. This is done by in-house experts when of the serial title is set up for Scopus coverage; the classification is based on the aims and scope of the title, and on the content it publishes. If the distribution of the scientific output by the All Science Journal Classification (ASJC) are analysed regarding the distribution in the four subject areas, the one that contributes most is physical sciences with 44%, followed closely by life sciences with 38%, in third place health sciences with 16%, in fourth place social sciences with less than 1% as expected. The works in the multidisciplinary category have not been attributed to any subject area, being overall 1%. Note that this scientific production refers to the whole, i.e., it includes articles, books, and proceedings.

If the studies are analyzed by subject area classifications, Figure 7 is obtained. The highest percentage of studies is biochemistry, genetics and molecular with 23%, followed by medicine with 15%, and then chemistry with 10%. This means, for example, that of the total number of Spanish scientific output cited in patents, 15% are classified in the field of medicine. The other categories are already below 10%. Figure 8 shows a cloud of words made with the subcategories of the ASJC in order to establish a visual comparison.

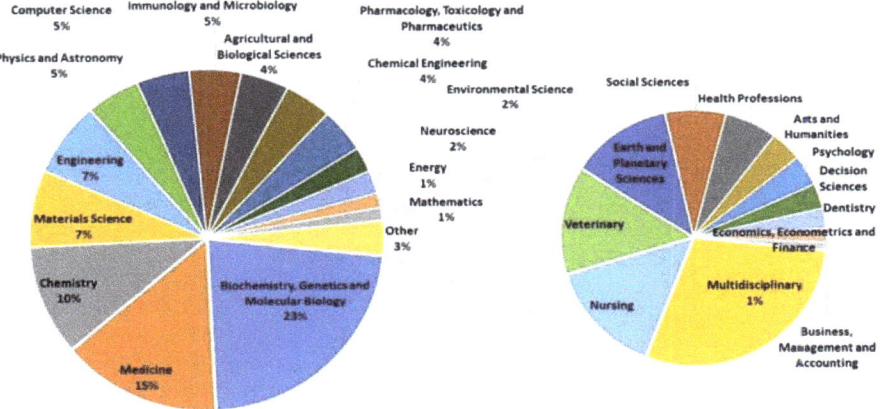

Figure 7. Distribution of the scientific output by ASJC (articles, books, and proceedings).

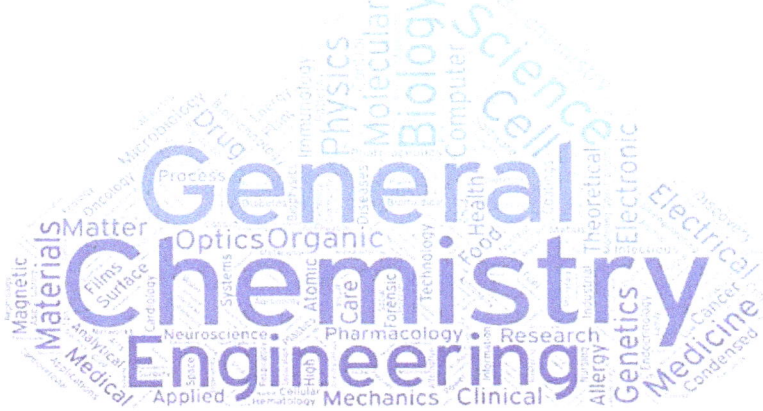

Figure 8. Cloud Word of Topic cluster names.

3.5. Topics of the Publications Cited in Patents

The topics covered in all these papers could be summarized by two indexing fields: topic cluster name, and topic name. Table 4 lists the first 20 Topic Cluster names and Topic names. In the Topic names, the topics of medicine and biochemistry are more present, but some of other areas such as algorithms, plants, or solar cells are present. On the other hand, in the Topic names no longer appears anything of these other areas, and they do appear diseases apart from neoplasms, appear terms like carcinoma, Alzheimer Disease, or HIV-1. To establish a visual comparison, the topic names have also been represented in a cloud of words in Figure 9.

Table 4. Top 20 Topic Cluster names and Topic names.

Topic Cluster Name	N	Topic Name	N
Neoplasms	3062	Neoplasms	1180
Patients	2743	Receptors	828
Catalysts	1614	Proteins	464
Synthesis (Chemical)	956	Cells	463
Models	883	Patients	374
Algorithms	842	Synthesis (chemical)	348
Genes	821	DNA	339
Hydrogenation	795	Carcinoma	336
Zeolites	795	Genes	312
Pharmaceutical Preparations	686	Mutation	304
Proteins	656	Pharmaceutical Preparations	294
Cells	641	Receptor	288
Catalysis	617	Peptides	284
T-Lymphocytes	596	T-Lymphocytes	276
Plants	586	Ligands	269
Bacteria	555	Breast Neoplasms	263
Solar Cells	551	Nanoparticles	258
Immunotherapy	535	Alzheimer Disease	236
Ligands	495	RNA	232
Breast Neoplasms	489	HIV-1	228

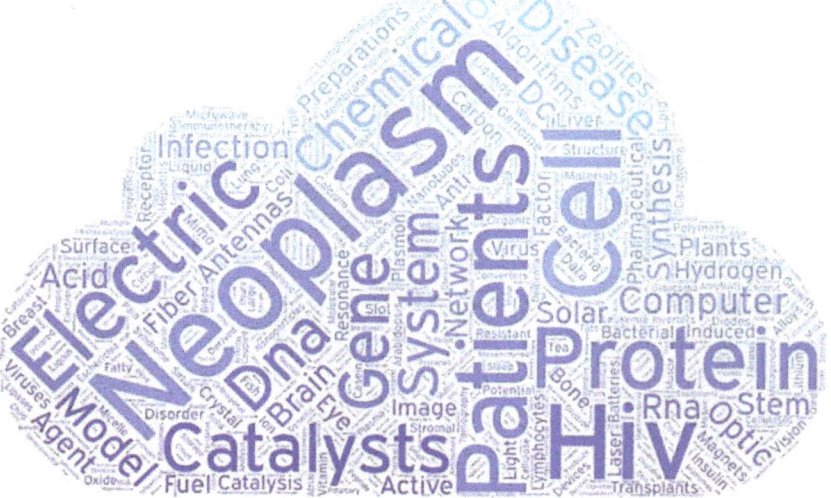

Figure 9. Cloud Word of Topic names.

4. The Contribution of Spanish Science to Patents: The Medicine Area

4.1. Temporal Trend in the Medicine Area

Although civil society is sometimes critical of medical patents, as universal access to medicines is understood from a human point of view. However, the WHO (World Health Organization) itself is in favor of this system, since it is clear that, after basic research, they have to be manufactured, and in order for them to be affordable, investment has to be made in their manufacture, which is determined by exclusivity or patents. Furthermore, the WHO itself makes it clear that it is possible to develop many medicines that are patentable (i.e., that meet the requirement of novelty and inventive step), but this does not mean that they add value to existing medicines. According to the data of the IQWiG (Institute for Quality and Efficiency in Health Care—Institut für Qualität und Wirtschaftlichkeit im Gesundheitswesen), of all the medicines that are patented annually, only 10% add great value to what already exists, and only 17% add considerable value, i.e., only 27% of these medicines should be incorporated into the health system.

In the previous sections, a ranking of universities has been established according to their transfer, but, although the Spanish university is not singularly specialized, except as mentioned for certain technical universities. It is necessary to establish a ranking by areas of knowledge. In this way it will be possible to know the transference and the relevance of a university in a specific area.

In this study, the publications classified within the category of medicine only are 11,287, but there are about 4100 that are also indexed in other categories. If we compare the field of medicine with the total, we can see that it has been very stable over the years. In Figure 10, it can be seen how scientific works classified in the category of medicine have always been at least 20% of the works cited by patents.

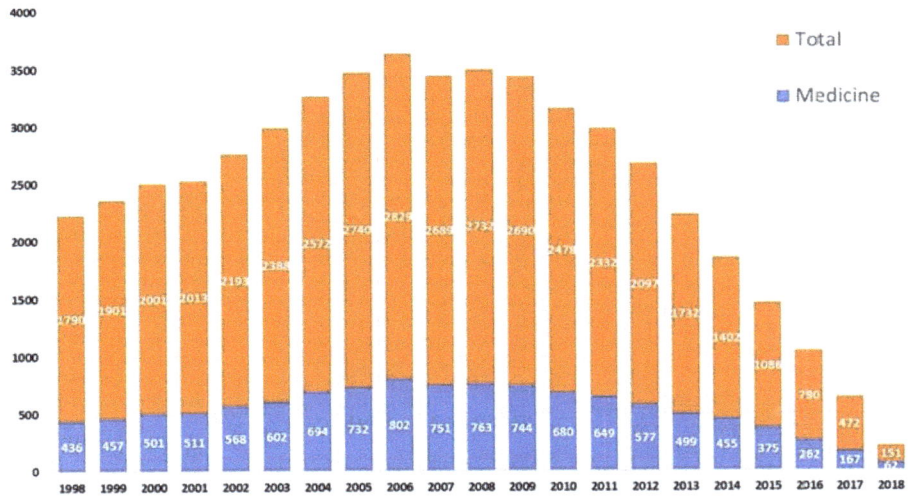

Figure 10. Medicine category display in relation to the total number of publications cited in patents.

4.2. Medicine Transference Index in Patents for Spanish Universities

The Spanish scientific output developed by the institutions in the field of medicine cited in patents is reflected in Table 5. Broadly speaking, it can be seen that they are basically the same institutions as the general transfer, with some exceptions of universities, which do not have medical faculties and do not appear in this ranking. If one observes the last column of the table, the explanation is easy: medical research accounts for a very high percentage of the publications cited in patents. The table has been ordered according to this percentage, with the University of Navarra reaching more than 50%. It can be seen that this percentage decreases in accordance with the vocation of each university, so that the last ones in this ranking are technical universities that do not have a medical faculty, and this scientific output is due to collaboration with other institutions.

Table 5. Medicine Transference Index in Patents (MED-TIP).

University	N-MED [1]	NCP [2]	N [3]	TIP [4]	TIP-MED [5]	% MED-TOT [6]
University of Navarra	566	1013	19,324	5.24	2.93	55.87
Autonomous University of Barcelona	1690	3384	65,910	5.13	2.56	49.94
University of Barcelona	2001	4089	68,392	5.98	2.93	48.94
Pompeu Fabra University	372	902	19,366	4.66	1.92	41.24
Complutense University	1223	3134	66,136	4.74	1.85	39.02
Polytechnic University of Valencia	568	1458	38,660	3.77	1.47	38.96
Universidad de Salamanca	223	650	19,411	3.35	1.15	34.31
Universidad Autónoma de Madrid	1207	3627	63,288	5.73	1.91	33.28
University of Valencia	568	1765	52,037	3.39	1.09	32.18
University of Santiago de Compostela	312	1146	32,766	3.50	0.95	27.23
University of Granada	235	949	43,755	2.17	0.54	24.76
University of Zaragoza	268	1122	32,863	3.41	0.82	23.89
University of Murcia	133	595	20,699	2.87	0.64	22.35
University of Valladolid	89	426	17,007	2.50	0.52	20.89
University of Oviedo	189	910	25,656	3.55	0.74	20.77
Universidad Rovira i Virgili	124	751	19,691	3.81	0.63	16.51
University of the Basque Country	159	1042	40,071	2.60	0.40	15.26
University of Seville	143	1274	37,233	3.42	0.38	11.22
Technical University of Madrid	52	859	37,155	2.31	0.14	6.05
Polytechnic University of Catalonia	69	1478	51,882	2.85	0.13	4.67

[1] N-MED Total number of publications classifies as Medicine category (ASJC) cited in patents; [2] NCP Total number of publications cited in patents; [3] N Total number of publications published by the institution in period 1998–2018; [4] TIP = NCP × 100/N; [5] TIP-MED = N-MED × 100/N; [6] % MED-TOT = N-MED × 100/NCP.

4.3. ASJC Clusters and Relationship Network

So, to this point, the above information is that which can be extracted more or less directly from the databases analysed. In this section, the aim is to detect in an independent way, and from the published studies, if the scientific fields of medicine described in previous sections, have any relation between them, that is to say, if they can be grouped in scientific communities or clusters. For this purpose, the bibliometric information of all these works have been downloaded with the Scopus API. If an analysis of data is made with the Gephi software of the network of relationships between the publications that are being analyzed on medicine. Figure 11 shows the relationship found between all the contributions, where each dot is a publication, and the line that joins two dots is the relationship it has for having been cited by that publication, the thickness of the dot indicates the number of times that publication is cited by the others. There is an outer circle of publications, which have no relationship with the others, that is, they would be publication that have been used in the references of some patents in the field of medicine, but which have no relationship with any other publication of this analysis. However, those that are linked to others, are publications that in addition to having been cited by patents, are related to others of this selection of publication. This means that these are more central publication that have been cited by patents, but they have also contributed to opening a line of work in this particular field for research itself since it is related to the other publication. In Figure 11, the publications have been colored according to the ASJR category assigned by Scopus. One can appreciate that they dominate oncology (11,78%), immunology and allergy (9.48%), infectious diseases (7.1%), cardiology and cardiovascular (6.63%), hematology (6.44%), neurology (clinical) (5.34%), and general medicine (4.74%). The oncology category has a central role in this relationship. On the other hand, it is seen that general medicine is widely spread throughout the network, as expected, since it has a direct relationship with all other medical disciplines. This is also the case, although to a lesser extent, with cardiology and cardiovascular.

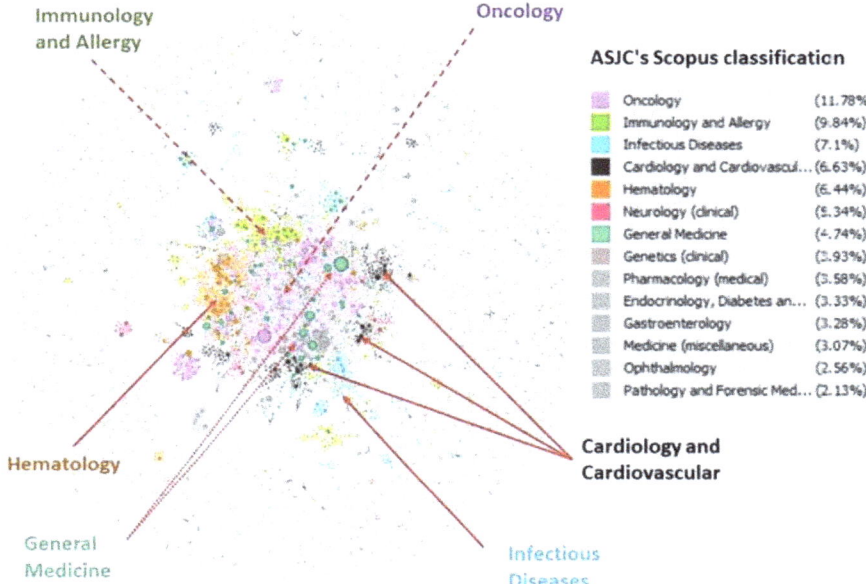

Figure 11. Relationship between publications that are cited in patents in the field of medicine according to the subcategories of medicine of the ASJC.

4.4. Cluster Detection Indenpent Analysis

In a second analysis, the relationships between the publications analysed will be detected. This analysis is independent of the ASJC's Scopus classification done in previous section. In this case the analysis was done with a cluster detection algorithm that contains the software Gephi. Thus, the clusters have been obtained according to the relationships that exist between the publications. Figure 12 shows a color-coded according to the twenty-two clusters cluster obtained. The weight of the cluster reflects in ratio the significance of this set of publications in the whole network of relations. Once the clusters are established, all the keywords are extracted from all the publications in that cluster. Then, the frequency of each keyword that is found in each cluster is calculated as an index of its importance within that cluster. Tables 6–11 show a list of the main keywords for the leading clusters found, up to 5% of weight. The proposed name for each cluster was made according to the keywords of this cluster.

Table 6. Neoplasms. Cluster (9), weigh 11.58%.

Topic Names	N = 335
Breast Neoplasms, Receptor, Epidermal Growth Factor, Adjuvant trastuzumab	27
Receptor, Epidermal Growth Factor, Neoplasms, Antibodies, Monoclonal	21
Multiple Myeloma, Patients, Diagnosed multiple	13
Activated-Leukocyte Cell Adhesion Molecule, T-Lymphocytes, Activated leukocyte	12
Colorectal Neoplasms, Drug Therapy, Colorectal cancer	11
Colorectal Neoplasms, Mutation, Anti-epidermal growth	10
Breast Neoplasms, Receptor, Epidermal Growth Factor, Immunohistochemistry (IHC)	9
Sirolimus, Neoplasms, Mammalian target	9
Breast Neoplasms, Neoplasms, HER3 expression	8

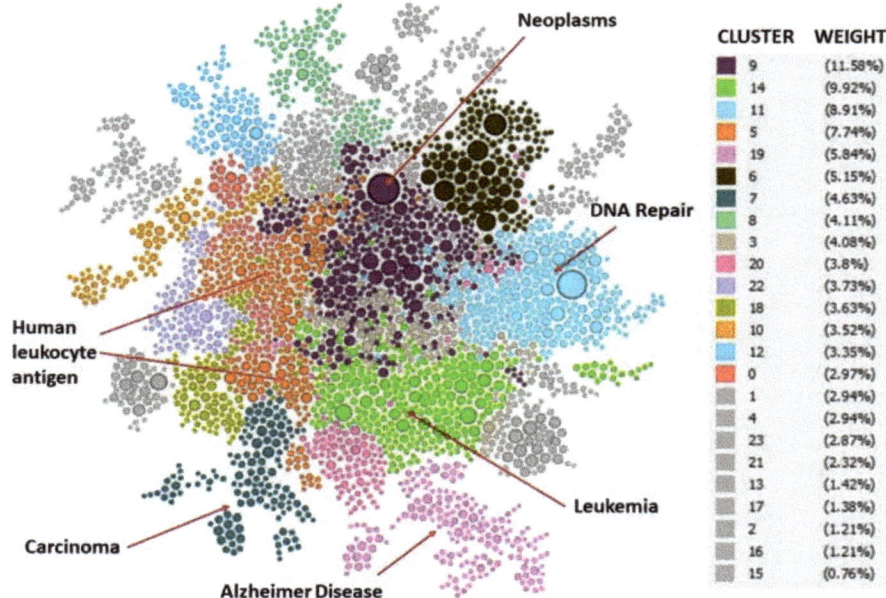

Figure 12. Network of the relationship between publications that are cited in patents in the field of medicine according to the subcategories of medicine of the ASJC.

Table 7. Leukemia. Cluster (14), weigh 9.92%.

Topic Names	N = 287
Leukemia, Lymphocytic, Chronic, B-Cell, Patients, Lymphocytic leukemia	19
Lymphoma, Large B-Cell, Diffuse, Lymphoma, Rituximab cyclophosphamide	18
Lymphoma, Mantle-Cell, Patients, MCL patients	16
Tetraspanins, Cells, Cell migration	10
T-Lymphocytes, B-Lymphocytes, XIAP (X-linked inhibitor of apoptosis protein) deficiency	8
Multiple Myeloma, Plasma Cells, Cytogenetic abnormalities	7
Leukemia, Precursor Cell Lymphoblastic Leukemia-Lymphoma, Phenotype acute	7
Lymphoma, Follicular, Lymphoma, Mantle cell	7
Precursor Cell Lymphoblastic Leukemia-Lymphoma, Neoplasm, Residual, Disease MRD (Minimal residual disease)	7
Liver Transplantation, Liver, Liver allograft	6

Table 8. DNA Repair. Cluster (11), weigh 8.91%.

Topic Names	N = 258
DNA, Neoplasms, Liquid biopsies	19
DNA Repair, Carcinoma, Non-Small-Cell Lung, Repair cross-complementation	18
Carcinoma, Non-Small-Cell Lung, Receptor, Epidermal Growth Factor, Lung cancers	16
Epithelial-Mesenchymal Transition, Neoplasms, Epithelial-to-mesenchymal transition	10
Breast Neoplasms, Methylation, Suppressor genes	8
Breast Neoplasms, Neoplasms, Cancer subtypes	7
DNA Methylation, Methylation, Whole-genome bisulfite	7
Methyltransferases, DNA, Temozolomide (TMZ)	7
Precursor Cell Lymphoblastic Leukemia-Lymphoma, DNA Methylation, Methylation	7
Urinary Bladder Neoplasms, Carcinoma, Bladder cancers	6

Table 9. Human leukocyte antigen (HLA). Cluster (5), weigh 7.74%.

Topic Names	N = 224
Neoplasms, HLA Antigens, HLA class	19
Fetal Blood, Transplantation, Blood UCB (Umbilical Cord Blood)	10
T-Lymphocytes, Neoplasms, Cancer immunotherapy	9
HLA-G Antigens, HLA Antigens, SHLA-G levels	8
Lectins, C-Type, T-Lymphocytes, T cells	8
Killer Cells, Natural, Receptors, Natural Killer Cell, Ly49 receptors	7
Receptors, Antigen, T-Cell, T-Lymphocytes, Antigen receptor	7
Dendritic Cells, T-Lymphocytes, Plasmacytoid DCs	5
Interleukin-12, Neoplasms, Gene therapy	5
Receptors, KIR (Killer Immunoglobulin-like Receptor), Killer Cells, Natural, Killer immunoglobulin-like	5

Table 10. Alzheimer Disease. Cluster (19), weigh 5.84%.

Topic Names	N = 169
Restless Legs Syndrome, Sleep, Patients	15
Tauopathies, Alzheimer Disease, Tau oligomers	12
Platelet-Rich Plasma, Blood Platelets, Intercellular Signaling Peptides and Proteins	10
Deep Brain Stimulation, Parkinson Disease, Microelectrode recording	8
Alpha-Synuclein, Parkinson Disease, Protein α-synuclein	7
Lipids, Lipolysis, Adipose triglyceride	6
Adrenoleukodystrophy, Fatty Acids, Acids VLCFA (Very Long Chain Fatty Acids)	5
Lewy Body Disease, Dementia, Probable DLB (Dementia with Lewy bodies)	5
Phenylketonurias, Phenylalanine, Phenylalanine levels	5
Alzheimer Disease, Amyloid, Amyloid plaques	4

Table 11. Carcinoma. Cluster (6), weigh 5.15%.

Topic Names	N = 149
Carcinoma, Hepatocellular, Survival, Sorafenib treatment	20
Hepatitis C, Chronic, Ribavirin, Hepacivirus	13
Carcinoma, Hepatocellular, Neoplasms, HCC (HepatoCellular Carcinoma) patients	10
HIV, Hepacivirus, HIV (Human Immunodeficiency Virus) /HCV (Hepatitis C Virus) co-infected	10
Hepatitis C, Liver Transplantation, Recurrent hepatitis	8
Elasticity Imaging Techniques, Fibrosis, Spleen stiffness	7
Hypertension, Portal, Fibrosis, Cirrhotic rats	6
Hemorrhage, Esophageal and Gastric Varices, Acute variceal	4
Hepacivirus, Ribavirin, Direct-acting antiviral	4
Carcinoma, Hepatocellular, Liver Transplantation, Microvascular invasion	3

The advantage of this second analysis is that it allows to detect which specific medical topics are being transferred to patents. Thus, the leading topics obtained were: neoplasms, leukemia, DNA repair, human leukocyte antigen, Alzheimer disease, and carcinoma.

4.5. Top Journals Used for the Spanish Medicine Publications Cited in Patents

Finally, these works have been published in specialized medical journals, and it is worth highlighting which have been the most used by patents in the field of medicine. Table 12 shows the most used journals, where the JCR categories and their ranking in 2018 and their five-year impact factor are also shown. The journals are mostly in the category of oncology (six of them) and Hematology (three of them). These journals mostly occupy relevant positions in their category, being 17 of them Q1, 2 of them Q3, and one Q4 (Drugs of the Future). This last journal is noteworthy because it is an atypical case, journals that are little valued by the scientific community, since the impact and position are based on the number of citations received for other scientific work, while here, they appear in a ranking of publications used in patents. Of course, the title of the journal itself has a strong emphasis on technology transfer. A bibliometric reflection on this work would be whether a ranking of journals cited in patents would be worthwhile, that is, as an indicator of scientific transfer fed by the sector itself and in which the university and research centres can also be involved.

Table 12. Top 20 journal in medicine category. Data 2018

Journal	N	SJR Category	Rank SJR	SJR Indicator	CiteScore Scopus	JCR Category	Rank JCR	Impact Factor (5 years) JCR
Blood	221	Biochemistry Cell Biology Immunology Hematology	9/446-Q1 19/288-Q1 10/216-Q1 2/133-Q1	6.065	7.27	Hematology	1/73-Q1	13.206
Cancer Research	181	Cancer Research Oncology	11/216-Q1 14/368-Q1	4.047	6.94	Oncology	21/230-Q1	9.062
New England Journal of Medicine	177	Medicine (miscellaneous)	3/2836-Q1	19.524	16.1	Medicine, General & Internal	1/160-Q1	70.331
Clinical Cancer Research	165	Cancer Research Oncology	7/216-Q1 10/368-Q1	4.965	8.32	Oncology	16/230-Q1	9.174
Drugs of the Future	155	Pharmacology (medical) Pharmacology	221/261-Q4 283/330-Q4	0.123	0.08	Pharmacology & Pharmacy	267/267-Q4	0.109
Journal of Immunology	147	Immunology Immunology and Allergy	28/216-Q1 21/203-Q1	2.521	4.41	Immunology	43/158-Q2	5.066
Vaccine	130	Molecular Medicine Immunology and Microbiology (miscellaneous) Infectious Diseases Public Health, Environmental and Occupational Health Veterinary (miscellaneous)	28/173-Q1 13/49-Q2 41/286-Q1 38/530-Q1 2/182-Q1	1.759	3.18	Immunolog Medicine, Research & Experimental	78/158-Q2 57/136-Q2	3.293
Journal of Clinical Microbiology	108	Microbiology (medical)	11/123-Q1	2.314	3.65	Microbiology	24/133-Q1	4.183
The Lancet	108	Medicine (miscellaneous)	5/2836-Q1	15.871	10.28	Medicine, General & Internal	2/160-Q1	54.664
Antimicrobial Agents and Chemotherapy	99	Infectious Diseases Pharmacology (medical) Pharmacology	29/286-Q1 11/261-Q1 21/330-Q1	2.096	4.34	Microbiology Pharmacology & Pharmacy	28/133-Q1 27/267-Q1	4.719
Hepatology	94	Hepatology Medicine (miscellaneous)	3/67-Q1 39/2836-Q1	5.096	6.87	Gastroenterology & Hepatology	5/84-Q1	12.795
Journal of Clinical Oncology	91	Cancer Research Medicine (miscellaneous) Oncology	2/216-Q1 9/2836-Q1 4/368-Q1	11.754	11.08	Oncology	5/230-Q1	22.565
Human Molecular Genetics	84	Genetics Molecular Biology Genetics (clinical) Medicine (miscellaneous)	27/338-Q1 47/409-Q1 8/100-Q1 75/2836-Q1	3.097	4.88	Biochemistry & Molecular Biology Genetics & Heredity	62/299-Q1 32/174-Q1	5.281
Annals of Oncology	78	Hematology Medicine (miscellaneous) Oncology	3/133-Q1 35/2836-Q1 8/368-Q1	6.047	8.44	Oncology	9/230-Q1	11.791
Leukemia	78	Cancer Research Anesthesiology and Pain Medicine Hematology Oncology	8/216-Q1 1/122-Q1 5/133-Q1 11/368-Q1	4.518	6.08	Oncology Hematology	14/230-Q1 4/73-Q1	9.679
Annals of the Rheumatic Diseases	72	Biochemistry, Genetics and Molecular Biology (miscellaneous) Immunology Immunology and Allergy Rheumatology	6/242-Q1 8/216-Q1 6/203-Q1 1/60-Q1	7.081	9.18	Rheumatology	2/31-Q1	12.692
Journal of Hepatology	72	Hepatology	2/67-Q1	6.274	9.32	Gastroenterology & Hepatology	3/84-Q1	14.265
Gastroenterology	71	Gastroenterology Hepatology	1/145-Q1 1/67-Q1	7.384	7.07	Gastroenterology & Hepatology	2/84-Q1	19.066
Haematologica	66	Hematology	6/133-Q1	3.077	4.07	Hematology	7/73-Q1	6.931
International Journal of Cancer	65	Cancer Research Oncology	18/216-Q1 24/368-Q1	3.276	6.93	Oncology	51/230-Q1	6.210

The analysis made to assess the articles published in the Top 20 journals cited in patents is now made in the case study of the category of medicine for Percentage of articles at Top 20 medicine journals: FWCI ≥ 1, top 10% topic and topic cluster. Figure 13 shows that the New England Journal of Medicine and the Lancet have all their articles above the expected citation value (100 % of FWCI ≥ 1). Four other journals also reach values between 90% and 100%, these are Gastroenterology, Journal of Clinical Oncology, Blood, and Annals of Oncology. Another eight journals are above 80% and all are above 50%, except Drugs of the Future with a very low percentage (4.52%).

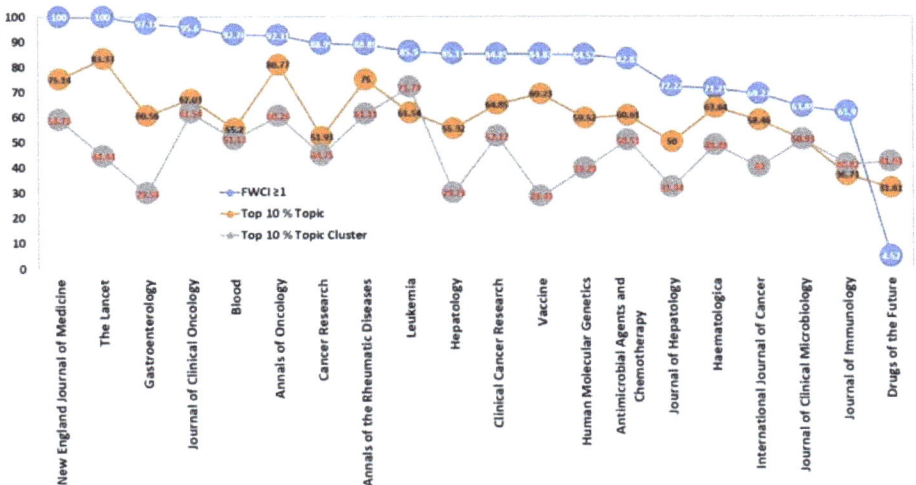

Figure 13. Percentage of articles at Topo 20 medicine journals: FWCI ≥ 1, Top 10% Topic and Topic Cluster.

According to the percentage of articles that are in the top 10% in topic, it is observed that there is a gradual increase among the journals, and that this ranking is led by journals with more than 75%, which are in order: The Lancet, Annals of Oncology, New England Journal of Medicine, and Annals of the Rheumatic Diseases. Then there are 13 journals with more than 50% and only two below 50%: Journal of Immunology, and Drugs of the Future. The topic cluster has an even lower grading, and there is no journal above 75 %. However, above 50% would be nine journals, where the first four are now: Leukemia, Journal of Clinical Oncology, Annals of the Rheumatic Diseases, and Annals of Oncology. This last journal is the only one that is among the first four in the three rankings analyzed FWCI ≥ 1, top 10% topic and topic cluster.

5. Conclusions

Universities and, by extension research centers or agencies, have the duty of producing knowledge, which is generally measured by their scientific production in the form of publications, which, if they are of good quality, are included in international databases that serve as a basis for future research or technological development. Today, this mission is intended to be extended to the solving of society's problems in general and specifically to the demands of the industrial segment. This new purpose has to date not been easily measured except in the form of patents that universities themselves have developed or applied for. However, this last aspect remains the most important aspect of basic research, which is probably the one that involves the greatest amount of funding. This study has been motivated by the need to understand the role of public research in the development of industry, which is reflected in the contribution to the number of patents. The aim is to address an important gap in the research system by proposing the dilemma of applied research versus basic research carried out in universities and research centres.

This study sets out a methodology to assess the impact of university research on the patent system by analysing the global impact of universities on international patents. In order to evaluate this parallelism, a methodology is established to relate the contribution of Spanish scientific production to international patents based on their citation in these patents. The study was carried out at a global level, but it has been reduced to the field of medicine since the high percentage (20%) of studies cited in patents related to this scientific field.

It has been observed that overall investment in research means an increase in the number of publications that have been cited in patents. Therefore, a direct relationship between funding and transfer is shown. At the same time, international collaboration amongst Spanish authors of these publications is a constant, as shown by the high level of collaboration with countries such as the USA. UK, or Germany at a global level and with France in the field of medicine. Apart from the leading role of the public research body (CSIC), the universities are the institutions that produce applied research and are cited in the patents. A method has been presented that allows the classification of universities based on the relationship between their overall scientific production and the production applied to patents. The results obtained allow to observe that the universities with a TIP (transference index in patents) higher than 5% (outstanding) are not those that have a mainly technological profile, as it would be reasonable to think. However, in the medicine transference index in patents (MED-TIP), it is the universities with medical schools that are positioned at the top of the table.

As an index of where Spanish science is standing out at the transfer level, the Topics and Topic Clusters have been considered. In addition, the highlighted Topics can be used for decision-making in future allocations to research funding. However, the fact that prominence (the topics) represents demand and general visibility should not be lost sight of. It is therefore necessary to support the top 10% topic and top 10% topic cluster indicators. The analysis of the topic and cluster topic has determined networks relating the publications cited in patents both at a general level and from the medical point of view. The clustering of outstanding topics translates directly into the visibility of these publications for the industry sector.

This study shows that public research is fundamental to industrial R&D, as reflected by the number of patents that are based on this knowledge and significantly to R&D in the field of medicine. The leading topics according the ASJC classification were oncology (11.78%), immunology and allergy (9.48%), infectious diseases (7.1%), cardiology and cardiovascular (6.63%), hematology (6.44%), neurology (Clinical) (5.34%), and general medicine (4.74%). In a more detailed and independent analysis, it allowed to determine the leading topics, which were: neoplasms, leukemia, DNA repair, human leukocyte antigen, Alzheimer disease, and carcinoma.

Contrary to the idea that university research generates abstract knowledge that is of poor use to society in general, this study reveals that public research and above all that carried out in universities suggests new products in the form of patents and therefore helps society to advance. Since patents are the basis for industries to develop a product, such research thus reaches society to improve our quality of life.

In short, from the bibliometric point of view, both databases such as Scopus or Web of Science, which provide quality indicators at the publication level, and databases such as JCR or SJR, which quantify the quality of the journals, lack specific indicators that measure the impact of both the publications and their sources in their R&D transfer aspect. Therefore, a ranking of journals cited in patents has been proposed as an indicator of scientific transfer, since it is fed by the industrial sector itself and in which the university and research centres can also be involved. Thus, for universities, the TIP (transference index in patents) has been proposed as a long-term indicator of scientific transfer in patents. In spite of the revealed complexity of the problem about the rates of return to R&D, this work opens new perspectives in the field of transfer of both basic and applied science by proposing a ranking for both journals and research centres, all based on the work cited in patents.

Author Contributions: M.C., A.A., J.A.G.-C. and F.M.-A. conceived the research, designed the search, and wrote the manuscript. All authors have read and agreed to the published version of the manuscript.

Funding: This research received no external funding.

Acknowledgments: The authors would like to thank to the CIAIMBITAL (University of Almeria, CeiA3) for its support.

Conflicts of Interest: The authors declare no conflict of interest.

References

1. Suresh, S. Research funding: Global challenges need global solutions. *Nature* **2012**, *490*, 337. [CrossRef] [PubMed]
2. Noll, H.-H. Social Indicators and Quality of Life Research: Background, Achievements and Current Trends. In *Advances in Sociological Knowledge*; Verlag für Sozialwissenschaften: Wiesbaden, Germany, 2004; pp. 151–181.
3. Katz, S. The science of quality of life. *J. Chronic Dis.* **1987**, *40*, 459–463. [CrossRef]
4. Meier, D.E.; Brawley, O.W. Palliative Care and the Quality of Life. *J. Clin. Oncol.* **2011**, *29*, 2750–2752. [CrossRef] [PubMed]
5. Garrido-Cárdenas, J.A.; Mesa-Valle, C.; Manzano-Agugliaro, F. Human parasitology worldwide research. *Parasitol.* **2017**, *145*, 699–712. [CrossRef]
6. Garrido-Cárdenas, J.A.; González-Cerón, L.; Manzano-Agugliaro, F.; Mesa-Valle, C. Plasmodium genomics: An approach for learning about and ending human malaria. *Parasitol. Res.* **2018**, *118*, 1–27. [CrossRef] [PubMed]
7. Nerkar, A.; Shane, S. Determinants of invention commercialization: An empirical examination of academically sourced inventions. *Strat. Manag. J.* **2007**, *28*, 1155–1166. [CrossRef]
8. Ramani, S.V.; De Looze, M.-A. Country-Specific Characteristics of Patent Applications in France, Germany and the UK in the Biotechnology Sectors. *Technol. Anal. Strat. Manag.* **2002**, *14*, 457–480. [CrossRef]
9. Ramani, S.V.; De Looze, M.-A. Using patent statistics as knowledge base indicators in the biotechnology sectors: An application to France, Germany and the UK. *Scientometrics* **2002**, *54*, 319–346. [CrossRef]
10. Stek, P.E.; Van Geenhuizen, M. Measuring the dynamics of an innovation system using patent data: A case study of South Korea, 2001–2010. *Qual. Quant.* **2014**, *49*, 1325–1343. [CrossRef]
11. Homma, A.; Tanuri, A.; Duarte, A.J.; Marques, E.T.A.; De Almeida, A.; Martins, R.; Silva-Junior, J B.; Possas, C. Vaccine research, development, and innovation in Brazil: A translational science perspective. *Vaccine* **2013**, *31*, B54–B60. [CrossRef]
12. Narin, F.; Noma, E. Is technology becoming science? *Scientometrics* **1985**, *7*, 369–381. [CrossRef]
13. Narin, F. Patent bibliometrics. *Sci.* **1994**, *30*, 147–155. [CrossRef]
14. Harhoff, D.; Narin, F.; Scherer, F.; Vopel, K. Citation Frequency and the Value of Patented Inventions. *Rev. Econ. Stat.* **1999**, *81*, 511–515. [CrossRef]
15. Collins, P.; Wyatt, S. Citations in patents to the basic research literature. *Res. Policy* **1988**, *17*, 65–74. [CrossRef]
16. Lewison, G. Gastroenterology research in the United Kingdom: Funding sources and impact. *Gut* **1998**, *43*, 288–293. [CrossRef] [PubMed]
17. Krauskopf, E. Cardiovascular disease: The Brazilian research contribution. *Braz. J. Cardiovasc. Surg.* **2019**, *34*. [CrossRef]
18. Xu, H.; Winnink, J.; Yue, Z.; Liu, Z.; Yuan, G. Topic-linked innovation paths in science and technology. *J. Inf.* **2020**, *14*, 101014. [CrossRef]
19. Xing, Z.; Yu, F.; Du, J.; Walker, J.; Paulson, C.B.; Mani, N.S.; Song, L.; Zhou, S.; Carvalho, D. Conversational Interfaces for Health: Bibliometric Analysis of Grants, Publications, and Patents. *J. Med Internet Res.* **2019**, *21*, e14672. [CrossRef]
20. Qin, Y.; Qin, Z.D.; Chen, J.; Cai, C.G.; Li, L.; Feng, L.Y.; Wang, Z.; Duns, G.J.; He, N.Y.; Chen, Z.S.; et al. From Antimicrobial to Anticancer Peptides: The Transformation of Peptides. *Recent Patents Anti-Cancer Drug Discov.* **2019**, *14*, 70–84. [CrossRef]
21. Plaza, L.G.; Albert, A.M. Biotechnology research and generation of patents of interest to the health system. *Med. Clin.* **2008**, *131* (Suppl. 5), 55–59.
22. Delfim FDrummond FCarmo IO Barroca AM Horta, T.; Kalapothakis, E. Evaluation of Brazilian Biotechnology Patent Activity from 1975 to 2010. *Recent Patents DNA Gene Seq.* **2012**, *6*, 145–159. [CrossRef]
23. Cogollos, L.C.; Costoya, A.S.; Domínguez, R.L.; Calatayud, V.A.; de Dios, J.G.; Benavent, R.A. Bibliometría e indicadores de actividad científica (XI). Otros recursos útiles en la evaluación: Google Scholar, Microsoft Academic, 1findr, Dimensions y Lens. org. *Acta pediátrica española* **2018**, *76*, 123–130.
24. Salmerón-Manzano, E.; Manzano-Agugliaro, F. The Electric Bicycle: Worldwide Research Trends. *Energies* **2018**, *11*, 1894. [CrossRef]

25. Salmerón-Manzano, E.; Manzano-Agugliaro, F. Worldwide Research on Low Cost Technologies through Bibliometric Analysis. *Invention* **2020**, *5*, 9. [CrossRef]
26. Salmerón-Manzano, E.; Manzano-Agugliaro, F. The Higher Education Sustainability through Virtual Laboratories: The Spanish University as Case of Study. *Sustainability* **2018**, *10*, 4040. [CrossRef]
27. Stek, P.E. Mapping high R&D city-regions worldwide: A patent heat map approach. *Qual. Quant.* **2020**, *54*, 279–296. [CrossRef]
28. Huang, M.-H.; Yang, H.-W.; Chen, D.-Z. Industry–academia collaboration in fuel cells: A perspective from paper and patent analysis. *Scientometrics* **2015**, *105*, 1301–1318. [CrossRef]
29. OPM (Oficina Española de Patentes y Marcas). 2020. Available online: https://www.oepm.es/export/sites/oepm/comun/documentos_relacionados/Memorias_de_Actividades_y_Estadisticas/estudios_estadisticos/Solicitudes_Patentes_Nacionales_Universidades_2007_2018.pdf (accessed on 15 May 2020).
30. Rodríguez, J.M.; Manzano-Agugliaro, F.; Garrido-Cárdenas, J.A. The state of global research on social work and disability. *Soc. Work. Health Care* **2019**, *58*, 839–853. [CrossRef]
31. Garrido-Cárdenas, J.A.; Manzano-Agugliaro, F.; González-Cerón, L.; Montoya, F.G.; Alcayde, A.; Novas, N.; Mesa-Valle, C. The Identification of Scientific Communities and Their Approach to Worldwide Malaria Research. *Int. J. Environ. Res. Public Health* **2018**, *15*, 2703. [CrossRef]
32. Garrido-Cárdenas, J.A.; Cebrián-Carmona, J.; González-Cerón, L.; Manzano-Agugliaro, F.; Mesa-Valle, C. Analysis of Global Research on Malaria and Plasmodium vivax. *Int. J. Environ. Res. Public Health* **2019**, *16*, 1928. [CrossRef]
33. Vardell, E.; Feddern-Bekcan, T.; Moore, M. SciVal Experts: A Collaborative Tool. *Med Ref. Serv. Q.* **2011**, *30*, 283–294. [CrossRef]
34. Scimago Journal & Country Rank Home Page. Available online: https://www.scimagojr.com/ (accessed on 1 May 2020).
35. Scopus: Access and use Support Center Home Page. Available online: https://service.elsevier.com/app/answers/detail/a_id/14880/supporthub/scopus/ (accessed on 1 May 2020).
36. Web of Science Group Home Page. Available online: https://clarivate.com/webofsciencegroup (accessed on 1 May 2020).
37. Wang, Q.; Waltman, L. Large-scale analysis of the accuracy of the journal classification systems of Web of Science and Scopus. *J. Inf.* **2016**, *10*, 347–364. [CrossRef]
38. Purkayastha, A.; Palmaro, E.; Falk-Krzesinski, H.; Baas, J. Comparison of two article-level, field-independent citation metrics: Field-Weighted Citation Impact (FWCI) and Relative Citation Ratio (RCR). *J. Inf.* **2019**, *13*, 635–642. [CrossRef]
39. Garrido-Cárdenas, J.A.; Mesa-Valle, C.; Manzano-Agugliaro, F. Genetic approach towards a vaccine against malaria. *Eur. J. Clin. Microbiol. Infect. Dis.* **2018**, *37*, 1829–1839. [CrossRef] [PubMed]
40. Garrido-Cárdenas, J.A.; De Lamo-Sevilla, C.; Cabezas-Fernández, M.; Manzano-Agugliaro, F.; Martínez-Lirola, M. Global tuberculosis research and its future prospects. *Tuberc.* **2020**, *121*, 101917. [CrossRef]
41. Pascual-Leone, A.; Tormos, J.M.; Keenan, J.; Tarazona-Santabalbina, F.J.; Ca??ete, C.; Catal??, M.D. Study and Modulation of Human Cortical Excitability With Transcranial Magnetic Stimulation. *J. Clin. Neurophysiol.* **1998**, *15*, 333–343. [CrossRef]
42. Fernández-García, A.; Juaidi, A.; Sutter, F.; Martínez-Arcos, L.; Manzano-Agugliaro, F. Solar Reflector Materials Degradation Due to the Sand Deposited on the Backside Protective Paints. *Energies* **2018**, *11*, 808. [CrossRef]

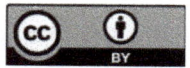 © 2020 by the authors. Licensee MDPI, Basel, Switzerland. This article is an open access article distributed under the terms and conditions of the Creative Commons Attribution (CC BY) license (http://creativecommons.org/licenses/by/4.0/).

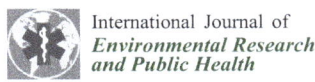
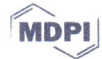

Article

A Scientometric Analysis of Global Health Research

Minxi Wang, Ping Liu, Rui Zhang, Zhi Li and Xin Li *

College of Management Science, Chengdu University of Technology, Chengdu 610059, China; wangminxi@mail.cdut.edu.cn (M.W.); liupingcdu@163.com (P.L.); ruizhang033@163.com (R.Z.); leannlee0618@gmail.com (Z.L.)
* Correspondence: lixin2012@cdut.cn

Received: 9 April 2020; Accepted: 22 April 2020; Published: 24 April 2020

Abstract: With the development and deepening of the process of global integration, global health is gaining increasing attention. An increasing number of studies have examined global health from diverse perspectives to promote the realization of global public health. The purpose of this research is to systematically and comprehensively evaluate the knowledge structure, knowledge domain, and evolution trend in the field of global health research. Based on the 14,692 document data retrieved from Web of Science Core Collection from 1996 to 2019, this article carried out a visual analysis of global health research from the perspective of scientific output characteristics, scientific research cooperation networks, keywords, and highly cited literature. The results show that scholars' interest in global health research is increasing, especially after the outbreak of SARS. USA, England, Canada, Australia, and China have the most prominent contributions to global health research. Significant authors, high impact journals and core institutions also identified. The study found that "global health governance", "global health diplomacy", "medical education", "global health education" and "antimicrobial resistance" are the research frontiers and hot spots. This study provides an overview and valuable guidance for researchers and related personnel to find the research direction and practice of global health.

Keywords: global health; public health; scientometric study; knowledge map; visualization analysis; CiteSpace

---

1. Introduction

Globalization has accelerated the spread of health risks, and the health threats of a certain country or region may become a global problem in a short time. Therefore, the health status of the public in one country is not only determined by the political, economic, and cultural development of the land but also affected by the health and safety status of other countries in the world [1]. Due to the globalization, complexity, and diversification of health influence factors, the development of global health requires all-round cooperation from all countries in the world. Global health, in a broad context, refers to improving public health worldwide, reducing disparities, and protecting against global threats that do not consider national borders [2].

Since the 21st century, infectious diseases, chronic diseases, climate change, resource depletion, ethnic conflicts, and poverty have continuously threatened the health of the global public [3]. Since the outbreak of the new coronavirus in 2019 (COVID-19), the number of people infected with the virus worldwide has reached more than 2.1 million, causing more than 145,000 deaths, and the epidemic has spread to 211 countries (as of 15 April 2020) [4]. The new coronavirus epidemic has brought tremendous harm and threat to the health of the global public and also exposed many problems in global health governance [5]. In this context, the global experts and scholars' attention to global health likely will further increase. To promote the deepening of research in global health, it is particularly essential to comprehensively summarize and review the current research results in the field of global health. Gostin et al. introduced the development history, framework, and deficiencies of global health law, and sought to establish domestic and global links in the field of health law [6]. Dieleman et al. examined the status and characteristics of fiscal health expenditures in 195 countries/regions and predicted the future development trend of global health spending [7]. García et al. revealed the severity and causes of corruption in the global health system, noting that policymakers, research scholars, and funders need to clarify their responsibilities and treat corruption as an essential area of research [8]. Herath et al. combed the research literature of interprofessional education in global health care and analyzed the main differences and features of global health education for undergraduates and postgraduates in developed and developing countries [9]. Other scholars have reviewed different aspects of global health, such as experience and progress in the prevention and control of infectious diseases [10], lessons learned and theoretical basis for the implementation of global health security [11], and mechanisms for international institutions to participate in global health governance [12]. Most of the existing studies started from a single perspective or focused on a specific research area of global health, which lacks a comprehensive and systematic review of global health research.

Science is not an independent activity. Therefore, the progress of science often needs to summarize previous research results [13]. In the past, the number of research literature on global health has multiplied [14,15]. Because global health research involves multiple disciplines and scattered research themes, it has brought a lot of difficulties for global health researchers to grasp this emerging research area and find research hotspots. Due to the development of technologies such as data mining, information analysis, and graphic drawing, the organic combination of computer technology and traditional mathematical statistics has made it possible for visual analysis of scientific metrology. Scientometrics can intuitively show the information panorama of each discipline through the knowledge map, and explore research hotspots and emerging trends in a particular field [16]. It is widely used in the areas of environmental ecology [17], public health [18,19], business economics, artificial intelligence [20], education research, resource science [21], and medicine.

From a new perspective, this study will use scientometric to comprehensively and systematically review the research in the field of global health. Specific analysis methods such as text mining, word frequency analysis, co-word analysis, cluster analysis, co-citation analysis, and network analysis will be adopted in this research to answer the following questions: (1) What are the changes in international experts' and scholars' attention to global health? (2) Which scholars, research institutions, countries, or regions have outstanding influence and contribution to the development of global health research? (3) Which journals have a high impact in the area of global health research? (4) What is the status of scientific research cooperation across global, multi-institution, and different authors in global health? (5) What is the evolutionary context, research frontiers, hot topics, and future trends in global health research?

2. Materials and Methods

2.1. Data Source

Literature databases commonly used by international experts and scholars include Google Scholar, Scopus, PubMed, and Web of Science. Each of these databases has advantages and disadvantages. Google Scholar has a broad coverage of literature data and plentiful literature types, but it has low data quality and many duplicate data [22]. PubMed is a free biomedical information retrieval system developed by the NCBI. PubMed has a rich literature in the medical field but lacks literature data in other subject areas. Scopus and Web of Science are comprehensive databases, and there is not much difference in data coverage between the two. However, some scholars have shown that when using CiteSpace software for visual analysis, the knowledge map made by the literature of the Web of Science database is better [23,24]. Therefore, this study uses the Web of Science to retrieve the literature data needed for analysis. To ensure the reliability of the scientific metrological analysis, we chose the Web of Science core collection, and the indexes are SCI-EXPANDED, SSCI, CCR-EXPANDED, and Index Chemicus. The detailed retrieval strategy is shown in Figure 1. After preliminary searching, 14,692 pieces of literature data were obtained. For some reason, there are differences and ambiguities in the expressions of author names, institution names, and country names in literature data. In response to this, before conducting scientific measurement analysis, we used CiteSpace's data deduplication and name merge functions to standardize the data. The literature search date is December 30 December 2019.

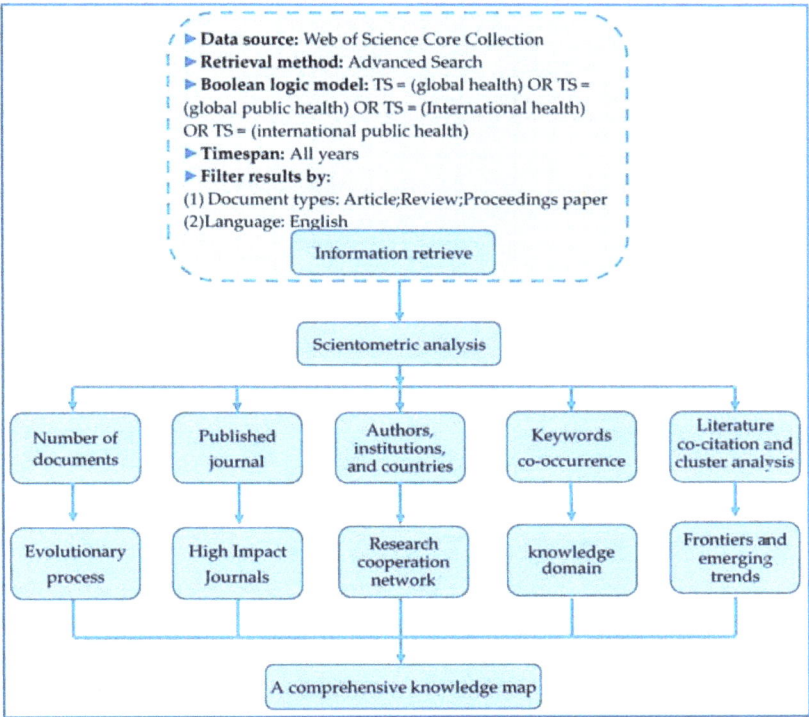

Figure 1. Research framework.

2.2. Data Visualization and Analysis

The software used in this article for scientometric analysis and visualization analysis is CiteSpace (5.6.R2). CiteSpace software is an information visualization software developed by Chen Chaomei, based on the Java language [25]. CiteSpace's theoretical basic system mainly includes five aspects: Kuhn's scientific development model theory, Price's scientific frontier theory, structural tree holes, the best information foraging theory of scientific communication, and the theory of discrete and reorganized knowledge units [26]. This article uses CiteSpace software to visualize the structure, regularity, and distribution of knowledge in the global health field, and analyze the co-citation of documents to mine the knowledge clustering and distribution of citation space. At the same time, we also performed co-occurrence analysis between other knowledge units in the global health field, such as cooperation between authors, institutions, and countries. Finally, we built a comprehensive knowledge map of global health research based on the results of scientific econometric analysis. Figure 1 shows the research framework of the article.

Some parameters and knowledge map identification methods will be involved in the results of the scientometric analysis, which will be explained uniformly here. The knowledge map shows the distance of time with warm and cold colors. When the time is closer to 2019, the colors become warmer. In the knowledge graph, the size of the nodes means the frequency of the authors, institutions, countries, and journals, and the connection between the nodes indicates that these nodes appear in the same article [27]. In general, when two or more authors (institutions, countries) appear in the same paper, it can be regarded as a scientific research cooperation relationship between these authors (institutions, countries) [28]. In the process of scientometric analysis, there are also some parameter indicators for a specific evaluation. H-index is a mixed quantitative index proposed by physicist George Hirsch of the University of California, USA, which is used to evaluate the amount of academic output and the level of the scholarly output of researchers and institutions. H-index indicates that h of the N papers published in the journal have been cited at least h times [29]. The Degree in the table indicates the number of connections between authors (institutions, countries) in the co-occurrence knowledge graph. A higher Degree value indicates more communication and cooperation between the authors (institutions, countries). Besides, intermediary centrality is an indicator that measures the importance of nodes in the research cooperation network, and the half-life is a parameter that represents the continuity of institutional research from a time perspective [25].

3. Results

3.1. Progression of Scientific Output

The change in the number of scientific research results reflects, to a certain extent, the changes in the attention paid by international experts and scholars to a specific subject area. A total of 14,692 literature data on global health research were recovered, including 12,012 articles, 1627 reviews, and 1053 proceedings papers. Figure 2 shows the details of the scientific output. The number of publications rose from 14 in 1996 to 1997 in 2019. On the whole, the scientific production in global health research shows a continuous upward trend. Specifically, the three types of documents (article, review, and proceedings paper) are also showing a growing trend.

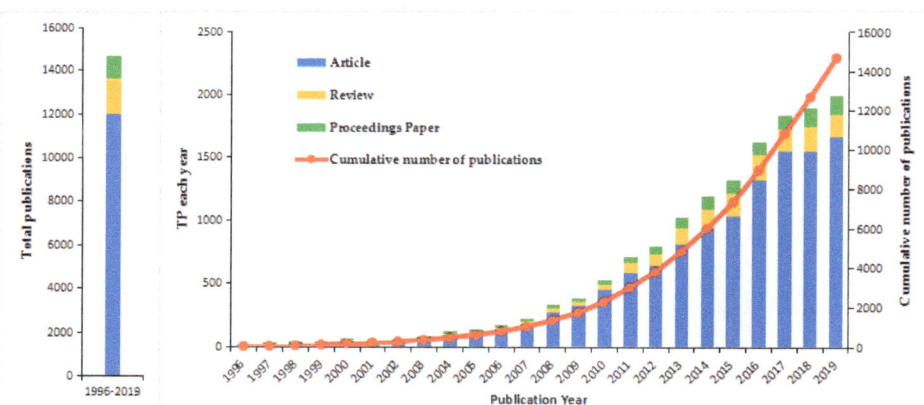

Figure 2. The scientific output from 1996–2019. The number of publications each year is based on the main ordinate axis (the left ordinate), and the cumulative number of publications is based on the secondary axis (right ordinate).

3.2. Analysis of Journals

Compared with the number of publications, the frequency of citations to the literature published by a journal can better reflect the influence and importance of the journal. Therefore, this article uses CiteSpace to analyze the quote of the journals, and produced a map of the cited journals, as shown in Figure 3. Based on the frequency of citations, we selectively counted the detailed information of the top 20 journals and drew Table 1. As can be seen in Figure 3 and Table 1, after careful consideration of citation frequency, impact factor, centrality, and H-index, the top five core journals are LANCET (IF:

59.10, H-index: 700), NEW ENGL J MED (IF: 70.67, H-index: 933), JAMA-J AM MED ASSOC (IF: 51.27, H-index: 622), SCIENCE (IF: 41.03, H-index: 1058) and NATURE (IF: 43.07, H-index: 1096). In Figure 3, the nodes of LANCET, NEW ENGL J MED, JAMA-J AM MED ASSOC, SCIENCE, NATURE, and P NATL ACAD SCI USA have relatively large node circles, and there are cool-tone areas in the node circles. However, node circles such as PLOS ONE, BMC PUBLIC HEALTH, LANCET INFECT DIS, and LANCET GLOBAL HEALTH are mostly warm colors. It shows that the critical early literature on global health research mainly came from the journals of LANCET, NEW ENGL J MED, JAMA-J AM MED ASSOC, SCIENCE, NATURE, and P NATL ACAD SCI USA. It is worth noting that the top five journals in the global health field are from the United States (NEW ENGL J MED, JAMA-J AM MED ASSOC, SCIENCE) and the United Kingdom(LANCET, NATURE).

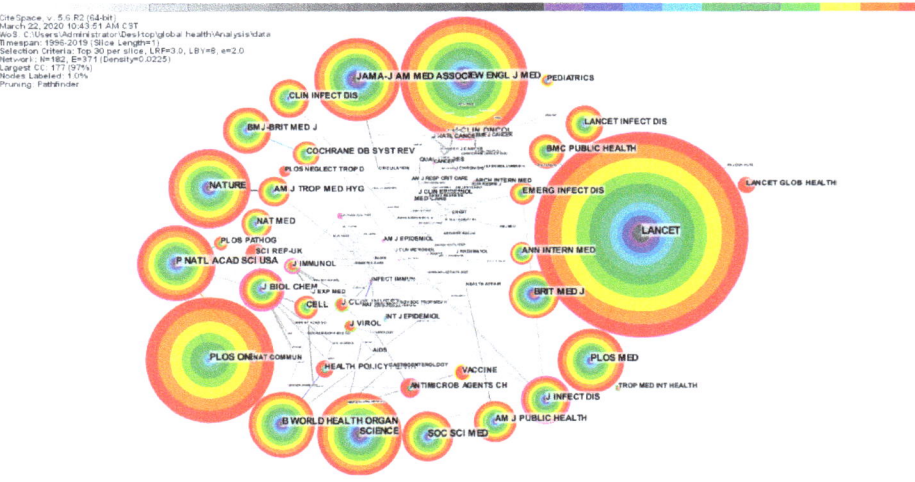

Figure 3. Visualization of co-citation journals.

Table 1. The top 20 journals.

Rank	Journal	Cited Frequency	Impact Factor	Centrality	H-index
1	LANCET	7316	59.10	0.14	700
2	NEW ENGL J MED	4552	70.67	0.17	933
3	PLOS ONE	4401	2.77	0.00	268
4	JAMA-J AM MED ASSOC	3121	51.27	0.09	622
5	SCIENCE	3039	41.03	0.00	1058
6	NATURE	2924	43.07	0.20	1096
7	P NATL ACAD SCI USA	2860	9.58	0.14	699
8	B WORLD HEALTH ORGAN	2445	6.81	0.09	148
9	PLOS MED	2393	11.04	0.02	184
10	BRIT MED J	1955	27.60	0.07	392
11	SOC SCI MED	1929	3.08	0.03	213
12	J INFECT DIS	1741	5.04	0.28	231
13	AM J PUBLIC HEALTH	1686	5.38	0.06	236
14	CLIN INFECT DIS	1536	9.05	0.00	303
15	J BIOL CHEM	1529	4.10	0.50	477
16	LANCET INFECT DIS	1432	27.51	0.00	201
17	BMC PUBLIC HEALTH	1263	2.56	0.00	117
18	NAT MED	1229	30.64	0.06	497
19	AM J TROP MED HYG	1224	2.31	0.05	135
20	ANN INTERN MED	992	19.31	0.00	359

3.3. Analysis of Scientific Cooperation Network

3.3.1. Co-author Analysis

As shown in Figure 4, the author's co-occurrence network knowledge graph has 830 nodes and 1171 connections. On the whole, the author's cooperation network density value is only 0.005, and the overall global cooperation and communication still need to be strengthened.

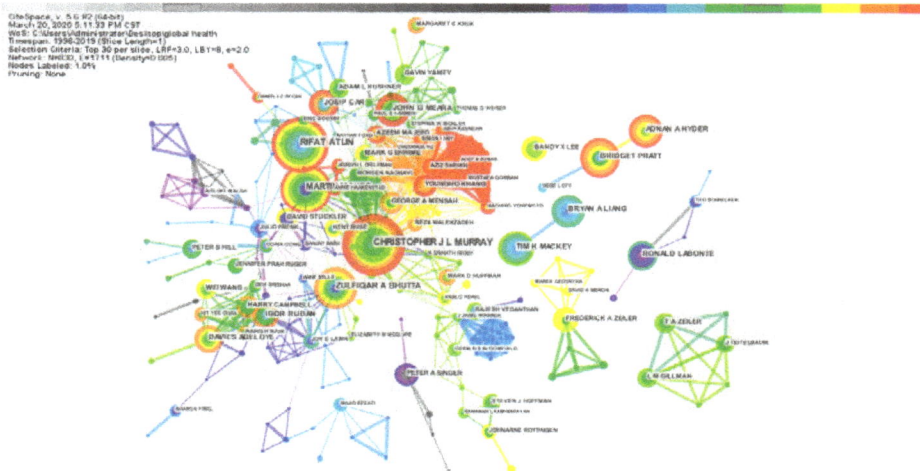

Figure 4. Knowledge map of co-author collaboration network.

The scientific research cooperation group centered on the authors of MURRAY C J L, ATUN R, MCKEE M, BHUTTA ZA, and MEARA JG has the closest communication. The details of the top 20 authors published papers are shown in Table 2.

Table 2. The Top 20 authors.

Code	Author	Quantity	H-index	Centrality	Degree
1	MURRAY C.J.L.	31	120	0.04	49
2	ATUN R.	28	46	0.01	7
3	MCKEE M.	25	94	0.04	29
4	BHUTTA Z.A.	22	18	0.03	18
5	PRATT B.	20	12	0.00	2
6	MACKEY T.K.	18	21	0.00	1
7	LIANG B.A.	17	19	0.00	1
8	HYDER A.A.	17	24	0.00	1
9	MEARA J.G.	17	36	0.00	10
10	CAR J.	15	46	0.00	7
11	LABONTE R.	15	27	0.00	3
12	ADELOYE D.	14	15	0.00	9
13	YAYA S.	13	14	0.00	1
14	LEE K.	13	11	0.00	3
15	CELLA D.	13	122	0.00	3
16	RUDAN I.	13	12	0.01	16
17	ZEILER F.A.	12	15	0.00	8
18	SINGER P.A.	12	58	0.00	3
19	KHANG Y.H.	11	27	0.00	41
20	CAMPBELL H.	11	104	0.00	8

In Table 2, MURRAY C.J.L. is the scholar with the most significant number of published papers in global health research, with a degree value of 49 and an H-index of 120. MURRAY C.J.L. mainly focuses on global health burden research, global health international assistance, global health finance, infectious disease prevention, global health professional education gap, etc. [30–32]. The research findings of ATUN R. are mainly related to the interaction between global health initiatives and national health systems, cancer control in low-income countries, measures to improve health systems in developing countries, and innovations in health financing [33–35]. The dialectical relationship between economic development and global health, global health diplomacy, and the strengthening of the global health system are the main concerns of MCKEE M. [36,37]. The two remaining core authors in the top five are BHUTTA Z.A. and PRATT B.

3.3.2. Co-institution Analysis

Figure 5 presents a co-institution network consisting of 167 nodes and 218 links. It can be seen from Figure 5 that there is a certain amount of collaboration and exchange between institutions in the world, but the cooperation between domestic institutions is closer than that between international institutions.

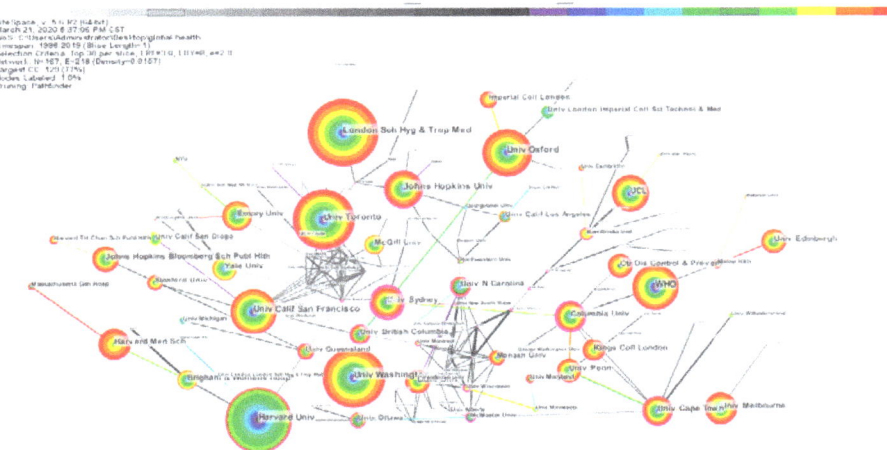

Figure 5. Knowledge map of co-institution collaboration network.

Combined with Figure 5, the top 20 institutions with published papers are listed in Table 3. The London Sch Hyg and Trop Med (433 articles, Harvard Univ (409 articles), Univ Toronto (396 articles), Univ Washington (385 articles), and Univ Oxford (327 articles). All of them made central contributions to the research on global health. It is worth noting that 12 of the top 20 institutions are from the USA, with 11 schools and one government agency. The second is the UK, with three institutions (London Sch Hyg and Trop Med, Univ Oxford, and UCL) in the top 20. It further demonstrates the outstanding contributions and leadership role of the USA and the UK in the field of global health research.

Table 3. The top 20 institutions.

Rank	Institutions	Publications	Centrality	Degree	HalfLife
1	London Sch Hyg and Trop Med (UK)	433	0.02	2	10
2	Harvard Univ (USA)	409	0.16	4	11
3	Univ Toronto (Canada)	396	0.18	11	17
4	Univ Washington (USA)	385	0.00	1	12
5	Univ Oxford (UK)	327	0.07	4	16
6	WHO	322	0.05	2	15
7	Univ Calif San Francisco (USA)	305	0.10	11	15
8	Johns Hopkins Univ (USA)	254	0.10	5	12
9	UCL (UK)	242	0.02	2	8
10	Univ Melbourne (Australia)	218	0.02	2	14
11	Emory Univ (USA)	206	0.06	3	9
12	Univ Sydney (Australia)	193	0.40	7	11
13	Columbia Univ (USA)	193	0.36	8	13
14	Univ Cape Town (South Africa)	191	0.12	7	11
15	Harvard Med Sch (USA)	186	0.02	2	2
16	Johns Hopkins Bloomberg Sch Publ Hlth (USA)	183	0.02	2	7
17	Ctr Dis Control and Prevent (USA)	180	0.00	1	15
18	Yale Univ (USA)	177	0.04	3	17
19	Univ Penn (USA)	167	0.06	3	12
20	Duke Univ (USA)	166	0.04	5	17

3.3.3. Co-country/Territory Analysis

In Figure 6, the country/territory cooperative network map has 203 nodes, 560 links, and the network density is 0.0273.

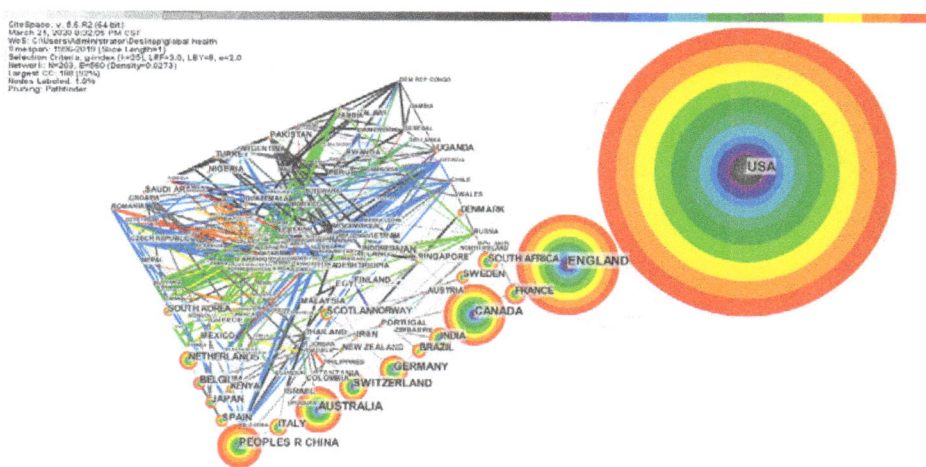

Figure 6. Knowledge map of the co-country/territory collaboration network.

From a global perspective, the network density of knowledge graphs is high, there are many connections between countries, and cooperation and exchanges between countries are relatively close. It also shows that global health has attracted the attention of various countries around the world. Due to the differences in the political, economic, and cultural development of each country, the coordination of global health and domestic health systems is that these countries also tend to solve problems in coordination and dialogue with other countries. In Table 4, it can be seen that the USA is the country with the most significant number of papers published in the global health field, with 6561 articles published accounting for 44.7% of the total.

Table 4. The top 20 countries.

Rank	Country	Publications	Percent%	Centrality	Degree	Burst	HalfLife
1	USA	6561	44.7	0.07	6	6.64	19
2	ENGLAND	2365	16.1	0.04	3	-	20
3	CANADA	1504	10.2	0.00	1	-	18
4	AUSTRALIA	1108	7.5	0.00	1	-	18
5	PEOPLES R CHINA	1086	7.3	0.01	3	-	17
6	GERMANY	759	5.2	0.00	2	7.05	18
7	SWITZERLAND	752	5.1	0.00	1	6.32	17
8	INDIA	635	4.3	0.00	1	-	16
9	SOUTH AFRICA	571	3.8	0.00	1	-	16
10	FRANCE	549	3.7	0.16	5	-	20
11	NETHERLANDS	527	3.6	0.00	2	-	19
12	ITALY	520	3.5	0.00	2	-	20
13	SWEDEN	425	2.8	0.02	4	7.61	19
14	BRAZIL	408	2.7	0.00	2	-	17
15	SPAIN	398	2.7	0.02	2	-	18
16	JAPAN	347	2.4	0.00	3	-	11
17	SCOTLAND	346	2.3	0.04	3	-	19
18	BELGIUM	333	2.3	0.17	7	-	19
19	SOUTH KOREA	308	2.1	0.00	2	-	16
20	KENYA	249	1.7	0.01	5	-	11

Note: Because of the scientific research cooperation between countries, two or more countries may appear in a paper. Therefore, when conducting a national cooperation network analysis, the total number of articles published in all countries is greater than 14692.

The remaining top five are the ENGLAND (2635 articles, 16.1%), CANADA (1504 articles, 10.2%), AUSTRALIA (1108 articles, 7.5%), and PEOPLES R CHINA (1086 articles, 7.3%). From Figure 6, the center of the circle of this node in PEOPLES R CHINA is mainly a warm tone, while the center of the circle of the node of the USA and ENGLAND has a cold tone. It shows that China, as a developing country, started research in the global health field later than developed countries such as the United States. Besides, although there are already 1086 articles published in China, among the top 20 authors and institutions, there are no authors and institutions from China. It indicates that although China started late in the global health field, it has developed rapidly.

3.4. Analysis of Co-occurring Keywords

After the vital co-occurrence network analysis, the keywords are summarized and classified according to the keyword frequency and research direction, as shown in Table 5.

These manually selected keywords are roughly divided into five main topics. The keywords of topic one mainly include "global health (2583)", "quality of life (933)"," mortality (712)", "public health (535)", "survival (200)", "health status (52)". Topic 1 is the main goal and direction of global health research, namely reducing global abnormal mortality through global health governance and international cooperation, meeting the minimum survival needs of people around the world, gradually enhancing the health status, and continuously improving the quality of life of the public. The second major topic in global health research is the threat factors that specifically affect global public health, including "infectious diseases (779)", "cancer (355)", "antibiotic resistance (39)", "mental health issues (50)", "obesity (348)", "climate change (56)", etc. The health prevention and treatment of some specific groups (children, women, students) is the third topic focused by scholars in the global health field. The keywords included in the fourth topic are "developing countries (399)", "Africa (384)", "middle-income country (62)", and the United States (348). The fifth is a relatively macro topic, mainly on the cooperation mechanism of global health, global health management, prevention of global health risks, and professional education of global health.

Table 5. List of keywords information.

Topic	Keyword	Frequency	Centrality	Degree	Burst
1	Global health	2583	0.26	13	-
	Quality of life	933	0.04	5	16.81
	Mortality	712	0.09	8	-
	Public health	535	0.12	7	-
	Survival	200	0.08	8	3.62
	Health status	52	0.20	6	13.38
2	Mental health	50	0.00	1	-
	Infection disease	779	0.11	10	-
	Hiv	368	0.11	8	-
	Cancer	355	0.07	8	-
	Obsity	348	0.02	3	-
	Tuberculosis	334	0.12	10	-
	Cardiovascular disease	149	0.05	3	14.94
	Mycobacterium tuberculosis	130	0.03	6	20.01
	Breast cancer	112	0.05	8	14.67
	Antibiotic resistance	39	0.00	1	-
	Human immunodeficiency virus	57	0.03	2	9.61
	Climate change	56	0.00	1	-
3	Children	518	0.00	1	-
	Woman	365	0.03	4	-
	Student	37	0.00	1	20.14
4	Developing country	399	0.06	6	11.81
	Afica	384	0.00	1	-
	United states	348	0.00	2	-
	Middle income country	62	0.00	1	-
5	Prevention	414	0.04	3	-
	Management	365	0.15	11	-
	Education	389	0.00	1	-
	Cooperation mechanism	244	0.00	1	-

3.5. Literature Co-citation Analysis

3.5.1. Analysis of Highly Cited Literature

Usually, scholars cite the research results of their predecessors in their papers and list them in the form of references. Mutual citations of scientific literature reflect the objective laws of scientific development [38]. In Figure 7, the early citation network is relatively sparse, and the middle and late citation networks are denser. At the same time, it can be seen from the location of some large nodes that highly cited documents also appear in the middle and late periods.

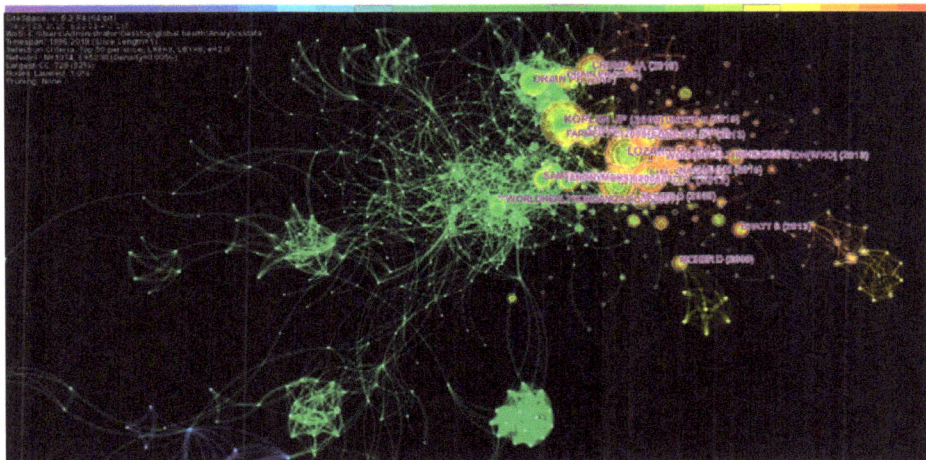

Figure 7. Knowledge map of co-citation literature. The selection criteria for the study of literature co-citation networks is top 50 per slice, and the largest citation sub-network is displayed.

With reference to Figure 7, this study selected the top ten documents cited by frequency and detailed information of these documents listed in Table 6. It should note that the citation frequency in this article is limited to the mutual citation between these 14,692 articles so that the specific citation frequency will be different from the statistics in Web of Science. The article "Towards a common definition of global health" published by Koplan J.P. is cited most frequently [2]. About the term "global health", the academic community has not unified its final definition. At present, the explanation given by Koplan J.P. scholars recognized by the academic community. The burst value in the last column of the table indicates that the literature has received significant attention for a certain time. The highest burst value is the article "Global and regional mortality from 235 causes of death for 20 age groups in 1990 and 2010" published by Lozano R. et al. [39]. The rest of the literature is mainly on global health disease burden research, global health status survey, medical education, and global surgical exploration. Eight of the top ten most frequently cited articles are from the Lancet journal.

Table 6. Top 10 cited documents.

Rank	Frequency	Author	Journal	Year	Burst
1	173	Koplan J.P. [2]	Lancet	2009	28.81
2	167	Lozano R. [39]	Lancet	2012	43.64
3	142	Murray C.J.L. [40]	Lancet	2012	38.32
4	130	Lim S.S. [41]	Lancet	2012	20.82
5	116	Frenk J. [42]	Lancet	2010	26.74
6	115	Crump J.A. [43]	AM J TROP MED HYG	2010	21.09
7	110	Drain P.K. [44]	ACAD MED	2007	29.31
8	105	Jamison D.T. [1]	Lancet	2013	22.87
9	92	Meara J.G. [45]	Lancet	2015	34.16
10	89	Naghavi M. [46]	Lancet	2015	25.82

3.5.2. Cluster Analysis of Literature Co-citation Network

As an exploratory data mining technology, cluster analysis used to analyze and determine important topics, content, and evolution trends. Cluster analysis of literature co-citation can effectively classify a large number of similar research documents into a single knowledge unit, and then objectively reflect the main content of each knowledge unit [47]. The literature clustering knowledge map is shown in Figure 8.

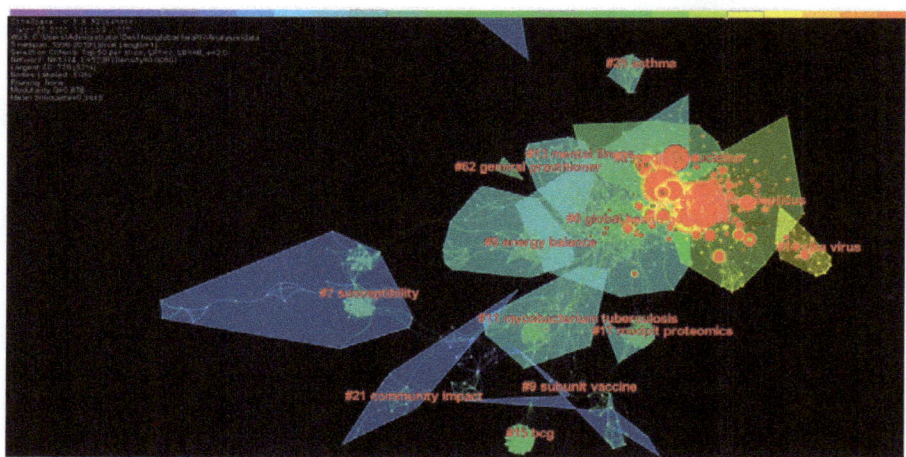

Figure 8. Knowledge map of literature cluster. In CiteSpace, clusters are named by citing the keywords of the literature, and the log-likelihood algorithm (LLR) used.

In Figure 8, the color of the cluster blocks from cold to warm represents the average time of clustering from far to near. The red nodes in the cluster color block represent the literature with burst value. The more red nodes in the cluster block, it shows that this clustering topic is the research frontier and hot spot. In order to further understand the clustering theme, we have summarized the detailed information of clustering and plotted it as Table 7.

Table 7. Summary table of cluster information.

Cluster ID	Size	Silhouette	Mean (Year)	Label (LLR)
0	162	0.719	2006	Global health governance; Global health diplomacy
1	127	0.827	2013	Status epilepticus; Antimicrobial resistance
2	66	0.889	2008	Medical education; Global health education
4	50	0.972	2001	Hepatitis c virus; Peptide inhibitors
5	47	0.999	1996	Quality of life;
7	44	0.981	2001	Susceptibility; Gene
8	41	0.943	2003	Energy balance; Adipose tissue; Appetite
9	40	0.963	2001	Subunit vaccine; Interferon-gamma
11	35	0.946	2005	Mycobacterium tuberculosis
13	23	0.967	2004	Mental illness; Mental health
14	20	0.991	2014	Zika Virus; Zika fever
15	20	0.997	2003	Bcg; Vaccine
17	18	0.98	2005	Mudpit proteomics; Egg secretome
21	14	0.994	2001	Community impact;
25	10	1	2005	Asthma; Rhintis
31	8	0.997	2000	Health services;
62	3	0.998	2007	General practitioner; Intervention strategies

Note: The silhouette value is the parameter used by CiteSpace software to evaluate the clustering effect. Specifically, the evaluation of clustering measuring the homogeneity of the network. The closer the silhouette value is to 1, the higher the homogeneity of the network and the clustering results with high reliability are greater than 0.7.

It can be seen from Table 7 that the silhouette values of all clustering results are greater than 0.7, indicating that there is no problem with clustering. According to Figure 8 and Table 6, currently, "global health governance", "global health diplomacy", "medical education", "global health education", "antimicrobial resistance" and "Zika Virus" are the research frontiers and hot spots in the global health field. In addition, "quality of life", "energy balance; adipose tissue; appetite", "subunit vaccine", "mental illness", "mental health", "community impact", "health services" and "interaction strategies" are important research topics and directions of global health.

3.6. Category Co-occurrence Analysis and a Knowledge Map

Co-occurrence analysis of subject categories allows us to intuitively understand the main subjects involved in a research field [48]. The classification of the categories in this study comes from the WOS database. In Figure 9, the purple circle on the edge of the node circle indicates that this node has a high intermediate centrality value. In Table 8, we list the top ten subject categories with co-occurrence frequency. Based on Figure 9 and Table 8, the subject categories of global health research are mainly "Public, Environmental and Occupational Health", "General and Internal Medicine", "Health Care Sciences and Services", "Medicine, General and internal" and "Infectious Diseases". It shows that global health research involves multiple disciplines and fields. Based on the analysis of the previous sections, we have drawn a comprehensive knowledge map of global health research, as shown in Figure 10.

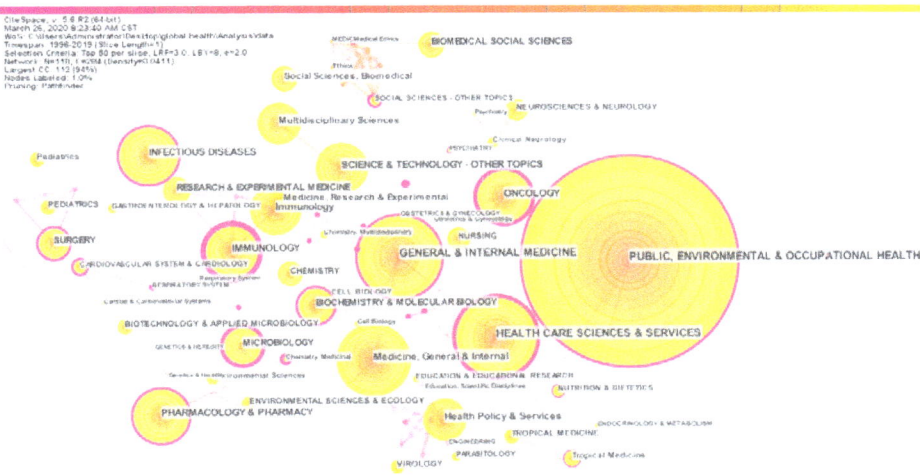

Figure 9. Knowledge map of co-occurrence categories.

Table 8. The top 10 subject categories.

Rank	Category	Frequency	Centrality	Burst
1	Public, Environmental, and Occupational Health	2670	0.21	-
2	General and Internal Medicine	1155	0.29	-
3	Health Care Sciences and Services	1105	0.43	7.06
4	Medicine, General, and Internal	1047	0.01	3.33
5	Infectious Diseases	867	0.19	7.75
6	Pharmacology and Pharmacy	815	0.28	-
7	Immunology	783	0.73	-
8	Science and Technology-other topics	776	0.03	-
9	Oncology	773	0.47	3.35
10	Health Policy and Services	683	0.03	-

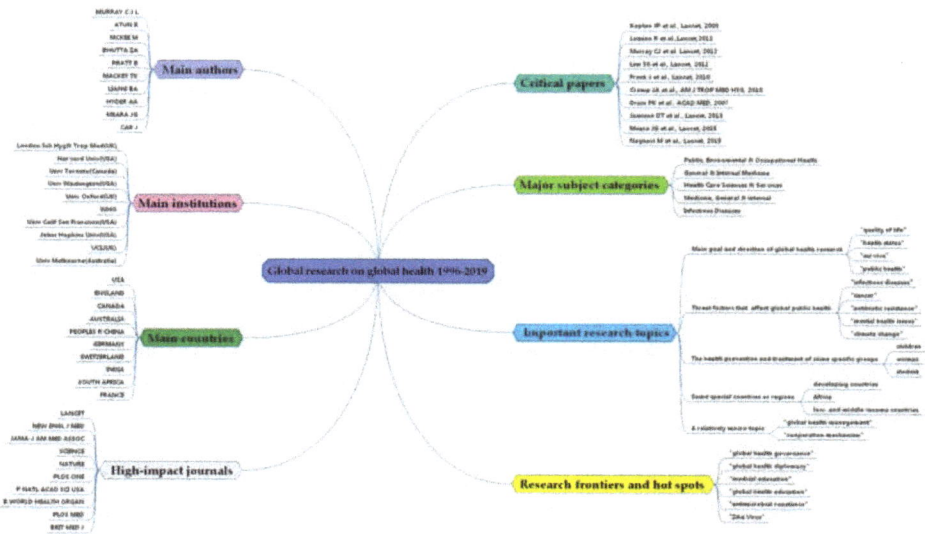

Figure 10. A comprehensive knowledge map in the global health research field: 1996–2019.

4. Discussion

4.1. General Information

In the analysis of scientific output, we find that the literature on global health research shows a trend of increasing nominally year by year. At the same time, the increase in the number of proceedings papers reflects, to a certain extent, the increase in international academic conferences in the global health field. It shows that international experts and scholars have paid continuous attention to the field of global health. In recent years, there were constant outbreaks of infectious diseases (Ebola Hemorrhagic Fever, MERS, Zika, etc.), increased mortality from chronic diseases, ethnic conflicts, and poverty. All of these have aroused widespread international concern and thinking about global health.

Among the five high-impact journals in the global health field, LANCET, NEW ENGL J MED, and JAMA-J AM MED ASSOC are three internationally recognized top journals in the medical field. These three journals have published for more than a century, and they have played a significant role in the history of human medicine. SCIENCE and NATURE are international comprehensive science magazines with a high reputation in academia. Most of the early basic literature and research hotspots in global health research come from these high-impact journals. Scholars in the global health field should pay attention to the scientific achievements published by these journals in real-time.

This article explores scientific research cooperation in the global health field from three perspectives: Micro-author cooperation network, meso-institutional cooperation network, and macro-national cooperation network. Although there are certain academic exchanges and cooperation between authors, institutions, and countries in the global health field, these scientific research collaborations mostly occur between different institutions in a certain country and between significant scholars in an institution. In this field, developed countries (USA, England, Canada, Australia, Germany, etc.) still hold the leading position, while some developing countries (China, India) with a relatively large number of articles have not yet appeared prominent research institutions and scholars. Therefore, more scientific research exchanges with developing countries will be more conducive to the development of global health compared with developed countries taking measures such as medical aid and financial contributions to some developing countries with severe public health problems.

4.2. Research Topics and Emerging Trends

This study explores the research topics and emerging trends in the global health area mainly from two aspects: Keyword co-occurrence analysis and literature co-citation analysis. Keywords can clearly and intuitively reflect the research theme, core research content, and main research direction of an article. Therefore, in the fields of scientific text mining and scientometrics, the co-occurrence analysis of keywords can quickly grasp the development trends and research topics of a specific research field [49]. From the results of keyword co-occurrence analysis, there are five main research topics in the global health field, including global health goals and directions, research on global health risk factors, research on specific groups and specific countries or regions, and research on cooperative communication mechanisms. The goal of global health is to improve the equity of global health and the quality of life of people worldwide [50]. The original intention of the rise of global health is based on its effective way of dealing with global health inequity, which provides a new perspective and approach for achieving the goal of global health equity [51]. Global health focuses on the fairness and health influencing factors of global health, not just the health status and influencing factors of people in a specific country or region. Global health also pays attention to the global distribution of health and disease and its determinants, attaches importance to the impact of globalization on health and changes in the nature of global health governance, and emphasizes interdependence and coping strategies that transcend national and policy sector boundaries [52,53].

After literature citation analysis and cluster analysis, we learned that "global health governance", "global health diplomacy", "medical education", "global health education", "antimicrobial resistance" and "Zika Virus" are the current research frontiers and hot spots. Global health governance is a tool for dealing with the determinants of a healthy society across sectors [54]. The theoretical research and practical aspects of global health reflect that poor governance at the national and international levels will undermine the achievement of global health goals [55]. The catalyst for global health implementation is global health diplomacy. An important change in the 2000 G-8 summit was the linking of foreign policy with global health issues, and global health began to become a major goal and strategy of foreign policy. Global health diplomacy promotes the participation of various actors in the global governance actions taken to solve global health and related issues [56]. Some sovereign countries have established bilateral or multilateral global health strategies with other countries or organizations through mechanisms such as foreign policy and negotiation and consultation, formulated global health plans, and provided relevant financial and technical assistance to low- and middle-income countries [57].

Besides, "quality of life", "energy balance; adipose tissue; appetite", "subunit vaccine", "mental illness", "mental health", "community impact", "health services" and "interaction strategies" are important research topics and directions of global health. Combined with real-time news and past development experience, the current global outbreak of the new coronavirus in 2019 (COVID-19) has exposed many global health problems. Therefore, the prevention and control of infectious diseases, epidemiological studies of infectious diseases, international collaboration on global health, and health assistance will be a new research hotspot and emerging trends.

Despite the positive findings of the study, there are still some limitations. From the perspective of literature data, the literature data in this article only come from the Web of Science core collection database. Moreover, we only selected documents written in English. Secondly, this article does not contain grey literature, such as non-publicly published government documents, dissertations, non-publicly issued conference documents, scientific reports, technical archives, etc. From the perspective of visual analysis, this article does not interpret all the information in the knowledge graph. It is also one of the problems and directions that the follow-up research needs to think of and explore further.

5. Conclusions

In this study, based on the 14,692 literature data on global health research retrieved from the WOS core collection from 1996 to 2019, we conducted a scientometric analysis of the knowledge structure and knowledge field of global health research. At the same time, a visual analysis of the knowledge unit in the global health field was conducted, and a comprehensive knowledge map was drawn. Research in the global health field is extensive, involving multidisciplinary theories and methods, and its development requires the participation of researchers and new scholars in various fields. Scientific research cooperation between developed and developing countries in the global health field is particularly important and needs to be further strengthened. The mechanism of global health governance, the prevention and control of various infectious diseases, and the cultivation of professionals require long-term attention and discussion. This study provides researchers with an overview of global health through a systematic and comprehensive analysis of scientific output, core authors, significant institutions and countries, high impact journals, research cooperation networks, research topics, and emerging trends in the field of global health research. By presenting a new, comprehensive, and holistic knowledge map, this research contributes to the existing global health knowledge system. It also provides valuable guidance for researchers and related personnel to find the research direction and practice of global health.

Author Contributions: Conceptualization, M.W.; Methodology, X.L. and P.L.; Validation, M.W.; Formal analysis, X.L.; Data curation, P.L; Syntax modification, R.Z.; Perfect chart, Z.L.; Writing—original draft preparation, P.L.; Writing—review and editing, M.W.; Supervision, X.L. All authors have read and agreed to the published version of the manuscript.

Funding: This work was supported by the Special Projects of Public Health Emergency Management for Chengdu University of Technology in 2020.

Conflicts of Interest: The authors declare no conflict of interest.

References

1. Jamison, D.T.; Summers, L.H.; Alleyne, G.; Arrow, K.J.; Berkley, S.; Binagwaho, A.; Bustreo, F.; Evans, D.; Feachem, R.G.A.; Frenk, J.; et al. Global health 2035: A world converging within a generation. *Lancet* **2013**, *382*, 1898–1955. [CrossRef]
2. Koplan, J.P.; Bond, T.C.; Merson, M.H.; Reddy, K.S.; Rodriguez, M.H.; Sewankambo, N.K.; Wasserheit, J.N. Towards a common definition of global health. *Lancet* **2009**, *373*, 1993–1995. [CrossRef]
3. Arie, S. Wins, losses, and draws in global health in past 10 years. *BMJ* **2019**, *367*, 1–2. [CrossRef]
4. Johns Hopkins University Coronavirus COVID-19 Global Cases. Available online: https://www.arcgis.com/apps/opsdashboard/index.html#/bda7594740fd40299423467b48e9ecf6 (accessed on 15 April 2020).
5. Thompson, R. Pandemic potential of 2019-nCoV. *Lancet Infect. Dis.* **2020**, *20*, 280. [CrossRef]
6. Gostin, L.O.; Meier, B.M. Introducing Global Health Law. *J. Law Med. Ethics* **2019**, *47*, 788–793. [CrossRef]
7. Chang, A.Y.; Cowling, K.; Micah, A.E.; Chapin, A.; Chen, C.S.; Ikilezi, G.; Sadat, N.; Tsakalos, G.; Wu, J.; Younker, T.; et al. Past, present, and future of global health financing: A review of development assistance, government, out-of-pocket, and other private spending on health for 195 countries, 1995–2050. *Lancet* **2019**, *393*, 2233–2260. [CrossRef]
8. García, P.J. Corruption in global health: The open secret. *Lancet* **2019**, *394*, 2119–2124. [CrossRef]
9. Herath, C.; Zhou, Y.; Gan, Y.; Nakandawire, N.; Gong, Y.; Lu, Z. A comparative study of interprofessional education in global health care: A systematic review. *Medicine* **2017**, *96*, e7336. [CrossRef]
10. Biesma, R.G.; Brugha, R.; Harmer, A.; Walsh, A.; Spicer, N.; Walt, G. The effects of global health initiatives on country health systems: A review of the evidence from HIV/AIDS control. *Health Policy Plan.* **2009**, *24*, 239–252. [CrossRef]
11. Meyer, D.; Cameron, E.E.; Bell, J.; Nuzzo, J.B. The Road to Achieving Global Health Security: Accelerating Progress and Spurring Urgency to Fill Remaining Gaps. *Health Secur.* **2020**, *18*, S1–S3. [CrossRef]
12. Piot, P. Governance for the future of global health. *Lancet* **2017**, *389*, 243–244. [CrossRef]
13. Mingers, J.; Leydesdorff, L. A review of theory and practice in scientometrics. *Eur. J. Oper. Res.* **2015**, *246*, 1–19. [CrossRef]
14. Rajaguru, P.P.; Premkumar, A.; Sheth, N.P. What happens to global health research: Analysis of the full-length publication rates of research abstracts presented at two major global health conferences. *Health Inf. Libr. J.* **2019**. [CrossRef]

15. Yao, Q.; Chen, K.; Yao, L.; Lyu, P.-H.; Yang, T.-A.; Luo, F.; Chen, S.-Q.; He, L.-Y.; Liu, Z.-Y. Scientometric trends and knowledge maps of global health systems research. *Health Res. Policy Syst.* **2014**, *12*, 26. [CrossRef] [PubMed]
16. Frenken, K.; Hardeman, S.; Hoekman, J. Spatial scientometrics: Towards a cumulative research program. *J. Informetr.* **2009**, *3*, 222–232. [CrossRef]
17. Xiang, C.; Wang, Y.; Liu, H. A scientometrics review on nonpoint source pollution research. *Ecol. Eng.* **2017**, *99*, 400–408. [CrossRef]
18. Chinchilla-Rodríguez, Z.; Zacca-González, G.; Vargas-Quesada, B.; Moya-Anegón, F. Latin american scientific output in public health: Combined analysis using bibliometric, socioeconomic and health indicators. *Scientometrics* **2015**, *102*, 609–628. [CrossRef]
19. Zacca-González, G.; Chinchilla-Rodríguez, Z.; Vargas-Quesada, B.; De Moya-Anegón, F. Bibliometric analysis of regional Latin America's scientific output in Public Health through SCImago Journal & Country Rank. *BMC Public Health* **2014**, *14*, 632.
20. Tran, B.X.; Latkin, C.A.; Vu, G.T.; Nguyen, H.L.T.; Nghiem, S.; Tan, M.X.; Lim, Z.K.; Ho, C.S.H.; Ho, R.C.M. The current research landscape of the application of artificial intelligence in managing cerebrovascular and heart diseases: A bibliometric and content analysis. *Int. J. Environ. Res. Public Health* **2019**, *16*, 2699. [CrossRef]
21. Garrido-Cardenas, J.A.; Esteban-García, B.; Agüera, A.; Sánchez-Pérez, J.A.; Manzano-Agugliaro, F. Wastewater treatment by advanced oxidation process and their worldwide research trends. *Int. J. Environ. Res. Public Health* **2020**, *17*, 170. [CrossRef]
22. Orduna-Malea, E.; Martín-Martín, A.; López-Cózar, E.D. Google Scholar as a source for scholarly evaluation: A bibliographic review of database errors. *Rev. Esp. Doc. Cient.* **2017**, *40*, 1–33.
23. Martín-Martín, A.; Orduna-Malea, E.; Thelwall, M.; Delgado López-Cózar, E. Google Scholar, Web of Science, and Scopus: A systematic comparison of citations in 252 subject categories. *J. Informetr.* **2018**, *12*, 1160–1177. [CrossRef]
24. Falagas, M.E.; Pitsouni, E.I.; Malietzis, G.A.; Georgios, P. Comparison of PubMed, Scopus, Web of Science, and Google Scholar: Strengths and weaknesses. *FASEB J. Off. Publ. Fed. Am. Soc. Exp. Biol.* **2008**, *22*, 338–342. [CrossRef] [PubMed]
25. Chen, C. CiteSpace II: Detecting and Visualizing Emerging Trends and Transient Patterns in Scientific Literature. *J. Am. Soc. Inf. Sci. Technol.* **2006**, *3*, 359–377. [CrossRef]
26. De Solla Price, D.J. *Little Science, Big Science*; Columbia University Press: New York, NY, USA, 1963.
27. Chen, C. Science Mapping: A Systematic Review of the Literature. *J. Data Inf. Sci.* **2017**, *2*, 1–40. [CrossRef]
28. Katz, J.S.; Martin, B.R. What is research collaboration? *Res. Policy* **1997**, *26*, 1–18. [CrossRef]
29. Hirsch, J.E. An index to quantify an individual's scientific research output. *Proc. Natl. Acad. Sci. USA* **2005**, *102*, 16569–16572. [CrossRef] [PubMed]
30. Ravishankar, N.; Gubbins, P.; Cooley, R.J.; Leach-kemon, K.; Michaud, C.M.; Jamison, D.T.; Murray, C.J.L.; Bill, F.; Foundation, M.G. Financing of global health: Tracking development assistance for health from 1990 to 2007. *Lancet* **2007**, *373*, 2113–2124. [CrossRef]
31. Ezzati, M.; Vander Hoorn, S.; Lawes, C.M.M.; Leach, R.; James, W.P.T.; Lopez, A.D.; Rodgers, A.; Murray, C.J.L. Rethinking the "Diseases of Affluence" Paradigm: Global Patterns of Nutritional Risks in Relation to Economic Development. *PLoS Med.* **2005**, *2*, e133. [CrossRef]
32. Hay, R.J.; Johns, N.E.; Williams, H.C.; Bolliger, I.W.; Dellavalle, R.P.; Margolis, D.J.; Marks, R.; Naldi, L.; Weinstock, M.A.; Wulf, S.K.; et al. The Global Burden of Skin Disease in 2010: An Analysis of the Prevalence and Impact of Skin Conditions. *J. Investig. Dermatol.* **2014**, *134*, 1527–1534. [CrossRef]
33. Pigott, D.M.; Atun, R.; Moyes, C.L.; Hay, S.I.; Gething, P.W. Funding for malaria control 2006–2010: A comprehensive global assessment. *Malar. J.* **2014**, *11*, 246. [CrossRef] [PubMed]
34. Atun, R.; Knaul, F.M.; Akachi, Y.; Frenk, J. Innovative financing for health: What is truly innovative? *Lancet* **2012**, *380*, 2044–2049. [CrossRef]
35. Swanson, R.C.; Atun, R.; Best, A.; Betigeri, A.; De Campos, F.; Chunharas, S.; Collins, T.; Currie, G.; Jan, S.; Mccoy, D.; et al. Strengthening health systems in low-income countries by enhancing organizational capacities and improving institutions. *Glob. Health* **2015**, *11*, 5. [CrossRef]

36. Risso-gill, I.; Mckee, M.; Coker, R.; Piot, P.; Legido-quigley, H. Health system strengthening in Myanmar during political reforms: Perspectives from international agencies. *Health Policy Plan.* **2014**, *29*, 466–474. [CrossRef] [PubMed]
37. Barlow, P.; Mckee, M.; Basu, S.; Stuckler, D. The health impact of trade and investment agreements: A quantitative systematic review and network co-citation analysis. *Glob. Health* **2017**, *13*, 13. [CrossRef]
38. Small, H. Co-citation in the scientific literature: A new measure of the relationship between two documents. *J. Am. Soc. Inf. Sci.* **1973**, *24*, 265–269. [CrossRef]
39. Lozano, R.; Naghavi, M.; Foreman, K.; Lim, S.; Shibuya, K.; Aboyans, V.; Abraham, J.; Adair, T.; Aggarwal, R.; Ahn, S.Y.; et al. Global and regional mortality from 235 causes of death for 20 age groups in 1990 and 2010: A systematic analysis for the Global Burden of Disease Study 2010. *Lancet* **2010**, *380*, 2095–2128. [CrossRef]
40. Murray, C.J.L.; Vos, T.; Lozano, R.; Naghavi, M.; Flaxman, A.D.; Michaud, C.; Ezzati, M.; Shibuya, K.; Salomon, J.A.; Abdalla, S.; et al. Disability-adjusted life years (DALYs) for 291 diseases and injuries in 21 regions, 1990–2010: A systematic analysis for the Global Burden of Disease Study 2010. *Lancet* **2014**, *384*, 582. [CrossRef]
41. Lim, S.S.; Vos, T.; Flaxman, A.D.; Danaei, G.; Shibuya, K.; Adair-rohani, H.; Almazroa, M.A.; Amann, M.; Barker-collo, S.; Baxter, A.; et al. A comparative risk assessment of burden of disease and injury attributable to 67 risk factors and risk factor clusters in 21 regions, 1990–2010: A systematic analysis for the Global Burden of Disease Study 2010. *Lancet* **2012**, *380*, 2224–2260. [CrossRef]
42. Frenk, J.; Chen, L.; Bhutta, Z.A.; Cohen, J.; Crisp, N.; Evans, T.; Fineberg, H.; Garcia, P.; Ke, Y.; Kelley, P.; et al. Health professionals for a new century: Transforming education to strengthen health systems in an interdependent world. *Lancet* **2010**, *376*, 1923–1958. [CrossRef]
43. Crump, J.A.; Sugarman, J.; Guidelines, E.; Training, H. Ethics and Best Practice Guidelines for Training Experiences in Global Health. *Am. J. Trop. Med. Hyg.* **2010**, *83*, 1178–1182. [CrossRef] [PubMed]
44. Drain, P.K.; Primack, A.; Hunt, D.D.; Fawzi, W.W.; Holmes, K.K.; Gardner, P. Global Health in Medical Education: A Call for More Training and Opportunities. *Acad. Med.* **2007**, *82*, 226–230. [CrossRef] [PubMed]
45. Meara, J.G.; Leather, A.J.M.; Hagander, L.; Alkire, B.C.; Alonso, N.; Ameh, E.A.; Bickler, S.W.; Conteh, L.; Dare, A.J.; Davies, J.; et al. Global Surgery 2030: Evidence and solutions for achieving health, welfare, and economic development. *Int. J. Obstet. Anesth.* **2016**, *25*, 75–78. [CrossRef] [PubMed]
46. Mortality, G.B.D.; Collaborators, D. Global, regional, and national age–sex specific all-cause and cause-specific mortality for 240 causes of death, 1990–2013: A systematic analysis for the Global Burden of Disease Study 2013. *Lancet* **2014**, *385*, 117–171.
47. Chen, C.; Ibekwe-SanJuan, F.; Hou, J. The Structure and Dynamics of Co-Citation Clusters: A Multiple-Perspective Co-Citation Analysis. *J. Am. Soc. Inf. Sci. Technol.* **2010**, *61*, 1386–1409. [CrossRef]
48. Hou, J.; Yang, X.; Chen, C. Emerging trends and new developments in information science: A document co-citation analysis (2009–2016). *Scientometrics* **2018**, *115*, 869–892. [CrossRef]
49. Chen, C.; Dubin, R.; Kim, M.C. Orphan drugs and rare diseases: A scientometric review (2000–2014). *Expert Opin. Orphan Drugs* **2014**, *2*, 709–724. [CrossRef]
50. Jacobs, M.; El-Sadr, W.M. Health systems and health equity: The challenge of the decade. *Glob. Public Health* **2012**, *7*, 63–73. [CrossRef]
51. Lo, S.; Horton, R. Transgender health: An opportunity for global health equity. *Lancet* **2016**, *388*, 316–318. [CrossRef]
52. Lopez, A.D.; Mathers, C.D.; Ezzati, M.; Jamison, D.T.; Murray, C.J. Global and regional burden of disease and risk factors, 2001: Systematic analysis of population health data. *Lancet* **2006**, *367*, 1747–1757. [CrossRef]
53. Lee, K. Shaping the future of global health cooperation: Where can we go from here? *Lancet* **1998**, *351*, 899–902. [CrossRef]
54. Gostin, L.O.; Mok, E.A. Grand challenges in global health governance. *Br. Med. Bull.* **2009**, *90*, 7–18. [CrossRef] [PubMed]
55. Gostin, L.O. Meeting the survival needs of the world's least healthy people: A proposed model for global health governance. *J. Am. Med. Assoc.* **2007**, *298*, 225–228. [CrossRef] [PubMed]

56. Kickbusch, I.; Silberschmidt, G.; Buss, P. Global health diplomacy: The need for new perspectives, strategic approaches and skills in global health. *Bull. World Health Organ.* **2007**, *85*, 230–232. [CrossRef] [PubMed]
57. Labonté, R.; Gagnon, M.L. Framing health and foreign policy: Lessons for global health diplomacy. *Glob. Health* **2010**, *6*, 14. [CrossRef]

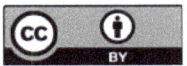

© 2020 by the authors. Licensee MDPI, Basel, Switzerland. This article is an open access article distributed under the terms and conditions of the Creative Commons Attribution (CC BY) license (http://creativecommons.org/licenses/by/4.0/).

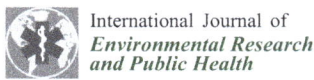

Article

A Bibliometric Analysis of the Health Field Regarding Social Networks and Young People

Pilar Aparicio-Martinez [1,2,3,*], Alberto-Jesus Perea-Moreno [4], María Pilar Martinez-Jimenez [4], María Dolores Redel-Macías [5], Manuel Vaquero-Abellan [1,3] and Claudia Pagliari [6]

1   Grupo Investigación epidemiológica en Atención primaria (GC-12) del Instituto Maimónides de Departamento de Enfermería, Campus de Menéndez Pidal, Universidad de Córdoba, 14071 Córdoba, Spain; mvaquero@uco.es
2   Usher Institute of Population Health Sciences and Informatics, University of Edinburgh, Edinburgh EH8 9YL, UK
3   Grupo Investigación epidemiológica en Atención primaria (GC-12) del Instituto Maimónides de Investigación Biomédica de Córdoba (IMIBIC), Hospital Universitario Reina Sofía, 14071 Córdoba, Spain
4   Departamento de Física Aplicada, Campus de Rabanales (ceiA3), Universidad de Córdoba, 14071 Córdoba, Spain; g12pemoa@uco.es (A.-J.P.-M.); fa1majip@uco.es (M.P.M.-J.)
5   Departamento Ingeniería Rural, Ed Leonardo da Vinci, Campus de Rabanales, Universidad de Córdoba, 14071 Córdoba, Spain; ig1remam@uco.es
6   eHealth Research Group, Usher Institute of Population Health Sciences and Informatics, University of Edinburgh, Edinburgh EH8 9YL, UK; Claudia.Pagliari@ed.ac.uk
*   Correspondence: n32apmap@uco.es; Tel.: +34-6-7972-7823

Received: 12 September 2019; Accepted: 18 October 2019; Published: 21 October 2019

Abstract: Social networks have historically been used to share information and support regarding health-related topics, and this usage has increased with the rise of online social media. Young people are high users of social media, both as passive listeners and as active contributors. This study aimed to map the trends in publications focused on social networks, health, and young people over the last 40 years. Scopus and the program VOSviewer were used to map the frequency of the publications, keywords, and clusters of researchers active in the field internationally. A structured keyword search using the Scopus database yielded 11,966 publications. The results reveal a long history of research on social networks, health, and young people. Research articles were the most common type of publication (68%), most of which described quantitative studies (82%). The main discipline represented in this literature was medicine, with 6062 documents. North American researchers dominate the field, both as authors and partners in international research collaborations. The present article adds to the literature by elucidating the growing importance of social networks in health research as a topic of study. This may help to inform future investments in public health research and surveillance using these novel data sources.

Keywords: social networks; health; young people; bibliometric study

1. Introduction

The creation of social groups to exchange information, share experiences, or provide support is a natural human impulse [1]. The growth of the internet has led to new channels for social networking, which have evolved and adapted to meet the needs and resources of the population [2].

In the digital era, online social networks have become a central node through which individuals connect and interact with other people [3], by sharing, viewing, or commenting on ideas and content posted by other users [4,5]. The use of social media has exponentially escalated since the late 1990s. The dynamic nature of these platforms has been the reason for their rapid growth, and the structure of these media has facilitated the creation of relationships among users [6,7]. Although individuals often use these networks to meet new people, there is a tendency to connect with those who hold similar expectations or preferences [8].

Additionally, one of the reasons for creating these social networks and exchanging information is to understand health, either from an individual or communal perspective [9]. Within these networks, young people are the most digitally connected members, both as active and passive users [10]. Nevertheless, adolescents and early adults are in a critical life stage, in which both self-identity and healthy or unhealthy behaviors are shaped [8,11]. Mental health issues such as depression, and physical disorders such as sexual infections, are more common in this group [11–15].

Recent research on this topic has focused on the relationship between social networks and health issues, both as prevention or educational tools, and as risk factors [6,16]. In this sense, researchers have explored the health-damaging effects of social media [5,15,17], or its side effects, such as isolation, depression, and eating disorders [18,19]. Different factors, such as gender or cultural background, have been linked to these side effects [10,12,20].

Other studies have explored the beneficial use of these networks for delivering health interventions [14,17], especially health education [21,22]. Engaging patients in health communities is also a topic of research, often focused on specific health problems or social support [22].

Overall, social media appears to have been used in different ways, depending on the user's health and behavior [23,24]. Based on this, a previous study was carried out in Scopus using the terms "social media", "health", and "young people". From this initial research (1785 documents), more recent publications and those published in journals with a high impact factor were used to represent the increase in the reach of social media and health (Table 1). Table 1 summarizes some of the latest publications regarding social networks as health problems or interventions. This research focused on the latest publications in major journals in the health field, such as the *Journal of Medical Internet Research* [25]. In this sense, the results showed that the health and education area tend to focus on the positive outcomes of using social networks. Meanwhile, the psychology area tends to study the side effects of using social media (Figure 1).

Table 1. Main areas of research on social networks related to health during the last 10 years.

Year	Relation with Health	Analysis	Positive/Negative Effect	Topic	Reference
2019	Cancer patients	Cross-sectional study	Positive outcome	Social networks as a means to improve young patients' health	[25]
2019	Kidney patients	Cross-sectional study	Positive outcome	Social media to support adolescent patients with disease	[26]
2019	Health and fitness	Interviews	Positive outcome	Social media as a pedagogical tool to understand or improve the wellbeing of young women	[27]
2019	Health education	Bibliometric	Positive outcome	Social networks as a pedagogical tool for education	[28]
2018	Suicide	Case report	Side effect	Social media as a negative factor in mental health	[29]
2018	Impulsive behavior and addiction	Cross-sectional study	Side effect	Addition to social media in young men	[30]

Table 1. *Cont.*

Year	Relation with Health	Analysis	Positive/Negative Effect	Topic	Reference
2018	Social distress	Interviews	Side effect	Stress in social media and the psychology health of young people	[31]
2018	Midwife study	Interviews	Positive outcome	Social media as an educational tool to enhance young people	[32]
2017	Emotional distress	Cross-sectional study	Side effect	Social media as a factor related to emotional distress	[33]
2017	Healthcare	Report	Positive outcome	Social media as an educational tool in health care	[34]
2017	Sexual healthcare	Experimental	Positive outcome	Social media as a mean to communicate sexual health	[35]

With this background, the principal objective of the present paper was to determine the tendencies of publications focused on social networks applied to health during the last 40 years (from 1978 to 2018). Additionally, the second objective of this study was to determine the link between social networks, health, and young people. The purpose of these objectives was to better understand the interaction of social networks in health, in order to assist the decision-making of health professionals and contribute to effective health education.

2. Research Approach

The analysis of previous works is an essential step in research in any field, though it is of great importance in the health field. This importance relates to the fact that new results contribute to the healthcare of patients. Additionally, this type of analysis has become a complementary tool to determine the quality of new scientific knowledge, and its impact on the health of the population. In this sense, it is possible to access the scientific data, and their effect on studies and sources [36].

Bibliometric studies provide essential information regarding the scientific data within a country, as well as in the international context. All of this information facilitates the decision-making of health professionals and will impact the future of social networking regarding health.

2.1. Database Selection

Prior to the analysis of the data from the research strategy, using the terms "social networks", "health", and "young people", a comparative analysis between different databases was conducted. The research strategy used was ALL = ("social networks" AND "health" AND "young people"). The databases included in this analysis were Scopus, Web of Sciences (WOS), PubMed, the Health and Medical Collection, and the Psychology Database. These databases were included based on their importance, use, and relevance in the health field, and were used to compare the results with the initial research.

The exclusion criteria used were the period of time from 1987 to 2018, terms in all cases and document types, and excluding papers with no scientific relevance such as news, obituaries, projects, or patents, available in journals.

The results show that for WOS, the number of documents was similar to the results obtained using Scopus. The results of the research using PubMed showed fewer publications than the number of documents. The results from the research using the Health and Medical Collection and Psychology Database show a higher number of documents than Scopus. The significant difference between these databases compared to Scopus or WOS may be caused by the nature of these resources. The Health and Medical Collection and Psychology Database were created to include all content in any form, so as to improve the learning, teaching, and research needs of institutions. Thus, these databases include both scientific and less scientific documents, such as medical reference eBooks, instructional videos, dissertations, and working papers. These platforms also include thousands of evidence-based articles and clinical trial records [37].

Overall, the documents obtained using Scopus included most of the scientific productions in the topic of health, social networks, and young people. This is based on the fact that, when it was used for the same strategy research, which focused on all fields, Scopus included more results than the other databases.

2.2. Data Collection

For this study, Elsevier's Scopus database was used to carry out the analysis. We identified studies from 1978 to 2018 that referred to social networks, health, or young people.

Scopus is a scientific bibliographic database of items from scientific journals. This database has been claimed as "the largest index database", including up to 65 million records and claims, many of which are in the health field, with titles providing complete coverage of Medline, Embase, and Compendex. In addition to articles, this database includes series, conferences, papers, books, and patents. The sources in the database date back to 1823, and it was established in 1996. Moreover, Scopus also provides the performance status of papers and authors according to the citations received for each work [38,39].

For this research, the inclusion criteria were the period from 1978 to 2018, and the theme of social media and health.

2.3. Statistical Analysis

The results from the research were analyzed, focusing on descriptive analyses, such as the frequencies of the types of document, the language, trends in scientific publications, primary sources, the field of the publication, the leading scientific institutions, associations among nations, the primary authors in the area, and the keywords used. In the case of keywords, a normalization of the terms was carried out, as many of the main keywords had both singular and plural forms. The keywords included in the manuscript were the author's keywords. In this sense, the keywords used were not MeSH terms.

Another aspect of the analysis was the identification of networks using the VOSviewer software [40]. This open-source program was created for constructing and viewing bibliometric maps by importing the data from several sources, including Scopus [41]. The criteria used to create the maps were a minimum of 10 connections between authors, fewer than 10 authors per document, and a minimum of five authors per document. This strategy was followed for the concurrency of keywords, connections between authors, and countries.

2.4. Exclusion and Inclusion Criteria

The inclusion criteria used for this study focused on the words "social networks" or "social media", "health", and "young people". These terms were used based on the objectives of this study, as the purpose was to analyze the intervention of social networks in health. With the results from the terms "social networks" or "social media" and "health", researchers looked for positive and negative interactions or applications of these networks to health. Additionally, the term "young people" was used to identify this specific population, determine implications, and find previous studies focused on this group.

Other terms, such as "youth" or "young adults", were not included, as it would result in the inclusion of more data that were not adequately focused on young people. The boolean operators used were "OR" and "AND", to link the three terms.

The exclusion criteria used were the period of time for the production of the documents, and the use of terms focusing on the title, abstract, or keywords. Additionally, the type of document was determined in order to exclude non-scientific productions, such as obituaries.

2.5. Sectional Analysis of the Initial Research Strategy

Before the use of the research strategy and the analysis of the data, the research strategy was divided into three sections. Each of these sections focused on the different relationships between health, social media, and young people.

The first section focused on the relationship between social media and the health of young people. The search used was (TITLE ({social networks}) OR ABS ({social networks}) OR AUTHKEY ({social networks}) OR TITLE ({social media}) OR ABS ({social media}) OR AUTHKEY ({social media}) AND TITLE ({young people}) OR ABS ({young people}) OR AUTHKEY ({young people}) AND TITLE ({health}) OR ABS ({health}) OR AUTHKEY ({health})) OR (TITLE ({social networks})). This strategy resulted in 262 documents, with the earliest publication in 1999. The most common theme in terms of the number of publications was medicine (166), followed by social sciences (83).

The second section was based on the interaction between social media and health. The search used was the following: (TITLE ({social networks}) OR ABS ({social networks}) OR AUTHKEY ({social networks}) OR TITLE ({social media}) OR ABS ({social media}) OR AUTHKEY ({social media}) AND TITLE ({health}) OR ABS ({health}) OR AUTHKEY ({health})). This second search resulted in 10,900 documents, with 5917 from the medicine area and 2750 from the social sciences thematic area.

The third section focused on the connection between social networks and young people. The search used was (TITLE ({social networks}) OR ABS ({social networks}) OR AUTHKEY ({social networks}) OR TITLE ({social media}) OR ABS ({social media}) OR AUTHKEY ({social media}) AND TITLE ({young people}) OR ABS ({young people}) OR AUTHKEY ({young people})). From this research, 1320 documents were found, with the first dated in 1997. The area with the most publications was social sciences (794), followed by medicine (305). Additionally, the results from this search were further analyzed using NOT (TITLE ("health") OR ABS ({health}) OR AUTHKEY ({health})). This deeper analysis showed that 25 documents did not include the term health, though the thematic areas were first medicine (17 documents), and then social sciences (11 documents).

Based on the results from each section, the final strategy was as follows: (TITLE ({social networks}) OR ABS ({social networks}) OR AUTHKEY ({social networks}) OR TITLE ({social media}) OR ABS ({social media}) OR AUTHKEY ({social media}) AND TITLE ({young people}) OR ABS ({young people}) OR AUTHKEY ({young people}) AND TITLE ({health}) OR ABS ({health}) OR AUTHKEY ({health})) OR (TITLE ({social networks}) OR ABS ({social networks}) OR AUTHKEY ({social networks}) OR TITLE ({social media}) OR ABS ({social media}) OR AUTHKEY ({social media}) AND TITLE ({health}) OR ABS ({health}) OR AUTHKEY ({health})) OR (TITLE ({social networks}) OR ABS ({social networks}) OR AUTHKEY ({social networks}) OR TITLE ({social media}) OR ABS ({social media}) OR AUTHKEY ({social media}) AND TITLE ({young people}) OR ABS ({young people}) OR AUTHKEY ({young people})). This, based on the health field, connected the terms "social networks", "health", and "young people".

The data obtained was a .csv file that contained the following: authors, title, author IDs, year, volume, issue, source title, article number, number of pages, cited by, digital object identifier system (DOI), link, document type, access type, source, and ID. Each item from the previous step was analyzed and studied separately; for instance, the number of documents per country, or the rate of publication of each author. Finally, the cluster determination of the thematic collections was examined with VOSviewer, resulting in diverse maps of global connections between authors and countries, as well as research tendencies, using keywords (Figure 1).

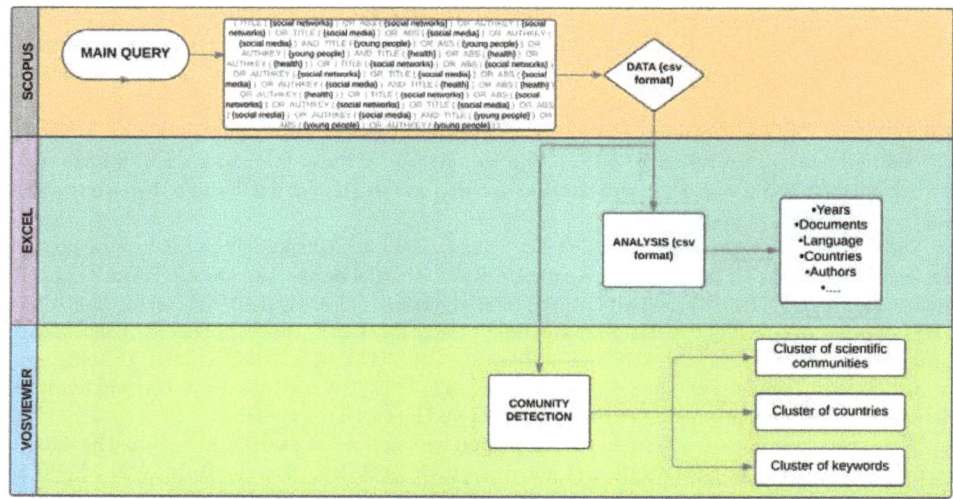

Figure 1. Methodology structure.

3. Results and Discussion

Article frequency, disciplinary focus, topics, authors' institutional affiliation, and country are all useful indicators of the popularity and type of research being undertaken in a scientific field, as well as its trends.

3.1. Type and Language of the Works

At total of 11,966 documents were obtained for the period of 1978–2018. Publications were diverse in type; the most common type of document was articles (68%), followed by conference papers (14%). The remaining types were reviews (8%); book chapters (4%); conference reviews (2%); and other types of documents (4%), such as books or notes (Figure 2). For the most common document, articles, the frequency was studied, and it was found that 82% were quantitative studies and 18% were qualitative studies. Most of the quantitative studies were cross-sectional studies (24%), followed by control trial studies (23%). These results are consistent with previous studies that have pointed out how quantitative articles are more common in the health field, with reviews or other documents being less commonly published [42]. As described by van Wesel M. (2016), the reasons for the higher number of articles may be related to a change of publication policy, author interest, or hot topic issues [43].

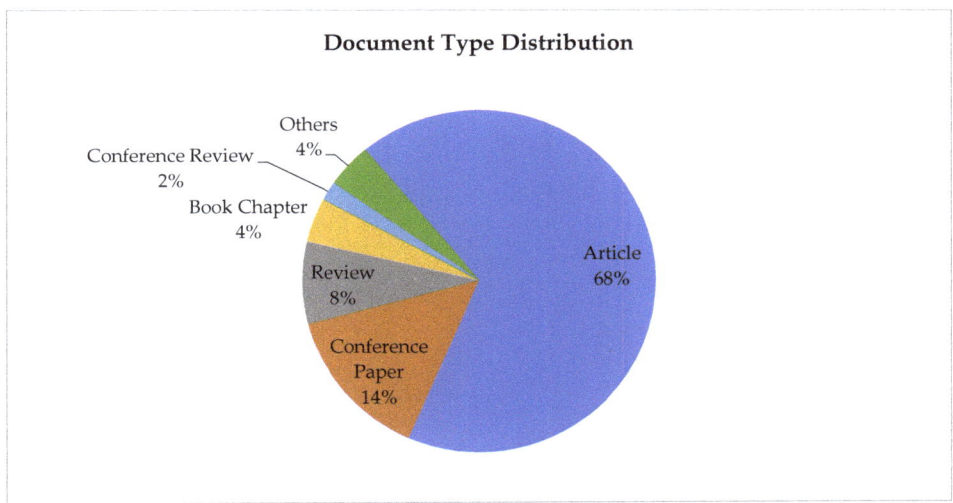

Figure 2. Frequency of the types of documents from 1978 to 2018.

Regarding the language used in the publications found in the search, the language most used was English in the different international journals (94.53%), followed by Spanish (2.03%), Portuguese (1.09%), and German (0.59%). Figure 3 shows the frequency of each language for the documents published over the last four decades, as found through the bibliometric examination.

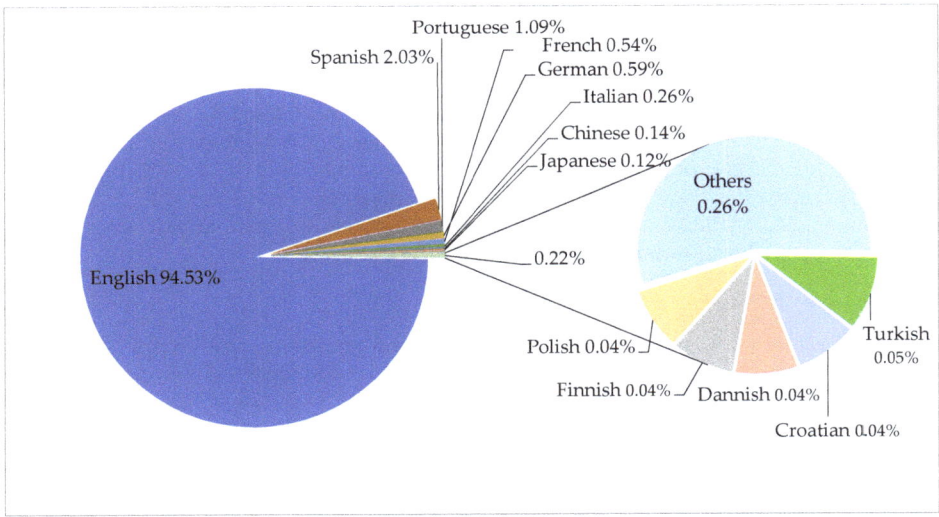

Figure 3. Languages of papers published over the period of 1978 to 2018.

The tendency to use English has been described in previous studies as the main language of publication [44], noting that researchers who write in English to communicate tend to have more opportunities [45].

3.2. Characteristics of Scientific Productions from 1978 to 2018

Figure 4 shows the frequency of academic publications focused on social networks, health, and young people, over the last four decades. The figure suggests an upward trend, implying that the number of annual outputs increased markedly from around 2002 to 2018.

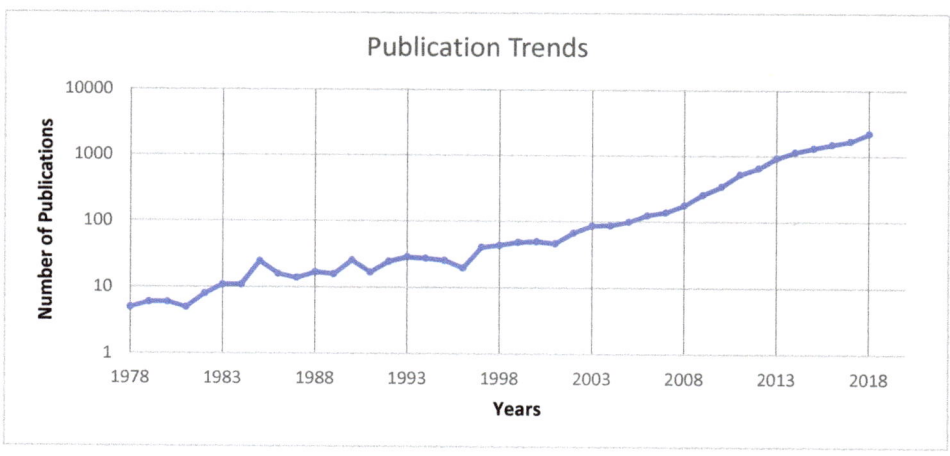

Figure 4. The trend of publications in social networks, health, and young people during the period of 1978–2018.

Based on this figure, the main observation is a rapid increase from the early 2000s, which coincides with the emergence of online social media and research exploring the interaction between social media and health.

These results are consistent with previous analyses showing increased research attention given to social networks related to the health field [34]. This interest highlighted the possibility of using these networks as tools, but also their negative effects on health [46]. Additionally, it is important to highlight that the increase of publications also affects other topics in the health field. In this sense, Kyvik S (2003) highlighted how the number of publications per researcher was higher in technology and the natural and medical sciences in 1998–2000. Additionally, this same author stated that the tendency for publication in such areas increased in the late 1990s [47].

3.3. International Dissemination of Publications

Figure 5 shows the production of relevant articles per country between 1978 and 2018. Colors indicate the number of papers, from red (highest) to grey (no publications). The country with most publications was the United States (5205), followed by the United Kingdom (1577), Australia (1058), Canada (811), and Spain (423). Within these countries, the use of social networks has increased, and has even been potentiated by governments and institutions in order to promote healthy lifestyles or to provide group support for patients [48]. In the case of Spain, the increase of publications related to social media and health might be linked to the growth in environmental performance, social performance, and corporate governance performance since 2002 [49].

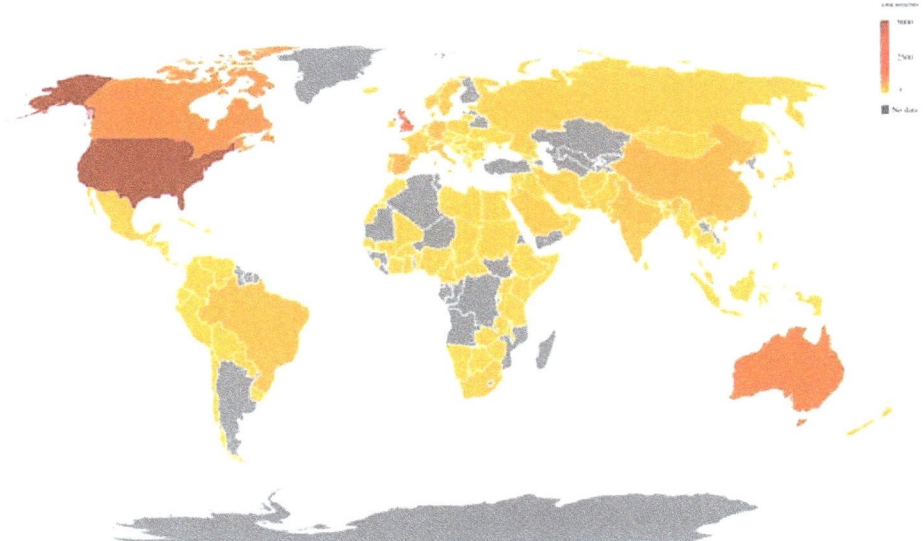

Figure 5. The trend of publications in each country during the period of 1978–2018.

Figure 6 shows the trajectory of research publications in each of the five countries with the highest production of papers on social networks, young people, and health, revealing the highest increase occurred in the United States.

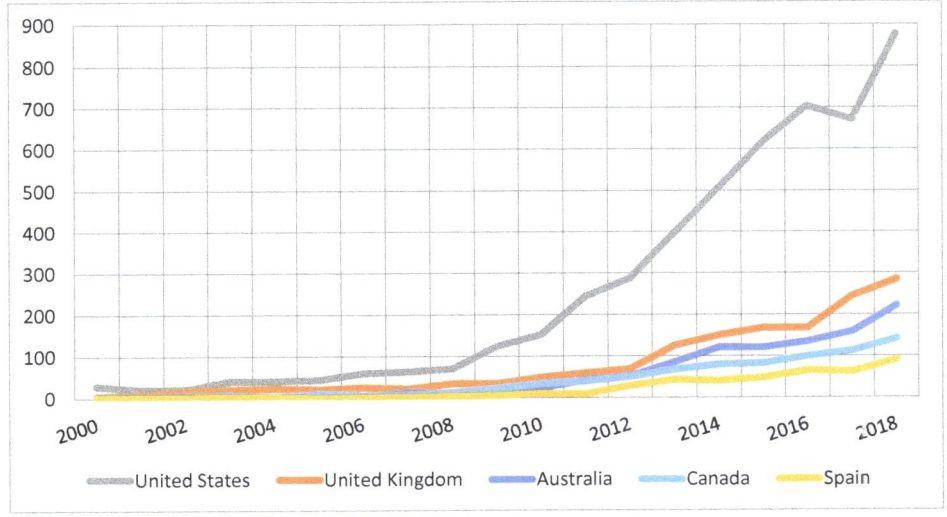

Figure 6. The trend of publications in the five countries with higher rates during the period of 1978–2018.

The social network map shown in Figure 7 illustrates the pattern of international collaboration between study authors. This figure was obtained after applying the software VOSviewer v.1 6.11. to a .csv file of the data extracted from Scopus during the literature search.

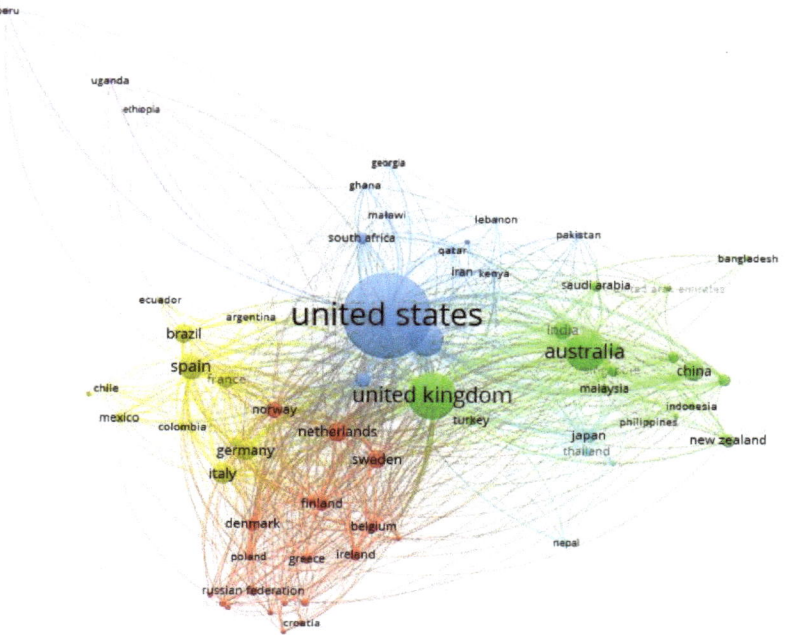

Figure 7. Collaboration among countries.

Three countries dominate in the six clusters seen in Figure 7 and Table 2, namely: the United Kingdom, the United States, and Australia. The first cluster comprises eastern European countries and Nordic countries, led by Finland. The green cluster, which is the second most crucial cluster, is led by the United Kingdom. The United Kingdom is the node of this cluster, because of the number of connections with other countries, and the number of publications. This cluster also includes Australia as the second most relevant nucleus, with a lower number of connections than the United Kingdom. All of the countries from this cluster seem to be connected via economic and political relationships.

Table 2. International collaborations in research on social media related to health and young people.

Cluster	Color	Countries	Geographic Area	%
1	Red	Netherlands–Denmark–Finland–Norway–Belgium–Poland–Sweden–Russia Federation	Nordic countries–East Europe–Russia	37.6
2	Green	United Kingdom–Australia–Hong Kong–China	United Kingdom–Australia–Asia	25.1
3	Blue	United States–Canada–Switzerland–South Africa	United States–Canada–Africa	24.2
4	Yellow	Spain–France–Italy–Germany–Colombia	Europe–Latin America	13.4
5	Purple	Cuba–Peru–Uganda–Ethiopia	Latin America–Africa	2.9
6	Pink	Japan–Nepal–Thailand–Vietnam	Asia	2.8

The blue cluster is third in importance, and is led by the United States, followed by Canada, and represents 24.2% of the publications. The yellow cluster is led by Spain, with connections to Latin America and Europe, representing 13.4% of publications on this topic. The purple cluster is linked to Latin America and African countries, led by Cuba. The last cluster is pink and is led by Japan, and is connected to a variety of different countries such as the United Kingdom, the United States, Australia, and New Zealand.

Of the countries that have published the most about social media in the health field, the United States stands out. Previous researchers have stated that the United States has dominated publications in different scientific fields, such as education. This tendency of publications to originate from the United States and a few other countries, such as the United Kingdom, has been attributed to a combination of factors, such as being English-speaking countries, authors coming from these countries, and the possible connections between researchers within the scientific community [50]. These results and previous works further support the idea of the United States being the leader of scientific productions in the health field, and therefore in the topic of social media connected to health and young people.

The essential and significant role of the United States is also shown by the connections between authors and affiliations, most of which belong to the United States (Table 3). Overall, these results might be explained by the fact that there may be economic, historical, geographical, and cultural influences between the groups, which can be applied to all of the clusters. In addition, the remaining clusters could be explained by specific topics relating to social networks, such as interventions or risks, and the type of young people that the research focused on.

3.4. Institutions Active in Relevant Research

In Table 3, the 10 organizations with the highest rates of publication in the field of social networks related to health and young people are presented. Additionally, the top three keywords used in each of these institutions are included in this table.

Table 3. Publications and keywords utilized by the top ten international institutions.

Affiliation	Country	Publications	Main Keywords Used		
			1	2	3
University of Toronto	Canada	158	Human/s	Female	Social media
The University of Sydney	Australia	157	Human/s	Social media	Female
University of Michigan, Ann Arbor	United States	155	Human/s	Article	Female
The University of North Carolina at Chapel Hill	United States	152	Human/s	Article	Female
University of Washington, Seattle	United States	143	Human/s	Social media	Female
University of Melbourne	Australia	140	Human/s	Social media	Article
Harvard Medical School	United States	132	Human/s	Article	Male
University of California, Los Angeles	United States	131	Human/s	Article	Female
Johns Hopkins Bloomberg School of Public Health	United States	126	Human/s	Female	Adult
University of California, San Francisco	United States	123	Human/s	Social media	Male

The University of Toronto is in first position, with 158 documents, which is not surprising, as the *Journal of Medical Internet Research* is based at this location. Next is the University of Sydney, in second position with 157 documents, and the University of Michigan in third position with 155. In positions four–six are the University of North Carolina at Chapel Hill with 152, the University of Washington with 143, and the University of Melbourne with 140 documents published. Finally, Harvard Medical School has 132, University of California has 131, Johns Hopkins Bloomberg School of Public Health has 126, and the University of California has 123. It should be highlighted that the keyword used most often by these institutions is "human/s", ranking in first place in all cases.

The increase of publications and the ranking of affiliations might be related to collaboration between authors. These collaborations have been previously studied by other authors, showing that, since 1997, collaborations in the United States or Canada have increased by 20% [51]. Moreover, these factors have been linked to collaborations between the United States and the other countries, showing a possible node of union [51].

Regarding the type of study implemented by each institution, according to Scopus, the results showed that all of the institutions focused on articles in the area of medicine, followed by the area of social sciences. The central countries with a higher number of publications were the United States, United Kingdom, and Canada. Finally, the most common keywords used according to Scopus were "human/s", "female", "articles", "male", and "social media."

3.5. Subject Categories and Journals Found using Scopus

The frequency of publications by each thematic area was acquired from the Scopus database. In Figure 8, the distribution of the main thematic areas is represented. This figure shows that the area with the highest percentage of documents was medicine (50.7%), followed by social sciences (28.9%), computer sciences (19.2%), and psychology (10%). Areas such as agricultural and biological sciences (1.3%); engineering (1.6%); or pharmacology, toxicology, and pharmaceutics (1.4%) were less common in the database. The "other" (5.9%) category represents unspecified areas.

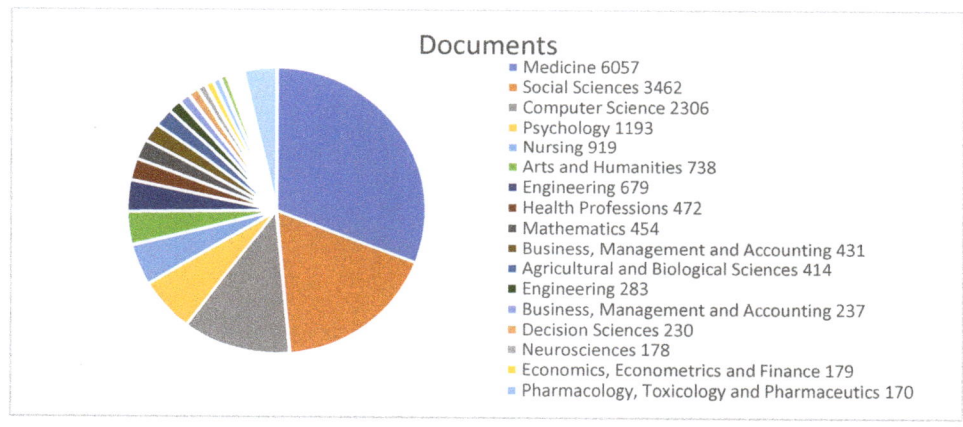

Figure 8. Distribution of scientific productions according to the main thematic areas.

These results show the two main thematic areas—medicine and social sciences (Table 4). Medicine is the central area of publication in the health field, as medicine is one of the most ancient areas of research [52]. The same could be said for social sciences, as social structures and social behavior have been studied for centuries [1].

Table 4. Main thematic areas concerning the total number of scientific productions found from the analysis.

Subject Area	Documents
Medicine	6057
Social Sciences	3462
Computer Science	2306
Psychology	1193
Nursing	919
Arts and Humanities	738
Engineering	679
Health Professions	472
Mathematics	454

Table 4. Cont.

Subject Area	Documents
Biochemistry, Genetics, and Molecular Biology	431
Business, Management, and Accounting	414
Agricultural and Biological Sciences	283
Environmental Science	237
Decision Sciences	230
Neurosciences	178
Economics, Econometrics, and Finance	179
Medicine	6057
Undefined	151
Other	705

The first quartile (Q1), Scimago Journal Rank (SJR), and Journal Citation Report (JCR) have been included in the table so as to present the importance and relevance of the major journals that have published more publications. These measures were chosen based on their quality and for being used worldwide in the scientific field. The quartiles are based on ranking each journal according to their subject, using the impact factor distribution the journal occupies for that subject category as a measure. In this sense, Q1 denotes the top 25% of the impact factor distribution. The Scimago Journal Rank measures the weighted citations received by the serial. Citation weighting depends on the subject field and the prestige of the citing serial. Finally, the Journal Citation Report is based on citations compiled from the Science Citation Index Expanded and the Social Sciences Citation Index [53].

The leading 11 journals that have published in this research field, and the number of publications in each according to the Scopus database, are shown in Table 5. As can be seen, most of the journals with the greatest number of documents published and the highest impact factors are from the United Kingdom (U.K.), Canada, and the United States (USA).

Table 5. Quartile, Scimago Journal Rank (SJR), and Journal Citation Report (JCR) of major worldwide journals.

Source	Quartile Score	SJR (2018)	JCR (2018)	Total Docs (2018)	Total Doc (3 Years)	Total Ref.	Total Cites (3 Years)	Cites/Docs (2 Years)	Country
Journal of Medical Internet Research	Q1	1.74	4.90	1281	2018	5419	3335	2.10	Canada
Lecture Notes In Computer Science Including Subseries Lecture Notes In Artificial Intelligence And Lecture Notes In Bioinformatics	Q4	0.28	1.06	22,590	63,930	445,801	68,303	1.06	Germany
Social Science and Medicine	Q1	2.03	3.08	509	1599	44,305	18,063	3.71	United Kingdom
Plos One	Q1	1.18	2.76	217,985	62,994	223,689	74,005	3.11	United States
ACM International Conference Proceeding Series	-	0.17	0.59	-	6788	53,752	1313	0.56	Canada
Studies In Health Technology And Informatics	-	2.03	0.25	1553	1599	16,001	2809	3.71	Germany
BMC Public Health	Q2	1.38	2.56	1322	3650	58,519	3335	2.94	United Kingdom
BMJ Open	Q2	1.32	2.37	13,753	7215	26,298	38,028	2.65	United Kingdom
Computers in Human Behavior	Q1	1.71	4.30	462	2247	6258	13,804	6.14	United Kingdom
Conference On Human Factors In Computing Systems Proceedings	-	0.30	-	-	1924	10,072	5621	2.92	United States
Journal of Health Communication	Q2	1.0	1.77	110	417	1972	1108	2.37	United States
American Journal of Public Health	Q1	2.51	5.38	611	1786	20,651	5861	3.12	United States

3.6. Determination of Scientific Groups and Utilization of Keywords

A further analysis was carried out based on the dominant authors in the field of social networks related to the health of the young. Table 6 and Figure 9 represent the scientific productions of the top five researchers focused on this subject during the last decade. De Choudhury, M. tops this field, with 35 documents over 10 years. Nevertheless, this author has an h-index of 28, lower than Christakis, N.A., with an h-index of 71, and Merchant, R.M., with an h-index of 32. Following this, according to the h-index, was Yang, C.C. with 23 and Young, S.D. with 22. Although De Choudhury, M. has a lower h-index compared to Christakis, N.A. or Merchant, R.M., the total number of documents published by this author, 2776, is higher than for any of the other authors.

Table 6. Progress of the top five authors' works during the last decade.

	De Choudhury, M.	Yang, C.C.	Young, S.D.	Christakis, N.A.	Merchant, R.M.	Total Documents
2008	0	0	0	3	0	3
2009	0	2	0	2	0	4
2010	0	0	0	2	0	2
2011	0	1	1	2	0	4
2012	0	4	3	2	0	9
2013	5	4	4	2	1	16
2014	4	8	2	1	5	20
2015	7	5	2	3	5	22
2016	6	5	1	1	5	18
2017	9	1	3	2	5	20
2018	4	4	9	3	2	22
Total Documents	35	34	25	23	23	140

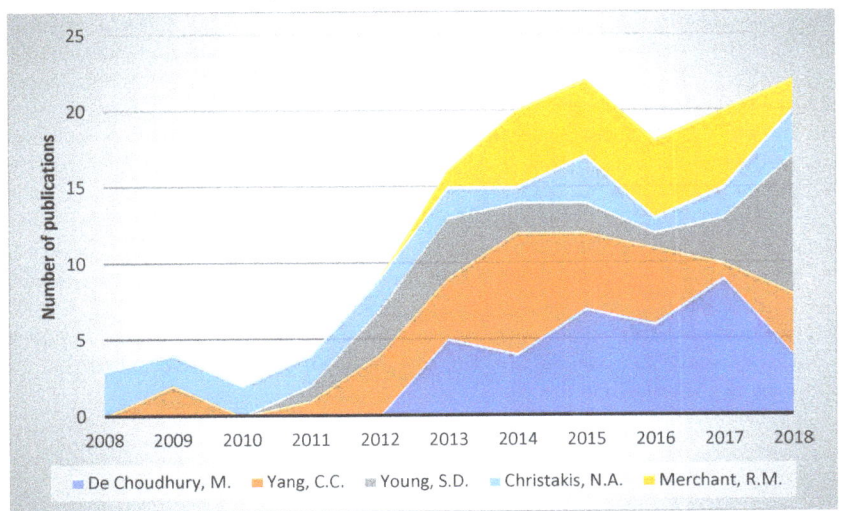

Figure 9. The top principal authors of the last decade.

All of the authors with the highest frequencies of publication are from the United States. These results match the previous results, which showed the high impact and leading role of the United States in research on social media applied to the health field.

However, possible critical authors in the field of health and social media, such as Eysenbach, G., with an h-index of 44, were not included in the previous analysis, based solely on the number of documents they authored on this topic. Table 7 shows the 10 top authors of documents on this topic, with h-index, citations, total publications, and the year of the first publication included. Moreover, the author ID has been included so as to differentiate the authors with the same name, as any other researcher may access these details.

Table 7. Top 10 authors published in the topic, with h-index, citations, and total publications.

Author	Publications	H-index	Total Citations	Total Publications	First Publication	Author ID
De Choudhury, M.	35	28	2776	97	2007	18433530100
Yang, C.C.	34	23	1959	191	2000	7407740308
Berkman, L.F.	28	97	43,285	348	1976	7005551894
Young, S.D.	25	78	1241	78	2009	34876005800
Christakis, N. A.	25	71	26,657	236	1985	7005400323
Kawachi, I.	25	113	51,266	1005	1988	7103096477
Merchant, R. M.	23	32	6441	127	1998	14028632100
Dredze, M.A.	22	35	4669	137	2003	14041686400
Fernandez-Luque, L.	21	18	1251	85	2006	35224861700
House, M.	20	16	865	146	2005	8667908000

This table shows how younger authors have fewer publications, a lower h-index, and fewer publications. This is important to highlight, as the number of publications in this topic is not fully representative of the relevance of the authors.

Like any community, the scientific community is deeply connected, creating an interactive and dynamic network. This type of community usually has a central nucleus that is cohesively connected to other elements from the community that are less representative. The scientific community is generally replicated by clusters from other groups.

Clustering is a significant issue in the current work. Recognizing these groups has relative importance to the topic of study, as determining them makes it possible to define the quantity and quality of the existing associations between the authors of different institutions and areas of knowledge. The existence of interactions between different thematic areas, such as medicine and engineering, has been established [54]. The algorithmic mapping technique used by the software VOSviewer [41] was applied in order to identify and measure the association between authors. VOSviewer's algorithm focused on the detection of items in a low-dimensional space, so that the distance between two items is a precise indicator of their affinity.

Figure 10 depicts the clusters of the scientific communities of the authors. This figure displays the interactions between the principal authors and remaining researchers in the field of social networks related to the health of young people. The first cluster, led by Young S.D., is the greatest, with 43 authors. The following cluster (green) comprises 27 authors, of which the top author is Moreno, M., with 21 documents. The top author in collaborations and publications is De Choudhury, M., with 35 publications and 22 collaborators. On this basis, the second author is Yang, C.C., with 434 publications and 34 collaborators.

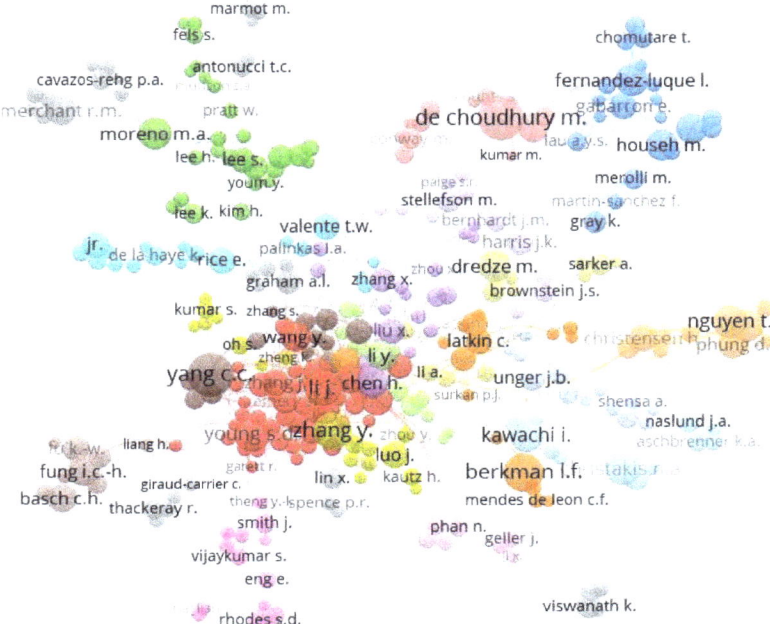

Figure 10. Scientific clusters of researchers focused on social networks in health.

Another analysis we carried out was the determination of the keywords used in the publications in this field. During the last four decades, from the 11,966 documents found, the most common author keywords used were "human/s", utilized in 10,936 items, followed by "social media" (3937 items), and "article" (3561 items). Table 8 illustrates the 40 most important keywords used in relevant documents during the last four decades.

Table 8. Forty critical keywords used in publications.

Order	Term	Documents	%
1	Human/s	10,936	91.4
2	Social media	3937	32.9
3	Article	3561	29.8
4	Female	3450	28.8
5	Male	3086	25.8
6	Adult	2665	22.3
7	Social network	2167	18.1
8	Social Support	2083	17.4
9	Social networks	1538	12.9
10	Social networking (online)	1535	12.8
11	Internet	1513	12.6
12	Adolescent	1387	11.6
13	Ageing	1346	11.2
14	Psychology	1208	10.1
15	Priority journal	1201	10.0
16	Aged	1187	9.9
17	Health	1065	8.9

Table 8. Cont.

Order	Term	Documents	%
18	Young adult	1064	8.9
19	United States	1004	8.4
20	Major clinical study	965	8.1
21	Procedures	964	8.1
22	Controlled study	900	7.5
23	Questionnaire	898	7.5
24	Mental health	800	6.7
25	Public health	799	6.7
26	Health promotion	717	6.0
27	Statistics and numerical data	706	5.9
28	Attitude to health	595	5.0
29	Health care	582	4.9
30	Qualitative research	572	4.8
31	Review	559	4.7
32	Social networking	541	4.5
33	Medical information	540	4.5
34	Health status	536	4.5
35	Cross-sectional study	534	4.5
36	Child	533	4.5
37	Education	527	4.4
38	Health behavior	527	4.4
39	Cross-sectional studies	507	4.2
40	Surveys and questionnaires	505	4.2

The analysis of the authors' keywords showed that most of the relevant keywords are commonly utilized for this topic. Nevertheless, it is essential to highlight that the term "human/s" was probably used to differentiate from animal research, rather than because of significance to the topic.

Based on these keywords, the results might imply the transversal inclusion of social media in the health field, from mental health to diabetes. However, it is essential to highlight that the keywords and topics of the studies also represented different points of view, such as on the side effects of using social media [55].

Overall, the study of keywords in scientific works is highly relevant, as this determines the trends of publications and the follow-up of these publications. In this sense, Table 7 shows how similar concepts are often written differently; for example, "social media", "Internet", or "adolescent". Figure 11 depicts a cloud of words, where the dimension of each word represents the significance of the keyword related to the number of documents in which it is used. The increased use of the term "social media" may be related to the increased use of platforms such as Facebook, Twitter, or Instagram [31,35,56]. The growth of other words, such as "health promotion" or "eHealth", might be related to the development of telemedicine and studies focused on new technologies and health [57–59].

Figure 12 displays the map of co-occurring keywords selected by researchers from the documents we analyzed that focused on social networks and the health of young people. The VOSviewer software with the Vos mapping technique was used to develop Figure 12. Each color symbolizes the separation between keywords, concerning the thematic area for which these colors have been selected. In addition, the dimension of the circles displays the frequency of use of each word, and the lines linking each circle show the associations among the different keywords used in the publications.

In this analysis, "human", "social media", and "article" are the most commonly used words. Table 8 shows the essential keywords used by the five top groups identified in the subject of social networks related to health and young people [60–62].

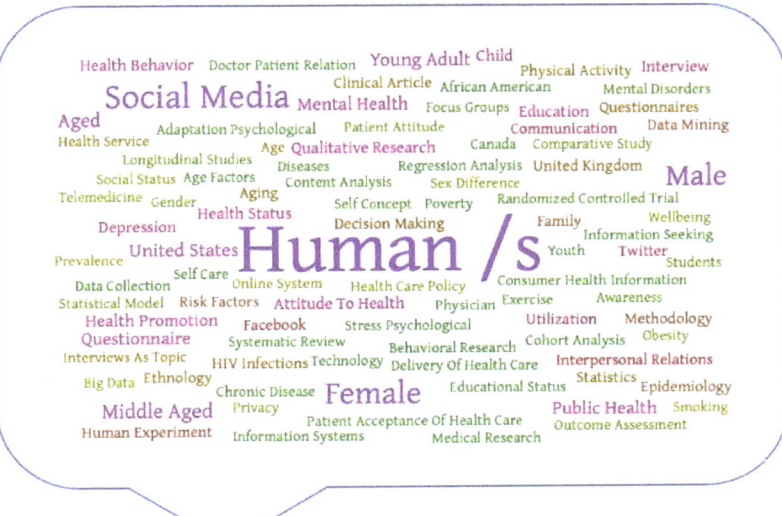

Figure 11. Cloud of the main keywords focused on social networks related to the health of young people.

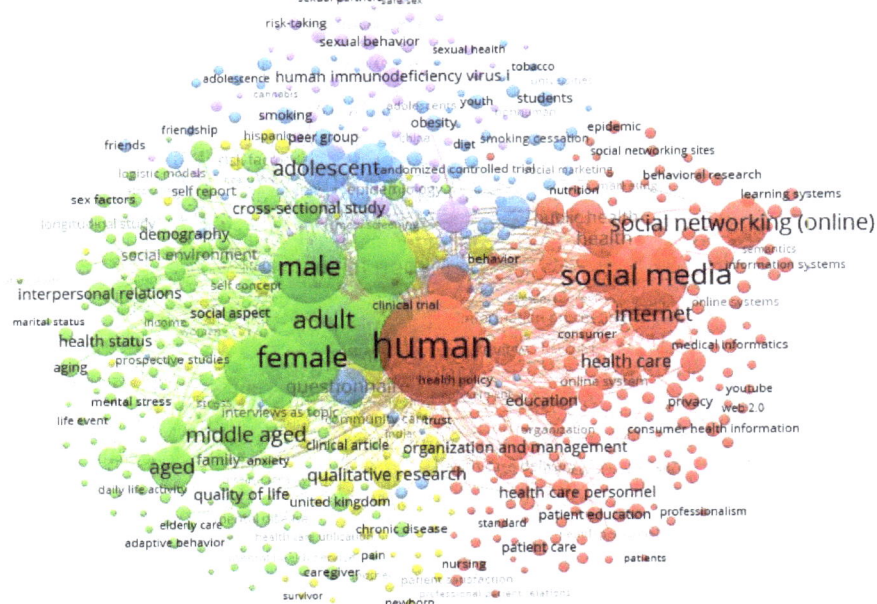

Figure 12. Clusters according to the co-occurrence of keywords.

Social networks are used for multiple reasons related to health, including feedback, creating a support group, health interventions, or to determine the influence of these interventions [63–65]. Table 9 shows the main characteristics of the clusters from Figure 12, showing how the five clusters were found. The most important, the red cluster, focuses on social media and health education. The green cluster focuses on social networks and mental health, which matches the latest studies focused on preventing mental health problems in children and teenagers [66–68]. The third cluster focuses on how social media may play an essential role in prevention programs for adolescents. A comparison of the findings from this cluster with those of other studies confirms the important role that social media may have in preventing health problems in younger people [67,69]. This is consistent with our earlier observations and previous research, which showed that social networks may be preventative and help-seeking tools for young people with mental health problems, such as drug use, depression, or addiction [70]. The fourth cluster points out the relationship between ethnicity and health aptitude from a qualitative perspective. These results reflect those of Sunil and Xu (2019), who found that ethnicity and cultural background play an important role in health [71,72]. The purple cluster is focused on young people and the relationship of social networks to sexual health. This influence has been previously studied as being both positive and negative; either being used as a health intervention in patients with human immunodeficiency virus (HIV), or studied as a factor that contributes to the increase of HIV [73–75].

Table 9. Keywords most utilized by the six top communities identified in the topic of social networks related to the health of young people.

Cluster	Color	Main Keywords	Topic	%
1	Red	Human–social media–medical information–eHealth–health education–public health	Social media–education	33.8
2	Green	Social network–age–epidemiology–gender–mental health–social support–psychological aspects	Mental health	28.9
3	Blue	Adolescent–young adults–health behavior–health promotion	Adolescents–health	14.0
4	Yellow	Qualitative research–interview–health attitude–ethnicity	Qualitative–health attitude	13.1
5	Purple	Health risk behavior–HIV infection–prevalence-risk assessment	Risk–prevention	10.3

Based on these connections, it could be concluded that the first objective of this study was accomplished, as the first, fifth, and sixth clusters focused on the positive use of these technologies in the health field in general. As previously stated, previous studies have corroborated the main perspectives of the recent trend of publications on using social media as education or prevention tools [76]. The second objective has been partially completed, as the second, third, and fourth clusters focused not only on young people, but also adolescents. These results may be because of the interconnection between being a young person and being an adolescent; young adults are between 18 and 24 years old, and are often partially included in the definition of adolescence [69].

4. Conclusions

This paper examines trends in research focused on social media related to health and young people, including prevalence, topics, global distribution, and the networks of researchers involved.

Although the trajectory of relevant research remained relatively stable over the first thirty years profiled in our analysis, a significant increase can be seen between 2003 and 2018, correlating with the popularity of online social networks, especially among young people [21]. In addition, during that decade, the idea of using technology for following or supporting patients at a distance emerged and increased [77]. In this sense, social media has been utilized for support systems for patients, such as cancer patients, or to receive feedback from patients [78,79].

It is also essential to highlight the types of research seen in the review. For example, in terms of the research from Scopus, most publications were original articles in the form of quantitative cross-sectional studies or controlled trials. Another significant result was the topics of the studies, which were based on keywords, and showed a variety of multiple sub-areas of the health field relating to social networks, such as mental health, education, or chronic diseases.

The second significant finding was that collaboration between authors and countries seems to be led by the United States, acting as the standard connection between countries and authors. Based on this, significant countries in terms of health prevention measures and the health system, as well as the number of inhabitants, might be linked to the prevalence of studies on the role of social networks in health interventions and as a risk factor [60,80,81].

Regarding the areas of studies undertaken in the field of social networks in health, the area of medicine (50.7%) stands out as the most relevant. As previously stated, the supremacy of this area might be related to its evolution and relevance [59].

This work also determined communities by using the collaborations between countries found in the bibliometric study. Five clusters were identified, with the most significant focused on the actual usability of the social networks for educational purposes. Moreover, these results have shown how most countries are connected to the United States. These results seem consistent with previous results in the health field about the leading role of the United States [52]. The clusters are formed by those countries with traditional political, historical, and economic relationships. In general, therefore, it seems that the use of social networks in the health field, especially for young people, continues to grow as a tool, particularly for educational purposes, in certain places.

Nevertheless, like any research, this study has limitations. One source of weakness in this study that could have affected the measurement of the data is the choice of keywords used to interrogate the databases. This research focused on including different terms for social networks, more than including other terms for young people, such as "youth". This was primarily to avoid the possible inclusion of publications not focused on any human population, such as those with the keyword "regenerative youth". Additionally, some critical authors in this topic have not been included, or their presence is less representative. Moreover, the study of keywords and, therefore, the topic of the documents, might not represent the totality of the research carried out in the health field, as the keywords used were not MeSH terms. Finally, the boolean operators used, which were "OR" and "AND", may have included some publications with the terms of the search, though the topic of study was different. However, based on the sample size, the number of the publications with different topic would produce an insignificant change in the result obtained in this study.

Overall, these findings have significant implications for the understanding of how the future of healthcare may lead to using social media in education and communication with patients. Additionally, this bibliometric analysis adds to the literature by elucidating the growing importance of social networks in health research, both as a topic of study and as a means of supporting scientific collaboration. This may help to inform future investments in public health research and surveillance using these different data sources, which may be particularly relevant for young people, who are a traditionally "hard to reach" group [82]. The bibliometric visualizations also provide an accessible means of communicating the key findings to researchers, policymakers, and those working in public health.

Author Contributions: Conceptualization, P.A.-M. and M.V.-A.; methodology, P.A.-M. and M.P.M.-J.; validation A.-J.P.-M.; formal analysis, P.A.-M. and A.-J.P.-M.; investigation, P.A.-M. and A.-J.P.-M.; resources, M.P.M.-J. and A.-J.P.-M.; data curation, M.D.R.-M.; writing—original draft preparation, P.A.-M., M.P.M.-J., and A.-J.P.-M.; writing—review and editing, M.V.-A. and C.P.; visualization, C.P.; supervision, M.D.R.-M., C.P., and M.V.-A.; project administration, M.V.-A. and M.P.M.-J.; funding acquisition, M.V.-A.

Funding: UCO Social Innova Project Galileo IV from the institution of OTRI of the University of Cordoba, Spain and the funding provided from "IDEP/Escuela de Doctorado" of the University of Cordoba.

Acknowledgments: We would also like to thank UCO Social Innova Project Galileo IV from the institution of OTRI of the University of Cordoba, Spain, and the funding provided from "IDEP/Escuela de Doctorado" of the University of Cordoba to one of the authors. The content is the responsibility of the authors, and does not necessarily represent the official views of the OTRI.

Conflicts of Interest: The authors declare no conflict of interest.

References

1. Anglade, C.; Dorze, G.L.; Croteau, C. Service encounter interactions of people living with moderate-to-severe post-stroke aphasia in their community. *Aphasiology* **2019**, *33*, 1061–1082. [CrossRef]
2. Erfani, S.S.; Abedin, B. Impacts of the use of social network sites on users' psychological well-being: A systematic review. *J. Assoc. Inf. Sci. Tech.* **2018**, *69*, 900–912. [CrossRef]
3. Penni, J. The future of online social networks (OSN): A measurement analysis using social media tools and application. *Telemat. Inform.* **2017**, *34*, 498–517. [CrossRef]
4. Anwar, M.M.; Liu, C.; Li, J. Discovering and tracking query oriented active online social groups in dynamic information network. *World Wide Web* **2019**, *22*, 1819–1854. [CrossRef]
5. Boyd, D.M.; Ellison, N.B. Social Network Sites: Definition, History, and Scholarship. *J. Comput. -Mediat. Commun.* **2007**, *13*, 210–230. [CrossRef]
6. Tajeuna, E.G.; Bouguessa, M.; Wang, S. Modeling and Predicting Community Structure Changes in Time-Evolving Social Networks. *IEEE Trans. Knowl. Data Eng.* **2019**, *31*, 1166–1180. [CrossRef]
7. Elbanna, A.; Bunker, D.; Levine, L.; Sleigh, A. Emergency management in the changing world of social media: Framing the research agenda with the stakeholders through engaged scholarship. *Int. J. Inf. Manage.* **2019**, *47*, 112–120. [CrossRef]
8. Dokuka, S.; Krekhovets, E.; Priymak, M. Health, Grades and Friendship: How Socially Constructed Characteristics Influence the Social Network Structure. In *Lecture Notes in Computer Science, Proceedings of the Analysis of Images, Social Networks and Texts, Moscow, Russia, 5–7 July 2018*; van der Aalst, W.M.P., Ignatov, D.I., Khachay, M., Kuznetsov, S.O., Lempitsky, V., Lomazova, I.A., Loukachevitch, N., Napoli, A., Panchenko, A., Pardalos, P.M., et al., Eds.; Springer International Publishing: Berlin/Heidelberg, Germany, 2018; pp. 381–391.
9. Romano, V.; Shen, M.; Pansanel, J.; MacIntosh, A.J.J.; Sueur, C. Social transmission in networks: Global efficiency peaks with intermediate levels of modularity. *Behav. Ecol. Sociobiol.* **2018**, *72*, 154. [CrossRef]
10. Cohen, R.; Newton-John, T.; Slater, A. 'Selfie'-objectification: The role of selfies in self-objectification and disordered eating in young women. *Comput. Hum. Behav.* **2018**, *79*, 68–74. [CrossRef]
11. Villanti, A.C.; Johnson, A.L.; Ilakkuvan, V.; Jacobs, M.A.; Graham, A.L.; Rath, J.M. Social Media Use and Access to Digital Technology in US Young Adults in 2016. *J. Med. Internet Res.* **2017**, *19*, e196. [CrossRef]
12. Błachnio, A.; Przepiórka, A.; Pantic, I. Internet use, Facebook intrusion, and depression: Results of a cross-sectional study. *Eur. Psychiatry* **2015**, *30*, 681–684. [CrossRef] [PubMed]
13. Ballester-Arnal, R.; Giménez-García, C.; Gil-Llario, M.D.; Castro-Calvo, J. Cybersex in the "Net generation": Online sexual activities among Spanish adolescents. *Comput. Hum. Behav.* **2016**, *57*, 261–266. [CrossRef]
14. Alhuwail, D.; Abdulsalam, Y. Assessing Electronic Health Literacy in the State of Kuwait: Survey of Internet Users From an Arab State. *J. Med. Internet Res.* **2019**, *21*, e11174. [CrossRef] [PubMed]
15. Shensa, A.; Escobar-Viera, C.G.; Sidani, J.E.; Bowman, N.D.; Marshal, M.P.; Primack, B.A. Problematic social media use and depressive symptoms among US young adults: A nationally-representative study. *Soc. Sci. Med.* **2017**, *182*, 150–157. [CrossRef]
16. Aiello, A.E. Invited Commentary: Evolution of Social Networks, Health, and the Role of Epidemiology. *Am. J. Epidemiol.* **2017**, *185*, 1089–1092. [CrossRef]
17. Ridout, B.; Campbell, A. The Use of Social Networking Sites in Mental Health Interventions for Young People: Systematic Review. *J. Med. Internet Res.* **2018**, *20*, e12244. [CrossRef]
18. Ainin, S.; Naqshbandi, M.M.; Moghavvemi, S.; Jaafar, N.I. Facebook usage, socialization and academic performance. *Comput. Educ.* **2015**, *83*, 64–73. [CrossRef]
19. Huang, Y.-T.; Su, S.-F. Motives for Instagram Use and Topics of Interest among Young Adults. *Future Internet* **2018**, *10*, 77. [CrossRef]
20. Sax, H.; Perneger, T.; Hugonnet, S.; Herrault, P.; Chraïti, M.-N.; Pittet, D. Knowledge of Standard and Isolation Precautions in a Large Teaching Hospital. *Infect. Control Hosp. Epidemiol.* **2005**, *26*, 298–304. [CrossRef]
21. Ilakkuvan, V.; Johnson, A.; Villanti, A.C.; Evans, W.D.; Turner, M. Patterns of Social Media Use and Their Relationship to Health Risks Among Young Adults. *J. Adolesc. Health* **2019**, *64*, 158–164. [CrossRef]
22. Shen, J.; Zhu, P.; Xu, M. Knowledge Sharing of Online Health Community Based on Cognitive Neuroscience. *NeuroQuantology* **2018**, *16*, 476–480. [CrossRef]

23. Barton, K.S.; Wingerson, A.; Barzilay, J.R.; Tabor, H.K. "Before Facebook and before social media . . . we did not know anybody else that had this": Parent perspectives on internet and social media use during the pediatric clinical genetic testing process. *J. Commun. Genet.* **2019**, *10*, 375–383. [CrossRef] [PubMed]
24. More, J.S.; Lingam, C. A SI model for social media influencer maximization. *Appl. Comput. Inform.* **2017**, *15*, 102–108. [CrossRef]
25. Keaver, L.; McGough, A.; Du, M.; Chang, W.; Chomitz, V.; Allen, J.D.; Attai, D.J.; Gualtieri, L.; Zhang, F.F. Potential of Using Twitter to Recruit Cancer Survivors and Their Willingness to Participate in Nutrition Research and Web-Based Interventions: A Cross-Sectional Study. *JMIR Cancer* **2019**, *5*, e7850. [CrossRef]
26. Haddad, R.N.; Mourani, C.C. Social Networks and Mobile Applications Use in Young Patients With Kidney Disease. *Front. Pediatr.* **2019**, *7*, 45. [CrossRef]
27. Camacho-Miñano, M.J.; MacIsaac, S.; Rich, E. Postfeminist biopedagogies of Instagram: Young women learning about bodies, health and fitness. *Sport Educ. Soc.* **2019**, *24*, 651–664. [CrossRef]
28. Song, Y.; Chen, X.; Hao, T.; Liu, Z.; Lan, Z. Exploring two decades of research on classroom dialogue by using bibliometric analysis. *Comput. Educ.* **2019**, *137*, 12–31. [CrossRef]
29. Aquila, I.; Sacco, M.A.; Gratteri, S.; Sirianni, M.; De Fazio, P.; Ricci, P. The "Social-mobile autopsy": The evolution of psychological autopsy with new technologies in forensic investigations on suicide. *Leg. Med.* **2018**, *32*, 79–82. [CrossRef]
30. Rothen, S.; Briefer, J.-F.; Deleuze, J.; Karila, L.; Andreassen, C.S.; Achab, S.; Thorens, G.; Khazaal, Y.; Zullino, D.; Billieux, J. Disentangling the role of users' preferences and impulsivity traits in problematic Facebook use. *PLoS ONE* **2018**, *13*, e0201971. [CrossRef]
31. Chang, P.F.; Whitlock, J.; Bazarova, N.N. "To Respond or not to Respond, that is the Question": The Decision-Making Process of Providing Social Support to Distressed Posters on Facebook. *Soc. Media + Soc.* **2018**, *4*. [CrossRef]
32. Nolan, S.; Hendricks, J.; Williamson, M.; Ferguson, S. Social networking sites (SNS) as a tool for midwives to enhance social capital for adolescent mothers. *Midwifery* **2018**, *62*, 119–127. [CrossRef] [PubMed]
33. Elmer, T.; Boda, Z.; Stadtfeld, C. The co-evolution of emotional well-being with weak and strong friendship ties. *Net. Sci.* **2017**, *5*, 278–307. [CrossRef]
34. Kotsilieris, T.; Pavlaki, A.; Christopoulou, S.; Anagnostopoulos, I. The impact of social networks on health care. *Soc. Netw. Anal. Min.* **2017**, *7*, 18. [CrossRef]
35. O'Donnell, N.H.; Willoughby, J.F. Photo-sharing social media for eHealth: Analysing perceived message effectiveness of sexual health information on Instagram. *J. Vis. Commun. Med.* **2017**, *40*, 149–159. [CrossRef]
36. Anderson, E.L.; Steen, E.; Stavropoulos, V. Internet use and Problematic Internet Use: A systematic review of longitudinal research trends in adolescence and emergent adulthood. *Int. J. Adolesc. Youth* **2017**, *22*, 430–454. [CrossRef]
37. BHM Regional Library. *Health & Medical Collection*; BHM Regional Library: Washington, NC, USA, 2018.
38. Burnham, J.F. Scopus database: A review. *Biomed. Digit. Libr.* **2006**, *3*, 1. [CrossRef]
39. Jenkins, D. Scopus—A Large Abstract and Citation Database for Research. 2017. The Orb. Available online: http://www.open.ac.uk/blogs/the_orb/?p=2062 (accessed on 12 September 2019).
40. Centre for Science and Technology Studies, Leiden University, VOSviewer. Available online: https://www.vosviewer.com (accessed on 12 September 2019).
41. van Eck, N.J.; Waltman, L. Software survey: VOSviewer, a computer program for bibliometric mapping. *Scientometrics* **2010**, *84*, 523–538. [CrossRef]
42. Sweileh, W.M. Research trends on human trafficking: A bibliometric analysis using Scopus database. *Glob. Health* **2018**, *14*, 106. [CrossRef]
43. van Wesel, M. Evaluation by Citation: Trends in Publication Behavior, Evaluation Criteria, and the Strive for High Impact Publications. *Sci. Eng. Ethics* **2016**, *22*, 199–225. [CrossRef]
44. Graddol, D. *The Future of English?* The British Council: London, UK, 1997.
45. Curry, M.J.; Lillis, T. Multilingual Scholars and the Imperative to Publish in English: Negotiating Interests, Demands, and Rewards. *TESOL Q.* **2004**, *38*, 663. [CrossRef]
46. Andreassen, C.S.; Pallesen, S.; Griffiths, M.D. The relationship between addictive use of social media, narcissism, and self-esteem: Findings from a large national survey. *Addict. Behav.* **2017**, *64*, 287–293. [CrossRef]

47. Kyvik, S. Changing trends in publishing behaviour among university faculty, 1980–2000. *Scientometrics* **2003**, *58*, 35–48. [CrossRef]
48. Błachnio, A.; Przepiorka, A.; Pantic, I. Association between Facebook addiction, self-esteem and life satisfaction: A cross-sectional study. *Comput. Hum. Behav.* **2016**, *55*, 701–705. [CrossRef]
49. Díaz Díaz, B.; García Ramos, R.; Baraibar Díez, E. Key Corporate Social Responsibility Initiatives: An Empirical Evidence from Spain. In *Key Initiatives in Corporate Social Responsibility: Global Dimension of CSR in Corporate Entities*; Idowu, S.O., Ed.; CSR, Sustainability, Ethics & Governance; Springer International Publishing: Berlin/Heidelberg, Germany, 2016; pp. 71–102. ISBN 978-3-319-21641-6.
50. Lee, M.; Wu, Y.; Tsai, C. Research Trends in Science Education from 2003 to 2007: A content analysis of publications in selected journals. *Int. J. Sci. Educ.* **2009**, *31*, 1999–2020. [CrossRef]
51. Barrios, C.; Flores, E.; Martínez, M.Á.; Ruiz-Martínez, M. Is there convergence in international research collaboration? An exploration at the country level in the basic and applied science fields. *Scientometrics* **2019**, *120*, 631–659. [CrossRef]
52. de Sio, F.; Fangerau, H. The Obvious in a Nutshell: Science, Medicine, Knowledge, and History. *Ber. Wissgesch.* **2019**, *42*, 167–185. [CrossRef]
53. Fundación Española Para la Ciencia y la Tecología Ínices de Impacto. Available online: https://www.recursoscientificos.fecyt.es/servicios/indices-de-impacto (accessed on 12 September 2019).
54. Kao, C.-K.; Liebovitz, D.M. Consumer Mobile Health Apps: Current State, Barriers, and Future Directions. *PM&R* **2017**, *9*, S106–S115.
55. Carrotte, E.R.; Prichard, I.; Lim, M.S.C. "Fitspiration" on Social Media: A Content Analysis of Gendered Images. *J. Med. Internet Res.* **2017**, *19*, e95. [CrossRef]
56. Houghton, J.P.; Siegel, M.; Madnick, S.; Tounaka, N.; Nakamura, K.; Sugiyama, T.; Nakagawa, D.; Shirnen, B. Beyond Keywords: Tracking the Evolution of Conversational Clusters in Social Media. *Sociol. Methods Res.* **2019**, *48*, 588–607. [CrossRef]
57. Di Lucca, G.A.; Fasolino, A.R. Testing Web-based applications: The state of the art and future trends. *Inf. Softw. Technol.* **2006**, *48*, 1172–1186. [CrossRef]
58. Patel, V.V.; Ginsburg, Z.; Golub, S.A.; Horvath, K.J.; Rios, N.; Mayer, K.H.; Kim, R.S.; Arnsten, J.H. Empowering With PrEP (E-PrEP), a Peer-Led Social Media-Based Intervention to Facilitate HIV Preexposure Prophylaxis Adoption Among Young Black and Latinx Gay and Bisexual Men: Protocol for a Cluster Randomized Controlled Trial. *JMIR Res. Protoc.* **2018**, *7*, e11375. [CrossRef] [PubMed]
59. Mathieson, K.; Leafman, J.S.; Horton, M.B. Access to Digital Communication Technology and Perceptions of Telemedicine for Patient Education among American Indian Patients with Diabetes. *J. Health Care Poor Underserved* **2017**, *28*, 1522–1536. [CrossRef] [PubMed]
60. Escoffery, C. Gender Similarities and Differences for e-Health Behaviors Among U.S. Adults. *Telemed. e-Health* **2018**, *24*, 335–343. [CrossRef] [PubMed]
61. Dini, A.A.; Saebo, O.; Wahid, F. Affordances and effects of introducing social media within eParticipation-Findings from government-initiated Indonesian project. *Electron. J. Inf. Syst. Dev. Ctries.* **2018**, *84*, e12035. [CrossRef]
62. Mansour, E. The adoption and use of social media as a source of information by Egyptian government journalists. *J. Libr. Inf. Sci.* **2018**, *50*, 48–67. [CrossRef]
63. Li, K.; Zhang, L.; Huang, H. Social Influence Analysis: Models, Methods, and Evaluation. *Engineering* **2018**, *4*, 40–46. [CrossRef]
64. Giles, S.J.; Reynolds, C.; Heyhoe, J.; Armitage, G. Developing a patient-led electronic feedback system for quality and safety within Renal PatientView. *J. Ren. Care* **2017**, *43*, 37–49. [CrossRef]
65. Hummel, A.C.; Smith, A.R. Ask and you shall receive: Desire and receipt of feedback via Facebook predicts disordered eating concerns. *Int. J. Eat. Disorder* **2015**, *48*, 436–442. [CrossRef]
66. Anderegg, W.R.L.; Goldsmith, G.R. Public interest in climate change over the past decade and the effects of the 'climategate' media event. *Environ. Res. Lett.* **2014**, *9*, 054005. [CrossRef]
67. Dowds, J. What do young people think about eating disorders and prevention programmes? Implications for partnerships between health, education and informal youth agencies. *JPMH* **2010**, *9*, 30–41. [CrossRef]
68. Frost, R.L.; Rickwood, D.J. A systematic review of the mental health outcomes associated with Facebook use. *Comput. Hum. Behav.* **2017**, *76*, 576–600. [CrossRef]

69. World Health Organization. Adolescent Health. Available online: http://www.who.int/topics/adolescent_health/en/ (accessed on 4 June 2018).
70. Evans, E.J.; Hay, P.J.; Mond, J.; Paxton, S.J.; Quirk, F.; Rodgers, B.; Jhajj, A.K.; Sawoniewska, M.A. Barriers to Help-Seeking in Young Women With Eating Disorders: A Qualitative Exploration in a Longitudinal Community Survey. *Eat. Disord.* **2011**, *19*, 270–285. [CrossRef] [PubMed]
71. Sunil, T.S.; Xu, X. Substance abuse and HIV/STD prevention at a Hispanic-serving institution in South Texas: A study of racial/ethnic and gender heterogeneity and intersectionality. *J. Ethn. Subst. Abus.* **2019**. [CrossRef] [PubMed]
72. Neupane, S.; Chimhundu, R.; Chan, K.C. Cultural values affect functional food perception. *Br. Food J.* **2019**, *121*, 1700–1714. [CrossRef]
73. Young, S.D. A "big data" approach to HIV epidemiology and prevention. *Prev. Med.* **2015**, *70*, 17–18. [CrossRef]
74. Janiszewska, E.; Pluta, D.; Dobosz, T. Knowledge of HIV/AIDS among young people. *Alerg. Astma Immunol.* **2019**, *24*, 24–29.
75. Vieira de Lima, I.C.; Gimeniz Galvão, M.T.; de Oliveira Alexandre, H.; Teixeira Lima, F.E.; de Araújo, T.L. Information and communication technologies for adherence to antiretroviral treatment in adults with HIV/AIDS. *Int. J. Med. Inform.* **2016**, *92*, 54–61. [CrossRef]
76. Mazzuoccolo, L.D.; Esposito, M.N.; Luna, P.C.; Seiref, S.; Dominguez, M.; Echeverria, C.M. WhatsApp: A Real-Time Tool to Reduce the Knowledge Gap and Share the Best Clinical Practices in Psoriasis. *Telemed. e-Health* **2018**. [CrossRef]
77. Hulsman, R.L.; van der Vloodt, J. Self-evaluation and peer-feedback of medical students' communication skills using a web-based video annotation system. Exploring content and specificity. *Patient Educ. Couns.* **2015**, *98*, 356–363. [CrossRef]
78. Li, S.; Yu, C.-H.; Wang, Y.; Babu, Y. Exploring adverse drug reactions of diabetes medicine using social media analytics and interactive visualizations. *Int. J. Inf. Manage.* **2019**, *48*, 228–237. [CrossRef]
79. Nereim, C.; Bickham, D.; Rich, M. A primary care pediatrician's guide to assessing problematic interactive media use. *Curr. Opin. Pediatr.* **2019**, *31*, 435–441. [CrossRef] [PubMed]
80. Masri, S.; Jia, J.; Li, C.; Zhou, G.; Lee, M.-C.; Yan, G.; Wu, J. Use of Twitter data to improve Zika virus surveillance in the United States during the 2016 epidemic. *BMC Public Health* **2019**, *19*, 761. [CrossRef]
81. Bond, W.F.; Deitrick, L.M.; Arnold, D.C.; Kostenbader, M.; Barr, G.C.; Kimmel, S.R.; Worrilow, C.C. Using Simulation to Instruct Emergency Medicine Residents in Cognitive Forcing Strategies. *Acad. Med.* **2004**, *79*, 438–446. [CrossRef] [PubMed]
82. Pilgrim, K.; Bohnet-Joschko, S. Selling health and happiness how influencers communicate on Instagram about dieting and exercise: Mixed methods research. *BMC Public Health* **2019**, *19*, 1054. [CrossRef] [PubMed]

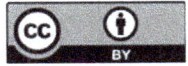 © 2019 by the authors. Licensee MDPI, Basel, Switzerland. This article is an open access article distributed under the terms and conditions of the Creative Commons Attribution (CC BY) license (http://creativecommons.org/licenses/by/4.0/).

MDPI
St. Alban-Anlage 66
4052 Basel
Switzerland
Tel. +41 61 683 77 34
Fax +41 61 302 89 18
www.mdpi.com

International Journal of Environmental Research and Public Health Editorial Office
E-mail: ijerph@mdpi.com
www.mdpi.com/journal/ijerph

www.ingramcontent.com/pod-product-compliance
Lightning Source LLC
LaVergne TN
LVHW070212100526
838202LV00015B/2037